MERRILL'S ATLAS OF
RADIOGRAPHIC POSITIONS and RADIOLOGIC PROCEDURES

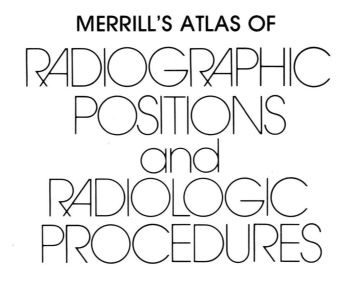

VOLUME ONE

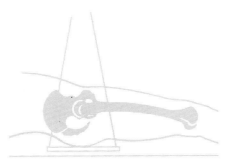

VOLUME ONE

MERRILL'S ATLAS OF

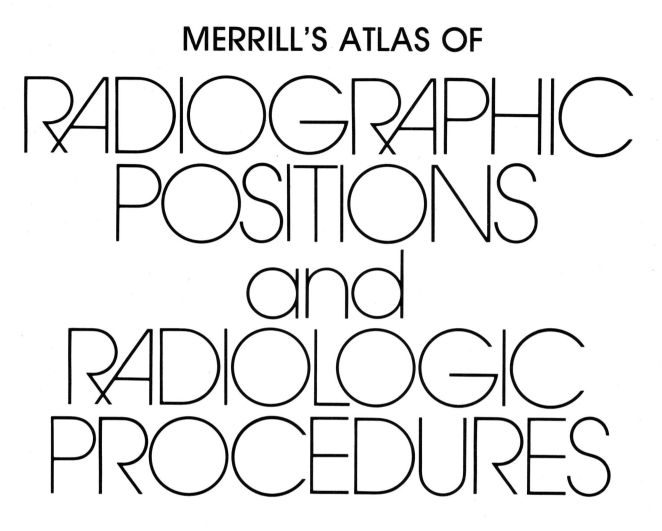

RADIOGRAPHIC POSITIONS and RADIOLOGIC PROCEDURES

Philip W. Ballinger, M.S., R.T.(R)

Director and Assistant Professor, Radiologic Technology Division,
School of Allied Medical Professions,
The Ohio State University,
Columbus, Ohio

FIFTH EDITION
with **2323** illustrations, including **11** in full color

The C. V. Mosby Company

ST. LOUIS • TORONTO • LONDON   1982

MOSBY

A TRADITION OF PUBLISHING EXCELLENCE

Editor: Don E. Ladig
Assistant editor: Rosa L. Kasper
Editing supervisor: Lin Dempsey Hallgren
Manuscript editors: Sally Gaines, Mary Wright, Jeanne L. Heitman
Design: Kay Kramer
Production: Linda Stalnaker, Jeanne Gulledge, Susan Trail,
Kathleen Teal, Mary Stueck, Barbara Merritt

FIFTH EDITION

The C.V. Mosby Company
11830 Westline Industrial Drive, St. Louis, Missouri 63141

Library of Congress Cataloging in Publication Data

Merrill, Vinita, 1905-
  Merrill's Atlas of radiographic positions and
radiologic procedures.

  Rev. ed. of: Atlas of roentgenographic positions
and standard radiologic procedures. 4th ed. 1975.
  Includes bibliographies and index.
  1. Radiography, Medical—Positioning—Atlases.
I. Ballinger, Philip W.   II. Title.   III. Title:
Atlas of radiographic positions and radiologic
procedures.   [DNLM: 1. Technology, Radiologic—
Atlases. WN 17 M5717a]
RC78.4.M47   1982   616.07'572   81-18854
ISBN 0-8016-3408-3   AACR2

TS/CB/B 9 8 7 6 5 4 3 2 1   02/B/221

Contributors

THOMAS J. BECK, M.S.

Senior Physicist,
Department of Radiology,
The Johns Hopkins Hospital,
Baltimore, Maryland

MARY J. BLOME, R.N.

Department of Radiology,
The Johns Hopkins Hospital,
Baltimore, Maryland

JEFFREY BOOKS, R.T.(R)

Supervisor, Tomography, Myelography,
 and Radiography of the Head and Neck,
Charlotte Memorial Hospital
 and Medical Center,
Charlotte, North Carolina

MICHAEL G. BRUCKNER, R.T.(R)

Division of Cardiovascular and Interventional
 Radiology,
Department of Radiology,
The Ohio State University Hospitals,
Columbus, Ohio

STEWART C. BUSHONG, Sc.D.

Professor of Radiological Science,
Department of Radiology,
Baylor College of Medicine,
Houston, Texas

JOHN MICHAEL CHUDIK, R.T.(R)

Division of Cardiovascular and Interventional
 Radiology,
Department of Radiology,
The Ohio State University,
Columbus, Ohio

DOROTHEA F. COOK, R.T.(R)

Division of Cardiovascular and Interventional
 Radiology,
Department of Radiology,
The Ohio State University Hospitals,
Columbus, Ohio

CHRIS DEMOCKO, R.T.(R)

Angiography Division,
Department of Radiology,
Saint Anthony Hospital,
Columbus, Ohio

JOHN P. DORST, M.D.

Director, Pediatric Radiology,
Department of Radiology,
The John Hopkins Hospital,
Baltimore, Maryland

ATIS K. FREIMANIS, M.D.

Professor and Chairman,
Department of Radiology,
The Ohio State University,
Columbus, Ohio

SANDRA L. HAGEN-ANSERT, B.A., R.D.M.S.

Educational Coordinator,
Clinical Science Center,
Department of Radiology/Section of
 Ultrasound,
University of Wisconsin–Madison,
Madison, Wisconsin

H. DALE HAMILTON, C.N.M.T.

Technical Director,
Department of Nuclear Medicine and
 Radiation Therapy,
Shawnee Medical Center Hospital;
Adjunct Assistant Professor,
Department of Radiologic Technology,
University of Oklahoma College of Health,
Oklahoma City, Oklahoma

ANN B. HRICA, R.T.(R)

Assistant Chief Technologist,
Department of Radiology,
Chief, Pediatric Radiology Section,
The Johns Hopkins Hospital,
Baltimore, Maryland

KENNETH C. JOHNSON, M.S.

Kenneth C. Johnson and Associates,
Columbus, Ohio

ROBERT A. KRUGER, Ph.D.

Medical Physics Division,
Department of Radiology,
University of Utah Medical Center,
Salt Lake City, Utah

CHARLES E. MARSCHKE, R.T.(T)

Program Director,
Radiation Therapy Technology Program,
School of Allied Health Sciences,
University of Vermont,
Burlington, Vermont

JOHN O. OLSEN, M.D.

Assistant Professor,
Department of Radiology,
The Ohio State University,
Columbus, Ohio

SHEILA ROSENFELD, M.A., C.N.M.T.

Education Coordinator and Program Director,
Nuclear Medicine Training,
Veteran's Administration Hospital,
St. Louis, Missouri

RONALD J. ROSS, M.D.

Cleveland, Ohio

DONALD L. SUCHER

Photographer and Graphic Illustrator,
Department of Radiology,
The Children's Hospital Medical Center,
Boston, Massachusetts

MICHAEL VAN AMAN, M.D.

Director, Division of Cardiovascular and
 Interventional Radiology,
Department of Radiology,
The Ohio State University,
Columbus, Ohio

JANE WARD, R.T.(R)

Program Director,
Radiologic Technology Program,
Weber State College,
Ogden, Utah

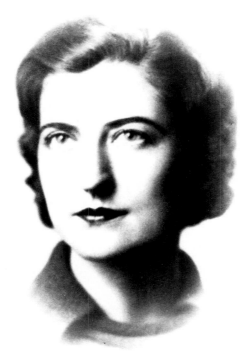

VINITA MERRILL

1905 - 1977

Seldom in any profession has a book met with such widespread acceptance as has
Vinita Merrill's *Atlas of Radiographic Positions and Radiologic Procedures*.
Those who worked with Vinita knew well her strength of personality,
which conceived, created, and sustained this atlas through 28 years.
Her contribution to her profession is monumental indeed, in no small part
the result of her dedication to accuracy and excellence.

Clark R. Warren

Preface

The purpose of the fifth edition of *Merrill's Atlas of Radiographic Positions and Radiologic Procedures* remains the same as that of the first edition—to provide a current source of reference for the student, technologist, and physician. In revising this edition the attempt was made to add recently described techniques and to selectively delete obsolete examinations or to combine discussions of similar examinations. The attempt was also made to organize and present the material in a concise, readable, and easy-to-use format.

Several changes have been made in this edition, including revisions of terminology. For instance, the title has been modified to reflect the profession's changes in terminology during recent years. In addition, the new chapter on radiographic terminology defines and illustrates the patient body positions by using the currently accepted terminology and abbreviations, which are in general agreement with those used in the profession, as well as with those used by The American Registry of Radiologic Technologists.

New chapters have been added, including those on computed tomography, diagnostic medical sonography, digital radiography, nuclear magnetic resonance, radiation protection, radiation therapy, and radiographic terminology. Extensive revisions were made in the chapters on the alimentary tract, mammography, nuclear medicine, pediatrics, and tomography and the section on visceral and peripheral angiography.

Most of the photographs for the radiographic positions have been replaced with new illustrations to show both the path of the central ray and a lighted collimator field. Selected illustrations show the use of gonad shielding, where appropriate.

Selected radiographs have been anatomically labeled in this edition. In general, the AP, PA, and lateral projections were not labeled, since line drawings corresponding to the anatomic structures were included in the anatomy section of the same chapter. Most labeling is included on oblique and axial projections in which the body parts may be distorted or the radiographic location altered in relation to the surrounding structures. I hope that this labeling will satisfy the requests made by numerous users of the text.

In earlier editions of this text numerous radiographic positions involving the cranium used specifically constructed angle platforms for positioning. Because of the increasing availability of specialty head units, most of these patient positions are shown using a head unit. In most cases, however, line drawings for the patient positions are included to demonstrate proper positioning of the patient for both horizontal and upright radiography.

The bibliographies in each of the three volumes have been extensively updated. Where possible, articles that have been published in the more widely circulated journals are cited. It is my belief that if an excellent article cannot be obtained easily, the value of such an article is not as great. To assist the user of the bibliography, an index is included on the first page of each bibliography.

Several items have been deleted from this edition. The chapter on dental radiography was deleted, and several projections requiring the use of accessory positioning devices no longer commercially available (e.g., Bullitt mastoid apparatus) were also deleted. Other projections were deleted to conform to NCRP regulations.

Mention of nonshockproof equipment was deleted from this edition because very few such installations remain in operation. Where such equipment is in use, extreme caution must always be exercised to ensure that the patient does not come close to or in contact with the x-ray tube or the overhead system.

During the revision of this edition it was a pleasurable experience to have received the cooperation and assistance of so many people. On several occasions problems seemed insurmountable. It was fortunate that at such times a resource person was always available, and I was gratified with the professional effort and support received.

For reviewing certain sections of the text and offering constructive criticism and thoughtful suggestions, I gratefully acknowledge my indebtedness to James Bland, C.N.M.T., Mary Pat Borgess, M.D., Steven K. Cho, M.D., Betsy A. Delzeith, R.T.(R), J. David Dunbar, M.D., Thomas R. Frye, M.D., Lawrence R. Fulmer, M.D., Howard D. Klosterman, M.D., Roscoe E. Miller, M.D., Charles F. Mueller, M.D., Jean R. Pacquelet, M.D., David J. Paul, M.D., Robert J. Ragosin, M.D., and Alfred E. Stockum, M.D.

My most sincere appreciation is extended to Picker International and specifically to Mr. Ron Ratliff for the prompt attention and action in loaning the radiographic unit used in photographing most of the patient positions. Without the unit the task of taking the hundreds of photographs would have been much more difficult and time consuming. Thanks are also extended to James W. Miller, R.T.(R), of E.G. Baldwin and Associates for the loan of the accessory equipment used in the photographs.

I owe special thanks to William F. Finney, R.T.(R), and Jeffrey L. Rowe, R.T.(R), for reviewing and offering valuable suggestions for selected specialty chapters and to J. James Jerele, D.O., for his time and effort in reviewing the manuscript on the alimentary tract.

For the careful reading of the manuscript to double-check for accuracy and clarity I thank Janie Moore, R.T.(R). I appreciate Ms. Sarah Mignery's secretarial assistance and responses to my many requests that the material was "needed yesterday."

To Elyse T. Massey, R.T.(R), I extend my sincere appreciation for her valuable assistance in updating the bibliography in all three volumes. Her competent and organized effort was indeed appreciated, and it was a pleasure to work with her.

I gratefully extend special thanks to Mr. Michael J. Keating and Mr. E. Brent Turner, who photographed and printed most of the new illustrations. During the shooting sessions many problems were overcome by their expertise and creativity. I truly appreciate their cooperation, support, and ability to meet almost impossible deadlines. Grateful appreciation is also extended to the staff of the Medical Illustration and Photography Department of The Ohio State University Hospitals for support provided in producing many new illustrations.

To Nina Massuros Kowalczyk, R.T.(R), and Alan J. Orth, R.T.(R), I extend my deepest appreciation and thanks for the more than full-time effort and competent assistance in planning, initiating, and seeing through to completion the changes in this edition. During our months of work I developed a greater respect for their abilities and for their dedication to accomplishing the objectives within the time allotted.

To the professional staff members of The C.V. Mosby Company I extend my deepest appreciation for all their help and assistance. It was indeed a pleasure to work with them and to learn of their sincere desire to produce a book of utmost quality.

Loving appreciation is given to my parents, D.W. and Mildred Ballinger, for encouraging me to pursue a career in radiography. Following my registration as an R.T., they encouraged me to pursue an undergraduate and graduate education for which I am profoundly grateful. I also extend my thanks to J. Robert Bullock, R.T.(R), for his valued support. I will always remember him as a teacher, supervisor, mentor, colleague, and friend. His valued opinions were often the basis for decisions affecting my career.

To my wife, Nancy, my thanks for her support and assistance in serving as chief errand runner, proofreader, clerk, bookkeeper, and general home manager during the time of my preoccupation with the text. I hope that my son, Eric, and my daughter, Monica, understand why I was not always available to them. Their often-asked question "Are you done with the book?" can now be answered, "Yes."

Philip W. Ballinger

Contents

Contents

VOLUME THREE

MERRILL'S ATLAS OF
RADIOGRAPHIC POSITIONS and RADIOLOGIC PROCEDURES

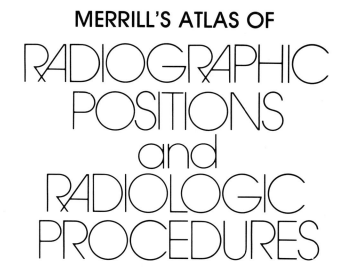

VOLUME ONE

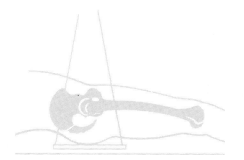

1

Preliminary steps
in
radiography

1. Radiograph
2. Clinical history needed by technologist
3. Initial examination
4. Diagnosis and the technologist
5. Ethics in radiologic technology
6. Care of radiographic examining room
7. Aseptic technique
8. Isolation unit
9. Disinfectants and antiseptics
10. Operating room
11. Minor surgical procedures in radiology department
12. Procedure book
13. Bowel preparation
14. Motion—its control
15. Structural relationship in positioning
16. Preparation instructions
17. Patient's dress, ornaments, and surgical dressings
18. Lifting and handling patients
19. Preexposure instructions
20. Foundation exposure technique
21. Adaptation of exposure technique to patient
22. Identification of radiographs
23. Film placement
24. English-metric conversion
25. Direction of central ray
26. Source-to-image receptor distance (SID)
27. Collimation of x-ray beam
28. Gonad shielding

1. RADIOGRAPH

A radiograph is the end result of an exacting technical procedure. Each phase of this procedure must be carried out with care to obtain the greatest possible information concerning the anatomic details of the structures for the purpose of demonstrating the absence of, or the presence and extent of, traumatic or pathologic changes. There is no examination in radiology in which accuracy and attention to detail are not essential.

The technologist should be thoroughly familiar with the radiographic shadows cast by normal structures. To develop the ability to properly analyze radiographs and to correct or prevent errors in technique, the technologist should study radiographs from the following standpoints:

a. The relationship of the structural shadows as to size, shape, position, and angulation must be reviewed.

b. The degree of detail in each structure must be compared with that of adjacent structures, such as the head of the humerus compared with the glenoid fossa and the acromion process.

c. The density of the radiograph must be within the useful density range. If a change in technique is necessary, the factors primarily controlling density are milliampere-seconds (mAs) and source-to-image receptor distance (SID).

d. The contrast of the radiograph must be sufficient to allow adjacent structures with different tissue densities to be distinguished radiographically. The primary controlling factor of radiographic contrast is the peak kilovoltage (kVp).

e. The image sharpness (definition) must be sufficient to clearly demonstrate the desired anatomic part. Image sharpness is controlled by several factors, which can be categorized as geometric factors, motion, and material.

f. The magnification in size of the body part must be evaluated and the controlling factors of object-film distance and SID considered. All radiographs possess some degree of magnification, since all body parts are three dimensional.

g. The shape distortion of the body part must be analyzed, and the controlling factors of direction of the central ray, central ray–film alignment, and part-film alignment must be studied. Shape distortion is often used to an advantage in radiography. An example of shape distortion is the axial projection of the cranium to demonstrate the occipital bone.

A sound knowledge of anatomy and the ability to analyze radiographs correctly are of particular importance to technologists who work where the radiologist is not in constant attendance. Under this condition the radiologist must be able to depend on the technologist to perform the technical phase of the examinations without aid.

2. CLINICAL HISTORY NEEDED BY TECHNOLOGIST

The technologist is responsible for performing radiographic examinations according to the standard procedure, except when contraindicated because of the condition of the patient. As the demands for the radiologist's time increases, less time is often available to devote to the technical phase of radiology. This circumstance makes it necessary for him to depend on the technologist to a greater extent in carrying out this phase of the patient's care. This places an additional responsibility on the technologist and makes it necessary for him to know (1) normal anatomy and normal anatomic variations, so that he can position the patient accurately, and (2) the radiographic characteristics of numerous pathologic conditions, that is, their effect on the normal radiopacity of structures, so that he can select the exposure factors accordingly. Although the technologist is not responsible for explaining the causation, diagnosis, or treatment of disease, he must know how to demonstrate the conditions radiographically to be a professional.

When the radiologist cannot see the patient, he depends on the technologist to take the necessary history and to observe any apparent abnormality that might affect the radiographic result, such as jaundice in gallbladder examinations and surface masses that might cast shadows that could be mistaken for internal changes. When the technologist assumes this responsibility, the radiologist will give specific instructions as to the information he desires.

The requisition received by the technologist should state the exact region desired and the condition present or suspected. The patient must be positioned and the exposure factors selected according to the region involved and the radiographic characteristics of the existent abnormality. These factors make it necessary for the technologist to understand the rationale behind the examination; otherwise it will not be possible for him to produce radiographs of the greatest possible diagnostic value. Having the information in advance saves both the delay and the expense of reexamination, not to mention the inconvenience and, of far greater importance, the unnecessary radiation exposure to the patient.

3. INITIAL EXAMINATION

The projections taken for the initial examination of each body part are based on the anatomy and/or function of the part and on the nature of the abnormality indicated by the clinical history. The projections utilized for the initial examination are usually held to the minimum number required to detect any demonstrable abnormality in the particular region. Supplemental studies for further investigation are then made as indicated. This method or routine of performing each examination is timesaving, eliminates unnecessary radiographs, and at the same time reduces radiation exposure to the patient.

4. DIAGNOSIS AND THE TECHNOLOGIST

It is quite natural for the patient to be anxious about the result of his examination and for him to ask questions. The technologist should tactfully advise him that his physician will receive the report as soon as the radiologist has interpreted the films. Referring physicians are also prone to ask questions of the technologist, and it is recommended not to discuss diagnostic problems; refer the physician to the radiologist.

5. ETHICS IN RADIOLOGIC TECHNOLOGY

Ethics is the term applied to the science of duty and right conduct toward others. The nature of the work in the medical profession requires that the rules of conduct be strict. The physician, being responsible for the welfare of the patient, must be able to depend on absolute honesty in his assistants in carrying out his orders and in reporting any mistakes.

The "Code of Ethics" developed and adopted by The American Society of Radiologic Technologists identifies the following 10 ethical principles[1]:

Principle 1. Radiologic technologists shall conduct themselves in a manner compatible with the dignity of their profession.

Principle 2. Radiologic technologists shall provide services with consideration of human dignity and the uniqueness of the patient unrestricted by considerations of sex, race, creed, social or economic status, personal attributes, or the nature of the health problem.

Principle 3. Radiologic technologists shall make every effort to protect all patients from unnecessary radiation.

Principle 4. Radiologic technologists shall exercise and accept responsibility for discretion and judgment in the performance of their professional services.

Principle 5. Radiologic technologists shall judiciously protect the patient's right to privacy, and shall maintain all patient information in the strictest confidence.

Principle 6. Radiologic technologists shall apply only the methods of technology founded upon a scientific basis and not accept those methods that violate that principle.

Principle 7. Radiologic technologists shall not diagnose, but in recognition of their responsibility to the patient, they shall provide the physician with all information that they have relative to radiologic diagnosis or patient management.

Principle 8. Radiologic technologists shall be responsible for reporting unethical conduct and illegal professional activities to the appropriate authorities.

Principle 9. Radiologic technologists should continually strive to improve their knowledge and skills by participating in educational and professional activities and sharing the benefits of their attainments with their colleagues.

Principle 10. Radiologic technologists should protect the public from misinformation and misrepresentation.

In 1981 Warner[2] analyzed the professional and legal implication of the ASRT Code. The article is recommended for those desiring additional information.

[1]"Code of Ethics," Radiol. Technol. **52**:520, 1981.
[2]Warner, S.L.: Code of ethics: professional and legal implications, Radiol. Technol. **52**:485-494, 1981.

6. CARE OF RADIOGRAPHIC EXAMINING ROOM

The radiographic examining room should be as scrupulously clean as any other room used for medical purposes. The mechanical parts of the x-ray machine, such as the table and tube stand, should be dusted with a clean, damp (not wet) cloth every day. The metal parts should be cleaned periodically with a disinfectant. The overhead system, x-ray tube, and other parts that conduct electricity should be cleaned with alcohol or a clean, dry cloth. Never use water to clean electrical parts.

Cones, collimators, compression devices, and other accessories should receive daily cleaning. The gummy residue left on cassettes and cassette stands by adhesive tape should be removed and the cassette then disinfected. The cassettes should be protected from bleeding, ulcerated, or other exudative lesions by using protective covers. Stained cassettes are revolting and inexcusable.

The radiographic room should be prepared for the examination before the patient is brought into the room. Fresh linen should be put on the table and pillow, and everything should be in place so that the room will look clean and fresh, not disarranged from the previous examination. The accessories to be used with the examination should be selected and placed nearby. These duties require only a few minutes, but they create a lasting impression on the patient.

7. ASEPTIC TECHNIQUE

Technologists are engaged in caring for the sick and therefore should be thoroughly familiar with aseptic technique. They should know how to handle patients who are on precaution or isolation without contaminating their hands, clothing, or apparatus, and they should know how to disinfect these things when they do become contaminated. As one of the first steps in aseptic technique, the technologist should keep his hands smooth, free from roughness or chapping, by the frequent use of soothing lotions. Any abrasion should be protected by a bandage to prevent the entrance of bacteria. The hands should be washed after each patient and should be kept away from the face and head.

For the protection of the health of the technologist as well as that of the patient, the laws of asepsis and prophylaxis must be obeyed. Scrupulous cleanliness should be used in handling all patients, whether they are known to have an infectious disease or not. If the patient's head, face, or teeth are to be examined, he should see the technologist wash his hands. If this is not possible, the technologist should wash his hands and then enter the room drying them with a fresh towel. If the patient's face is to come in contact with the cassette front, he should see the technologist clean the front with alcohol, or it should be covered with a clean drape.

A sufficient supply of gowns and disposable gloves should be kept in the radiology department to care for infectious patients. After known or suspected infectious patients, the technologist must wash his hands in running warm water and soapsuds, rinse them, and dry them thoroughly. If the washbasin is not equipped with a knee control for the water supply, the valve of the faucet should be opened through a paper towel when the hands are contaminated.

Before bringing isolation patients to the radiology department, the transporter should drape the stretcher or wheelchair with a clean sheet to prevent contamination of anything they might touch. When it is necessary to transfer these patients to the radiographic table, it should first be draped with a sheet. The edges of the sheet may then be folded back over the patient so that the technologist can position him through the clean side without becoming contaminated.

For the protection of the cassettes when using a non-Bucky technique, a folded sheet should be placed over the end of the stretcher or table. The cassette is then placed between the clean fold of the sheet, and, with his hands between the clean fold, the technologist can position the patient through the sheet. If it is necessary for the technologist to handle the patient directly, an assistant should position the tube and operate the equipment to prevent contamination.

When the examination is finished, the contaminated linen should be folded with the clean side out and returned to the unit with the patient, where it will receive the special attention given to linen used for these patients.

8. ISOLATION UNIT

When doing bedside work in an isolation unit, obtain a gown, cap, mask, and, if necessary, gloves. If more than one film is to be used, stand the additional cassettes on paper towels outside the patient's room. Take the machine into the room and manipulate it into position, being careful not to let it touch the bed. Put the cassette in a clean pillowcase (a clean case for each cassette used), and have an assistant technologist who can do the contamination work of adjusting the cassette and patient, or ask for an assistant who can do this work under direction. If it is not possible to have an experienced technologist to assist when the position is an exacting one, make the necessary adjustments on the control panel and tube, and operate the machine through a clean cloth, being careful not to let the contaminated side of the cloth come in contact with the equipment.

When the exposures have been finished, remove the mask, cap, and gown, place them in the precaution hamper, and wash the hands before leaving the room. The cable of the x-ray machine, which has of necessity been on the floor, must be wiped with a disinfectant solution.

9. DISINFECTANTS AND ANTISEPTICS

Chemical substances that will kill pathogenic bacteria are classified as *germicides* or *disinfectants*. Chemical substances that inhibit the growth of, without necessarily killing, pathogenic microorganisms are called *antiseptics*. *Sterilization,* which is usually performed by means of heat, is the destruction of all microorganisms. Thus sterilization is the killing of all microorganisms, whereas disinfection is the process of killing only those that are pathogenic. The objection to many chemical disinfectants is that to be effective they must be used in solutions so strong that they damage the material being disinfected.

Since alcohol is commonly used in medical facilities, it should be noted that alcohol has antiseptic but not disinfectant properties.

10. OPERATING ROOM

Carrying out aseptic technique is a fixed habit with nurses, but technologists who have not had extensive nursing education must exercise constant watchfulness to avoid doing anything that will contaminate sterile objects in the operating room. After putting on scrub clothing, cap, and mask it is advisable to step into the operating room to survey the particular setup before taking the x-ray machine in. By taking this precaution the technologist can make sure that he will have sufficient room to bring the machine in and do his work without danger of contaminating anything. If necessary, ask the circulating nurse to move such items as the sterile-bowl stand. Because of the danger of contamination of the sterile field, of sterile supplies, or of persons who are scrubbed for the operation, the technologist should never approach the operative side of the table.

After the setup has been checked, the technologist should take the x-ray machine in on the free side of the operating table, that is, the side opposite the surgeon, scrub nurse, and sterile layout. The machine should be maneuvered into a position that will make the final adjustments easy when the surgeon is ready to proceed with the examination. Needless to say, the x-ray machine should be thoroughly dusted with a damp (not wet) cloth before it is taken into the operating room. The cassette is placed in a sterile pillowcase or in other sterile covering, depending on the type of examination to be done. The surgeon or one of the assistants will hold the sterile case open while the technologist gently drops the cassette into it, being careful not to touch the sterile case. The technologist may then give directions for placing, adjusting, and holding the cassette for the exposure.

The technologist should make the necessary arrangements with the operating room supervisor when doing work in the operating room that requires the use of a tunnel or other special equipment. The cassette tunnel or grid should be placed on the table when it is being prepared for the patient, with the tray opening to the free side of the table. With the cooperation of the surgeons and operating room supervisor, a system can be worked out whereby radiographic examinations can be performed in the operating room accurately and quickly, without moving the patient and without endangering the sterile field.

11. MINOR SURGICAL PROCEDURES IN RADIOLOGY DEPARTMENT

Many procedures that require a rigid aseptic technique, such as cystography, intravenous pyelography, gallbladder injections, spinal punctures, angiography, and angiocardiography, are often carried out in the radiology department. Although in certain of these procedures the radiologist needs the assistance of a nurse, the technologist can make the necessary preparations and give sufficient assistance in others.

For the procedures that do not require a nurse, the technologist should know what surgical instruments and supplies are needed and how to prepare and sterilize them. It is advisable for nonnurse technologists to make arrangements with the surgical supervisor for the training necessary to equip them to carry out these procedures. Adequate training in both aseptic technique and dressings can be given in a rather short time.

12. PROCEDURE BOOK

There should be a procedure book covering each specialized examination performed in the radiology department. Under the appropriate heading, each procedure should be outlined and should state the staff required and the duties of each member of the team, and there should be a listing of the sterile and nonsterile items. A copy of the sterile instruments required should be given to the supervisor of the central supply room to facilitate preparation of the trays for each of the different procedures.

13. BOWEL PREPARATION

Radiographic examinations involving the abdomen often require that the entire colon be cleansed before the examination to obtain diagnostic quality radiographs. The patient's colon may be cleansed by one or any combination of the following: limited diet, laxatives, and enemas. The technique used to cleanse the patient's colon is generally selected by the medical facility or the physician.

14. MOTION—ITS CONTROL

Motion plays a large role in radiography. Since motion is the result of muscle action, it is important to know something of the function of muscles to eliminate or control motion for the period of time necessary for a satisfactory examination. There are three types of muscular tissue: smooth, cardiac, and striated. The first two types are classified as involuntary muscles and the third as voluntary.

Involuntary muscles. The visceral muscles are composed of smooth muscular tissue and are controlled partially by their inherent characteristic of rhythmic contractility and partially by the autonomic nervous system. By their rhythmic contraction and relaxation these muscles perform the movements of the internal organs. The rhythmic action of the muscular tissue of the alimentary tract, called peristalsis, is normally more active in the stomach (about three or four waves per minute) and gradually diminishes along the intestine. The specialized cardiac muscular tissue functions by contracting the heart to pump blood into the arteries and by expanding or relaxing to permit the heart to receive blood from the veins. The normal rhythmic actions of cardiac muscular tissue are independent of nerve stimulus and thus are said to be myogenic in origin or to be an inherent characteristic of the muscle tissue. The phase of contraction is termed *systole,* and the phase of relaxation is termed *diastole.* One phase of contraction and one phase of relaxation, that is, a systole and a diastole, are called a complete cardiac cycle. The pulse rate of the heart varies with emotions, exercise, and food, as well as with size, age, and sex.

Involuntary motion is caused by the following:

Heart pulsation	Chills
Peristalsis	Tremor
Spasm	Pain

Control. Speed of exposure is the only recourse against involuntary motion.

Voluntary muscles. The voluntary, or skeletal, muscles are composed of striated muscular tissue and are controlled by the central nervous system. These muscles perform the movements of the body initiated by the will. Each skeletal muscle has a name that was derived from its position, shape, structure, action, direction, or points of attachment. Each muscle con-

sists of a body, or belly, and two tendinous extremities for attachment.

The body of the muscle is made up of cylindrical fibers that are covered with a thin membrane and bound together into primary bundles called fasciculi. The covering sheaths of the individual fibers, the fasciculi, and that of the muscle are prolonged into round, fibrous cords called tendons or into flattened tendons called aponeuroses. The tendons serve to attach the muscles to bone. When the muscle contracts, one end is moved toward the other. Although most of the striated muscles can be made to act from either extremity, the less movable attachment is called the origin of the muscle, and the more movable is called the insertion. The contraction acts in the direction of the tendinous attachments.

The skeletal muscles never work singly. A combination of muscles is brought into play in any movement. One set acts as the prime movers; one set, called synergists, acts to inhibit movements not required; one set acts as fixation muscles in steadying the point from which the force is being applied; and, lastly, one set, the antagonists of the prime movers, relax to remove resistance to the action. In radiography the patient's body must be positioned in such a way that the synergetic, antagonistic, and fixation muscles can perform their part of the work; otherwise the action of the prime movers will be hampered. The patient's comfort is a good index to the success of the position.

Voluntary motion resulting from lack of control is caused by the following:

Nervousness	Discomfort
Excitability	Mental illness
Fear	Age (child)

Control. Voluntary motion can be controlled by giving clear instructions, providing for comfort of the patient, and correctly applying and adjusting support and immobilization. Immobilization for extremity work can often be obtained for the duration of the exposure by having the patient phonate an m—m—m sound with the mouth closed or an ah—h—h sound with the mouth open.

NOTE: The voluntary motion caused by the last two classifications, mental illness and age, can be controlled only by speed of exposure.

15. STRUCTURAL RELATIONSHIP IN POSITIONING

The position and relationship of the organs of the trunk vary considerably with the position of the body. The technologist must know not only the size, shape, position, and relationship of the organs when the body is in the anatomic position but also the change in the relationship when the body is moved from the erect to the recumbent position and to the sitting position.

For example, the diaphragm lies in an oblique plane on a level with the sixth costal cartilage anteriorly and with the tenth rib posteriorly when the body is erect. When the body is placed in the dorsal recumbent, or supine, position, the diaphragm is situated from 2 to 4 inches higher than when erect. The exact elevation depends on the curvature of the spine and the pressure of the abdominal viscera and muscles. The elevation will be less in thin patients. When the body is placed in the ventral recumbent, or prone, position, the diaphragm will be from 2 to 4 inches lower than in the erect position because of relaxation of pressure from the abdominal viscera and muscles and removal of the tilting caused by the spinal curvature. The depression of the diaphragm will be greater in thin patients.

When the body is placed in a seated position, the diaphragm assumes its lowest position because of lung pressure, relaxation of the abdominal muscles, and relaxation of pressure from the abdominal viscera. When the body is placed in a lateral recumbent position, the upper half of the diaphragm assumes a position lower than when seated, and the lower half assumes a position higher than when supine because of unequal pressure from the abdominal viscera. Here the two halves of the diaphragm cease to function in unison with breathing; the lower half has a greater excursion than the upper half. The original height of the diaphragm varies constantly during respiration. Its excursion between deep inspiration and deep expiration is approximately 1 inch, the right cupola having a slightly greater excursion than the left cupola.

The thoracic and abdominal viscera vary in location along with the diaphragm through all its movements. Likewise the anterior bony structures of the trunk vary in their relation to posterior structures as the position of the body is changed. For this reason the surface landmark for any given body position cannot be relied on when the body is placed in any position other than the one specified. Nor can surface landmarks be depended on to hold for one position on all patients. Landmarks are based on the average, and although they are applicable to a majority of patients, they cannot be used when a patient's form varies considerably from the normal.

If all patients were average in size and shape, the technologist would have few problems. Since this is not the case, he must study anatomy from the standpoint of relationship and mechanics. With a reasonable knowledge of normal anatomy, the mechanics of body movement, and the usual deviations from the normal, the element of error in positioning is reduced to a minimum.

16. PREPARATION INSTRUCTIONS

When the examination is one that requires preparation, as in kidney and gallbladder examinations, instruct the patient carefully. Although the particular routine may be an "old story" to us, it is new to the patient. Frequently, judged stupidity really results from lack of sufficiently explicit directions. Be sure that the patient understands not only what he is to do but also why he is to do it. Patients are more likely to follow instructions correctly if they see reason for them. If the instructions are complicated, write them out. For example, because few patients know how to take an enema correctly, it is advisable to question the patient and when necessary to take the time to explain the correct procedure to him. This will often save film, radiation exposure to the patient, and the time consumed in giving another enema in the radiology department.

17. PATIENT'S DRESS, ORNAMENTS, AND SURGICAL DRESSINGS

Have the patient dressed in a gown that, with the use of a sheet where necessary, will allow the region under examination to be exposed. *Never expose a patient unnecessarily.* Have only the area under examination uncovered, and be sure to cover the rest of the patient's body well enough to keep him warm. For examining parts that must be covered, cotton is the preferred gowning material and it should not be starched; starch is somewhat radi-

opaque. Straighten out any folds in the cloth to prevent confusing shadows. It is important to remember that a material that will not cast a shadow on a heavy exposure, such as that used on an adult abdomen, may show clearly on a light exposure, such as that used on a child's abdomen.

Ask the patient to remove any ornament that is worn in the region to be examined or that might be projected into the region by central ray angulation. When examining the skull be sure that *dentures, removable bridgework, earrings, and all hairpins are removed.*

Examine surgical dressings for radiopaque substances, such as metallic salves, oiled silk, and adhesive tape. If permission to remove the dressings has not been obtained or if the technologist does not know how and the radiologist is not present, the surgeon or nurse should be asked to accompany the patient to the radiology department to remove them. When dressings are removed, always make sure that open wounds are adequately protected by a cover of sterile gauze.

18. LIFTING AND HANDLING PATIENTS

All patients deserve an explanation of the procedure to be performed if they are coherent and capable of understanding. See that the patient understands just what is expected of him, make him comfortable, and alleviate his fears if he is apprehensive about the examination. However, if the procedure is one that will hurt or be unpleasant, as in cystoscopy and intravenous injections, do not tell the patient that it will not hurt or be unpleasant. Explain the procedure calmly. Tell him that it will hurt a little or be unpleasant, as the case may be, but that since it is a necessary part of his examination his full cooperation is needed. If the patient sees that everything is being done for his comfort, he will usually respond favorably.

Because the whole procedure is new to him, the patient usually works in reverse when given more than one order at a time; that is, when he is instructed to get up on the table and lie on his abdomen, he will usually get onto the table in the most awkward possible manner and lie down on his back. Instead of asking him to get onto the table in a specific position, first have him sit on the table and then instruct him to assume the desired position. If he sits on

the table first, he will be able to assume the position with less strain and with fewer awkward movements. *Never rush a patient.* If he feels hurried, he will be under a nervous strain and therefore unable to relax and cooperate. In moving and adjusting a patient into position, handle him gently but firmly. A too light touch can be as irritating as one that is too firm. Instruct the patient and let him do as much of the moving as possible.

Regardless of what part is being examined, the entire body must be adjusted to avoid muscle pull against the part being examined, with resultant motion or rotation. When the patient is in an oblique position, apply support and adjust it so that he is relieved of strain in holding the position. Use immobilization devices and compression bands whenever necessary, but not to a point of discomfort to the patient. Use care in releasing a compression band over the abdomen; it should be released slowly.

In making the final adjustments on a position, the technologist should stand with this eyes in line with the position of the focal spot, visualize the internal structures, and adjust the part accordingly. The rules of positioning are few and simple, and many repeat examinations can be eliminated by following the rules.

Great care must be exercised in handling trauma patients, particularly those who have skull, spinal, and long bone injuries. Because of the possibility of fragment displacement, any necessary manipulation should be performed by the surgeon or radiologist, never by the technologist. Adapt the positioning technique to the patient so that he may be moved as little as possible. If the tube-part-film *relationship* is maintained, the resultant projection will be the same regardless of the position.

When it is necessary to move a patient who is too sick to help himself, the following considerations must be kept in mind:
  a. To protect the patient, move him as little as possible.
  b. Never try to lift a helpless patient alone.
  c. To avoid straining the muscles of your back when lifting a heavy patient, flex the knees, straighten the back, and bend from the hips.
  d. When lifting a patient's shoulders, support his head. While holding the head with one hand, slide the oppo-

site arm under the shoulders and grasp the axilla in such a way that the head can rest on the bend of the elbow when the patient is raised.

e. When it is necessary to move the patient's hips, first flex his knees. In this position the patient may be able to raise himself. If not, it is easier to lift the body when the knees are bent.

f. When a helpless patient must be transferred to the radiographic table from a stretcher or bed, he should be moved on a sheet by at least four, preferably six, people. Place the stretcher parallel to and touching the table. Two people should be stationed on the side of the stretcher and two on the far side of the radiographic table to grasp the sheet at the shoulder and hip levels. One person should support the patient's head and another his feet. When the signal is given, all six should lift and move the patient in unison.

Many hospitals now have a specially equipped radiographic room adjoining the emergency receiving room. These units usually have special radiographic equipment and stretchers with radiolucent tops, so that severely injured patients can be examined in the position in which they arrive. Where this ideal setup does not exist, the trauma patient is conveyed to the main radiology department, where he must be given precedence over nonemergency patients.

19. PREEXPOSURE INSTRUCTIONS

Instruct the patient in breathing, and practice with him until he understands exactly what he is to do. After he is in position, before leaving him to make the exposure, have him practice the breathing once more. This procedure requires a few minutes, but it saves much time, radiation, and many films. There are definite reasons for the phase of breathing used in examinations of the trunk. The correct phase and the reason for its use are given under the positioning instructions on each region within the trunk area.

Inspiration depresses the diaphragm and the abdominal viscera, lengthens and expands the lung fields, elevates the sternum and pushes it anteriorly, and elevates the ribs and reduces their angle near the spine. Expiration elevates the diaphragm and the abdominal viscera, shortens the lung fields, depresses the sternum, and lowers the ribs and increases their angle near the spine.

When exposures are to be made during breathing, have the patient practice slow, even breathing, so that only the structures above the one being examined will move. When lung motion, but not rib motion, is desired, have the patient practice slow, deep breathing after the compression band has been applied across the chest.

20. FOUNDATION EXPOSURE TECHNIQUE

Specific exposure techniques are not included in this text. Too many variable factors are involved, not only from one department to another but from one unit to another within the same department. Only by familiarity with the characteristics of the particular equipment and accessories employed and a knowledge of the radiologist's preference in film quality can a satisfactory technique be established. The electrical current available (three phase or single phase), the kilowatt rating of the generator and tube, the radiation characteristics (whether hard or soft), the filtration used, the type of film, the type of screens, the grid, and the type of processing solutions must all be taken into account in establishing the correct foundation technique for each unit. With these data available, the exposure factors can be selected for each region of the body and balanced in such a way that they will produce films having the greatest possible amount of detail and a quality that exceeds the prescribed standard.

21. ADAPTATION OF EXPOSURE TECHNIQUE TO PATIENT

It is the responsibility of the technologist to select the combination of exposure factors that produce the desired quality of radiograph for each region of the body and to standardize this quality. Once the standard quality is established, there should be as little deviation as possible. The foundation factors should be adjusted to the individual patient to maintain uniform quality throughout the range of patients. However, correctly balanced factors cannot be expected to produce the same amount of detail on all subjects any more than one combination of exposure factors can be expected to produce the same contrast standard on all subjects. Just as some people are blond and others are brunet or redheaded, some patients have fine, distinct trabecular markings and others do not. Congenital and developmental changes from the normal, age changes, and pathologic changes must all be considered when one is judging the quality of the film.

Certain pathologic conditions require the technologist to compensate when establishing an exposure technique. Selected conditions requiring a decrease in patient radiation exposure include age (infants, children, and the elderly), emphysema, degenerative arthritis, atrophy, multiple myeloma, active osteomyelitis, and sarcoma. Other patient conditions require increased radiation exposure to penetrate the part. Such conditions include atelectasis, advanced carcinoma, edema, pleural effusion, pneumoconiosis, and osteopetrosis.

22. IDENTIFICATION OF RADIOGRAPHS

The identification marker should include (1) the patient's name and/or identification number or case number, (2) the date, and (3) the side marker, right or left. The importance of correct identification bears stressing and restressing. There is no instance in which it is not important, but it becomes vital in comparison studies on follow-up examinations and in medicolegal and compensation cases. It is advisable to develop the habit of rechecking the identification marker just before placing it on the film.

Numerous methods of marking films for identification are available. They range from the direct method of radiographing it along with the part, to "flashing" it onto the film in the darkroom before development, to writing it on the film after it has been processed, to perforating the information on the film, and to specialty cassette-marking systems designed for accurate and efficient operation.

23. FILM PLACEMENT

The part is always centered to the center point of the cassette or to where the angulation of the central ray will project it there. The film should always be adjusted in such a way that its long axis will lie parallel with the long axis of the part being examined. Although having a long bone angled across the film does not impair its diagnostic value, such an arrangement is aesthetically distracting.

Even though the lesion may be known to be at the midshaft area, use a film large enough to include at least one joint on all long bone studies. This is the only means of determining the position of the part and of localizing the lesion. Always use a film large enough to cover the region under examinatin, but not larger. In addition to being extravagant, large films include extraneous parts that detract from the appearance of the radiograph and, of greater importance, unnecessary radiation exposure is delivered to the patient. When examining the abdominal area, flex the elbows and place the hands on the upper chest so that the forearms will not be in the exposure field.

The rule of "place the part as close to the film as possible" might better read "place the part as close to the film as possible for accurate anatomic projection." Although there is greater magnification, less distortion is obtained by increasing the part-film distance in such examinations as lateral projections of the middle and ring fingers so that the part will lie parallel with the film, and there is less structural distortion and superimposition if oblique projections of the ribs are made with the injured side elevated. Magnification can be reduced in these examinations by increasing the source-to-image receptor distance to compensate for the increase in part-film distance. In certain instances gross magnification is desirable, and it is obtained by positioning and supporting the part exactly midway between the film and the focal spot of the tube. This procedure is known as *enlargement* or *magnification technique.*

For ease of comparison, bilateral examinations of small parts should be placed on one film. However, exact duplication of the location of the images on the film is difficult if the cassette or film holder is not accurately marked. Mark the cassette face in half both longitudinally and transversely, and then mark the center point of each half. If three projections are to be placed on one film, mark the cassette face in half in the longitudinal direction and in thirds in the transverse direction.

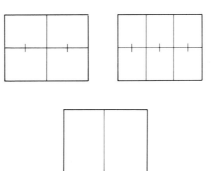

When masks are used, it is advisable to mark the outline of the masks on the cassette face. By doing this, the part can be accurately centered. After the exposures have been made, alternately covering each part of the film with a lead blocker, place the masks in position to protect the exposed areas, center the identification marker, and make an exposure just heavy enough to radiograph the marker onto the film and to blacken the background.

One word of caution on this system at this point: The parts should always be placed on the film in the same manner, either facing or backing each other, according to established routines. The identification marker should be placed so that it will read from left to right or from bottom to top of the film. For frontal projections it should face with the part; that is, it should face the tube for AP projections and should face the film for PA projections. Even when the side markers (right and left) are radiographed onto the film with the patient, the screens should be marked in such a way that it will not be possible to make an error in side identification.

24. ENGLISH-METRIC CONVERSION

In the past few years efforts have been made to convert all English measurements to the world standard metric system. These efforts have been met with some resistance. Nevertheless, in the near future total conversion to the metric system most likely will occur.

In the procedures described in this text the English linear measurements have been retained, since this remains the terminology most commonly used. The following information is provided to assist the radiographer in converting measurements from the English to the metric system and vice versa:

1 inch = 2.54 centimeters (cm)
1 centimeter (cm) = 0.3937 inch
40 inches SID (source-to-image receptor distance) = 1 meter (m) (approximately)

Cassette and film sizes with approximately the same dimensions are the following:

Inches	Centimeters
8 × 10	18 × 24
10 × 12	24 × 30
11 × 14	30 × 35
14 × 14	35 × 35
14 × 17	35 × 43
7 × 17	18 × 43
9 × 9	24 × 24

25. DIRECTION OF CENTRAL RAY

The central or principal beam of rays, simply referred to as the central ray, is always centered to the film unless film displacement is being used for the inclusion of an adjacent area. The central ray is angled through the part under the following conditions:

a. When it is necessary to avoid the superimposition of overlying structures

b. When it is necessary to avoid stacking a curved structure on itself, such as the sacrum and coccyx

c. When it is necessary to project angled joints such as the knee joint and the lumbosacral junction

d. When it is necessary to project angled structures without foreshortening or elongation, such as a lateral projection of the neck of the femur

The aim is to have the principal beam of rays at right angles to the structure. Accurate positioning of the part and accurate centering of the central ray are of equal importance in securing a true structural projection.

26. SOURCE-TO-IMAGE RECEPTOR DISTANCE (SID)

The rule of "Use the greatest distance possible consistent with the electrical energy required" does not apply in all examinations. For example, in certain skull examinations, such as of the mastoids and of the paranasal sinuses, it is desirable to use a distance short enough to magnify the opposite table of the skull to make the detail of the side being examined more visible. A more accurate and inclusive rule to follow, therefore, might be as follows: "Consistent with the electrical energy required, use the distance that will give the sharpest detail of the structure being examined."

It must be noted that the technologist is not permitted to use a technique that places the source of the radiation (x-ray tube) closer than 12 inches from the nearest patient body surface. The source-to-part distance is recommended to be 15 or more inches.

A general rule for the placement of the tube might be as follows: "Adjust the tube so that the central ray is at right angles to the structure and the focal spot at a distance that will project the best definition of the structure."

27. COLLIMATION OF X-RAY BEAM

The beam of x-radiation must be so delimited to irradiate only the area under examination. This restriction of the x-ray beam serves a twofold purpose. First, it minimizes the amount of radiation to the patient and reduces scatter radiation in the room and thus able to reach the film. Second, it serves the purpose of obtaining radiographs showing clear structural delineation and increased contrast by (1) reducing scatter radiation and thereby producing a shorter-scale radiograph and (2) preventing secondary radiation from unnecessarily exposing surrounding tissues, with resultant film fogging from this source.

The area of the beam of radiation is reduced to the required area through the use of collimators or appropriately apertured sheet diaphragms or shutters that are constructed of lead or other metal that has high radiation absorption power. By so confining the beam, the peripheral radiation strikes and is absorbed by the intervening metal, while only the rays in line with the exit aperture are transmitted to the exposure field. Cones or diaphragms can be attached to the collimator and their effectiveness depends on their close proximity to the x-ray source.

28. GONAD SHIELDING

The patient's gonads may be irradiated when radiologic examinations of the pelvis and hip areas are performed. When practical, gonad shielding should be used to protect the patient. The Bureau of Radiological Health recommends that gonad shielding be used in three instances[1]: (1) when the gonads lie within the primary x-ray field or within close proximity (about 5 cm), despite proper beam limitation, (2) if the clinical objective of the examination will not be compromised, and (3) if the patient has a reasonable reproductive potential. The technologist must evaluate the above criteria in regard to the patient and decide whether gonad shielding is appropriate.

Gonad shielding is included in selected illustrations in this text. For additional information on the rationale of gonad shielding, see Chapter 4.

[1]Gonad shielding in diagnostic radiology, Pub. No. (FDA) 75-8024, Rockville, Md., 1975, Bureau of Radiological Health.

2

Radiographic terminology

Radiographic terminology developed in a haphazard fashion. Attempts to analyze the usage often lead to confusion, because the manner in which the terms are used does not follow one specific rule. The terminology used in this text is consistent with that used in the profession and is in confirmed agreement with "Positioning and Projection Terminology" adopted by The American Registry of Radiologic Technologists.[1]

BODY POSITIONS

Body positions are the manner in which the patient is placed in relation to the surrounding space. The following terms are used to describe body positions:

decubitus (L. *decumbere*, to lie down) Act of and position assumed in lying down; position assumed is described according to dependent surface: **dorsal decubitus,** lying on back (supine); **ventral decubitus,** lying face down (prone); **left lateral decubitus,** lying on left side; **right lateral decubitus,** lying on right side.

dorsal recumbent Supine.

lateral recumbent Lying on side.

prone Lying face down.

recumbent or **decubitus** Lying down.

supine Lying on back.

ventral recumbent Prone.

[1]McGowan, R.C.: Personal communication, June 1981.

PART AND POSITION

Following are the standard terms to describe part location or position:

anterior and **ventral** Refer to forward part of body or to forward part of an organ; superior surface of foot is referred to as **dorsum** or **dorsal** surface.

central Refers to midarea or main part of an organ.

distal Designates part away from source, or beginning, of a structure, generally used in describing lower part of an extremity.

external Refers to superficial structures, those near periphery, or outer limits, of a part.

inferior and **caudal** Refer to parts away from head end of body.

internal Refers to deep structures, those near center of a part.

lateral Refers to parts away from median plane of body or away from middle of a part to right or left.

medial and **mesial** Refer to parts toward median plane of body or toward middle of a part; opposite of lateral.

parietal Refers to walls of a cavity.

periphery and **peripheral** Refer to parts away from central mass of an organ and toward its outer limits.

posterior and **dorsal** Refer to back part of body or to back part of an organ; inferior surface of foot is referred to as **plantar** surface or **sole.**

superior, cranial, and **cephalic** Designate parts toward head end of body.

proximal Designates nearness to source, or beginning, of a structure; generally used to describe upper part of an extremity.

visceral Refers to organs contained within a cavity.

RADIOGRAPHIC POSITIONING
Projection

Projection is the process of recording a body part on an image receptor (film). Projection usually describes the path of radiation as it goes from the x-ray tube through the patient to the image receptor.

View

View describes the representation of an image as seen from the vantage of the image receptor. In comparing the definitions of *view* and *projection,* it must be noted that they are exact opposites. For many years view and projection were often used interchangeably, which led to confusion. View is no longer an acceptable term to describe a patient position and has been eliminated from this text.

Method

Some radiologic procedures are named after individuals (for example, Chassard-Lapiné or Towne) in recognition of their having developed a *method* to demonstrate a specific anatomic part. The method describes the position of the body in reference to established anatomic landmarks. In addition, the method describes the position of the film and central ray in relation to the body position. In this text a method is also described by using the standard anatomic projection terminology; for example, the Caldwell method for demonstrating the frontal and ethmoid sinuses is called a *PA projection* when the central ray is angled 23 degrees caudal to the glabellomeatal line.

11

PROJECTIONS
Frontal projections (AP or PA)

The patient is depicted in the supine or dorsal recumbent body position. The x-ray beam is shown entering the front (anterior) body surface and exiting the back (posterior) surface. This position correctly prepares the patient for an *AP (anteroposterior) projection.*

The patient is shown in the upright or erect body position with the central ray entering from the posterior body surface. This patient is properly positioned for a *PA (posteroanterior) projection.*

Lateral projections

Lateral projections are always named by the side of the patient that is placed closest to the film. Some individuals may describe the *left lateral projection* more completely as a right-to-left lateral projection. However, in this text the right or left sides are not routinely indicated on lateral projections, because either side of the patient may be placed adjacent to the image receptor. The side selected will vary, depending on the condition of the patient, the anatomic structure of clinical interest, and the purpose of the examination.

Oblique projections

The term *oblique* refers to a position in which the body part is rotated so that it does not produce a frontal (AP or PA) or a lateral projection.

The patient can be described as having been prepared for a left posterior to right anterior projection, in the *oblique* body position, or a PA (posteroanterior) oblique position with the side indication (right or left) being named by the side of the patient closest to the film. It must be noted, however, that the vast majority of radiographers in the United States refer to

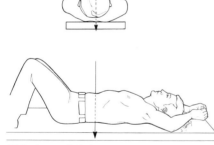

AP (anteroposterior)

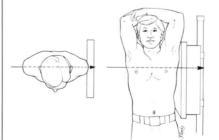

Left lateral

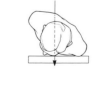

Right PA oblique (RAO)

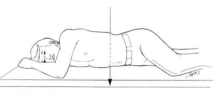

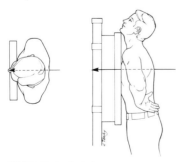

PA (posteroanterior)

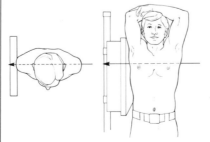

Right lateral

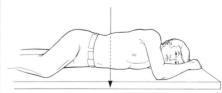

Left PA oblique (LAO)

this as the *right anterior oblique (RAO) position*. It is so named by the side (right or left) and the body surface (anterior or posterior) that are closest to the film. This text uses the term *PA oblique projection* with the commonly referred to abbreviation in parentheses.

Similar to the previous oblique projection, the body position is called a *left PA oblique projection (LAO)*, as illustrated on the preceding page.

Following the same principle for all oblique projections, the AP oblique positions are named as indicated below.

Decubitus projections

Decubitus projections are so named to indicate that the patient is lying down and that the central ray is parallel to the horizon. In most radiographic decubitus positions the patient is lying on his lateral body surface. Similar to lateral and oblique positions, decubitus positions are named by the body surface on which the patient is lying.

The patient is in the *left lateral decubitus position*. It must be noted that this position results in an AP radiographic projection of the body part that is most useful

in the diagnosis of air-fluid levels in the chest and abdomen.

The patient is placed in a *dorsal decubitus position*, and the resulting radiographic image is a right lateral projection.

The prone patient is in the *ventral decubitus position*, which yields a left lateral projection.

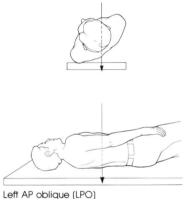

Left AP oblique (LPO)

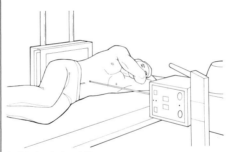

Left lateral decubitus

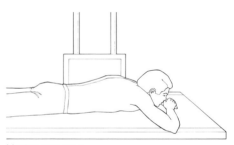

Ventral decubitus

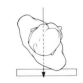
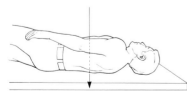

Right AP oblique (RPO)

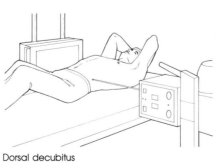

Dorsal decubitus

Tangential projections

A projection in which the central ray skims between body parts to profile a bony structure and project it free of super-imposition is a *tangential projection*.

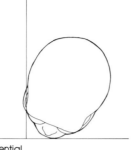
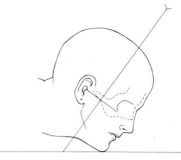

Tangential

Axial projections

In an *axial projection* there is longitudinal angulation of the central ray with the long axis of the body part.

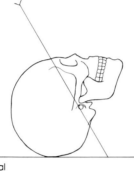

Axial

ANATOMIC TERMS

Processes or **projections** that extend beyond or jut out from the main body of a structure are designated by the following terms:

condyle A rounded projection at an articular extremity.
coracoid or **coronoid** A beaklike process.
crest A ridgelike projection.
epicondyle A projection above a condyle.
facet A small, smooth-surfaced process for articulation.
head Expanded end of a long bone.
malleolus A club-shaped process.
protuberance or **process** General terms for a projection.
spine A sharp projection.
styloid A long, pointed process.
trochanter Either of two large, rounded processes (greater, or major, and lesser, or minor) located at junction of neck and shaft of femur.
tubercle A small, rounded process.
tuberosity A large, rounded process.

Depressions are hollow, or depressed, areas and are described by the following terms:

fissure A cleft or groove.
foramen A hole in a bone for transmission of blood vessels and nerves.
fossa A pit, fovea, or hollow.
groove A shallow, linear depression.
sinus A recess, groove, cavity, or hollow space:
    1. A recess or groove in bone, as used to designate a channel for venous blood on inner surface of cranium.
    2. An air cavity in bone or a hollow space in other tissue; used to designate a hollow space within a bone as in paranasal sinuses.
    3. A fistula or suppurating channel in soft tissues.
sulcus A furrow, trench, or fissurelike depression.

Movement of the body can be described by the following terms:

abduction Movement of a part away from central axis of body.
adduction Movement of a part toward central axis of body.
evert or **eversion** To turn outward.
extension Straightening of a joint; stretching of a part; also, a backward bending movement; opposite of flexion.
flexion A bending movement of a joint whereby angle between contiguous bones is diminished; also, a forward bending movement; opposite of extension.
invert or **inversion** To turn inward.
pronate To turn arm so that palm of hand faces backward.
supinate To turn arm so that palm of hands faces foward.

3

General anatomy

Anatomy is the term applied to the science of the *structure* of the body. *Physiology* is the term applied to the science of the *function* of the body organs. Technologists need to study anatomy and physiology thoroughly, giving increased attention to a few particular body systems. Technologists also need to study the structure of the body, with particular reference to the mechanics of joint action. However, technologists often concentrate their attention on one system or region when studying. This habit can result in failure to position the body as a unit and may account for the greatest number of repeat examinations that result from to motion or rotation.

According to anatomists, there is no such thing as isolated muscle action; many muscles are brought into play by even the simplest movement. This also means that there is an interdependence of joint action, that the rotation of any joint results in compensatory reaction in remote joints to allow muscle correlation in performing the first action. No part can be pushed, pulled or twisted into a position without placing the muscles of both the immediate and the remote regions under a mechanical stress too great for them to bear. The result is either a quivering motion caused by strain or rotation to a more comfortable position to relieve the strain. Therefore it is important for the technologist to study anatomy from the standpoint of mechanics, so that he can position the body as a related whole.

This text includes the anatomy and physiology considered necessary to equip the technologist to position the body correctly for the examination of the various regions.

SKELETON

In the adult the skeleton is normally composed of 206 bones and, in certain places, pieces of cartilage. The bones and cartilage are united by ligaments in such a way that they form the supporting framework of the body, afford places of attachment for muscles, and protect the delicate visceral organs.

Bones are composed of an inner spongy, or trabeculated, portion called cancellous tissue and an outer layer of compact bony tissue called the cortex. The comparative amount of cancellous and compact tissue composing the different bones varies widely depending on their location and function, the cortex being thicker where protection or stength is required. Long bones have a central cylindrical cavity called the medullary canal. The medullary canal of long bones and the spaces of the cancellous bone are filled with marrow, which contains immature blood cells and blood vessels. Except where covered by articular cartilage, the bones are covered by a tough fibrous membrane called the periosteum. The surfaces of the bones are smooth at points of articulation, are roughened by projections at points of muscle and ligament attachment, and present depressions for the passage of blood vessels and nerves. Depending on their shape, the bones are classified as long, short, flat, or irregular.

Long bones consist of a shaft, or body, and two articular extremities. These bones are curved for strength and narrowed to accommodate muscles. Until full growth is attained, the articular ends are separated from the shaft by a layer of cartilage. The shaft is referred to as the *diaphysis*, and the articular ends as the *epiphyses*. Long bones are found only in the extremities.

Short bones consist mainly of cancellous tissue and have only a thin outer layer of compact tissue. They are found where compactness, elasticity, and laminated motion are required. The carpals and tarsals of the wrists and ankles are short bones.

Flat bones consist largely of compact tissue in the form of two plates, or tables, that enclose a layer of cancellous tissue, or diploë. Flat bones provide protection, as in the bones of the cranium, or broad surfaces for muscular attachment, as in the shoulder blades.

Irregular bones, because of their peculiar shape, cannot be classified in any of the foregoing groups. The vertebrae, the bones of the base of the skull, and the pelvis are typical bones of this group.

The bones begin to develop in small areas of the membrane (membrane bones) and the cartilage (cartilage bones) at about the second month in embryonic life. These areas of bone formation are termed *centers of ossification.* The time required for the bones to reach full development varies for the different regions of the skeleton and is somewhat less in the female than in the male. The illustration below shows the normal development of the bones, the time of the radiographic appearance of various centers of ossification, and the time of union between the epiphyses and diaphyses of the bones arising from two or more centers of ossification.

The bony framework of the body is divided into two main groups termed the *appendicular skeleton* and the *axial skeleton.* The appendicular skeleton consists of the upper and lower extremities and their girdles, the shoulders, and the pelvis. The axial skeleton includes the skull, the vertebral column, the sternum, and the ribs. The anatomy of each of these divisions is considered in the chapter dealing with the positioning of the particular region.

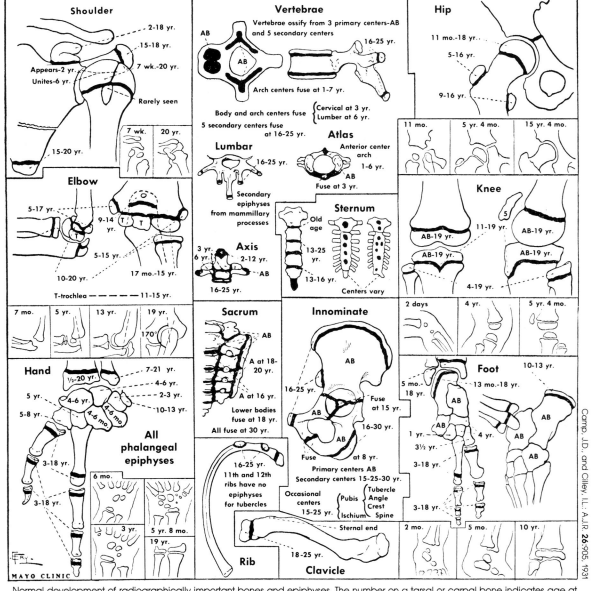

Normal development of radiographically important bones and epiphyses. The number on a tarsal or carpal bone indicates age at which calcification is radiographically visible. Two numbers, for example, 16-25, indicate visible ossification at 16 years and union at 25 years of age. The number at a cartilaginous junction indicates age at which ossification occurs. There is considerable normal variation at any given age. A, Appears; AB, ossification visible at birth.

BODY PLANES AND POSITIONS

The *anatomic position* of the body is erect, with the arms at the sides and the palms turned forward. Many of the terms established to describe location or position of parts are based on this body position. There are three fundamental planes of the body.

1. The *midsagittal*, or *median sagittal*, *plane* passes vertically through the midline of the body from front to back, dividing it into equal right and left portions. Any plane passing through the body parallel with the midsagittal plane is termed a sagittal plane.

2. The *midcoronal*, or *midfrontal*, *plane* passes vertically through the midaxillary region of the body and through the coronal suture of the cranium at right angles to the midsagittal plane, dividing the body into anterior, or ventral, and posterior, or dorsal, portions. Any plane passing vertically through the body from side to side is called a coronal, or frontal, plane.

3. A *transverse*, or *horizontal*, *plane* passes crosswise through the body at right angles to its longitudinal axis and to the sagittal and coronal planes, dividing it into superior, or cranial, and inferior, or caudal, portions. Any plane passing through the body at right angles to its longitudinal axis is called a transverse, or horizontal, plane.

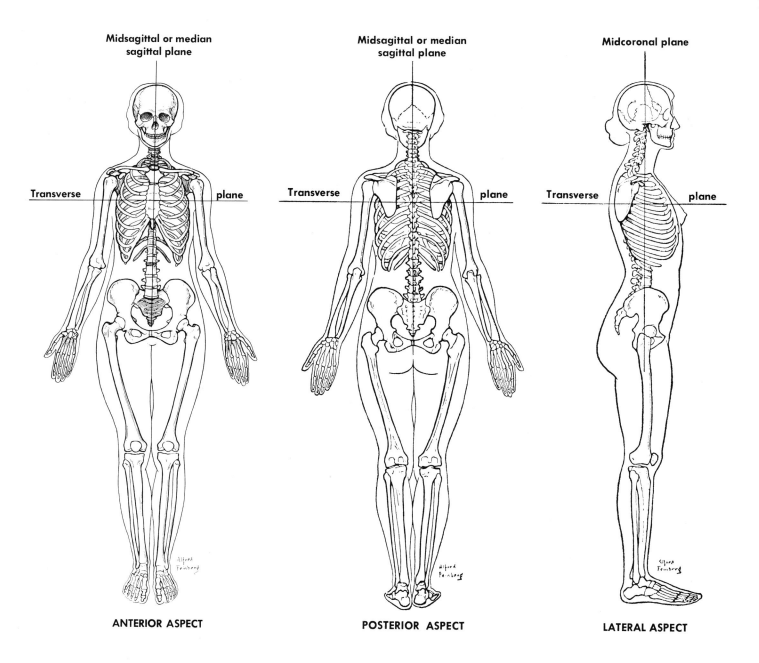

Midsagittal or median sagittal plane

Transverse plane

ANTERIOR ASPECT

Midsagittal or median sagittal plane

Transverse plane

POSTERIOR ASPECT

Midcoronal plane

Transverse plane

LATERAL ASPECT

JOINTS

The bones of the skeleton are joined together by ligaments, capsules, cartilages, or the dovetailing of bone, as in the sutures of the cranium. The joints, or articulations, are classified according to their movability. The three main classes are as follows:

1. *Synarthrosis* is the term applied to immovable joints. The opposing surfaces of the bones forming these joints are separated only by a thin layer of fibrous tissue or by a layer of cartilage. Epiphyseal articulations are considered synarthrodial joints, and, with the exception of the mandible, the articulations of the skull are synarthrodial joints. The latter are called *sutures*.

2. *Amphiarthrosis* is the term applied to joints having limited motion. The articular surfaces of the bones are connected by disks of fibrocartilage, as between the vertebral bodies, the pubes, and the sacroiliac joints, or by fibrous bands, as in the lower tibiofibular articulation.

3. *Diarthrosis* is the term applied to freely movable joints. The articular surfaces of the bones are reciprocally shaped for the movement required of the joint, are covered by articular cartilage, and are enclosed in a fibrous envelope called a capsule. The capsule consists of two layers of tissue—an outer fibrous layer and an inner fluid-secreting layer called synovial membrane. In certain joints an articular disk, or meniscus, is interposed between the articular cartilages to give further protection to the joint. The greatest number of the articulations of the body are diarthrodial joints. The articulations of the extremities, the mandible, and between the vertebral arches are examples of diarthrodial joints.

Depending on the shape of the articular surfaces of the contiguous bones, four kinds of movement are possible in diarthrodial joints. These movements are circumduction, rotation, angular, and gliding movements, and they are combined in many of the body actions to produce the great variety of movements.

Where the joint action is such that muscles or tendons slide over underlying parts, fluid-containing sacs called *bursae* are interposed between the sliding surfaces to prevent friction. Bursae are lined with synovial membrane. Important bursae are located at such joints as the shoulder, the elbow, the hip, and the knee and under such muscles as the deltoid and the trapezius.

4

Radiation protection

STEWART C. BUSHONG

INTRODUCTION
Early injuries

Perhaps no other event in our technologic history caused as much feverish scientific activity by so many as the accidental discovery of x rays by Wilhelm Roentgen in November of 1895. Because Roentgen was so amazingly thorough in his investigations, within a few short weeks he was able to characterize the nature of x rays to nearly the level of understanding that we have today. This early work gained him the first Nobel prize for physics in 1902. Roentgen immediately recognized the potential diagnostic medical applications of his new "X-light." He produced the first radiograph, that of his wife's hand.

During 1896, the first year following Roentgen's discovery, the scientific literature of the world was flooded with reports of experiments with x rays. Very soon thereafter reports appeared relating cases of radiodermatitis, in some instances severe enough to require surgery. These reports had two immediate effects: (1) to speed the experimentation and application of x rays in radiation therapy and (2) to suggest that radiation protection methods were necessary to ensure the safety of both the operator and the patient during diagnostic procedures. However, it was to be more than 30 years later before even moderately consistent radiation protection measures were universally applied.

By 1910 several hundred cases of severe x-ray burns, many leading to death, had been reported. To illustrate this early tragedy of radiation pioneers, consider the case of Clarence Daley, Thomas Edison's friend and principal assistant. Within a couple of days after the cable announcement of the discovery of x rays,

Edison had an x-ray apparatus operating and was deeply involved in his own investigations. Within months several of his assistants experienced a radiodermatitis. Clarence Daley's condition was mild at first but, because of continued exposure, progressed rapidly and resulted in several amputation operations. He died in 1904 and is considered the first radiation fatality in the United States. When Daley died, Edison discontinued his work with x rays. He had already discovered calcium tungstate as an intensifying phosphor and had developed the fluoroscope. Who knows what additional contributions Edison might have made to radiology had he continued his investigations.

Present suspected radiation responses

In the 1930s a consensus was reached on the need for radiation protection devices and procedures. These radiation protection activities were principally in response to the reported radiation injuries to early radiologists. In the 1950s scientific reports began to appear that suggested that even the low levels of radiation exposure experienced in diagnostic radiology could be responsible for late radiation responses and injury to patients. Current radiation protection practices are prompted by concern for late effects in patients and radiation workers.

Following high doses of radiation exposure, a number of acute early responses may appear. Whole body radiation in excess of 200,000 mrads can result in death within weeks. Partial body irradiation to any organ or tissue can cause atrophy (shrinking) and dysfunction (improper metabolism). Whole body exposure as low as 25,000 mrads can produce a measurable hematologic depression (a reduction in the number of cells of the peripheral blood) that may require months for recovery. These early effects result from high doses of radiation and therefore are of no concern in diagnostic radiology.

Concern today is for the late effects of radiation exposure. Such effects follow low exposures and may not occur for years. They fall into two natural categories—genetic effects and somatic effects. Late genetic effects of radiation exposure are suspected; they have not been measured in humans. However, data from a considerable number of studies of animals indicate that such effects may occur.

Somatic effects refer to the response to radiation by all cells of the body except the germ (genetic) cells. The principal late somatic effects following low-dose irradiation have only been measured in humans by the use of rather sophisticated epidemiologic and statistical methods. No individual has ever been identified as a radiation victim following low-dose exposure. A low dose is generally considered to be a whole body dose less than about 25,000 mrads, and for partial body irradiation it is somewhat higher. Such effects are detectable only when observations are made on thousands and even hundreds of thousands of irradiated individuals.

The shortening of life resulting from nonspecific premature aging was observed many years ago in American pioneer radiologists. This effect is rare today, but studies of animals have demonstrated that life shortening is a true late effect. It has been suggested that this late effect may occur to the extent of 10 days of life lost for every 1000 mrads of exposure; however, the principal cause of life shortening is now considered to be the accelerated induction of malignant disease. Local tissues can also experience late radiation effects of a nonmalignant nature. The most prominent late effect and one that has some significance in diagnostic radiology is radiation-induced cataracts. However, this is a late effect that does not follow low-dose irradiation; it requires approximately 200,000 mrads of exposure to the lens.

Radiation-induced malignant disease is the delayed somatic effect of primary concern. Leukemia and cancers of nearly every type involving nearly every organ have been implicated by animal investigations and by large-scale observations of humans. Leukemia is a rare disease and therefore is more readily observed in a heavily irradiated population than is cancer. The most accurate estimate for the induction of leukemia by irradiation suggests that if 1 million persons received 1000 mrads, up to 55 additional cases of leukemia would be produced during the 25 years following irradiation. Without irradiation the incidence of leukemia is approximately 80 cases/1 million persons/yr.

Cancer is not uncommon, and therefore radiation-induced cancer is difficult to detect, even statistically. Of every 1 million persons, 167,000 will die of cancer. If that 1 million persons received an annual dose of 1000 mrads for life, approximately 8000 additional cancers would be induced.

Need for radiation protection

Radiologic technologists receive an average of 500 mrads per year, nearly all of which is received during fluoroscopy and portable radiography, during which protective apparel is worn. Consequently, exposures, although identified as whole body on the exposure report, are actually partial body exposures. Although exposure levels are low and the possibility of a late effect is remote, it is prudent to keep radiation exposure to technologists and patients ALARA (as low as reasonably achievable).

Following low-dose irradiation, late genetic effects and the late somatic effects of importance are considered to be possible at any dose, regardless of how small. There is no dose threshold for such effects. Exposures that technologists experience because of their occupation result in a very small and indeterminate probability, and therefore such effects are very rare. In all cases in which radiologic technologists have been studied no such late effects have been observed.

RADIATION UNITS

A special set of units is used to express the quantity of ionizing radiation. These units, the roentgen, the rad, and the rem, have been developed and defined over many years and are familiar to radiologic workers. Unfortunately, those in training and in practice at this time must become familiar with a new set of special radiation units derived from the international system of weights and measures (SI). The SI units associated with classical radiation units and the appropriate conversions are shown in Table 1. Although they are only referred to superficially in this chapter, technologists should be aware that they exist and should be prepared to implement them in the future.

Table 1. Conventional radiation units, SI radiation units, and conversion factors

Quantity	Conventional unit	SI unit	Conversion factor
Exposure	R	C/kg	2.58×10^{-4} C/kg/R
Absorbed dose	rad	gray (Gy)	10^{-2} Gy/rad
Dose equivalent	rem	seivert (Sv)	10^{-2} Sv/rem
Activity	curie (Ci)	becquerel (Bq)	3.7×10^{10} Bq/Ci

Unit of exposure

When an x-ray tube is energized, x rays are emitted in a collimated beam as light from a flashlight. This useful beam of x-rays causes ionization of the air through which it passes. This is called exposure and the unit of exposure is the roentgen (R). An exposure of 1 R will produce 2.08×10^9 ionizations in a cubic centimeter of air at standard temperature and pressure. The official definition of the roentgen is 2.58×10^{-4} coulombs per kilogram (C/kg) of air, and this is equivalent to the previous quantity. The SI unit of radiation exposure has no special name; it is simply the C/kg.

Unit of radiation dose

When a radiation exposure occurs, the resulting ionizations deposit energy in the air. If an object such as a patient is present at the point of exposure, then energy will be deposited by ionization in the patient. This deposition of energy by radiation exposure is called radiation absorbed dose, or simply absorbed dose, and it is measured in rads. One rad is equivalent to the deposit of 100 ergs of energy in each gram of the irradiated object. The SI unit of absorbed dose is the gray (Gy), and 1 Gy = 100 rads = 1 joule/kg. The erg and joule are units of energy.

Unit of dose equivalent

If the irradiated object is a radiologic technologist or other radiation worker, then the radiation dose resulting from an occupational radiation exposure is said to result in a radiation dose equivalent. The dose equivalent is measured in rems (radiation equivalent man), and 1 rem = 100 ergs/gm. The SI unit of dose equivalent is the seivert (Sv), and 1 Sv = 1 joule/kg. Note that the rad and the rem (gray and seivert) are expressed in similar units. The basic difference between the rem and the other radiation units is that the rem is used only for radiation protection purposes; it is the unit of occupational exposure.

In diagnostic radiology 1 R can be considered to be equal to 1 rad and to 1 rem. This simplifying assumption is accurate to within about 15% and therefore is sufficiently precise for nearly all considerations of exposure and dose in diagnostic radiology. Radiation workers in the nuclear power industry and in some other industrial and research activities may be exposed to different kinds of radiation, in which case this simplifying assumption does not apply.

Application of radiation units

Although all three units (the roentgen, the rad, and the rem) are used interchangeably in diagnostic radiology, such use is incorrect, because each unit has a precise application. One roentgen, 1 rad, and 1 rem are all rather large quantities. In practice, quantities that are 1000 times smaller, the milliroentgen (mR), the millirad (mrad), and the millirem (mrem), are used. When a medical physicist calibrates or surveys a radiographic or fluoroscopic x-ray tube, the radiation intensity is expressed in milliroentgens. The radiation intensity will be measured by any one of a number of various types of radiation detectors and the output expressed in milliroentgens or sometimes as milliroentgens per milliampere-seconds (mR/mAs) at some given kilovolt peak (kVp). When a patient is irradiated during an examination and the amount of radiation received by the patient is of concern, it is expressed in millirads. If a pregnant patient is irradiated (a rare occurrence), fetal dose is also expressed in millirads. The radiation dose to any of the patient's organs would likewise be expressed in millirads. Often, however, the skin dose will be expressed as an exposure in milliroentgens and called an entrance exposure.

Exposure received by technologists is measured with a personnel radiation monitor. The source of their occupational exposure is nearly always scattered radiation from the patient. The monitor measures exposure, but the radiation report indicates the dose equivalent in millirems. The millirem is reserved exclusively for use in radiation protection and therefore is a unit not only of occupational exposure but also sometimes used to express the dose received by populations as the consequence of medical, industrial, and research applications of radiation.

The useful x-ray beam is measured in milliroentgens, the patient dose in millirads, and occupational exposure in millirems.

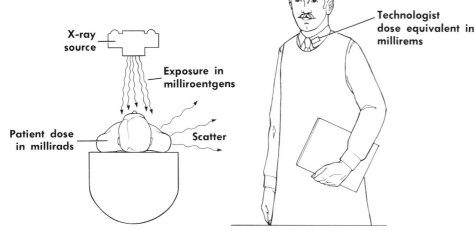

X-ray source

Exposure in milliroentgens

Patient dose in millirads

Scatter

Technologist dose equivalent in millirems

RADIATION SOURCES AND LEVELS

We are exposed to ionizing radiation in our daily lives from multiple sources. The largest source is natural background radiation, something over which we have no control. Other sources are medical diagnostic and therapeutic procedures and radiation applications associated with industry, research, and consumer products. To place in perspective the radiation exposures and risks associated with being a radiologic technologist, one should know something about the radiation levels associated with these other sources (Table 2).

Natural background

Human beings have inhabited this planet for perhaps 100,000 years and have evolved in the presence of a constant radiation exposure called natural background radiation. This natural background radiation comes from three principal sources: (1) terrestrial radiation resulting from naturally occurring radionuclides in the earth and from products made from earth, (2) cosmic radiation resulting from sources outside the earth, principally the sun but also sources outside our solar system and galaxy, and (3) internal exposure from radionuclides naturally deposited in the human body. In the United States these sources produce a whole body dose of 75 to 300 mrads/yr depending on location and diet. Table 2 includes these components of the natural background radiation and their quantities.

Terrestrial radiation

At the time of the earth's formation some elements (principally uranium and thorium) were created that were slightly radioactive, having a radioactive half-life of billions of years. As these radionuclides decay, they emit radiation, and this source contributes to the total natural background radiation level. The terrestrial radiation level is very dependent on geographic location and particularly the type of soil or rock present. Along the Atlantic and Gulf coasts the terrestrial doses range from 15 to 35 mrads. In the northeastern, central, and far western portions of the United States the terrestrial radiation ranges from 35 to 75 mrads. In the Colorado plateau area the range is from 75 to 140 mrads. By applying the appropriate terrestrial radiation dose rate to the resident population, the average U.S. rate is estimated to be 40 mrads.

Table 2. Radiation in our daily lives: sources and average annual levels

Source	Level (mrads/yr)
Natural background	96
Terrestrial	40
Cosmic	31
Internal	25
Medical exposure	93
Diagnostic x rays	77
Dental x rays	1
Radiopharmaceuticals	14
Radiation therapy	1
Nuclear weapons testing	4
Nuclear power generation	<1
Research activities	<1
Consumer products	4
Air travel	0.5
TOTAL (approximate)	200

Cosmic radiation

The sources of cosmic radiation are many. Photons and particles are emitted by the sun and by sources outside of our solar system—even outside of our galaxy. Since this radiation is incident on the earth, its intensity is influenced by the shielding of the overlying atmosphere and by the geomagnetic latitude. In general, radiation intensity is lower at the equator than at the poles because of the deflection of particles by the earth's magnetic field. The intensity increases with increasing altitude, so that 1 mile above the earth's surface the cosmic intensity is approximately twice that at sea level. When all of these influences are considered, the U.S. population receives an estimated 31 mrads of cosmic radiation per year.

Internally deposited radionuclides

The air we breathe, the water we drink, and the food we eat all contain small quantities of naturally occurring radionuclides. Some of these radionuclides are metabolized and incorporated permanently into the tissues of the body. The radionuclides of principal importance are ^3H, ^{14}C, ^{40}K, ^{226}Ra, and ^{210}Po. Collectively, these internally deposited radionuclides result in an average estimated annual dose of 25 mrads.

Medical diagnostic and therapeutic radiation

Patients receive radiation exposure from radiographic examinations, fluoroscopic procedures, dental diagnosis, radioisotope procedures, and radiation therapy. By far, most radiation exposure is received from medical radiographic procedures. It is difficult to assign precise dose values to such procedures because of the many associated complications. Approximately 65% of the U.S. population is exposed to radiation each year for medical or dental purposes. Medical applications of radiation represent the second most intense source of radiation exposure.

Two measures of patient dose are important in assessing the extent of medical radiation exposure on the population: the genetically significant dose (GSD) and the mean marrow dose (MMD). The GSD is a genetic dose index. It is the gonad dose that, if received by every member of the population, would be expected to produce the sum total effect on the population as the sum of the individual doses actually received. In the United States at this time the GSD is estimated to be 20 mrads. The GSD indicates nothing about possible or probable genetic effects. It is only an attempt to estimate the dose received by the population gene pool.

There is a similar index for somatic effects—the MMD; it too is expressed in millirads per year. The MMD to the U.S. population is currently estimated to be 77 mrads. Like the GSD, the MMD is a weighted average over the entire population, including those who are and those who are not irradiated. It takes into account the fraction of anatomic bone marrow irradiated as a function of each type of examination and averages this by the total active bone marrow. Since bone marrow irradiation is considered to be responsible for radiation-induced leukemia, the MMD is a somatic dose index for leukemia. The mean marrow dose is a measure of radiation dose and not of late radiation effect.

Industrial applications

Industrial applications of ionizing radiation result in average occupational exposures of up to several hundred millirems per year in some groups such as nuclear power plant workers. In addition to these workers, others who are employed in the mining, refining, and fabrication of nuclear fuel, in industrial radiography, and in the handling of radioisotopes for a large number of industrial applications receive occupational exposure. Included in these industrial applications is the transportation of radioactive material, particularly as it pertains to the air freight of nuclear medicine radiopharmaceuticals. When prorated over the entire U.S. population these industrial activities add approximately 0.2 mrad/yr to the population dose.

Research applications

Research applications of ionizing radiation include particle accelerators, other radiation-producing machines, and radionuclides. Particle accelerators, such as cyclotrons, synchrocyclotrons, Van de Graaff generators, and linear accelerators, are employed in university and industrial research laboratories, and, although they can generate intense fields of radiation, they are always shielded and protected. X-ray diffraction units and electron microscopes are common research tools employed to investigate the structure of matter. The x-ray diffraction unit generates an intense field of highly collimated and very soft radiation. It does not normally represent a whole body hazard but rather a danger to hands if they are accidentally placed in the useful beam. Electron microscopes likewise produce low-energy x rays, but these are well shielded and do not represent a significant occupational radiation hazard nor a population

radiation hazard. Many research activities employ radionuclides, but mostly low-energy beta-emitting radionuclides such as ^{3}H and ^{14}C are used. Although there is a small occupational hazard from these activities, the population exposures are nil. Collectively, these research activities contribute no more than 0.1 mrad/yr to the population dose.

Consumer products

Surprisingly, many consumer products incorporate x-ray devices or radioactive material. Television receivers, video display terminals, and airport surveillance systems are three devices that produce x rays. In the case of the first two the x-rays produced are of a very low energy and very low intensity and pose no hazard to the consumer. Surveillance systems likewise emit low levels of x-radiation, and these units are well shielded and are provided with safety interlocks. Radioactive material is incorporated into various luminous products, such as instrument gauges, clocks, and exit signs. Radioactive material is also incorporated into such devices as check sources, static eliminators, and smoke detectors. Collectively, these devices may contribute an additional 0.5 mrad/yr to the population dose. Many consumer products consist of natural radioactive materials, such as tobacco, building materials, highway and road construction materials, combustible fuels, glass, and ceramics. Under some circumstances use of these naturally occurring materials can enhance the existing natural background radiation dose by as much as 5 mrads/yr.

RADIATION PROTECTION GUIDES

Most radiation biology research, dealing with experimental animals or observations on humans, has been devoted to describing the quantitative relationship between the radiation dose and the biologic effect. Such dose-response relationships have been described with great precision for the early effects of radiation following high doses. Most early effects, such as skin erythema, hematologic depression, and lethality, exhibit a threshold type of dose-response relationship. Such a dose threshold indicates that there is a dose level below which no response will occur.

This is not true for the late effects of low-level radiation exposure. Late effects are considered to have no dose threshold and are linear; that is, there is considered to be no radiation dose below which such an effect will occur. This type of dose-response relationship suggests that no radiation dose, regardless of how small, is considered absolutely safe. At zero dose a small but measurable response may be observed. This represents the natural incidence of effect under observation.

Basis for radiation protection standards

This linear, nonthreshold type of dose-response relationship is the basis for current radiation protection standards. The late effects of principal concern are leukemia, cancer, and genetic effects, and they have been shown with reasonable accuracy to follow this dose-response model. More recent data and a more refined analysis of previous data have shown that the

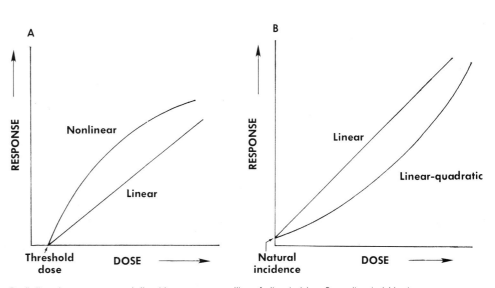

Radiation dose–response relationships appear as either, **A**, threshold or, **B**, nonthreshold in shape.

linear quadratic dose-response model probably better represents the actual experience of these effects. If this is true, then the adoption of the linear model results in an overestimation of the true radiation effects at low dose levels. Nevertheless, it is conservative and prudent to hold to the linear dose-response model as the basis for radiation protection guides.

This basis for radiation protection guidance was first enunciated in 1931 when the National Council for Radiation Protection and Measurements (NCRP) recommended a whole body maximum permissible dose (MPD) of 50,000 mrems/yr. Since that time there have been numerous revisions of the MPD down to the present level of 5000 mrems/yr. Thousands of occupationally exposed persons have been observed, and very few have been exposed to a dose that exceeded the present MPD. For instance, in diagnostic radiology approximately 70% of radiologic technologists receive less than 100 mrems/yr. Only 3% are exposed to dose levels greater than 1000 mrems/yr. These observations of occupationally exposed technologists have not resulted in a single observed case of radiation effect.

It should be clear that any attempt to establish an MPD is highly judgmental and requires value assessments beyond the realm of science. The present maximum permissible dose has been in effect for more than 20 years and remains a prudent and safe level.

The development of the MPD and other radiation protection guidelines acknowledges that there is some risk involved in all radiation exposure. The task is to set these standards at a level of radiation exposure associated with an acceptable risk, recognizing that what may be an acceptable risk for one individual is unacceptable for another. The MPD is considered to be an acceptable risk to all radiation workers. Therefore it is that dose which, if received each year for a 50-year working lifetime, would not be expected to produce any harmful effect. The MPD for the population at large is one tenth of that for occupationally exposed persons, or 500 mrems/yr.

The phrase *maximum permissible dose* is used in preference to earlier statements of dose limitations such as *tolerance dose* or *allowable dose*. This is intended to emphasize the possible but unobserved low-dose radiation effects and the fact that the specified dose limits are acceptable. In

Table 3. Maximum permissible doses

Subject exposed	Dose
Occupationally exposed persons	
Whole body	
Prospective annual limit	5 rems in any 1 year
Long term accumulation to age n years	$(n\text{-}18) \times 5$ rems
Skin	15 rems in any 1 year
Hands	75 rems in any 1 year (25 rems/3 mo)
Forearms	30 rems in any 1 year (10 rems/3 mo)
Other organs, tissue, and organ systems	15 rems in any 1 year (5 rems/3 mo)
Pregnant women (with respect to fetus)	0.5 rem in gestation period
General population	
Individual or occasional exposed persons	0.5 rem in any 1 year
Students	0.1 rem in any 1 year
Population dose limit	0.17 rem per year (average)

addition, radiation protection programs must be consistent with the ALARA concept.

Specific radiation protection concepts

In addition to the specification of a whole body MPD for occupationally exposed persons and for the population at large, several tissues and organs of the body are considered for their individual radiosensitivity. Specific individuals in the population are likewise accorded attention in specifying the MPD. Table 3 is a summary of all of these applicable MPDs and other dose-limiting recommendations.

The whole body MPD includes not only the whole body but also the head and neck, the lenses of the eyes, the trunk of the body, the gonads, and the blood-forming organs. Each of these parts of the body when irradiated by external means should be restricted to the same MPD, 5000 mrems/yr. Irradiation of the gonads of course is considered separately because of concern about possible genetic effects. Irradiation of blood-forming tissue is associated with the possible development of leukemia, and irradiation of the lenses of the eyes is associated with the possible induction of cataracts. This level of 5000 mrems/yr is the prospective annual MPD.

There may be occasions when the prospective MPD will be exceeded, but this should rarely if ever occur in diagnostic radiology. In such a situation, if the individual's previous occupational exposure was low, then a retrospective MPD of 12,000 mrems/yr may be permitted.

The retrospective MPD may be acceptable in some circumstances, but only if the accumulative lifetime exposure does not exceed $5(n\text{-}18)$ rems, where n is the age in years. This statement of MPD is known as the long-term accumulation to age n years. This MPD dictates that no one under age 18 be employed as a radiation worker. Students may be under age 18, but a different MPD applies to them. Use of the terms *prospective, retrospective,* and *accumulated dose equivalent* serves to emphasize that these MPD's are guides only and that exceeding a numerical MPD may be acceptable under some circumstances.

Other regions of the body have different MPDs. The MPD for the skin of the body is 15,000 mrems/yr. This MPD applies to exposure to nonpenetrating radiation such as electrons and low-energy photons. In diagnostic radiology, mammography is the only type of procedure in which exposure of the skin of the technologist can reach its limit before the whole body MPD becomes applicable.

During fluoroscopy it is often necessary for the hands or forearms to be in the useful beam. Usually these parts are protected by lead gloves. However, during certain procedures the use of such protective apparel is not possible. The MPD for the hands is 75,000 mrems/yr, but not more than 25,000 mrems can be received in any one calendar quarter. The MPD for the forearms is 30,000 mrems/yr, and not more than 10,000 mrems can be received in any quarter.

The MPD for any other organ not previously mentioned is 15,000 mrems/yr.

This includes the thyroid gland, which in some radiologic situations could be exposed to external beams as well as to internal irradiation by radioiodine. In such a situation, to apply the dose-limiting recommendations rigorously the technologist would add the internal and the external exposure and specify that the thyroid gland not receive a combined total of 15,000 mrems/yr.

The unborn child is known to be particularly sensitive to the effects of ionizing radiation; consequently, an MPD of 500 mrems/9 mo is applied. This presents a special problem in diagnostic radiology. In the case of the pregnant technologist, it is rare that the MPD for the fetus would ever be approached, much less exceeded, because of the use of protective apparel during fluoroscopy and portable radiography. Nevertheless, rigorous radiation protection methods may be required during pregnancy.

Under some circumstances students under age 18 may be involved in educational experiences and therefore are granted a separate MPD of 100 mrems/yr. This level is in addition to the 500 mrems/yr that they may receive as members of the general population. This MPD is directed particularly to high school and college students of any age but also to radiologic technology students under age 18.

MEDICAL RADIATION DOSE AND EXPOSURE

The output intensity of an x-ray beam from any given radiographic or fluoroscopic unit can vary widely depending on the type of equipment and techniques employed. There may even be a sizable variation among x-ray units of the same manufacture and model when identical techniques are employed. The output intensity of any x-ray unit of course determines the radiation dose not only to the patient but also to the technologist. Consequently, several methods are used to determine x-ray output to estimate doses to patient and technologist.

The tabletop output intensity during fluoroscopy is difficult to estimate by computation with even moderate precision; it must be measured. Modern fluoroscopes have beam intensities limited to 10 R/min at the tabletop. Experience has shown that when operated at a technique of about 100 kVp/1 mA most fluoroscopes will produce an approximate tabletop exposure of 1 to 2 R/min.

Radiographic output intensities are also difficult to estimate by computation unless at least a single measurement is available. For a properly calibrated radiographic system the output intensity will vary directly with the milliampere-seconds and directly with the square of the kVp. It will also vary inversely as the square of the distance from the target. Mathematically this is represented as follows:

$$\text{Output intensity} = \frac{k(mAs)\,(kVp)^2}{d^2}$$

where: k = empirically determined constant
mAs = x-ray tube current multiplied by the exposure time
kVp = tube potential
d = distance from the source to the entrance surface of the patient (SSD)

Using this formulation and one measurement of k, a reasonably accurate estimate of radiographic output intensity can be made for any technique. Usually this one measurement is made at 70 kVp and expressed in milliroentgens per milliampere-seconds at a source-to-image receptor distance (SID) of 40 inches. Experience shows this value to range from about 2 to 8 mR/mAs depending on the age, manufacture, and adequacy of calibration of the radiographic unit. With this measured value, the output intensity at any other radiographic technique can be computed by using the following expression:

Output intensity (mR) =
$$k(mR/mAs)\,(mAs^1) \left(\frac{kVp^1}{70}\right)^2 \left(\frac{40 \text{ inches}}{d'}\right)^2$$

where: k = measured value at 70 kVp/40 inches SID
mAs^1 and kVp^1 = the desired technique
d' = SSD

EXAMPLE: The physicist's report shows the radiographic output to be 4.8 mR/mAs at 70 kVp/40 inches SID. The technique chart calls for 76 kVp/80 mAs for a KUB examination. If the SSD is 32 inches, the skin exposure will be as follows:

Skin exposure
$$= (4.8 \text{ mR/mAs})\,(80 \text{ mAs}) \left(\frac{76}{70}\right)^2 \left(\frac{40}{32}\right)^2$$
$$= 707 \text{ mR}$$

Some investigators have produced nomograms for ease in estimating radiographic output intensity.

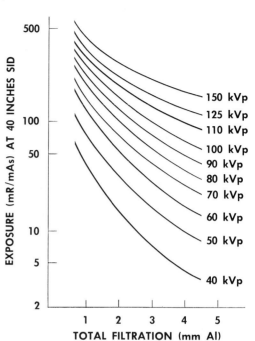

A graphic relationship of radiographic output intensity (mR/mAs) as a function of kVp and added filtration at a source-to-image receptor distance (SID) of 40 inches.

Redrawn from E.C. McCullough, Mayo Clinic, Rochester, Minn.

Patient dose

The dose received by patients during diagnostic radiologic examinations is usually expressed in one of three ways: skin exposure, organ dose, or fetal dose. Each has a specific application in assessing the risk to the patient, but skin exposure is the easiest to estimate.

Skin exposure

The exposure to the entrance surface of the patient during any radiographic examination can be measured directly or estimated by using the techniques previously described. Skin exposure during fluoroscopy usually must be measured, although it too can be estimated from a tabletop exposure measurement at the technique under investigation.

Two methods are generally employed to measure skin exposure. Small ion chambers can be placed on the entrance surface of the patient and exposed during any clinical procedure. Ion chambers have a sufficiently wide range and are sensitive and accurate. However, they are difficult to position and use, and therefore their application is very limited. Most current

Table 4. Representative skin exposures and maximum recommended entrance skin exposures for several routine examinations

Examination	Skin exposure (mrads per projection)	
	Normal	Maximum recommended
Chest (PA)	10-20	30
Skull (lateral)	100-200	300
Abdomen (AP)	250-500	750
Cervical spine (AP)	<5-150	250
Thoracic spine (AP)	300-600	900
Intraveneous pyelogram	300-600	900
Extremity	50-200	300
Dental (bite-wing and periapical)	200-500	700

Table 5. Representative skin exposure and tissue midline dose for the three types of mammography examinations

Examination	Skin exposure per projection (mR)	Midline dose per projection (mrad)
Direct exposure	6000-15,000	1000-4000
Xeromammography	500-1500	100-600
Screen/film	200-1000	20-250

Table 6. Representative bone marrow doses for selected radiographic examinations

X-ray examination	Mean marrow dose (mrads)
Skull	50
Cervical spine	20
Full-mouth dental	25
Chest	10
Stomach and upper gastrointestinal	400
Gallbladder	300
Lumbar spine	400
Intravenous pyelography	400
Abdomen	80
Pelvis	100
Extremity	10

Table 7. Approximate gonad doses resulting from various radiographic examinations

X-ray examination	Gonad dose (mrad)	
	Male	Female
Skull	<0.5	<0.5
Cervical spine	<0.5	<0.5
Full-mouth dental	<0.5	<0.5
Chest	1	<0.5
Stomach and upper gastrointestinal	2	150
Gallbladder	1	75
Lumbar spine	225	700
Intraveneous pyelography	200	600
Abdomen	100	225
Pelvis	375	210
Upper extremity	<0.5	<0.5
Lower extremity	15	<0.5

estimates of skin exposure are made with thermoluminescent dosimeters (TLD). TLDs are equally sensitive and precise, and they have a much wider range of response. Furthermore, they are very easy to use and because of their small size can be positioned in multiple units on the entrance surface of the skin. TLDs are nearly tissue equivalent and therefore will not be imaged except at a very low kVp.

Measurements of exposure to skin have been made by a number of investigators. Table 4 shows the average skin exposure during certain specific radiographic examinations.

In recent years there has been an attempt by some government agencies to restrict the radiation exposure to patients during routine radiographic examinations. Table 4 indicates these maximum recommended skin exposures for specific examinations. These suggested maximum levels are rather generous in light of the techniques and image receptors currently employed.

Organ dose

Sometimes the radiation dose received by a specific organ or tissue is of primary importance. Of course, organ doses for the most part cannot be measured directly but must be estimated. The breast, for example, is a tissue of primary concern because of the relatively high dose of radiation received during mammography. Table 5 shows the approximate skin exposures and midline doses received by the breast as a function of the type of image receptor employed. Direct exposure examination is no longer used because of the high patient dose. The total breast dose during a given examination can be estimated by simply adding each estimated midline dose.

Another organ of particular concern is the bone marrow. Bone marrow dose is used to estimate the population MMD as an index of the somatic effect of radiation exposure. Table 6 relates some average bone marrow doses associated with various radiographic exposures. Each of these doses is averaged over the entire body even though partial body exposure exists.

The gonads are other organs of concern in diagnostic radiology because of the possible genetic effects of ionizing radiation. Table 7 indicates average gonad doses received during various procedures. The large difference between male and female is because of the shielding of the ovaries by overlying tissue. The weighted average gonad dose to the general population is used to estimate the GSD.

Fetal dose

Like most organ doses, fetal dose cannot be measured; it must be estimated. Such estimates are usually obtained from phantom measurements or by computer-generated calculations. Table 8 shows the results of an analysis by The Bureau of Radiological Health and reports fetal doses as a function of the normalized skin exposure. To use this table, first the skin exposure for the type of examination in question must be measured. The fetal dose is given in millirads per 1000 milliroentgens of skin exposure. Obviously the fetal dose is highest when the uterus is in the useful beam, such as during abdominal and pelvic examinations. During examination of distal parts of the body, the fetal dose will be very low, often not exceeding 1 mrad.

Table 8. Approximate fetal dose (mrads) as a function of entrance exposure (1000 mR)

X-ray examination	Fetal dose (mrad/R)
Skull	< 0.01
Cervical spine	< 0.01
Full-mouth dental	< 0.01
Chest	2
Stomach and upper gastrointestinal	25
Gallbladder	3
Lumbar spine	250
Intraveneous pyelography	265
Abdomen	265
Pelvis	295
Extremity	< 0.01

Technologist exposure

During the course of normal x-ray examinations, the technologist receives at least 95% of occupational exposure during fluoroscopy and portable radiography. However, during fluoroscopy and portable radiography the technologist wears protective apparel, so that only part of the body is exposed.

Adjacent to the examination table exposure rates may approach 500 mR/hr. The protective curtain draping the image intensifier tower will usually reduce the exposure to less than 5 mR/hr. The technologist exposure can be estimated by assuming a position near the table and determining the x-ray beam on-time. For example, if a barium enema requires 3 minutes of x-ray tube on-time and the technologist is positioned in a 100 mR/hr field, then the occupational exposure to the unshielded part of the technologist would be as follows:

$$100 \text{ mR/hr} \times \frac{3}{60} \text{ hr} = 5 \text{ mR}$$

Protective apparel usually provides an exposure reduction factor of at least one tenth, so that in the above example the exposure to the trunk of the body of the technologist would be less than 1 mR.

During fixed conventional radiography, the technologist is positioned behind a protective barrier, which often may be a secondary barrier. In such cases the useful beam is never directed at the technologist. A useful way to estimate exposure to the technologist during radiography is to apply the rule of thumb that the exposure level 1 m (meter) laterally from the patient is approximately 0.1% of the entrance exposure. For example, in the illustration on p. 21 the technologist is positioned 2 m from the patient. If the examination were of the chest, the skin exposure would be approximately 25 mR. The scatter radiation 1 m laterally would be 0.1% of the entrance exposure or 0.025 mR. According to the inverse square law, at 2 m the scatter radiation intensity would be 0.006 mR or 6 μR.

PROTECTION OF PATIENT

The patient is protected from unnecessary radiation during diagnostic x-ray examinations by two general methods. Certain design features of x-ray equipment and of specially fabricated auxiliary apparatus are principally for patient protection. Special administrative procedures will also help to avoid unnecessary patient dose.

Equipment and apparatus design

Usually those features of radiographic and fluoroscopic equipment that are designed to reduce patient dose will also reduce technologist exposure. This aspect of radiation control should be kept in mind when considering patient protection.

Filtration

A minimum of 2.5 mm Al equivalent total filtration is required on all fluoroscopic tubes and for those radiographic tubes operating above 70 kVp. The purpose of filtration is to reduce the amount of low-energy radiation (soft x rays) reaching the patient. Since only penetrating radiation is useful in producing an x-ray image, nonpenetrating soft radiation is absorbed in the patient and contributes only to patient dose and not to the radiographic or fluoroscopic image. In general, the higher the total filtration, the lower will be the patient dose.

Collimation

Collimation is extremely important in patient protection. The x-ray beam should always be collimated to the region of anatomic interest. The larger the useful x-ray beam the higher will be the patient dose. Restricting the x-ray beam by collimation reduces not only the volume of tissue irradiated but also the absolute dose at any point because of the accompanying reduction in scatter radiation. Reduction of scatter radiation also contributes to increased image quality by increasing radiographic contrast.

Specific area shielding

In specific area shielding part of the primary beam is absorbed during the examination by shielding a specific area of the body. Gonad shielding is a good example of specific area shielding and can be applied in two ways—with shadow shields and contact shields. Shadow shields are attached to the radiographic tube head and positioned with the aid of the light localizer midway between the tube and the patient. Contact shields are usually fabricated of vinyl lead cut into various shapes and are simply laid on the patient. Gonad shielding should be used under the following conditions: (1) on all patients of reproductive age, (2) when the gonads lie in or near the useful beam, and (3) when the use of such shielding will not compromise the required diagnostic information. Gonad shielding will protect the patient from unnecessary radiation by reducing the gonad dose to near zero.

Image receptors

The speed of an image receptor can greatly influence patient dose. Newly developed rare earth screens in conjunction with matched photographic emulsions show relative speeds of up to eight times of that for a conventional calcium tungstate screen-film combination. Rare earth screen-film combinations that will reduce patient dose in half can be used with no loss of diagnostic information. Higher patient dose reductions are possible, but the quality of the image may be compromised somewhat by radiographic noise. Newer fluoroscopic image intensifier tubes also incorporate more efficient input phosphorus that can result in a 25% to 50% reduction in patient dose. Use of these newer imaging modalities has been responsible for the most significant reduction in patient dose in many years.

Radiographic technique

Radiographic technique not only is important in the production of a quality image but also greatly influences patient dose. Ideally, the higher the kVp the lower will be the patient dose, because a large reduction in mAs must accompany an increase in kVp. However, as kVp is raised, the image contrast is reduced and for some examinations this reduction in contrast may be unacceptable. For example, mammography could be done at far lower patient doses if the operating kVp were increased. However, the radiographic contrast would be very poor and the image would contain less diagnostic information. In general, the highest practicable kVp with an appropriate low mAs should be employed in all examinations.

Administrative procedures

Patient selection and examination selection are two areas in which technologists can provide procedures for reducing unnecessary patient dose.

Pregnancy

To ensure that an unknown pregnancy is not irradiated, procedures should be implemented that satisfy the 10-day rule. The 10-day rule states that women of childbearing age who are referred for x-ray examinations of the abdomen and pelvis should have such examinations performed only during the first 10 days following the onset of menstruation, when it is certain that there is no pregnancy.

Three techniques can be employed that satisfy the 10-day rule. In small community hospitals in which there is good communication between the clinician and the radiologist, elective booking can be instituted. This requires that the clinician determine the patient's last menstrual period and schedule her accordingly. Alternatively, in any facility a positive response by the patient may be required. If this type of procedure is too bothersome, the waiting area and examination room should be conspicuously posted with signs to alert the patient.

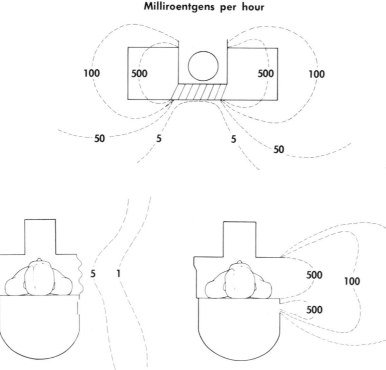

Milliroentgens per hour

100   500   500   100

50   5   5   50

Approximate isoexposure contours during fluoroscopy.

5   1

500   100   50

500

**With protective curtain and
Bucky slot cover**

Without protective devices

X-RAY CONSENT FOR WOMEN OF CHILDBEARING AGE

X-ray examinations of abdomen and pelvis exposing the uterus to radiation are:

Abdomen (KUB)	Colon (barium enema)	Pyelograms (IVP & retrograde)
Stomach (UGI)	Gallbladder	Cystograms
Small intestine (S.I.)	Hips, sacrum, coccyx	Lumbar spine & pelvis
All nuclear medicine studies		

The 10 days following onset of menstrual period are generally considered safe for x-ray examinations.

Onset of last menstrual period, Date:_____ Date today:_____

I am pregnant   Yes_____ No_____ Don't know
I have had a hysterectomy   _____ _____
I use an IUD (intrauterine device)   _____ _____

I recognize that if I am pregnant and have radiation to the abdomen, there is a possibility of injury to the fetus. However, I understand that the likelihood of such injury is slight and that my physician feels that the information to be gained from this examination is important to my health. I therefore wish to have this x-ray examination performed now.

_____
Name of examination

_____   _____
Witness   Signature of patient

Dr. V.P. Collins

Sample of a patient questionnaire useful in guarding against irradiating an unknown pregnancy

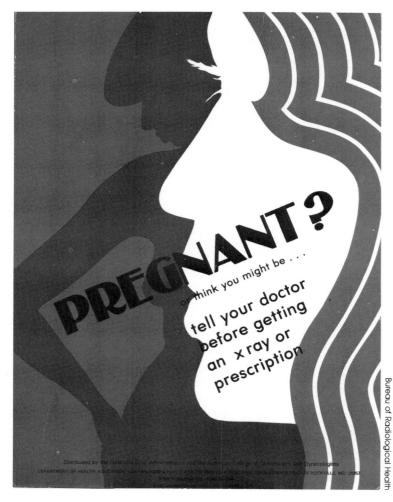

One of many signs available to alert patient to possibility of irradiating an unknown pregnancy

Bureau of Radiological Health

Patient and examination selection

Certain aspects of administrative control for reduction of unnecessary patient dose are generally the responsibility of the radiologist, not the technologist. Patient and examination selection are two such situations. Patients selected for x-ray examination fall into two categories: patients who have symptoms and those who do not. Patients with symptoms usually require x-ray examinations to evaluate any previous clinical management and to provide the physician with information to plan the patient's future clinical management. Patients without symptoms usually are referred for x-ray examination to provide baseline information for possible future problems or to satisfy certain legal, insurance, or employment requirements.

When accepting a patient with symptoms for x-ray examination, the radiologist must be certain that the type of examination prescribed can provide the information necessary for proper medical management of the patient's condition. Furthermore, even if the findings of the examination are negative or normal, the performance of the examination should be beneficial and should significantly influence the course of management. For example, a skull series following trauma should be carefully evaluated by the radiologist and the clinician. Several investigational series have reported that skull examinations are helpful in influencing the medical management of less than 10% of patients. Similarly, the efficacy of x-ray pelvimetry is limited, particularly with the emergence of diagnostic ultrasound. Investigations of other types of examinations, intravenous pyelography and barium enema, for example, have likewise shown a low yield of significant diagnostic information affecting the medical management of the patient.

Selection of patients without symptoms for x-ray examination involves mass screening and routine procedures, many of which may not be medically justified. Mammography, lumbar spine examinations, and routine chest examinations are just three that require considerable evaluation of the patient by the radiologist and clinician before the examinations are performed. Each of these examinations is the subject of heated controversy at this time, and future restrictions on their use for patients without symptoms are likely.

PROTECTION OF TECHNOLOGIST
Equipment and apparatus design

The principal source of radiation exposure to the technologist occurs during fluoroscopy and portable radiography. Consequently, particular care and attention should be exercised by technologists during such situations.

Protective apparel

For both types of procedures protective apparel is used, and it should be used faithfully. Table 9 shows the degree of protection provided by the principal sizes of protective lead (Pb) aprons available. Most find the 0.5 mm Pb apron perfectly adequate. Aprons of 1.0 mm Pb often are much too heavy for technologists who are engaged in a heavy fluoroscopy schedule. Each portable x-ray unit should have assigned to it a protective apron, and the apron should remain with the unit at all times.

Protective barriers

During conventional radiography the technologist is positioned behind the control booth barrier or other fixed protective barrier. Mobile protective screens should be avoided whenever possible. Although most protective barriers consist of a certain thickness of lead, not all do, and it is not necessary that all contain lead. Table 10 shows the British, metric, and construction equivalences of common thicknesses of lead employed in diagnostic radiology. Rarely is it necessary to exceed 4 pounds per square foot.

Newer x-ray equipment and faster image receptors are significantly reducing the intensity of radiation during diagnostic x-ray procedures; therefore the amount of shielding required today is not what it was in years past. Although it is unnecessary for the technologist to know how to compute the barrier thickness, some of the considerations that enter into that computation should be understood.

Primary versus secondary barriers

A primary barrier is any barrier that is likely to intercept the useful x-ray beam. A secondary barrier is one that intercepts only leakage and scatter radiation. The floor is nearly always considered a primary barrier and anywhere from one to four walls may also be primary barriers. The ceiling is always considered a secondary

Table 9. X-ray attenuation values for the common lead (Pb) equivalent thicknesses of protective aprons

Equivalent thickness (mm Pb)	Percent of x-ray attenuation		
	50 kVp	75 kVp	100 kVp
0.25	97	66	51
0.5	99	88	75
1.0	99	99	94

Modified from Bushong, S.C.: Radiologic science for technologists: physics, biology, and protection, ed. 2, St. Louis, 1980, The C.V. Mosby Co.

Table 10. British, metric, and construction equivalences of common thicknesses of lead employed in diagnostic radiology*

British (inches)	Metric (mm)	Construction (pounds/square foot)
1/64	0.4	1
1/32	0.8	2
3/64	1.2	3
1/16	1.6	4
5/64	2.0	5
3/32	2.4	6

*Protective lead shielding is usually computed in British or metric units, but it is given to the builder in pounds per square foot.

barrier. In addition, the control booth barrier is often considered a secondary barrier. During fluoroscopy all fixed barriers are considered secondary, because the image intensifier tower is designed as a built-in primary barrier.

Maximum permissible dose

The maximum permissible dose (MPD) expressed as a weekly intensity is determined for each barrier on the basis of the use of the area being protected. If the adjacent area, such as another x-ray examination room or the darkroom, is to be occupied only by radiation workers and patients, it is identified as a controlled area. The MPD for a controlled area is 0.1 R/wk. If the adjacent area is a laboratory, an office, or an area occupied by persons in the general population, it is called an uncontrolled area, and the MPD is 0.01 R/wk.

Distance

The distance from the x-ray tube to the area being protected is important because the radiation intensity decreases rapidly with an increase in distance. If the barrier is designated as a primary barrier, then the distance can hardly be less than 3 feet and is usually much more. The distance to a secondary barrier is often shorter. Obviously, for larger examination rooms, the respective distances will be larger and the required shielding less.

Workload

Workload is an expression of the total intensity of radiation employed during 1 week. It is described in units of milliampere-minutes per week and takes into account the number of patients examined, the number of projections per patient, and the average mAs per projection. Rarely will the radiographic workload of a busy room exceed 1000 mA-min/wk. Special-purpose radiographic units such as chest, head, and pediatric units may have considerably lower workloads. Less shielding is required for low-workload facilities.

Use factor

Under normal conditions, during most of the time that a general-purpose radiographic tube is energized it is pointed toward the floor. During some fraction of its beam on-time it may be pointed toward any vertical barrier. The fraction or percent of time that the useful beam is directed to a barrier while energized is the use factor. The floor is generally assigned a use factor of 1 and each wall a use factor of ¼. The use factor is 1 for all secondary barriers, since at all times while the tube is energized, scatter and leakage radiation are generated.

Occupancy factor

The occupancy factor is an expression of the extent to which the area being protected is occupied. Obviously an area that is always occupied will require more shielding than one that is rarely occupied. The recommended occupancy factors range from full occupancy for an adjacent office or laboratory to partial occupancy for a hallway or restroom to occasional occupancy for outside areas, elevators, and stairwells.

These factors are all taken into consideration when the required protective barrier thickness is computed. Although lead is the usual shielding material for most diagnostic x-ray applications, other types of building material may be acceptable, particularly for secondary barriers. Clay brick, concrete block, gypsum board, and conventional plate glass are sometimes suitable. Frequently, multiple thicknesses of gypsum board may be used instead of lead-lined wallboard. Plate glass that is ½ to 1 inch thick may sometimes be substituted for leaded glass, as in the viewing window of a control booth console. A block wall, brick wall, or concrete wall will often satisfy the requirements for a primary barrier. A 4-inch concrete slab floor will likewise usually provide adequate protection as a primary barrier. If the slab is thin, it is sometimes permissible to position additional protective lead under the examination table with an appropriate overhang.

Administrative procedures

Every radiologic technologist should be familiar with the cardinal principles of radiation protection—time, distance, and shielding: (1) The time of exposure to a radiation source should be kept to a minimum; (2) The distance between the radiation source and the technologist should be as great as possible; and (3) When appropriate and practicable, protective shielding material should be positioned between the source and the technologist. A finer example of adherence to these cardinal principles occurs in fluoroscopy. During fluoroscopy the maximum exposure rate exists adjacent to the table, as shown on p. 28. Since the primary beam is emitted by the under-table tube and intercepts the patient, the patient becomes the radiation source because of scatter radiation. The radiologist must minimize the exposure time by activating the foot or hand control intermittently for minimum beam on-time. The technologist can help by making certain that the 5-minute fluoroscopic reset timer is functioning and is used properly. The technologist can minimize occupational exposure by taking one step back from the edge of the fluoroscopic table when it is not absolutely essential to remain there. Both the radiologist and the technologist wear protective lead apparel during fluoroscopy, and this is perhaps the most effective method for reduction of occupational exposure.

Personnel monitoring

Perhaps the single most important aspect of a radiation control program in diagnostic radiology is the conduct of a properly designed personnel radiation monitoring program. Three types of radiation measuring devices are used as personnel monitors—pocket ionization chambers, film badges, and thermoluminescent dosimetry badges.

Pocket ionization chambers can be used for personnel monitoring, although they seldom are in diagnostic radiology. These devices have the singular advantage that they can be evaluated daily. However, the record keeping required with pocket chamber dosimeters is great; thus their use in diagnostic radiology is generally restricted to monitoring occasional visitors.

Photographic film has been successfully used for nearly half a century as a personnel radiation monitor. The design of the film badge has undergone many refinements and enables it to measure not only the quantity of radiation but also the type of radiation, the approximate energy, and the direction. Consequently it is very important that such a monitor be properly handled and worn.

Thermoluminescent dosimetry (TLD) has been used for approximately 10 years as a personnel radiation monitor. TLD badges have many of the same performance characteristics of film badges. The TLD sensitive material is reusable, and although the initial cost is high the long-term expense is comparable to that of film badges. Because of the nature of this detector, it can be used for lengths of time exceeding the monthly interval limits placed on film badges. Under some circumstances it is not only permissable but advisable to monitor x-ray workers for calendar quarter intervals rather than for monthly or biweekly intervals. The principal advantage to this mode of radiation monitoring is the reduced amount of record keeping that is required.

Regardless of the type of monitor employed there are certain important aspects to the conduct of a successful personnel radiation monitoring program. Each shipment of personnel monitors will be accompanied by a control badge. The control badge should normally be stored in some location distant from any radiation source, such as the chief technologist's office. Individual radiation monitors should not leave the hospital. A rack or other holding device should be available, so that technologists can store their badges at the hospital at the end of the day. This will help to ensure that the monitors are not inadvertently damaged or exposed to environmental elements outside of the hospital. Of course, the holding rack should be positioned distant from any radiation source.

Since technologists receive most of their occupational exposure during fluoroscopy and portable radiography during which protective apparel is worn, the anatomic position of the personnel monitor is important. However, there is not complete agreement among experts about monitor position. Consensus and most state regulations suggest that the monitor be positioned above the protective apron, unshielded, at the collar region. This region of the body is restricted to the same MPD (5000 mrems/yr) as the protected trunk of the body. Because the collar region, including the head, neck, and lenses of the eyes, is unprotected it will receive at least 10 times the radiation exposure of the trunk of the body. Therefore it is prudent to monitor the collar region, since it will receive the highest percentage of the applicable MPD; this is the most restrictive and conservative procedure. Regardless of the position of the personnel radiation monitor, a notation of where it is worn should be a part of each radiation monitoring report and of departmental rules and regulations.

A personnel monitoring program is not complete unless proper documentation is provided. Most commercial vendors of personnel radiation monitors will provide the user with a periodic computer-generated report containing all of the required information. For this report to be complete, all of the requested information on each individual must be supplied. This includes name, social security number, birthdate, sex, and previous radiation exposure. The last quantity may sometimes be difficult to obtain. Documentation of efforts initiated to obtain this information must be generated and filed.

Pregnant technologists

Special administrative procedures are required for handling pregnant technologists. It is the responsibility of each technologist to inform her supervisor when she discovers or suspects that she is pregnant. A supervisor should then consult with the technologist and review completely the ongoing radiation control program of the department. Under normal circumstances a technologist will receive less than 1000 mrems annually, as recorded by the personnel monitor. Consequently, the exposure under the protective apron should not exceed 100 mrems annually, and the resulting fetal dose should not exceed 50 mrems. This compares with the MPD to the fetus of 500 mrems for the gestation period. Consequently, under most circumstances additional radiation protective measures may not be necessary. However, two measures that are easy to carry out are usually in order. First, if possible, the pregnant technologist should not be assigned to fluoroscopy or portable radiography. If this is not possible, a review of proper technique during these procedures is necessary. Second, the pregnant technologist should be provided with a second personnel radiation monitor and should be instructed to wear it at waist level under the protective apron. The radiation monitoring report associated with this badge should reflect that it is a fetal dose monitor.

5

Lower extremity

The bones of the lower extremities together with their girdle, the pelvis, which will be considered in Chapter 8, are divided into four parts: (1) the foot, (2) the leg, (3) the thigh, and (4) the hip. These bones are so composed, shaped, and placed that they can carry the body in the erect position and transmit its weight to the ground with a minimum amount of stress to the individual parts.

FOOT

The foot consists of 26 bones, which are subdivided into three parts: (1) the tarsus, or bones of the ankle, (2) the metatarsus, or bones of the instep, and (3) the phalanges, or bones of the toes. For descriptive purposes, the foot is sometimes divided into (1) the forefoot, which includes the metatarsals and toes, (2) the midfoot, which includes the cuneiforms, the navicular, and the cuboid, and (3) the hindfoot, which includes the talus and the calcaneus. The bones of the foot are so shaped and jointed together that they form a series of longitudinal and transverse arches. This results in a considerable variation in the thickness of the component parts of the foot. To overcome the resulting difference in radiopacity, it is necessary to balance the exposure factors in such a way to obtain the greatest possible range of tissue density.

Phalanges. There are 14 phalanges in the toes—two in the great toe and three in each of the other toes. The phalanges of the great toe are termed the first, or proximal, and the second, or distal. The phalanges of the other toes are termed the first, second, and third, or the proximal, middle, and distal. Each phalanx is composed of a shaft and two expanded ends. The distal phalanges are small and flattened and have a roughened rim of cancellous tissue at their distal end for the support of the nail. The interphalangeal articulations are of the hinge type.

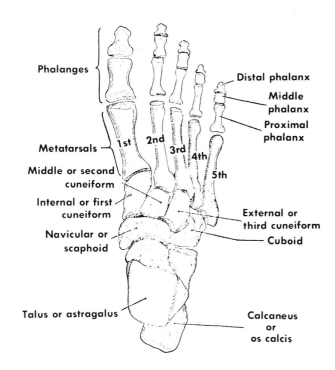

ANTERIOR (DORSAL) ASPECT OF FOOT

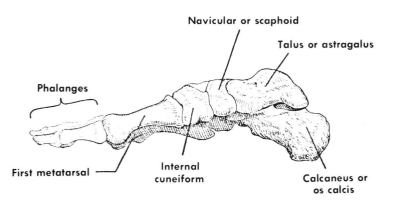

MEDIAL ASPECT OF FOOT

Metatarsus. The five metatarsals are numbered beginning at the medial side of the foot. The metatarsals consist of a body, or shaft, and two articular extremities. The distal extremities of the metatarsus, called the heads, form the ball of the foot and articulate with the proximal phalanges to form joints having the movements of flexion, extension, adduction, and abduction. Their proximal extremities articulate with one another and with the tarsals, forming joints that have only slight gliding movements. The first metatarsal is the shortest and thickest of these bones, the second metatarsal is the longest, and the fifth presents a prominent tuberosity at the lateral side on its base. Two sesamoids are always present on the plantar surface of the first metatarsophalangeal joint, and occasionally there are more. Frequently sesamoids are found on the plantar surface at one or more of the other metatarsophalangeal joints and at the interphalangeal joints of the first and second toes. These sesamoids begin to appear between the ages of 8 and 12 years.

Tarsus. There are seven tarsals in the ankle—the *calcaneus* or *os calcis,* the *talus,* or *astragalus,* the *navicular,* or *scaphoid,* the *cuboid,* and three *cuneiforms.* The cuneiform bones are termed, beginning at the medial side of the foot, the first, or internal, the second, or middle, and the third, or external.

The calcaneus is the largest bone of the tarsus, is more or less cuboidal in shape, and projects posteriorly and medially at the lower posterior part of the foot. It is also directed inferiorly, so that its long axis forms an angle of approximately 30 degrees, open forward, with the sole of the foot. The calcaneus supports the talus above, articulating with it by an irregularly shaped, three-faceted joint known as the subtalar joint, and articulates with the cuboid in front. The talus is the second largest bone of the tarsus. It is irregular in form and occupies the highest position. It rests on the calcaneus, articulates with the navicular anteriorly, supports the tibia above, and articulates with the malleoli of the tibia and fibula at its sides.

The cuboid lies on the lateral side of the foot between the calcaneus and the fourth and fifth metatarsals. The navicular lies on the medial side of the foot between the talus and the three cuneiforms. The cuneiforms lie at the central and medial sides of the foot between the navicular and the first, second, and third metatarsals. The first cuneiform is the largest and the second is the smallest of the three cuneiforms.

The intertarsal and tarsometatarsal articulations allow only slight gliding movements between the bones. The joint spaces are narrow and are obliquely situated. Those lying in the transverse plane slant inferiorly and posteriorly at an angle of approximately 15 degrees to the vertical. The joints lying in the longitudinal plane slant inferiorly and medially at an angle of approximately 15 degrees to the vertical. When the joint surfaces of these bones are in question, it is necessary to angle the tube or adjust the foot to place the joint spaces parallel with the central ray. Several positions with varying central ray angulations are required for the demonstration of the subtalar joint. Each of the three parts of the joint is formed by reciprocally shaped facets situated on the inferior surface of the talus and the superior surface of the calcaneus. Study of the superior and medial aspects of the calcaneus (left, illustrated below) will help the student technologist to better understand the problems involved in radiography of this joint.

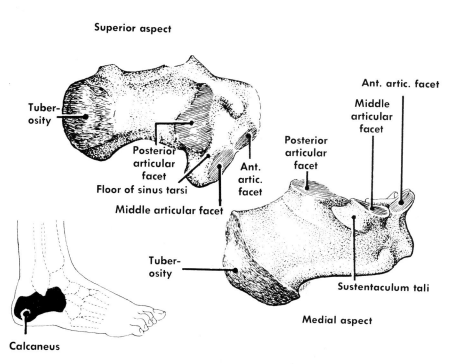

ARTICULAR FACETS OF CALCANEUS

LEG

The leg has two bones—the tibia and the fibula. The tibia is the second longest bone in the body and is situated on the medial side of the leg slightly anterior in position to the fibula, which is located on the lateral side of the leg.

Tibia. The tibia is the larger of the two bones of the leg. It consists of a shaft and two expanded extremities. The upper end of the tibia presents two prominent processes, the medial and lateral condyles. The upper surfaces of the condyles form smooth facets for articulation with the condyles of the femur. Between the two articular surfaces is a sharp projection, the intercondyloid eminence, or tibial spine, which terminates in two peaklike processes called tubercles. The lateral condyle has a facet at its lower posterior surface for articulation with the head of the fibula. On the anterior surface of the tibia, just below the condyles, is a prominent process that is called the tuberosity. Extending along the anterior surface of the shaft from the tuberosity to the medial malleolus is a sharp ridge called the anterior crest, or border. The lower end of the tibia is broad, and its medial surface is prolonged into a large process called the medial malleolus. Its lateral surface is flattened and presents a triangular depression for the inferior tibiofibular articula-

tion. Its undersurface is smooth and shaped for articulation with the talus.

Fibula. The fibula is slender in comparison to its length. It consists of a shaft and two articular extremities. The upper end of the fibula is expanded into a head, which articulates with the posteroinferior surface of the lateral condyle of the tibia. At the lateral and posterior part of the head is a conical projection called the apex or styloid process. The enlarged distal end of the fibula is the lateral malleolus. The lateral malleolus is pyramidal in shape, articulates with the talus at its medial surface, and is marked by several depressions at its inferior and posterior surfaces.

Ankle joint. The ankle joint is formed by the articulation of the talus with the tibia and the fibula. It is a diarthrosis of the hinge type, which permits the movements of flexion and extension only. Other movements at the ankle are largely dependent on the gliding movements of the intertarsal joints, particularly that between the talus and calcaneus.

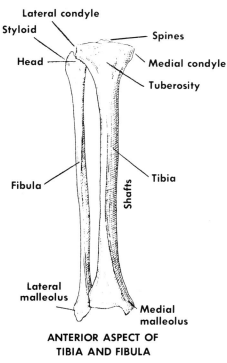

ANTERIOR ASPECT OF TIBIA AND FIBULA

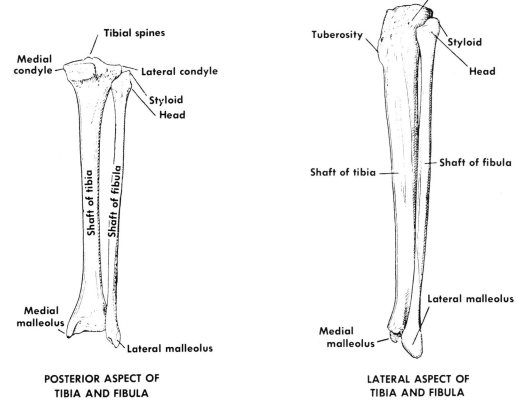

POSTERIOR ASPECT OF TIBIA AND FIBULA

LATERAL ASPECT OF TIBIA AND FIBULA

THIGH

The femur, or thigh bone, is the longest, strongest, and heaviest bone in the body. It consists of a shaft and two articular extremities. The shaft is cylindrical in form and slightly convex anteriorly. The shaft slants obliquely inferiorly and medially, the degree of the medial inclination depending on the breadth of the pelvic girdle. The upper extremity of the femur will be considered with the hip.

The lower end of the femur is broadened and presents two large eminences—the larger medial condyle and the smaller lateral condyle. Anteriorly the condyles are separated by a shallow, triangular depression, the patellar surface, which articulates with the patella. Posteriorly the condyles are separated by a deep depression called the intercondyloid fossa, or notch. The inferior surfaces of the condyles articulate with the tibia. A slight prominence, the medial and lateral epicondyles, is above each condyle.

The patella, or kneecap, is the largest and most constant sesamoid bone in the body. It is a flat, triangular bone situated at the lower anterior surface of the femur with its apex directed inferiorly. The patella develops in the tendon of the quadriceps femoris muscle between the ages of 3 and 5 years. The tip of the apex lies slightly above the joint space of the knee and is attached to the tuberosity of the tibia by the patellar ligament. The patella articulates with the patellar surface of the femur and functions to protect the front of the knee joint. When the knee is extended in a relaxed state, the patella is freely movable over the patellar surface of the femur. When the knee is flexed, the patella is locked in position in front of the intercondyloid fossa.

Knee joint. The knee joint, a diarthrosis of the hinge type, is the largest joint in the body. Two menisci, one medial and one lateral, are interposed between the articular surfaces of the tibia and the condyles of the femur. The joint is enclosed in an articular capsule and held together by numerous ligaments. There are many bursae around the anterior, lateral, and medial surfaces of the joint.

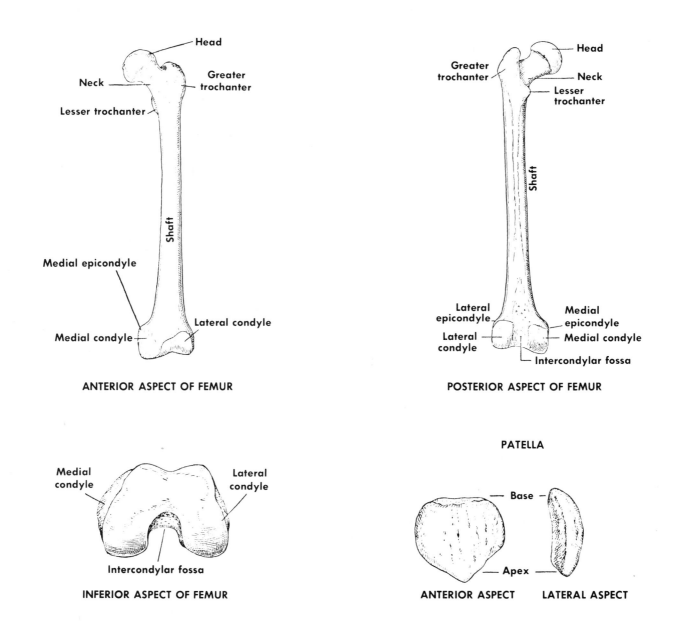

ANTERIOR ASPECT OF FEMUR

POSTERIOR ASPECT OF FEMUR

INFERIOR ASPECT OF FEMUR

PATELLA

ANTERIOR ASPECT   LATERAL ASPECT

✳ ### Toes
PLANTODORSAL (PA) AND
✳ ### DORSOPLANTAR PROJECTIONS

Film: 8″ × 10″ for two projections on one film.

Position of patient

Because of the natural curve of the toes, demonstration of the interphalangeal joint spaces and of the phalanges without foreshortening requires that the foot be adjusted in the plantodorsal position or from the dorsoplantar position. The dorsoplantar position requires that the toes be elevated on a 15-degree foam wedge. The patient may be placed in the prone or supine position.

Position of part

Plantodorsal projection. With the patient in the prone position, elevate the toes on one or two small sandbags and adjust the support to place the toes in the horizontal position.

Place the cassette under the toes with the midline parallel with the long axis of the foot, and center it to the second metatarsophalangeal joint.

Dorsoplantar projection. With the patient in the supine position, it is best to have him flex his knees, separate his feet about 6 inches, and rest his knees together for immobilization.

Place a 15-degree foam wedge well back under the foot to rest the toes near the elevated base of the wedge. Adjust the

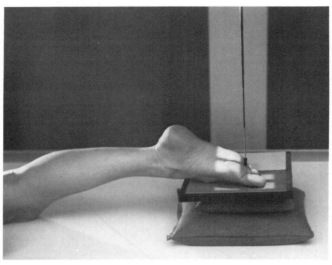

Plantodorsal

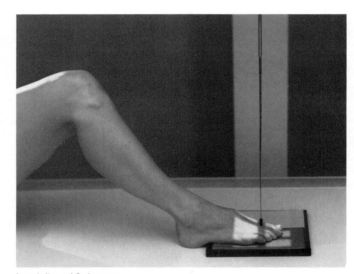

Angulation of 0 degrees

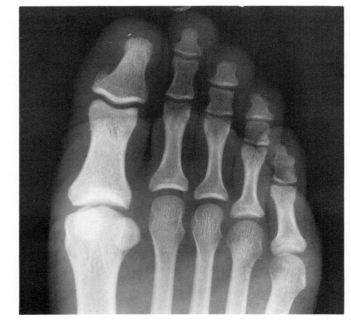

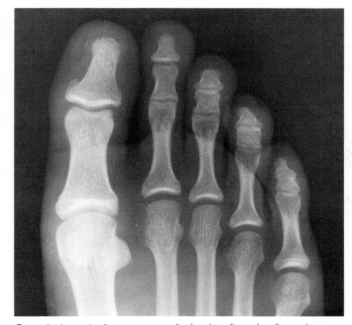

Dorsoplantar projection on same patient as in adjacent radiograph

cassette under the wedge with its midline parallel with the long axis of the foot, and center it to the second metatarsophalangeal joint.

Central ray

Direct the central ray vertically to the midpont of the film.

When a wedge is not used the central ray may be directed vertically, or for the delineation of the joint spaces a 15-degree posterior angle may be used.

Structures shown

A frontal projection (plantodorsal or dorsoplantar) demonstrates the 14 phalanges of the toes, the interphalangeal joints, and the lower ends of the metatarsals.

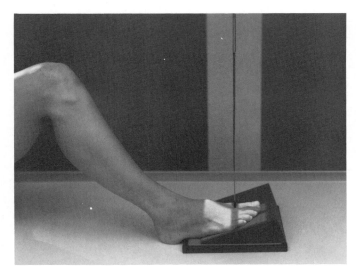

Wedge of 15 degrees

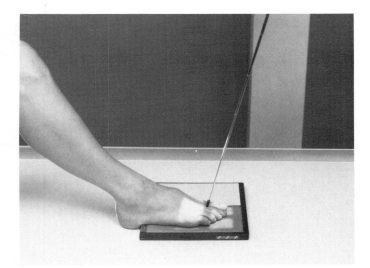

Angulation of 15 degrees

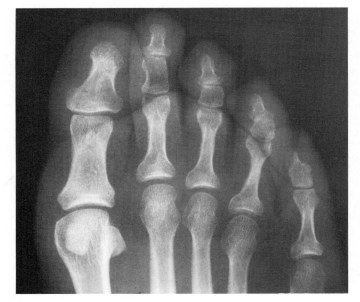

Toes on wedge

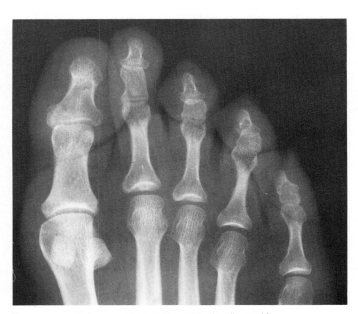

Toes on cassette (same patient as in adjacent radiograph)

OBLIQUE AND LATERAL PROJECTIONS

PLANTODORSAL OBLIQUE (PA) PROJECTION

Film: 8″ × 10″ for two projections on one film.

Position of patient

Have the patient lie in the lateral recumbent position on his affected side.

Position of part

Adjust the affected extremity in a partially extended position. Have the patient turn toward the prone position until the ball of the foot forms an angle of approximately 30 degrees with the horizontal, or have him rest his foot against a foam wedge or sandbag.

Center the cassette to the second metatarsophalangeal joint and adjust it so that its central line is parallel with the long axis of the foot.

Central ray

Direct the central ray vertically to the second metatarsophalangeal joint.

Structures shown

An oblique projecton of the phalanges shows the toes and the distal portion of the metatarsals.

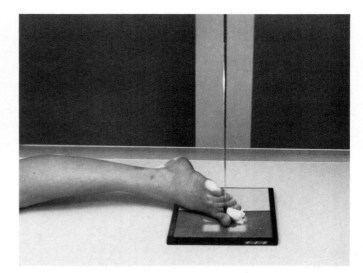

Oblique

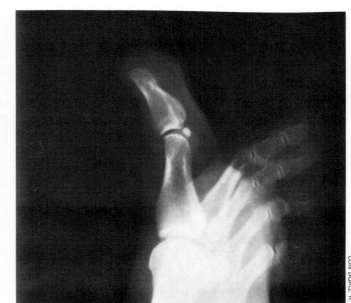

Lateral

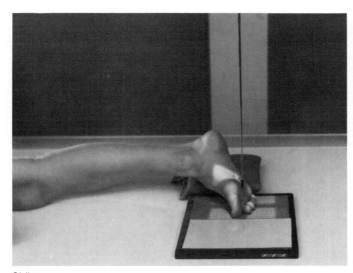

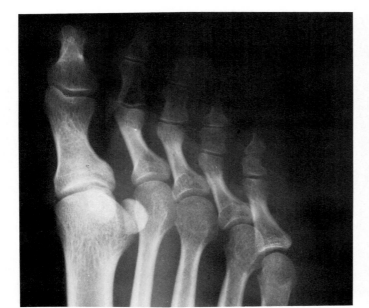

Lois Baird, R.T.

✳ LATERAL PROJECTION

Film: 8″ × 10″ or occlusal.

Position of patient

Have the patient lie in the lateral recumbent position on his unaffected side. Support the affected extremity on sandbags and adjust it in a comfortable position.

To prevent superimposition, tape the toe or toes above the one being examined into a flexed position. A 4″ × 4″ gauze pad may also be used to separate the toes.

Position of part

Great toe. Place an 8″ × 10″ cassette under the toe and center to the proximal phalanx. Grasp the extremity by the heel and knee and adjust its position to place the great toe in a true lateral position. Adjust the cassette so that its center line is parallel with the long axis of the great toe (opposite page).

Lesser toes. Depending on the size of the film available, select an occlusal film or an 8″ × 10″ cassette. If the occlusal film is used, place it pebbled surface up between the toe being examined and the subadjacent toe. For occlusal film or a cassette adjust the position of the extremity to place the toe and film in a parallel position. Support the elevated heel on a sandbag.

Central ray

With the central ray perpendicular to the plane of the film, direct it to the proximal interphalangeal joint.

Structures shown

A lateral projection of the phalanges of the toe and the interphalangeal articulations, projected free of the other toes, is demonstrated.

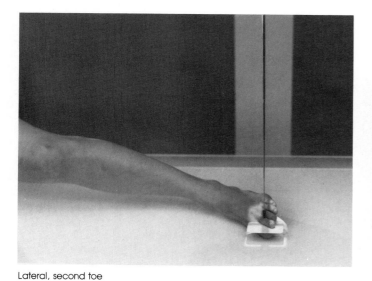

Lateral, second toe

Second toe

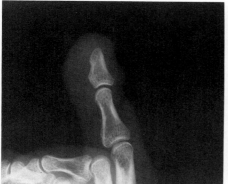

Third toe

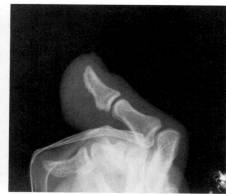

Fourth toe

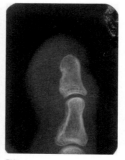

Fifth toe

Sesamoids (metatarsophalangeal)
TANGENTIAL PROJECTION
LEWIS METHOD[1]

Film: Occlusal lengthwise.

Position of patient

Place the patient in the prone position. Elevate the ankle of the affected side on sandbags and put a folded towel under the knee for comfort.

Position of part

Rest the great toe on the table in a position of dorsiflexion and adjust it to place the ball of the foot perpendicular to the horizontal. Place an 8″ × 10″ cassette crosswise and center it to the second metatarsal.

[1]Lewis, R.W.: Non-routine views in roentgen examination of the extremities, Surg. Gynecol. Obstet. **69**:38-45, 1938.

Central ray

Direct the central ray vertically to the second metatarsophalangeal joint.

Structures shown

A tangential projection of the metatarsal heads and sesamoids is shown.

NOTE: Holly[2] described a position that he believes is more comfortable for the patient. With the patient seated on the table, the foot is adjusted so that the medial border is vertical and the plantar surface is at an angle of 75 degrees with the plane of the film. The patient holds the toes in a flexed position with a strip of gauze bandage. The central ray is directed vertically to the head of the first metatarsal bone.

[2]Holly, E.W.: Radiography of the tarsal sesamoid bones, Med. Radiogr. Photogr. **31**:73, 1955.

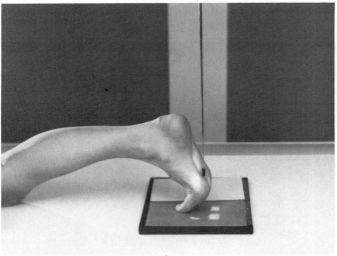

Lewis method

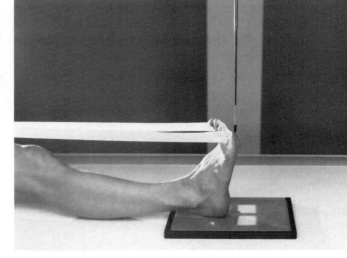

Holly method

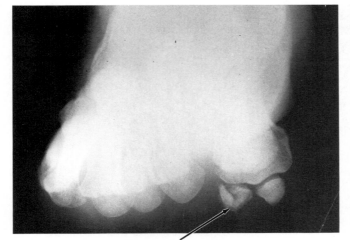

Fractured sesamoid

Toes against cassette

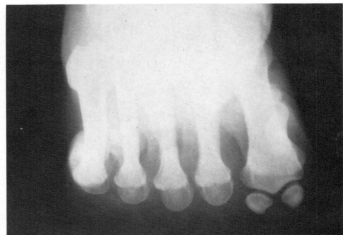

Heel against cassette

Dr. Hudson J. Wilson, Jr.

LATEROMEDIAL TANGENTIAL PROJECTION
CAUSTON METHOD[1]

Film: 8″ × 10″.

Position of patient

Place the patient in the lateral recumbent position on his unaffected side and flex the knees.

Position of part

Partially extend the extremity being examined and put sandbags under the knee and foot. Adjust the height of the sandbag under the knee to place the foot in the *lateral position* with the first metatarsophalangeal joint perpendicular to the horizontal.

Place the cassette under the lower metatarsal region and adjust it so that the midpoint will coincide with the central ray.

Central ray

Direct the central ray to the prominence of the first metatarsophalangeal joint at an angle of 40 degrees toward the heel.

Structures shown

This oblique projection separates the shadows of the first metatarsophalangeal sesamoids.

Occlusal film technique

For improved detail a similar projection may be taken using an occlusal film. The film is placed on a sandbag as illustrated.

[1]Causton, J.: Projection of sesamoid bones in the region of the first metatarsophalangeal joint, Radiology **9**:39, 1943.

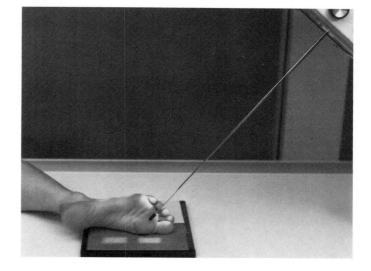

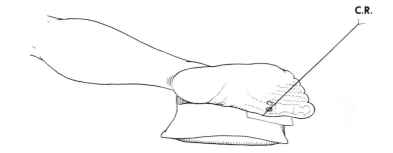

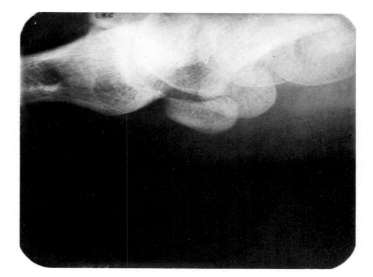

Foot

✳ DORSOPLANTAR PROJECTION

Similar radiographs may be obtained by directing the central ray perpendicularly to the plane of the film or by angling the central ray 10 degrees posteriorly. The joint spaces between the metatarsals and the midfoot are usually demonstrated better when using a posterior angulation.

Film: 8″ × 10″ or 10″ × 12″, depending on the length of the foot.

Position of patient

Place the patient in the supine position. Flex the knee of the affected side enough to have the sole of the foot rest firmly on the table.

Position of part

Position the cassette under the foot, center to the base of the third metatarsal, and adjust it so that its midline is parallel with the long axis of the foot. The leg can be held in the vertical position by having the patient flex his opposite knee and lean it against the knee of the affected side.

In this foot position the entire plantar surface rests on the cassette; thus it is necessary to take precautions against the cassette slipping.

Central ray

Direct the central ray one of two ways: (1) vertically to the base of the third metatarsal or (2) 10 degrees posteriorly to the base of the third metatarsal.

Structures shown

The dorsoplantar projections of the tarsals anterior to the talus, the metatarsals, and the phalanges are presented. These projections are used for foreign body localization, for determining the positions of fragments in fractures of the metatarsals and anterior tarsals, and as a general survey of the bones of the foot.

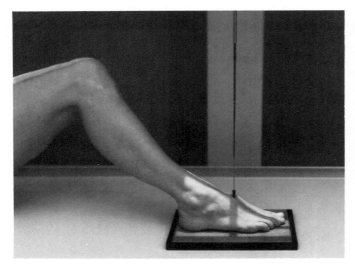

Angulation of 0 degrees

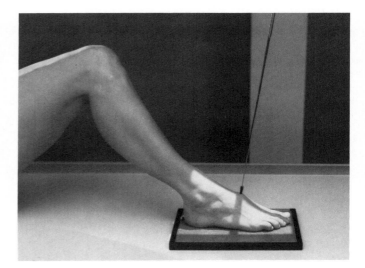

Posterior angulation of 10 degrees

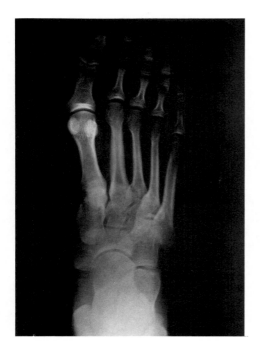

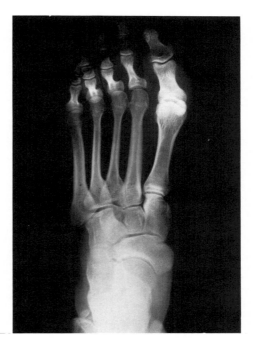

PLANTODORSAL OBLIQUE PROJECTIONS
GRASHEY METHODS

Film: 8″ × 10″ or 10″ × 12″, depending on the length of the foot.

Position of patient

Place the patient in the prone position. Elevate the affected foot on sandbags. A folded towel may be placed under the knee.

Position of part

Adjust the elevation of the foot to place its dorsal surface in contact with the cassette. Position the cassette under the foot, parallel with its long axis, and center it to the base of the third metatarsal.

1. To demonstrate the interspace between the first and second metatarsals, rotate the heel medially approximately 30 degrees.

2. To demonstrate the interspaces between the second and third, the third and fourth, and the fourth and fifth metatarsals, adjust the foot so that the heel is rotated laterally approximately 20 degrees.

Central ray

Direct the central ray perpendicularly to the midpoint of the film.

Structures shown

An oblique plantodorsal projection of the bones of the foot and of the interspaces of the proximal ends of the metatarsals is demonstrated.

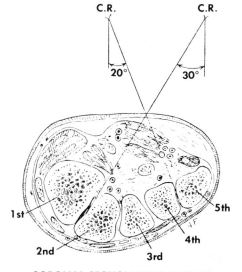

CORONAL SECTION NEAR BASE OF METATARSALS OF RIGHT FOOT

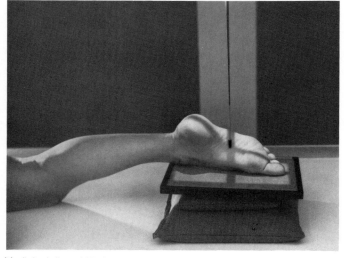

Medial rotation of 30 degrees

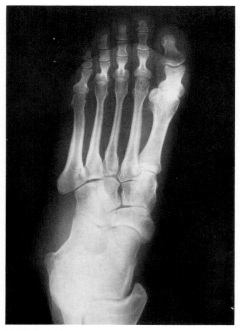

Medial rotation

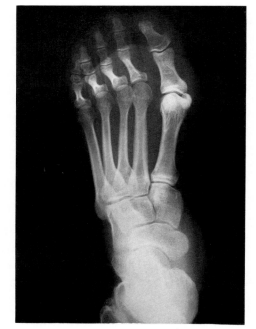

Lateral rotation

✳ MEDIAL AND LATERAL OBLIQUE PROJECTIONS

Film: 8″ × 10″ or 10″ × 12″, depending on the length of the foot.

Position of patient

With the patient in the supine position, flex the knee of the affected side enough to have the sole of the foot rest firmly on the table.

Position of part

Place the casette under the foot, parallel with its long axis, and center it to the midline of the foot at the level of the base of the fifth metatarsal.

Medial oblique projection. Rotate the leg medially until the sole of the foot forms an angle of 30 degrees to the plane of the film.

Lateral oblique projection. Rotate the leg laterally until the sole of the foot forms an angle of 30 degrees to the film.

The elevated side of the foot should be supported on a 30-degree foam edge to ensure consistent results.

Central ray

Direct the central ray perpendicularly to the midpoint of the film.

Structures shown

Medial oblique projection. The interspaces between the cuboid and calcaneus, between the cuboid and the fourth and fifth metatarsals, between the cuboid and the third cuneiform, and between the talus and the navicular are demonstrated. The sinus tarsi is also well shown in this projection.

Lateral oblique projection. The interspaces between the first and second metatarsals and between the first and second cuneiforms are demonstrated.

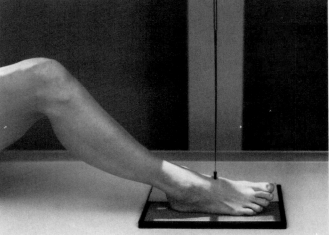

Medial oblique

Lateral oblique

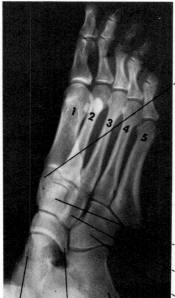

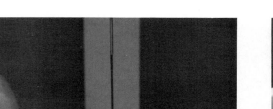

First cuneiform

Metatarsals

Second cuneiform

Third cuneiform

Cuboid

Talus   Navicular   Calcaneus

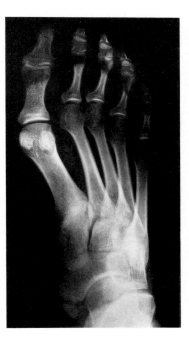

PLANTODORSAL OBLIQUE PROJECTION

Film: 8″ × 10″ or 10″ × 12″, depending on the length of the foot.

Position of patient

Place the patient in the lateral recumbent position on the affected side and have him flex his knees.

Position of part

Fully extend the leg of the side being examined. Have the patient turn toward the prone position until the sole of the foot forms an angle of about 45 degrees to the plane of the film. Center the cassette opposite the base of the fifth metatarsal and adjust it so that its midline is parallel with the long axis of the foot. To obtain uniform results the dorsum of the foot may be rested against a foam wedge. The general survey study is usually made with the foot at an angle of 45 degrees.

Central ray

Direct the central ray perpendicularly to the midpoint of the film.

Structures shown

This projection presents an oblique image of the bones of the foot. The articulations between the cuboid and the adjacent bones—the calcaneus, the third cuneiform, and the fourth and fifth metatarsals—are clearly shown. The articulations between the talus and the navicular, between the navicular and the cuneiforms, and between the sustentaculum tali and the talus are usually shown.

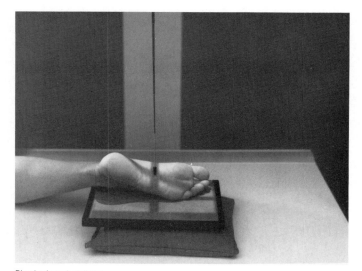

Plantodorsal oblique

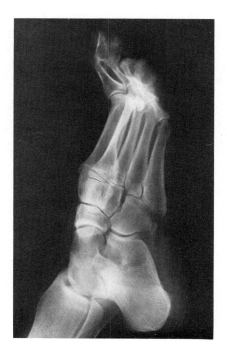

LATERAL PROJECTIONS

Film: $8'' \times 10''$ or $10'' \times 12''$, depending on the size of the foot.

Position of patient

Whenever possible, lateral projections of the foot should be made with its medial side in contact with the cassette. In the absence of an unusually prominent medial malleolus, hallux valgus, or other deformity, the foot assumes an exact or nearly exact lateral position when resting on its medial side. Therefore true lateral projections are more easily and consistently obtained with the foot in this position.

LATEROMEDIAL PROJECTION

Position of part

Have the supine patient turn away from the affected side until the leg and foot are laterally placed. Elevate the knee enough to place the patella perpendicular to the horizontal, and support the knee on a sandbag or sponge.

Center the cassette to the midarea of the foot and adjust it so that its midline is parallel with the long axis of the foot. Adjust the foot so that the plantar surface is perpendicular to the film.

Central ray

Direct the central ray perpendicularly to the midpoint of the film.

Structures shown

A true lateral projection of the foot, the ankle joint, and the distal ends of the tibia and fibula is presented.

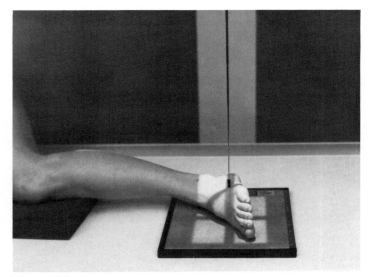

Lateromedial

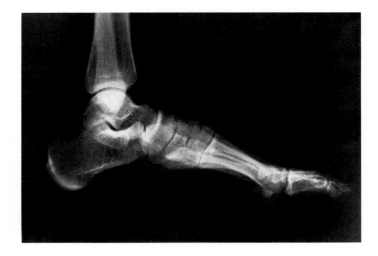

MEDIOLATERAL PROJECTION

Position of part

Place the patient on the table and have him turn toward the affected side until the leg and foot are lateral. Elevate the knee enough to place the patella perpendicular to the horizontal and adjust a sandbag support under the knee.

Center the cassette to the midarea of the foot and adjust it so that the midline is parallel with the long axis of the foot.

Dorsiflex the foot enough to rest it on its lateral surface, and adjust it so that the plantar surface is perpendicular to the film.

Central ray

The central ray is directed perpendicularly to the midpoint of the film.

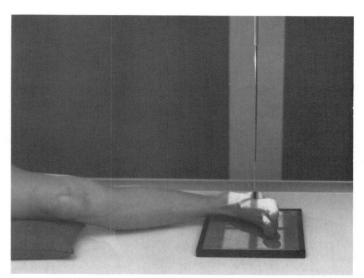

Mediolateral

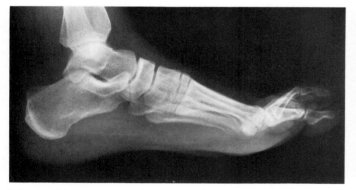

Lateromedial

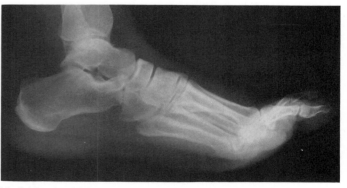

Mediolateral projection on same patient as in adjacent radiograph

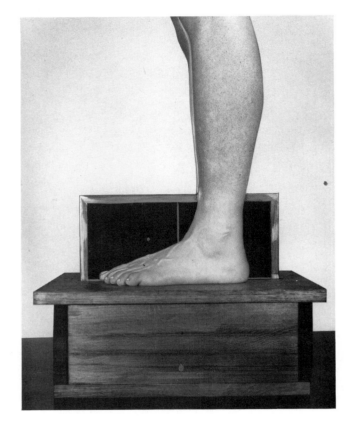

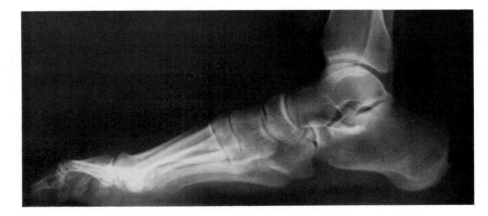

LONGITUDINAL ARCH
LATERAL PROJECTION
WEIGHT-BEARING POSITION

Film

Select an 8″ × 10″ or a 10″ × 12″ film, depending on the length of the foot and whether a unilateral or a bilateral examination is being done.

Position of patient

The patient is placed in the erect position, preferably on a low bench that has a film well such as that described by Gamble.[1] If such a bench is not available, blocks can be used to elevate the feet to tube level and to support the lead mat for the protection of the lower half of the cassette.

Position of part

Place the cassette in the film well of the bench or between blocks with a sheet of leaded rubber to protect its lower half.

Have the patient stand in a natural position, one foot on each side of the projecting film holder, with the weight of the body equally distributed on the feet. Adjust the cassette so that it is centered to the base of the fifth metatarsal.

After the first exposure has been made, lift the cassette out of the film well, turn it over to face the opposite foot, and place it back into the film well, being careful to center to the same point. Swing the tube around to the opposite side and make the second exposure.

Central ray

Direct the central ray perpendicularly to a point just above the base of the fifth metatarsal.

Structures shown

A lateral projection of the bones of the foot in their weight-bearing position is shown. This position is used to demonstrate the structural status of the longitudinal arch. Both sides are examined for comparison.

[1]Gamble, E.O.: A special approach to foot radiography, Radiogr. Clin. Photogr. 19:78-80, 1943.

COMPOSITE DORSOPLANTAR PROJECTION

☀ WEIGHT-BEARING, AXIAL PROJECTION OF ENTIRE FOOT

Film: 8″ × 10″ or 10″ × 12″, depending on the length of the foot.

Position of patient

The patient is placed in the standing-erect position. A mobile unit is often used for this examination, because it allows the patient to stand at a comfortable height on a low bench or on the floor.

Position of part

With the patient standing erect, adjust the cassette under the foot and center its midline to the long axis of the foot.

To prevent superimposition of the leg shadow on that of the ankle joint, have the patient place the opposite foot one step backward for the exposure of the forefoot and one step forward for the exposure of the calcaneus.

Central ray

To utilize the masking effect of the leg the central ray must be directed along the plane of alignment of the foot in both exposures.

1. With the tube in front of the patient and adjusted for a posterior angulation of 15 degrees, center to the scaphoid for the first exposure.

Caution the patient to carefully maintain the position of the affected foot and then have him place the opposite foot one step forward in preparation for the second exposure.

2. Place the tube behind the patient, adjust it for an anterior angulation of 25 degrees, and direct the central ray to the posterior surface of the ankle. The central ray emerges on the plantar surface at the level of the lateral malleolus.

Structures shown

A weight-bearing, axial projection of all of the bones of the foot is shown. The full outline of the foot is projected free of the shadow of the leg.

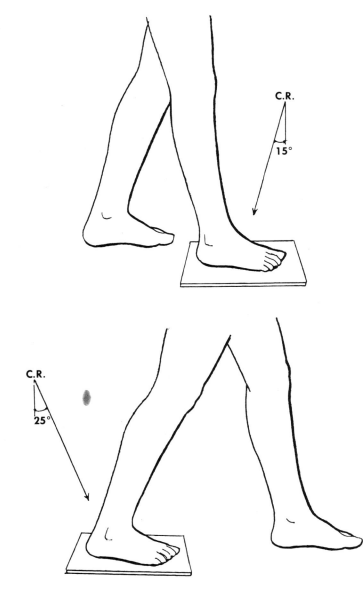

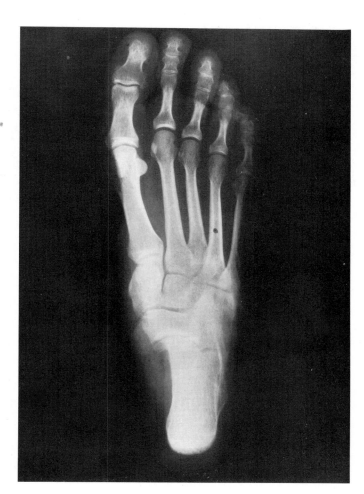

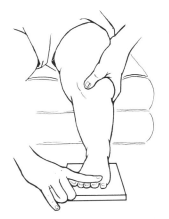

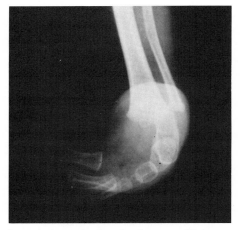

Dorsoplantar projection showing near 90-degree adduction of forefoot

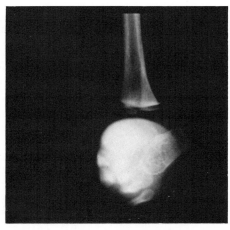

Lateral projection showing pitch of calcaneus, but other tarsals obscured by adducted forefoot

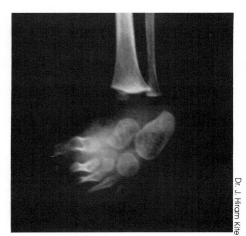

Oblique

Dr. J. Hiram Kite

Congenital clubfoot

The typical clubfoot, called talipes equinovarus, shows three deviations from the normal alignment of the foot in relation to the weight-bearing axis of the leg. These deviations are plantar flexion and inversion of the calcaneus (equinus), medial displacement of the forefoot (adduction), and elevation of the medial border of the foot (supination). There are numerous variations of the typical clubfoot and varying degrees of deformity in each of the typical abnormalities described above.

KITE METHODS

The classic Kite[1,2] methods—exactly placed dorsoplantar and lateral projections—for radiography of the clubfoot are employed to demonstrate the anatomy of the foot and the bones or ossification centers of the tarsus and their relation to one another. *A primary objective makes it essential that no attempt be made to change the abnormal alignment of the foot when placing it on the cassette.* Kite[3] and Davis and Hatt[4] have stated that even slight rotation of the foot can show marked alteration in the radiographically projected relation of the ossification centers.

Dorsoplantar projection

The dorsoplantar projection demonstrates the degree of adduction of the forefoot and the degree of inversion of the calcaneus.

Position of patient

Place the infant in the supine position, with the hips and knees flexed to permit the foot to rest flat on the cassette. Elevation of the body on firm pillows to knee height simplifies both gonad shielding and leg adjustment.

Position of part

The feet are rested flat on the cassette, with the ankles extended slightly to prevent superimposition of the leg shadow. Hold the knees together or in such a way that the legs are exactly vertical, that is, so that they do not lean medially or laterally. Also, hold the toes by using a lead glove. When the adduction deformity is too great

to permit correct placement of the legs and feet for bilateral projection without overlap of the feet, they must be separately examined.

Central ray

The central ray is directed *vertically* to the tarsus, midway between the tarsal areas for a bilateral projection. Kite stresses the importance of directing the central ray vertically for the purpose of projecting the true relationship of the bones and ossification centers.

Lateral projection

The lateral radiograph demonstrates the anterior talar subluxation and the degree of plantar flexion (equinus).

Position of patient

Place the infant on his side in as near the lateral position as possible. The uppermost extremity is flexed, drawn forward, and so held in place.

Position of part

After adjusting the cassette under the foot, place a support having the same thickness as the cassette under the knee to prevent angulation of the foot. The infant's toes must be held in position with tape or a protected hand.

Central ray

The central ray is directed vertically to the midtarsal area.

NOTE: For the demonstration of the degree of equinus deformity and of the relationship and concentricity of the opposing surfaces of the tibia and the talus, Marique[1] recommends that lateral studies of the ankle joint be made before and after treatment. For these studies the foot should be dorsiflexed as much as possible without causing discomfort to the infant.

Freiberger, Hersh, and Harrison[2] recommend that dorsiflexion of infant feet be obtained by pressing a small plywood board against the sole of the foot. Older children and adults are placed in the erect position for a horizontal projection, with the patient leaning the leg forward to dorsiflex the foot.

Conway and Cowell[3] recommend tomography for the demonstration of coalition at the middle facet and particularly for the hidden coalition involving the anterior facet.

[1]Kite, J.H.: Principles involved in the treatment of congenital clubfoot, J. Bone Joint Surg. 21:595-606, 1939.
[2]Kite, J.H.: The clubfoot, New York, 1964, Grune & Stratton, Inc.
[3]Kite, J.H.: Personal communication.
[4]Davis, L.A., and Hatt, W.S.: Congenital abnormalities of the feet, Radiology 64:818-825, 1955.

[1]Marique, P.: La réintégration non sanglante de l'astragale, Rev. d'Orthop. 28:37-50, 1942.
[2]Freiberger, R.H., Hersh, A., and Harrison, M.O.: Roentgen examination of the deformed foot, Semin. Roentgenol. 5:341-353, 1970.
[3]Conway, J.J., and Cowell, H.R.: Tarsal coalition: clinical significance and roentgenographic demonstration, Radiology 92:799-811, 1969.

KANDEL METHOD
Dorsoplantar projection

Kandel[1] recommends the inclusion of a dorsoplantar (suroplantar) projection in the examination of clubfeet.

For this method the infant is held in a vertical or a bending-forward position. The sole of the foot should rest on the cassette, although a moderate elevation of the heel is acceptable when the equinus deformity is well marked. The central ray, at an anterior angulation of 40 degrees, is directed through the lower leg, as for the usual dorsoplantar projection of the calcaneus.

Freiberger states that sustentaculum talar joint fusion cannot be assumed on one projection, since the central ray may not have been parallel with the articular surfaces. He recommends that three films be obtained with varying central ray angulations (35, 45, and 55 degrees).

[1]Kandel, B.: The suroplantar projection in the congenital clubfoot of the infant, Acta Orthop. Scand. 22:161-173, 1952.

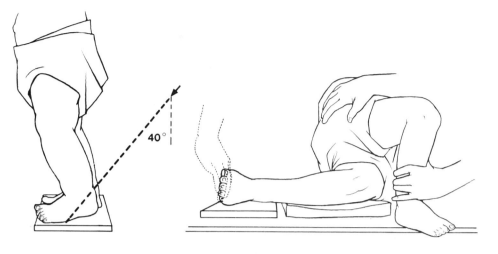

40°

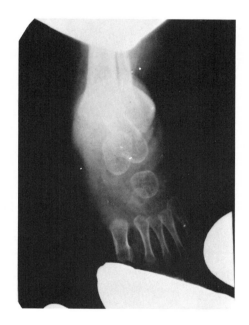

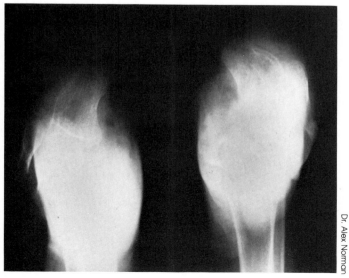

Dorsoplantar

Dr. Alex Norman

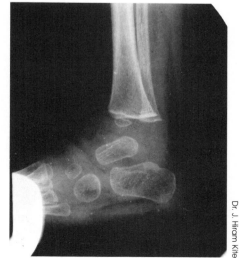

Dr. J. Hiram Kite

Dorsoplantar and lateral studies after correction of clubfoot deformity shown on facing page

Tarsus: calcaneus

✳ AXIAL (PLANTODORSAL) PROJECTION

Film: 8″ × 10″.

Position of patient

Place the patient in the supine position or in a seated position with the legs fully extended.

Position of part

Place the cassette under the ankle and center it midway between the ankle joints.

A long strip of gauze may be placed around the ball of the foot. Have the patient grasp the gauze to hold the ankles in right-angle dorsiflexion. If the ankles cannot be flexed enough to place the plantar surface of the foot perpendicular to the horizontal, elevate the leg on sandbags to obtain the correct position.

Central ray

Direct the central ray to the midpoint of the film at a cephalic angle of 40 degrees to the long axis of the foot. The central ray will enter the plantar surface of the foot at the level of the bases of the fifth metatarsals and emerge just proximal to the ankle joint.

Structures shown

An axial projection of the calcaneus from the tuberosity to the sustentaculum tali and trochlear processes is shown.

LATERAL PROJECTION

Use an 8″ × 10″ film for a lateral projection of the calcaneus. Center it to the midportion of the heel, about 1 to 1½ inches distal to the medial malleolus. Adjust the cassette so that the long axis is parallel to the plantar surface of the heel.

AXIAL – 10x12
LAT. – Both positions on film (crosswise)

Center film ankle jt.
Flex foot
cephald 40°
Enter plantar surface of foot (middle)
5th base (level)

LAT. – center 1½" below medio malai
os calcus center of film
(position just like foot)
Include ankle jt.

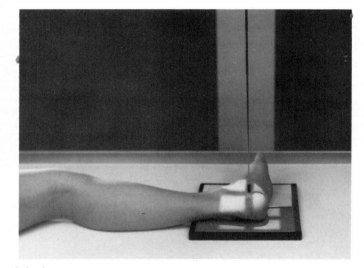

Axial (plantodorsal)

Lateral

Sustentaculum tali

Trochlear process

Lateral process

Tuberosity

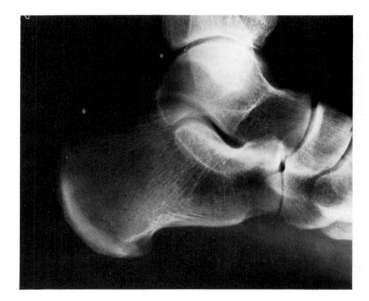

✳AXIAL (DORSOPLANTAR) PROJECTION

Film: 8″ × 10″.

Position of patient

Place the patient in the prone position.

Position of part

Elevate the ankle on sandbags. Adjust the height and position of the sandbags under the ankle in such a way that the patient can dorsiflex his ankle enough to place the long axis of the foot perpendicular to the horizontal. Place the cassette against the plantar surface of the foot and support it in position with sandbags or a portable cassette holder.

Central ray

Direct the central ray to the midpoint of the film at a caudal angle of 40 degrees to the long axis of the foot. The central ray will enter the dorsal surface of the ankle joint and emerge on the plantar surface at the level of the base of the fifth metatarsal.

Structures shown

An axial projection of the body of the calcaneus is demonstrated from the tuberosity to the sustentaculum tali and trochlear process.

WEIGHT-BEARING "COALITION VIEW"

This method, described by Lilienfeld[1] (cit. Holzknecht), has come into use for the demonstration of calcaneotalar coalition.[2-4] For this reason, it has been called the "coalition view."[2]

[1]Lilienfeld, L.: Anordnung der normalisierten Röntgenaufnahmen des menschlichen Körpers, ed. 4, Berlin, 1927, Urban & Schwarzenberg, p. 36.
[2]Harris, R.I., and Beath, T.: Etiology of peroneal spastic flat foot, J. Bone Joint Surg. **30-B:**624-634, 1948.
[3]Coventry, M.B.: Flatfoot with special consideration of tarsal coalition, Minnesota Med. **33:**1091-1097, 1950.
[4]Vaughan, W.H., and Segal, G.: Tarsal coalition, with special reference to roentgenographic interpretation, Radiology **60:**855-863, 1953.

Place the patient in the standing-erect position. Center the cassette to the long axis of the calcaneus with the posterior surface of the heel at the edge of the cassette. To prevent superimposition of the leg shadow, ask the patient to place the opposite foot one step forward.

With the central ray at an anterior angle of exactly 45 degrees, direct it through the posterior surface of the flexed ankle to a point on the plantar surface at the level of the base of the fifth metatarsal.

Handwritten notes:
Enter in ankle jt.
exit through level base of the 5th
So your exit area will be centered to film
lean forward with other Foot
CR - dorsal surface of Ankle Jt.
45° wt. bearing cauldad
40° regular
(for weight bearing pt will need to stand up)

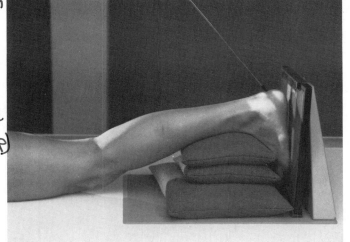

Axial (dorsoplantar)

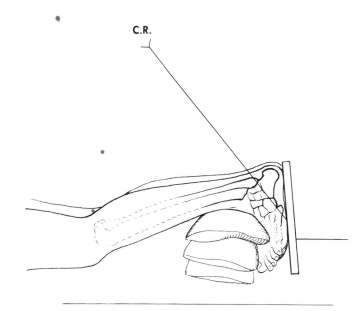

C.R.

45°

C.R.

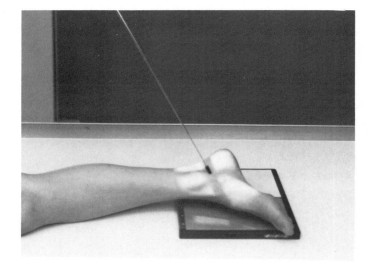

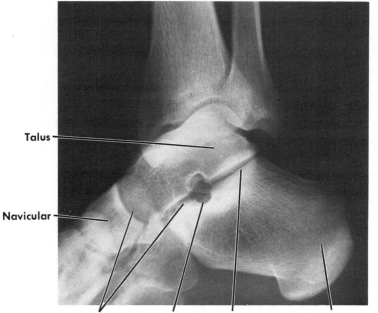

Talus

Navicular

Talonavicular joint   Sinus tarsi   Talocalcaneal articulation   Calcaneus

Subtalar joint
ANTERIOR AND POSTERIOR ARTICULATIONS
SUPEROINFERIOR OBLIQUE PROJECTION

Film: 8″ × 10″ lengthwise.

The subtalar joint consists of the two articulations between the calcaneus and the talus. The anterior articulation forms the talocalcaneonavicular joint. The posterior or talocalcaneal articulation is formed between the calcaneus and the talus on the posterior surface.

Position of patient

Have the patient lie on the affected side in the lateral position. Flex the uppermost knee to a comfortable position and support it on sandbags to prevent too much forward rotation of the body.

Position of part

Ask the patient to extend the affected extremity. Let it roll slightly forward from the lateral position. Center the cassette 1 to 1½ inches distal to the ankle joint and adjust it so that its midline is parallel with the long axis of the leg.

Adjust the obliquity of the foot so that the heel is elevated about 1½ inches from the exact lateral position. The ball of the foot (the metatarsophalangeal area) will be angled forward approximately 25 degrees.

Central ray

Direct the central ray to the ankle joint at an eccentric angle of 5 degrees anteriorly and 23 degrees distally.

Structures shown

This projection demonstrates the anterior and posterior articulations of the subtalar joint and gives an "end-on" image of the sinus tarsi and an unobstructed image of the lateral malleolus.

POSTERIOR ARTICULATION
BRODEN METHODS

Broden[1] recommends these right-angle oblique projections for the demonstration of the posterior articular facet of the calcaneus to determine the presence of joint involvement in cases of comminuted fracture.

Film: $8'' \times 10''$.

Position of patient

Place the patient in the supine position. Adjust a small sandbag under each knee and under the unaffected ankle.

Position of part

Place the cassette under the lower leg and heel with its midline parallel with and centered to the leg. Adjust the film so that the lower edge will be about 1 inch distal to the plantar surface of the heel.

A strip of bandage may be looped around the ball of the foot. Ask the patient to grasp the ends of the bandage and to dorsiflex his foot enough to obtain right-angle flexion at the ankle joint. Ask him to maintain the flexion for the exposure.

Lateromedial oblique projections

Position of part

With the patient's ankle joint maintained in right-angle flexion, rotate the leg and foot 45 degrees medially and rest the foot against a 45-degree foam wedge.

[1]Broden, B.: Roentgen examination of the subtaloid joint in fractures of the calcaneus, Acta Radiol. **31**:85-91, 1949.

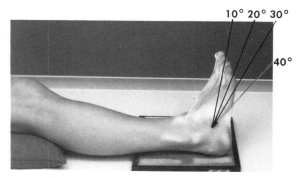

Lateromedial

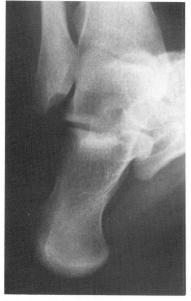

Projection of 40 degrees

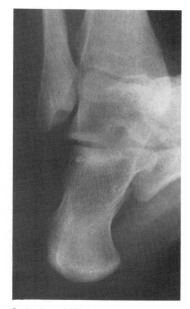

Projection of 30 degrees

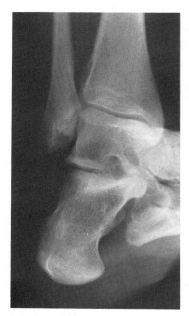

Projection of 20 degrees

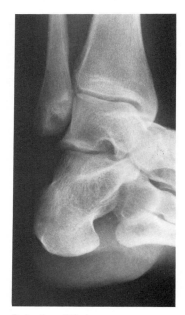

Projection of 10 degrees

57

Central ray

Four projections are taken with the central ray angled cephalad at 40, 30, 20, and 10 degrees, respectively. For each of the projections the central ray is directed to a point 2 or 3 cm caudoanteriorly to the lateral malleolus, to about the midpoint of an imaginary line extending between the most prominent point of the lateral malleolus and the base of the fifth metatarsal.

Structures shown

The 40-degree projection shows the anterior portion of the posterior facet to the best advantage. The 10-degree projection shows the posterior portion. The articulation between the talus and the sustentaculum tali is usually shown best in one of the intermediate projections.

Mediolateral oblique projections
Position of part

With the ankle joint held in right-angle flexion, rotate the leg and foot 45 degrees laterally and rest the foot against a 45-degree foam wedge.

Central ray

Two or three studies may be made with a 3- or 4-degree difference in central ray angulation. The central ray is directed to a point 2 cm distal and 2 cm anterior to the medial malleolus, at a cephalic angulation of 15 degrees for the first exposure.

Structures shown

The posterior facet of the calcaneous is shown in profile. The articulation between the talus and the sustentaculum tali is usually shown.

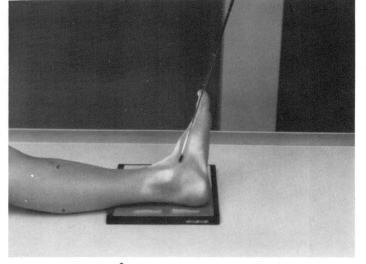

Mediolateral

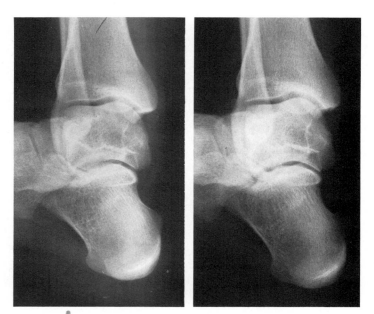

Projection of 15 degrees   Projection of 18 degrees

ISHERWOOD METHODS

Isherwood[1] devised a method for each of the three separate articulations of the subtalar joint—an *oblique lateral* projection for the demonstration of the anterior articulation, a *medial oblique* projection for the middle articulation, and a *lateral oblique* projection for the posterior articulation. Feist[2] later described a similar projection.

Film: 8″ × 10″ for each projection.

Oblique lateral projection
Position of patient

Place the patient in a semisupine or seated position and have him turn away from the side being examined. Ask him to flex his knee enough to place the ankle joint in near right-angle flexion and then to lean the leg and foot medially.

Position of part

With the medial border of the foot resting on the cassette, place a 45-degree foam wedge under the elevated lateral side. Adjust the leg so that its long axis is coextensive with that of the foot. Place a support under the knee.

Central ray

Direct the central ray perpendicularly to a point 1 inch distal and 1 inch anterior to the lateral malleolus.

Structures shown

The anterior subtalar articulation and an oblique image of the tarsus are demonstrated. The Feist-Mankin method produces a similar image representation.

[1]Isherwood, I.: A radiological approach to the subtalar joint, J. Bone Joint Surg. **43-B:**566-574, 1961.
[2]Feist, J.H., and Mankin, H.J.: The tarsus: basic relationships and motions in the adult and definition of optimal recumbent oblique projection, Radiology **79:**250-263, 1962.

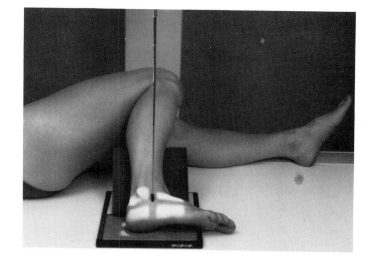

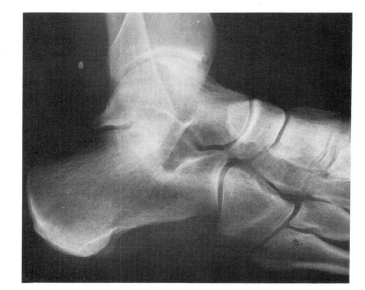

Anterior articulation

Medial oblique projection
Position of patient

Have the patient assume a seated position on the table and turn with his weight resting on the flexed hip and thigh of the unaffected side. The patient may be adjusted in a semilateral recumbent position if it is more comfortable.

Position of part

Ask the patient to rotate the leg and foot medially, enough to rest the side of the foot and ankle against a 30-degree foam wedge. Place a support under the knee and, if the patient is recumbent, place another under the greater trochanter. Dorsiflex the foot, invert it when possible, and have the patient maintain the position by pulling on a strip of 2- or 3-inch bandage looped around the ball of the foot if needed.

Central ray

Direct the central ray to a point 1 inch distal and 1 inch anterior to the lateral malleolus at an angle of 10 degrees cephalad.

Structures shown

The middle articulation of the subtalar joint and an "end-on" projection of the sinus tarsi are shown.

Lateral oblique projection
Position of patient

The patient may be placed in the supine or the seated position.

Position of part

Ask the patient to rotate the leg and foot laterally until the side of the foot and ankle rests against a 30-degree foam wedge. Dorsiflex the foot, evert it when possible, and have the patient maintain the position by pulling on a broad bandage looped around the ball of the foot if needed.

Central ray

Direct the central ray to a point 1 inch distal to the medial malleolus at an angle of 10 degrees cephalad.

Structures shown

The posterior articulation of the subtalar joint is projected in profile.

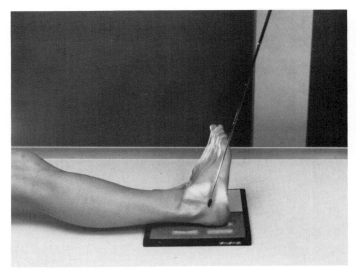

Medial oblique

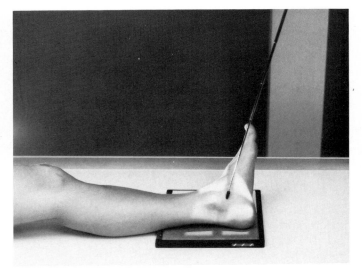

Lateral oblique

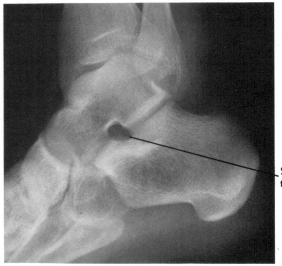

Sinus tarsi

Middle articulation

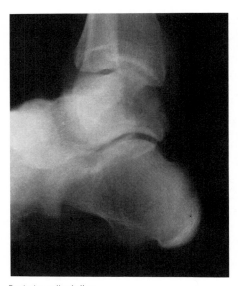

Posterior articulation

Ankle

* AP PROJECTION

Film: 8″ × 10″ lengthwise; 10″ × 12″ crosswise for two projections on one film.

Position of patient

Place the patient in the supine position and place a small sandbag under each knee to relieve strain.

Position of part

Adjust the ankle joint in the AP position by flexing the ankle and pronating the foot enough to place its long axis in the vertical position. Slight inversion of the
* foot, using care not to rotate the leg, will open the talofibular articulation, as shown in the right radiograph (arrow).

Ball and Egbert[1] state that the appearance of the ankle mortise will not be appreciably altered by moderate plantar flexion or dorsiflexion as long as the leg is rotated neither laterally nor medially.

If a larger area of the leg is desired, use a larger cassette and position the plantar surface of the heel to the lower edge of the film. However, if the joint is involved, *always* direct the central ray to the joint.

[1]Ball, R.P., and Egbert, E.W.: Ruptured ligaments of the ankle, A.J.R. **50:**770-771, 1943.

Central ray

Direct the central ray vertically to the ankle joint at a point midway between the malleoli.

Structures shown

An AP projection of the ankle joint, the lower ends of the tibia and fibula, and the upper portion of the astragalus is demonstrated. Neither the inferior tibiofibular articulation nor the inferior portion of the lateral malleolus is well demonstrated in this projection.

AP   10 × 12   Lengthwise
Obliq.
Lat.   8 × 10

AP -
center Film to ankle
invert Foot med. not the leg
dorso flex foot - perpendicular to
film
CR - perpendicular to film right between
malli oli (ankle jt.)

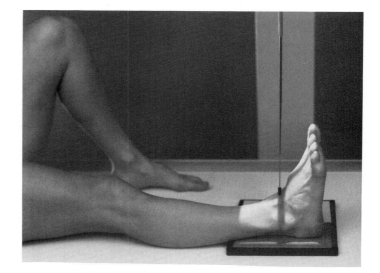

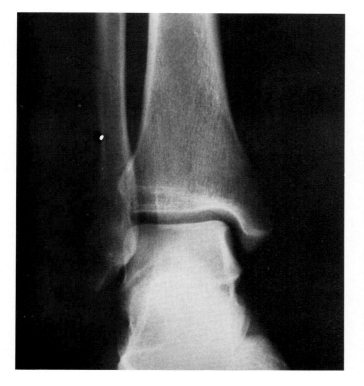

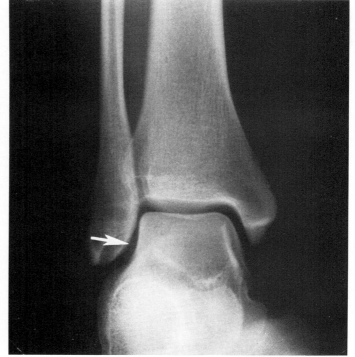

long axis of leg to
long axis of film
want pattella perpendicular
To table

CR - Right over malli di
(ankle)

dorsal Flex Foot

✳ LATERAL PROJECTION

Film: 8″ × 10″.

It is often recommended that lateral projections of the ankle joint should be made with the medial side of the ankle in contact with the cassette. This position places the joint closer to the film and thus provides an improved image. A further advantage is that exact positioning of the ankle is more easily and more consistently obtained when the extremity is rested on its comparatively flat medial surface.

Lateromedial projection

Have the supine patient turn away from the affected side until the leg is approximately laterally placed.

Position of part

Center the cassette to the ankle joint and adjust the cassette so that its midline is parallel with the long axis of the leg. Adjust the foot in the lateral position. Have the patient turn anteriorly or posteriorly as required to place the patella perpendicular to the horizontal. If necessary, place a support under the knee.

Mediolateral projection

Have the supine patient turn toward the affected side until the leg is approximately lateral.

Position of part

With the midline of the cassette parallel with the long axis of the leg, center it to the ankle joint. Have the patient turn anteriorly or posteriorly as required to place the patella perpendicular to the horizontal and place a support under the knees. Dorsiflex the foot and adjust it in the lateral position; dorsiflexion is required to prevent lateral rotation of the ankle.

Central ray

Direct the central ray perpendicularly through the ankle joint.

Structures shown

A true lateral projection of the lower third of the tibia and fibula, of the ankle joint, and of the tarsus is demonstrated.

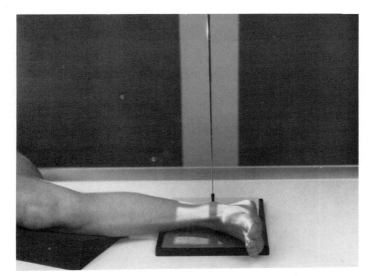

Mediolateral

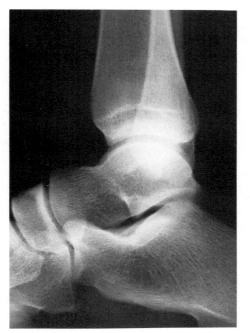

Mediolateral

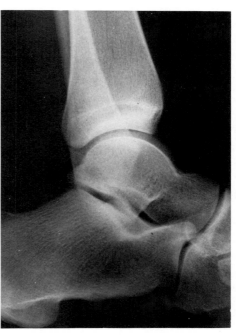

Lateromedial

OBLIQUE PROJECTIONS

Film: 8″ × 10″ lengthwise; 10″ × 12″ crosswise for two projections on one film.

Position of patient

The patient is examined in the recumbent position.

Position of part

The leg as well as the foot must be rotated for oblique projections of the ankle, and, since the knee is a hinge joint, rotation of the extremity can come only from the hip joint.

An increase in the normal anteversion of the femoral neck rolls the extremity laterally when the body is supine. Positioning for a lateral oblique projection requires that the side of the ankle and foot be rested against a 45-degree foam wedge and that the foot be adjusted in dorsiflexion.

To rotate the extremity medially, the femoral neck must also be rotated.

Center the cassette to the ankle joint midway between the malleoli, and adjust it so that its midline is parallel with the long axis of the leg. Adjust the support under the hip so that the medial side of the ankle and foot rests against a 45-degree foam wedge. Place a sandbag support under the knee.

Dorsiflex the foot enough to prevent superimposition of the lateral malleolus and the calcaneous and enough to place the ankle at near right-angle flexion. The ankle may be immobilized with sandbags placed against the sole of the foot or by having the patient hold the ends of a strip of bandage looped around the ball of the foot.

Central ray

Direct the central ray perpendicular to the ankle joint.

Structures shown

This oblique projection demonstrates the distal ends of the tibia and fibula. The lateral malleolus is particularly well shown in the medial oblique projection. The projection obtained of the talus and the talocalcaneal articulation depends on the degree of dorsiflexion of the foot.

*have patient rotate Foot, ankle, leg 45°
Central Ray perpendicular to film
centered at ankle jt.*

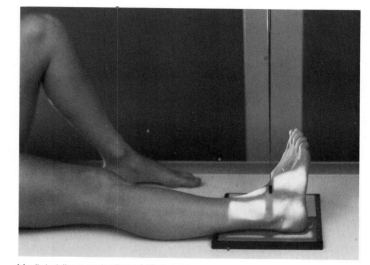

Medial oblique projection of 45 degrees

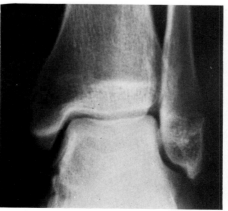

AP

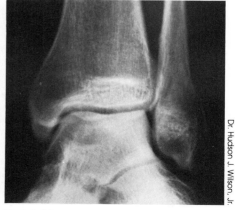

Medial oblique

Dr. Hudson J. Wilson, Jr.

AP STRESS STUDIES

Stress studies of the ankle joint are made, usually following an inversion or eversion injury, to verify the presence of a ligamentous tear. Rupture of a ligament is demonstrated by widening of the joint space on the side of the injury when, with the ankle kept in the AP position, the foot is forcibly turned toward the opposite side.

When the injury is recent and the ankle is acutely sensitive to movement, the orthopedic surgeon may inject a local anesthetic into the sinus tarsi preceding the examination. The physician adjusts the foot when it must be turned into extreme stress and holds or straps it in position for the exposure. Under local anesthesia or when the ankle is not too painful, the patient can usually hold the foot in the stress position by asymmetrical pull on a strip of bandage looped around the ball of the foot.

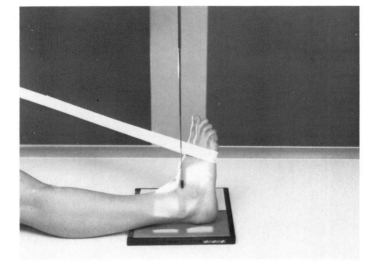

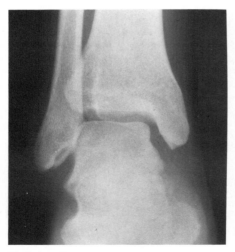

Neutral position

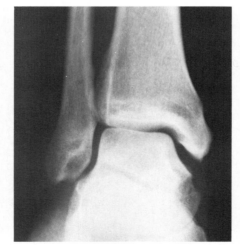

Eversion stress: no damage to medial ligament indicated

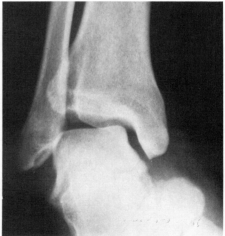

Inversion stress with change in joint and rupture of lateral ligament

Dr. William H. Shehadi

✳ Leg

AP, LATERAL, AND OBLIQUE PROJECTIONS

Film: 7″ × 17″; 14″ × 17″ for two projections on one film.

For each of these projections, the cassette is placed parallel with the long axis of the leg and centered to the midshaft. Unless the leg is unusually long, the film will extend beyond the knee and ankle joints enough to prevent their being projected off the film by the divergency of the x-ray beam. The film should extend from 1 to 1½ inches beyond the joints. When the leg is too long for these allowances and the site of the lesion is not known, two radiographs should be taken. Place the longer film high enough to include the knee joint and use a small film for the distal end of the leg. If the site of the lesion has been localized, adjust the film to include the nearer joint.

Position of patient

The patient is placed in the supine position.

Position of part

AP projection. With the patient supine, adjust the body so that there is no rotation of the pelvis. Adjust the leg in the AP position; invert the foot slightly, but do not rotate the leg. Place a sandbag against the sole of the foot to immobilize it in the correct position if necessary.

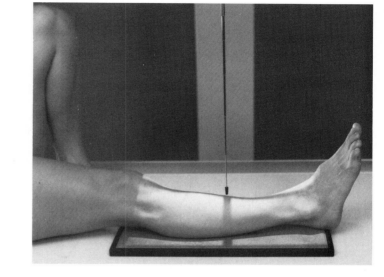

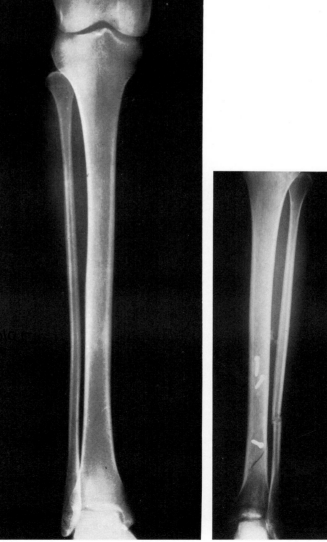

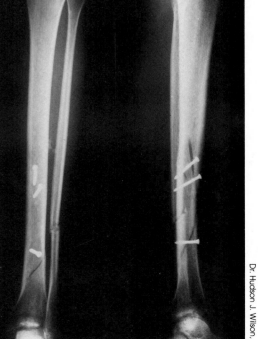

AP - include both knee and
    Ankle Jt. slight invert
    Foot.

If you can't get Jts. on film
as far as CR - Turn tube
So it will open up to 14 X 17

diag. And lead sides perpendicular
CR - to center of leg.

AP   AP   Lateral

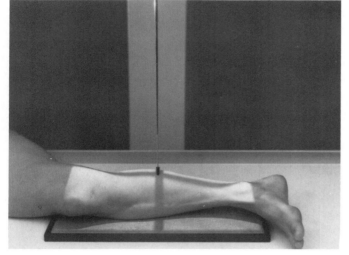

Lateral

Lateral projection. From the supine position, the patient may be turned toward or away from the affected side. Adjust the rotation of the body to place the patella perpendicular to the horizontal, and place sandbag supports where needed for the patient's comfort and to stabilize the body position.

After the placement of the cassette, check the position to make sure that the patella is perpendicular to the plane of the film.

When the patient cannot be turned from the supine position, the lateral projection must be made by cross-table projection. Lift the leg just enough for an assistant to slide a rigid support under the leg. The film may be placed between the legs and the central ray directed from the lateral side.

Oblique projections. Oblique projections of the leg are taken by alternately rotating the extremity 45 degrees laterally and medially. Because of the increased anteversion of the femoral neck in the supine position, the adjustment of the leg for the mediolateral oblique projection usually requires that the lateral side of the foot and ankle be rested against a 45-degree foam wedge. For the lateromedial oblique projection, elevate the affected hip enough to rest the medial side of the foot and ankle against a 45-degree foam wedge and place a support under the greater trochanter.

Central ray

The central ray is directed perpendicularly to the midpoint of the film.

Structures shown

AP, lateral, and 45-degree oblique projections of the bones and soft tissues of the leg and one or both of the adjacent joints are shown.

LAT –
patella perpendicular
To film
Slightly ~~Bent~~ Flex Knee
Include Ankle Jt. & Knee
CR – perpendicular to film
Centered of leg.

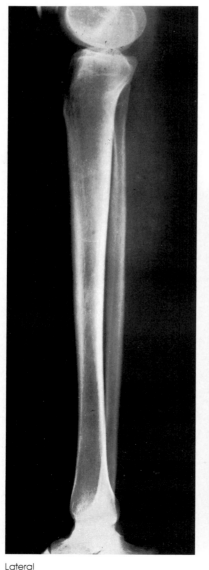

Lateral   Oblique projections of 45 degrees

Dr. Hudson J. Wilson, Jr.

✳ Knee

Radiographs of the knee may be taken with or without the use of a grid. The size of the patient's knee and the preference of the technologist and physician are the factors considered in reaching a decision. Most medical facilities establish a policy for the routine knee procedure, and, whether or not the policy is to use a grid or nongrid technique, the positioning of the body part remains the same.

Attention is again called to the need for gonad shielding in examinations of the lower extremities.

AP PROJECTION

Film: 8" × 10".

Position of patient

Place the patient in the supine position and adjust the body so that there is no rotation of the pelvis.

Position of part

With the cassette under the patient's knee, flex the joint slightly, locate the apex of the patella, and as the patient extends the knee center the cassette about ½ inch below the patellar apex. This will center the cassette to the joint space.

Adjust the leg in a true AP position. The patella will lie slightly off center to the medial side. If the knee cannot be fully extended, a curved cassette may be used.

Central ray

When radiographing the joint space, angle the tube so that the central ray is directed to the joint at an angle of 5 to 7 degrees cephalad.

When radiographing the distal end of the femur or the proximal ends of the tibia and fibula, the central ray may be directed perpendicularly to the joint.

Structures shown

An AP projection of the knee structures is shown. If the position is correct and the knee is normal, the interspace between the medial tibial plateau and the medial femoral condyle will be equal in width to the interspace between the lateral femoral condyle and the lateral tibial plateau.

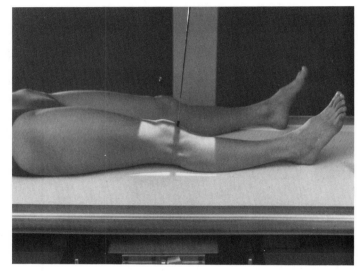

Angulation of 5 degrees

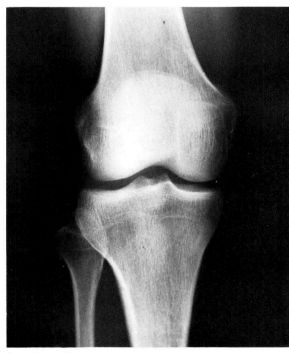

Angulation of 5 degrees

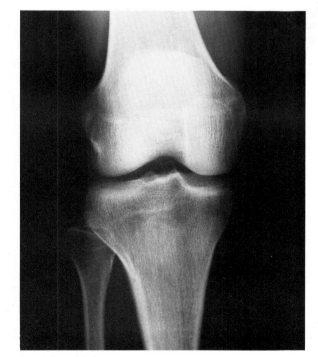

Angulation of 0 degrees

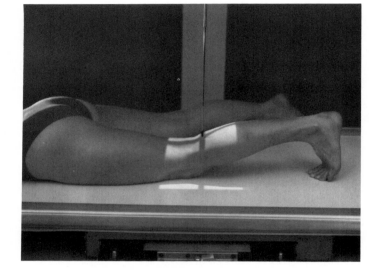

PA PROJECTION

Film: 8″ × 10″.

Position of patient

Place the patient in the prone position with the toes resting on the table, or place sandbags under the ankle for support.

Position of part

Center a point ½ inch below the patellar apex to the center of the film and adjust the leg in a true PA position. Because the knee is balanced on the medial side of the obliquely located patella, care must be used in adjusting the knee.

Central ray

Direct the central ray perpendicularly to the film. Since the tibia and fibula are slightly inclined, the central ray will be parallel with the tibial plateau.

Structures shown

A PA projection of the knee is demonstrated. If the position is correct and the knee is normal, the interspaces between the medial femoral condyle and the medial tibial plateau and between the lateral femoral condyle and the lateral tibial plateau will be equal in width.

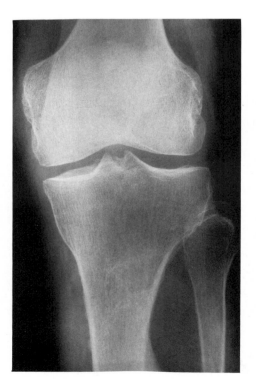

✳ LATERAL PROJECTION

Film: 8″ × 10″ lengthwise.

Position of patient

Ask the patient to turn onto his affected side. When the knee is to be adjusted in right-angle flexion, have the patient bring it forward and extend the other extremity behind it, as shown. When the knee is to be examined in extension or partial flexion, the opposite extremity may be brought forward and the flexed knee supported to prevent forward rotation of the pelvis.

A flexion of 20 to 30 degrees is usually preferred for survey studies because, as pointed out by Scheller,[1] this position relaxes the muscles and shows the maximum volume of the joint cavity.

To prevent fragment separation in new or unhealed patellar fractures, the knee should not be flexed more than 10 degrees.

Position of part

Flex the knee to the desired angle and center the film to the knee joint. The joint can be easily located by palpating the depression between the femoral and tibial condyles on the medial side of the knee just below the level of the patellar apex.

Place a support under the ankle, grasp the medial and lateral borders of the patella between the thumb and index finger of one hand, and adjust the support to place the long axis of the leg in a horizontal position. The patella will be perpendicular to the plane of the film.

Central ray

Direct the central ray to the knee joint at an angle of 5 degrees cephalad. This slight angulation of the central ray will prevent the joint space from being obscured by the magnified shadow of the medial femoral condyle.

Structures shown

A lateral projection of the lower end of the femur, the patella, the knee joint, the upper ends of the tibia and fibula, and the adjacent soft tissue is presented. If the position is correct and there is no rotation, the interspace between the patella and the femoral condyles will be well demonstrated.

[1]Scheller, S.: Roentgenographic studies on epiphyseal growth and ossification in the knee. Acta Radiol. **195** (suppl.): 12-16, 1960.

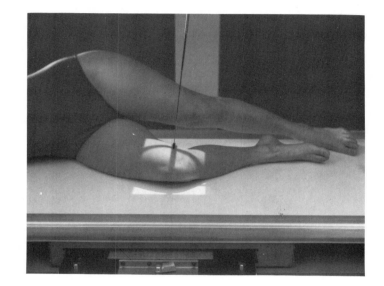

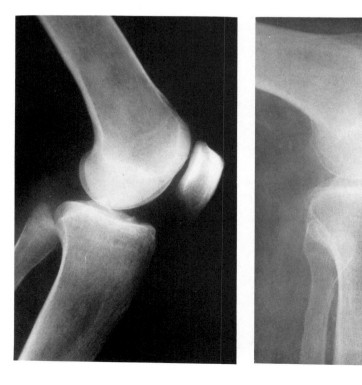

Dr. Henry K. Taylor

Arthritic knee
WEIGHT-BEARING AP PROJECTION

Leach, Gregg, and Siber[1] recommend that a bilateral weight-bearing AP projection be routinely included in the radiographic examination of arthritic knees. They found that a weight-bearing study often reveals narrowing of a joint space that appears normal on the non-weight-bearing study. They state that the weight-bearing film also permits more accurate estimation of the degree of lower extremity varus or valgus deformity, and this aids in preoperative and postoperative evaluation of knees undergoing osteotomy.

Film: $10'' \times 12''$ or $11'' \times 14''$ crosswise for bilateral projection.

Position of patient

The patient is placed in the erect position before and with his back toward a vertical grid device. Center the film at the level of the apices of the patellae.

Position of part

Have the patient adjust his position and center the knees to the film. Ask him to place his toes straight ahead, with the feet separated enough for good balance. Ask the patient to stand straight with his knees fully extended and his weight equally distributed on the feet.

Central ray

Direct the central ray horizontally and center it midway between the knees at the level of the apices of the patellae.

NOTE: For a weight-bearing study of a single knee, have the patient put his full weight on the affected side. He may balance himself with slight pressure on the toes of the unaffected side.

[1]Leach, R.E., Gregg, T., and Siber, F.J.: Weight-bearing radiography in osteoarthritis of the knee, Radiology **97**:265-268, 1970.

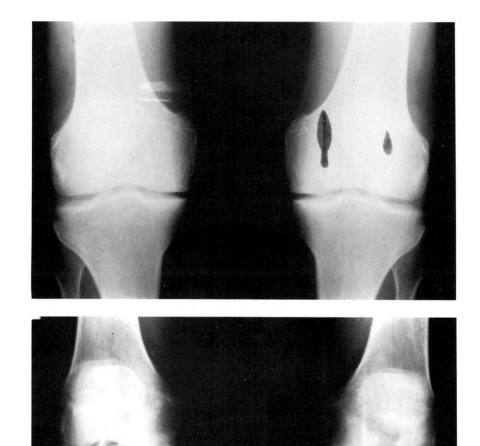

Dr. R.E. Leach

Sixty-eight-year-old man with 4-year history of painful knees. Non-weight-bearing (upper) film shows no abnormalities. Weight-bearing film shows narrowing of medial joint space and varus of tibia of both knees.

Knee

PA OBLIQUE PROJECTIONS

Film: 8″ × 10″ lengthwise.

Position of patient

Place the patient on the table in the prone position.

Position of part

Posteromedial oblique projection. Elevate the hip of the affected side enough to rotate the extremity medially 45 degrees, and support the hip. Center the cassette to the joint space.

Posterolateral oblique projection. Reverse the above position by elevating the unaffected hip enough to rotate the affected extremity laterally about 45 degrees. Support the elevated hip.

Holmblad[1] has recommended that the knee be flexed about 10 degrees on both of these projections.

Central ray

Direct the central ray perpendicularly through the knee joint.

[1]Holmblad, E.C.: Improved x-ray technic in studying knee joints, Southern Med. J. **32:**240-243, 1939.

Structures shown

The oblique projections of the femoral condyles, the patella, the tibial condyles, and the fibular head are shown. The head of the fibula and the proximal tibiofibular articulation are particularly well shown with the posterolateral oblique projection.

11 X 14 crosswise split
Table top

IF someone has a lg. knee you do knee bucky
2 8X10 lengthwise (without bucky
IF youdid screen on lg pt. (knee)
you would lose your bone detail
And you would have more grays. →

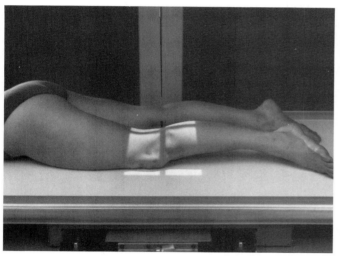

Posteromedial

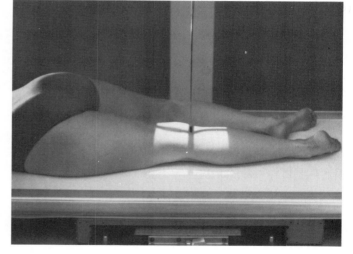

Posterolateral

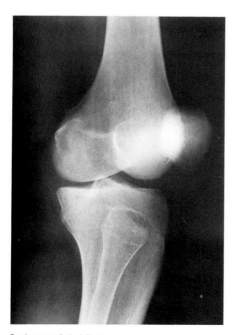

Posteromedial oblique

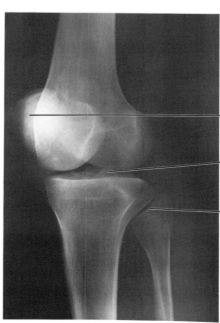

Posterolateral oblique

— Patella

— Intercondyloid eminence

— Proximal tibiofibular articulation

AP—Extend leg have Knee in a true AP posit. CR—perpendicular to center Knee jt. center of film. 1/2" below the apex. Angle 5-7° cephalad for opening of Knee jt.

mediolateral—Bend Knee 20-30° Have patella at a right angle to the film.

Place foot that is affected on unaffected foot as Rest Angle tube 5° cephalad 8x10 - 11x14

AP OBLIQUE PROJECTIONS

Film: 8″ × 10″ lengthwise.

Position of patient

Place the patient on the table in the supine position and support the ankles.

Position of part

Anterolateral oblique projection. If necessary, elevate the hip of the unaffected side enough to rotate the affected extremity 45 degrees laterally. Support the elevated hip and knee of the unaffected side.

With the cassette parallel with the long axis of the knee, center the cassette approximately ½ inch below the apex of the patella.

Anteromedial oblique projection. Reverse the above position by inverting the foot and elevating the hip of the affected side enough to rotate the extremity 45 degrees medially; place a support under the hip if needed.

Central ray

Direct the central ray perpendicularly to the knee joint.

Structures shown

This projection demonstrates an anterior oblique projection of the femoral condyles, the patella, the tibial condyles, and the head of the fibula. The proximal tibiofibular articulation is well demonstrated in the anteromedial oblique projection.

lateral obliq. + medio obliq. — Rotate leg 45° CR-1½" below apex perpendicular to film for both obliq.

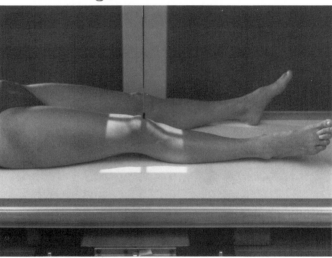

Anterolateral

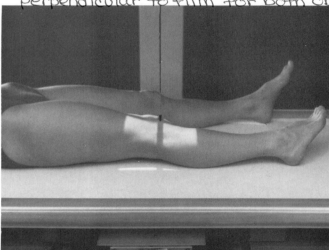

Anteromedial

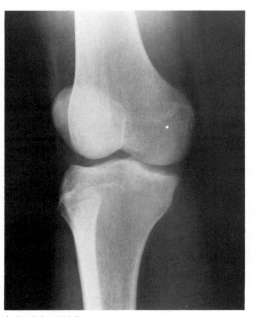

Anterolateral oblique

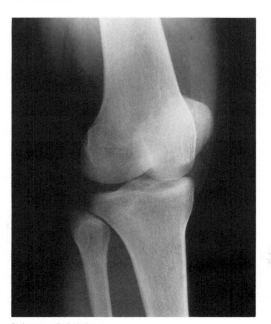

Anteromedial oblique

Intercondyloid fossa

AXIAL PA PROJECTION
CAMP-COVENTRY METHOD[1]

Film: 8″ × 10″ lengthwise.

Position of patient

With the patient in the prone position, adjust the body so that there is no rotation.

[1]Camp, J.D., and Coventry, M.B.: Use of special views in roentgenography of the knee joint, U.S. Naval Med. Bull. **42:**56-58, 1944.

Position of part

Flex the knee to an approximate 40-degree angle and rest the foot on a suitable support. Center the proximal half of the cassette to the knee joint; the central ray angulation projects the joint to the center of the film.

According to the preferred angle, set the protractor arm at an angle of either 40 or 50 degrees from the horizontal and place it beside the leg. Adjust the position of the foot support to place the anterior surface of the leg parallel with the arm of the protractor. Adjust the leg so that there is no medial or lateral rotation of the knee.

Central ray

Tilt the tube to direct the central ray perpendicularly to the long axis of the leg and center to the popliteal depression. The central ray will be angled 40 degrees when the knee is flexed 40 degrees, and 50 degrees when the knee is flexed 50 degrees.

Structures shown

This superoinferior projection gives a more "open" image of the intercondyloid fossa than that obtained with the positions described on the following pages.

NOTE: An intercondyloid fossa projection is usually included in routine examinations of the knee joint for the detection of loose bodies (joint mice). The projection is also used in evaluating split and displaced cartilage in osteochondritis dissecans and flattening or underdevelopment of the lateral femoral condyle in congenital slipped patella.

Pt. proneposition
eleuate lower leg to 40-50°
Knee jt. proxmial half of film
CR- perpendicular to lower leg cauldad centered to popliteal depression 40-50°

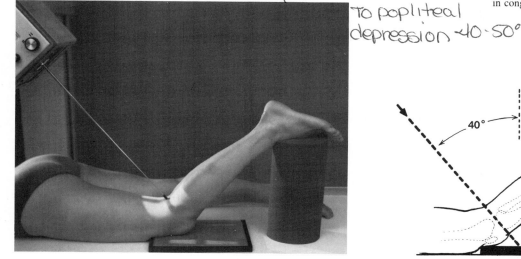

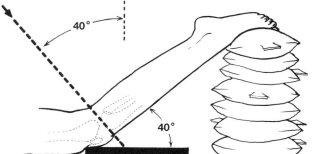

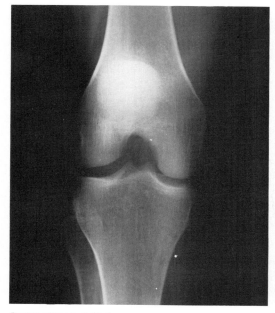

Flexion of knee at 40 degrees

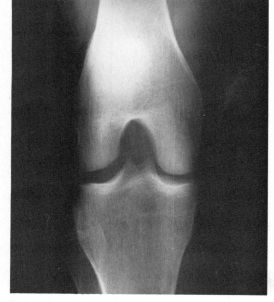

Flexion of knee at 50 degrees

You should really use curve cassette
center knee jt. to center of cassette
CR-perpendicular to lower leg
    centered at knee jt.
    angle to knee jt.

Shows: Intercondyloid space

have pt. angle at 1ˢᵗ 90° and then go down
30° which the lower leg and femur would then
have a 120° angle.

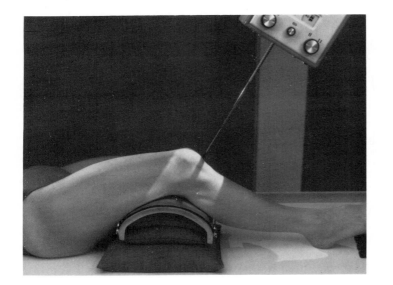

AP AXIAL PROJECTION
BÉCLÈRE METHOD

Film

A curved cassette is preferred to obtain a closer part-film distance. An 8″ × 10″ transverse cassette may also be used.

Position of patient

Place the patient in the supine position and adjust the body so that there is no rotation.

Position of part

Flex the affected knee enough to place the long axis of the femur at an angle of 60 degrees to the long axis of the tibia, open posteriorly. Support the knee on sandbags.

Place the cassette under the knee and position it so that the center point will coincide with the central ray. Adjust the leg in the AP position and immobilize the foot with sandbags.

Central ray

Direct the central ray perpendicularly to the long axis of the tibia and center to the knee joint.

Structures shown

This projection gives a profile image of the intercondyloid fossa, the tibial spine, and the knee joint.

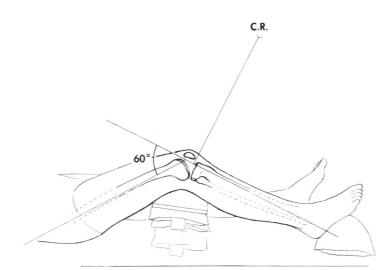

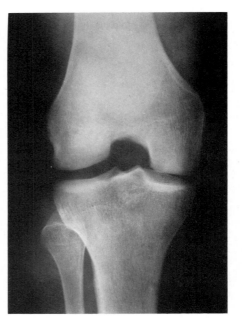

PA AXIAL PROJECTION
HOLMBLAD METHOD[1]

Film: 8″ × 10″ lengthwise.

Position of patient

Place the patient on the table in a kneeling position so that the long axes of the legs will be parallel with the table. Have the patient lean forward on his hands.

Position of part

Place the cassette under the knee, parallel with the long axis of the tibia, and center to the apex of the patella.

Adjust the position of the body, that is, the degree of leaning, so that the long axes of the femora form an angle of 70 degrees from the horizontal (20 degrees to the vertical). Adjust the legs in a true PA position and immobilize them.

Central ray

Direct the central ray perpendicularly to the midpoint of the film.

Structures shown

The intercondyloid fossa of the femur and the tibial spine are shown in profile. Holmblad[1] states that the degree of flexion used in this projection widens the joint space between the femur and tibia and gives a better image of the joint and of the surfaces of the tibia and femur.

[1]Holmblad, E.C.: Postero-anterior x-ray view of the knee in flexion, J.A.M.A. **109:**1196-1197, 1937.

Pt. get on all 4
Pt. Bend forward 20°
Cassete under knee
CR- perpendicular centered to poptieal depression

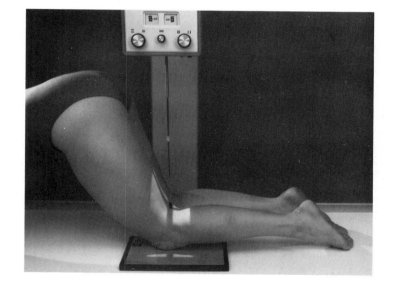

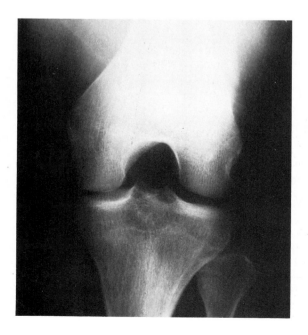

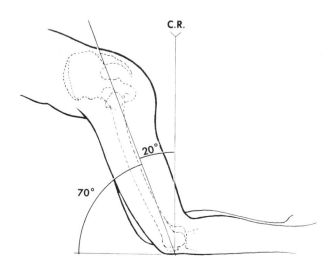

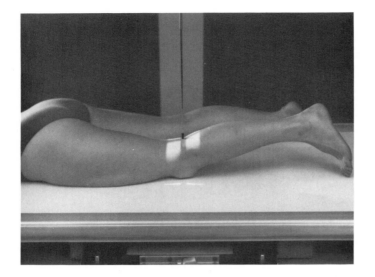

Patella
PA PROJECTION

Film: 8″ × 10″ lengthwise.

Position of patient

Place the patient in the prone position. If the knee is painful, place one sandbag under the thigh and another under the leg to relieve pressure on the patella.

Position of part

Center the cassette to the patella. Adjust the position of the leg to place the patella parallel with the plane of the film. This usually requires that the heel be rotated 5 to 10 degrees laterally.

Central ray

Direct the central ray perpendicularly to the midpoint of the film.

Structures shown

A PA projection of the patella provides sharper detail than can be obtained in the AP position, because of a closer part-film distance.

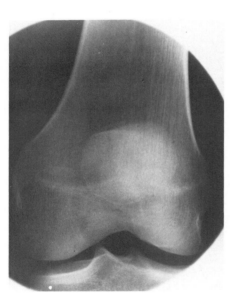

PA

PA in prone position
rstate heel lat. 5-10°
CR-perpendicular to film
going through patella
(also use cone) if you don't
have cone collimate
if you do xray pattella manual
you must up your KV 10 for
Better detail

Lat.- no angle
CR-perpendicular to film
have pt in position for
lat. Knee

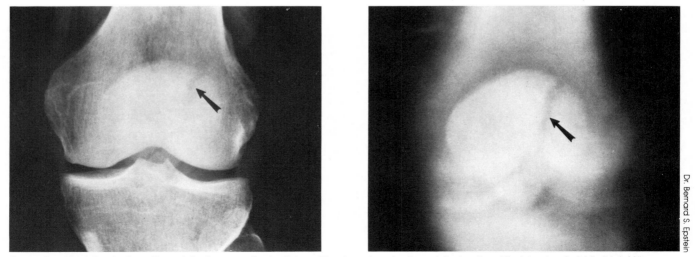

Conventional frontal projection of the patella shows a vertical radiolucent line *(arrow)* passing through the junction of the lateral and middle thirds of the upper patella. On tomography this defect is seen to extend from the superior to the inferior margin of the patella. It is a bipartite patella and not a fracture.

Dr. Bernard S. Epstein

TANGENTIAL PROJECTION
KUCHENDORF METHOD

Film: 8″ × 10″ lengthwise.

Position of patient

Place the patient in the prone position. Elevate the hip of the affected side 2 or 3 inches. Place a sandbag under the ankle and foot and adjust it so that the knee will be slightly flexed, approximately 10 degrees, to relax the muscles.

Position of part

Center the cassette to the patella. With the knee turned slightly laterally from the PA position, place the index finger against the medial border of the patella and press it laterally. Rest the knee on its anteromedial side to hold the patella in a position of lateral displacement.

Central ray

Direct the central ray to the joint space between the patella and the femoral condyles at an angle of 25 to 30 degrees caudad. It enters the posterior surface of the patella.

Structures shown

A slightly oblique PA projection of the patella is demonstrated, showing most of the patella free of superimposed structures.

This position is more comfortable for the patient than the direct PA position, since no pressure is placed on the injured kneecap. The slight pressure required to displace the patella laterally is rarely objectionable to the patient.

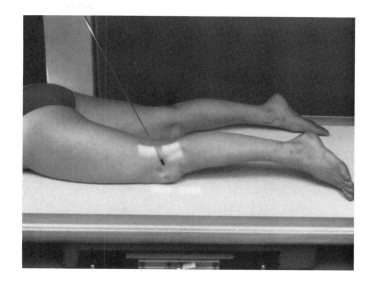

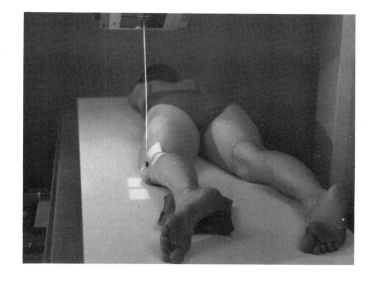

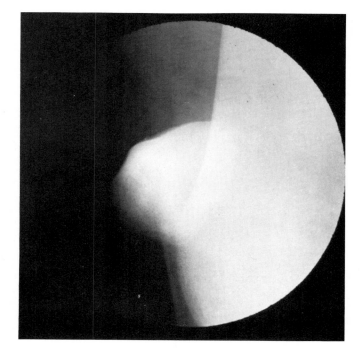

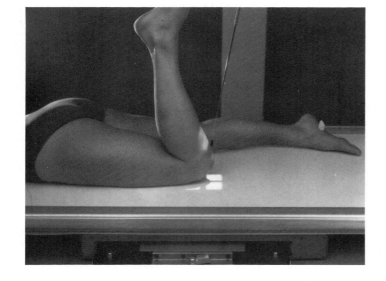

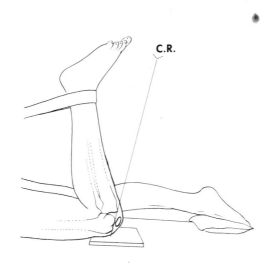

C.R.

TANGENTIAL PROJECTION
SETTEGAST METHOD

Because of the danger of fragment displacement by the acute flexion of the knee required for this projection, it should not be attempted until a transverse fracture of the patella has been ruled out with a lateral projection.

Film: 8″ × 10″.

Position of patient

The patient may be placed in the supine or the prone position. The latter is preferable, because the knee can usually be flexed to a greater degree and immobilization is easier. When the supine position is used, the cassette must be securely held in position.

Position of part

With the patient in the prone position, flex the knee *slowly* as much as possible or until the patella is perpendicular to the film. *By slow, even flexion, the patient will be able to tolerate the position, whereas quick, uneven flexion may cause too much pain.*

A long strip of bandage may be looped around the ankle or foot, and have the patient grasp the ends over his shoulder to hold the leg in position. Adjust the leg so that its long axis is vertical.

AXIAL or settegast)
Screen
2 methods:

PA- have pt. lying in prone position
center knee center of film
flex knee slowly as much as possible

Jt. space perp. to film

CR- parrallel through
the Jt. space determine
Angulation

IF pt. can't flex knee
use tape around foot
To help.

IF pt. can't flex After
doing the above
angle tube.

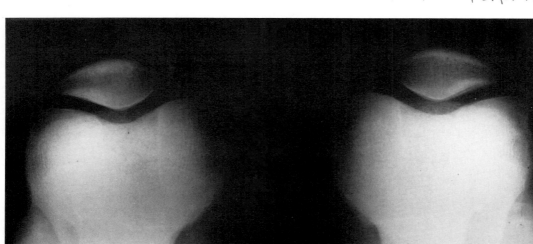

Place the cassette transversely under the knee and center to the joint space between the patella and the femoral condyles.

By maintaining the same part-film and tube-film relationships, this projection can be obtained with the patient in the lateral or in a seated position, as illustrated.

Central ray

Direct the central ray perpendicularly to the joint space between the patella and the femoral condyles. The degree of central ray angulation will depend on the degree of flexion of the knee.

Structures shown

This projection of the patella is used to demonstrate vertical fractures of bone and to investigate the articulating surfaces of the femoropatellar articulation.

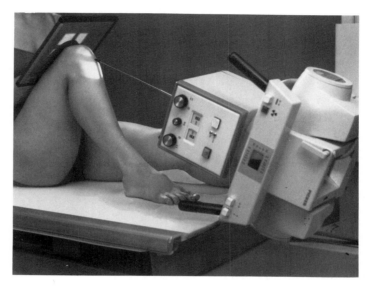

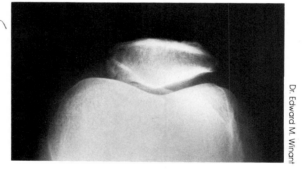

Dr. Edward M. Winant

have pt. sitting up to Edge of table
have pt. flex Knee as much as possible
angle tube through Jt. Space.

(this is just like the Prone position but Pt is Supine position)

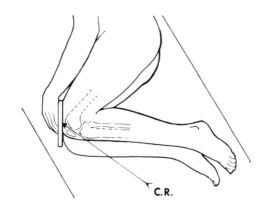

C.R.

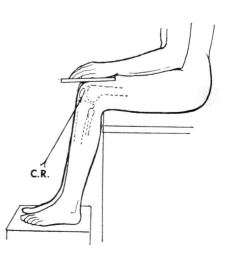

C.R.

TANGENTIAL PROJECTION
HUGHSTON METHOD[1,2]

Film: 8″ × 10″ for unilateral; 10″ × 12″ crosswise for bilateral examination.

Position of patient

The patient is placed in a prone position with the foot resting on the radiographic table. The body is adjusted so that there is no rotation.

Position of part

With the patient prone, slowly flex the affected knee so that the tibia and fibula form a 50- to 60-degree angle from the table. The foot may be rested against the collimator or supported in position.

Adjust the leg so that there is no medial or lateral rotation from the vertical. Place the cassette under the knee.

Central ray

The x-ray tube is angled 45 degrees cephalad and directed through the patellofemoral joint.

Structures shown

This tangential projection of the patella demonstrates subluxation of the patella and patellar fractures and allows radiologic assessment of the femoral trochlea and condyles. Hughston recommends that both knees be examined for comparison purposes.

NOTE: Care must be taken to ensure that the foot does not come in contact with the hot collimator housing heated by the light. It is also essential that the x-ray tube and support mechanism be properly grounded.

[1]Hughston, J.C.: Subluxation of the patella, J. Bone Joint Surg. **50A:**1003-1026, 1968.
[2]Kimberlin, G.E.: Radiological assessment of the patellofemoral articulation and subluxation of the patella, Radiol. Technol. **45:**129-137, 1973.

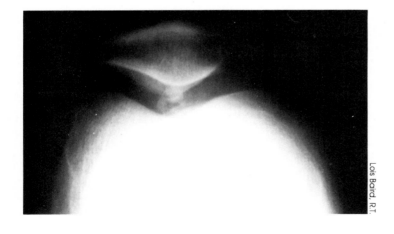

Lois Baird, R.T.

✳ Femur

AP PROJECTION

Film: $7'' \times 17''$, $14'' \times 17''$ for a bilateral examination.

If the femoral heads are separated by an unusually broad pelvis, the shafts will be more strongly angled toward the midline.

Position of patient

Place the patient in the supine position and adjust the body in a true AP position.

Position of part

For a bilateral examination center the midsagittal plane of the body to the midline of the table. For a unilateral examination center the affected thigh to the midline of the table.

Invert the toes approximately 15 degrees to overcome the anteversion of the femoral necks.

Apply a gonad shield according to the criteria outlined in Chapter 4.

Central ray

Direct the central ray perpendicularly to the midpoint of the film.

Structures shown

An AP projection of the femur, including the hip and/or the knee joint, is presented.

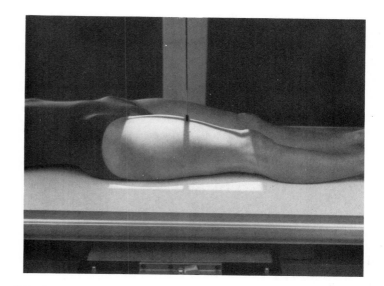

AP-hip jt. usually at Inguinal fold or make a STRAIGHT line hip jt. (draw line between ASIS and symphis then draw 1" line perpendicular to middle of that line

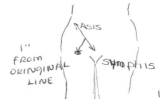

ASIS

1" FROM ORINGINAL LINE

symphis

INVERT Foot 15° medially
CR- to center of leg or center of film

Done bucky lengthwise clips down
Using 4 films 14 X17 10X12 for each leg
may use 1 14X17 for children

Must include both jts unless followup
Then include jt. clossest to fracture on a 14X17

<u>Distal</u> - overlap 2 Films - include knee in AP

<u>Medial tat:</u> - pt. lay lat c̄ unaffected
leg over affected leg

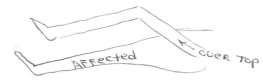

AFFECTED   over top

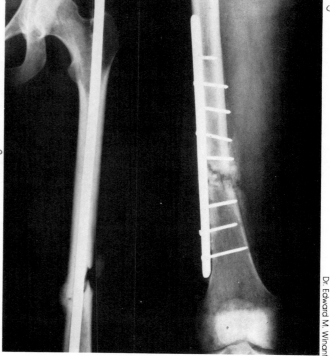

patella perpendicular to Film (depending how far
pt. raises leg is whether or not you use a 14 or 10)

✳ LATERAL PROJECTION

Film: 7″ × 17″ lengthwise.

Position of patient

Ask the patient to turn onto his affected side. Adjust the body position, and center the dependent thigh to the midline of the table. Have the patient grasp the side of the table with the upper hand to aid in maintaining the position.

Position of part

1. If the hip joint is to be included, draw the upper extremity posteriorly and support it. Adjust the pelvis so that it is rolled posteriorly just enough to prevent superimposition; 10 to 15 degrees from the lateral position is sufficient.

2. If only the knee joint is to be included, draw the uppermost extremity forward and support it at hip level on sandbags. Adjust the pelvis in a true lateral position.

Flex the dependent knee somewhat, place a sandbag under the ankle, and adjust it and the body rotation to place the patella perpendicular to the horizontal.

Adjust the position of the Bucky tray so that the film will project approximately 2 inches beyond the joint to be included.

Central ray

Direct the central ray perpendicularly to the midpoint of the film.

Structures shown

A lateral projection of about three fourths of the femur and of the adjacent joint is presented. Two films must usually be taken for the demonstration of the entire length of the adult femur.

NOTE: Because of the danger of fragment displacement, the above position is not recommended for fracture cases, nor should it be used if there is a question of destructive disease. These subjects should be examined in the supine position by placing the cassette vertically along the medial or the lateral aspect of the thigh and knee and directing the central ray horizontally. A wafer grid or a grid-front cassette should be used to minimize secondary radiation.

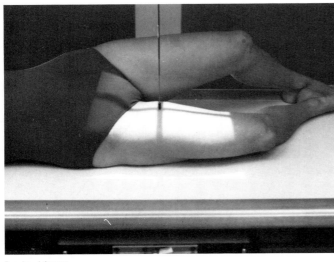

Proximal femur

Superimpose leg lat.
Rotate hips 10-15° lat.
then place unaffected leg back from affected leg
bend knee a little (affected leg)
you want femur in lat. position as much as possible

CR - at center of film (closer to medtain collimate c̄ lead)

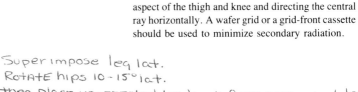

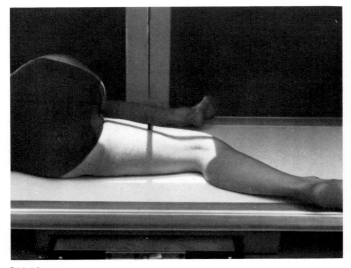

Distal femur

Dr. Edward M. Winant

6

Long bone
measurement

Radiography provides the most reliable means of obtaining accurate measurements of the length of long bones, specifically of length differences between the two sides. Measurement studies are made of the upper extremities, but the procedure is most frequently applied to the lower extremities. Various radiographic methods have been devised for long bone measurement, only a few of which are considered here. For a detailed description of the different procedures and their modifications, see the bibliography for a listing of original papers.

RADIATION PROTECTION

Extremity length differences, which are more common in children, result from any one of a variety of disorders. Patients usually require yearly examinations for evaluation of any inequality in growth. More frequent examinations may follow surgical intervention to equalize length by controlling the growth of the normal side. This is usually done by means of a diaphysial-epiphysial fusion at the distal femoral or proximal tibial level. Patients have interval checkups extending over a period of years. It is therefore necessary to guard their well-being by the application of local gonad shielding and by avoiding repeated exposures through careful positioning, secure immobilization, and accurate centering of a closely collimated beam of radiation.

POSITION OF PATIENT

The patient is placed in the supine position for all methods, and both sides are examined for comparison. When a soft tissue abnormality (swelling or atrophy) is causing rotation of the pelvis, the low side must be elevated on a radioparent support to overcome the rotation and thereby place the upper femora equidistant from the film for a comparable-sized projection.

POSITION OF PART

The upper extremities are alternately adjusted and immobilized in the AP position for a unilateral projection.

The lower extremities are extended and immobilized in the AP position with the ankles separated 5 or 6 inches. When the knee of the abnormal side cannot be fully extended, the normal knee must be flexed to the same degree and each knee supported on one of a pair of *identical-sized* supports to ensure that the joints are flexed to the same degree and are equidistant from the film.

LOCALIZATION OF JOINTS

For the methods that require centering over the joints, each joint must be accurately localized and marked to indicate the centering point. Both sides are examined for comparison, and, since there is usually a bone-length discrepancy, the joints of each side must be marked. This is done with a skin-marking pencil after the patient is placed in the supine position.

For the upper extremity, the mark for the shoulder joint is placed over the head of the humerus near its upper border; for the elbow joint, midway between the epicondyles of the humerus; and for the wrist, midway between the styloid processes of the radius and ulna.

For the lower extremity, the *hip joint* is localized by placing a mark, ½ to 1 inch, according to the age and size of the patient, laterodistally at exact right angles to the midpoint of an imaginary line extending from the anterior superior iliac spine to the pubic symphysis. The *knee joint* is located just below the apex of the patella at the level of the depression between the femoral and tibial condyles. The *ankle joint* is located directly under the depression midway between the malleoli.

Orthoroentgenographic method

Orthoroentgenography was introduced by Hickey[1] in 1924. He used a cassette long enough for the inclusion of the entire length of the extremities and made a single exposure at an SID of 7 feet. This method, now with the use of a long, finely graduated metal ruler and usually a 6-foot SID, is still widely used.

Modifications of the orthoroentgenographic method vary. In one method a Bucky tray is used. A metal ruler is taped to the top of the table so that part of it is included in the exposure field, which records the position of each joint. Measurements can then be quickly determined. A cassette is placed in the Bucky tray and is shifted for centering at the three joint levels without moving the patient. Three exposures are made on one 14″ × 17″ film.

The midsagittal plane of the patient's body is centered to the midline of the cassette or table. The cassette and the tube are successively centered at the previously

marked level of the hip joints, the knee joints, and the ankle joints for simultaneous bilateral projections. When there is a difference in level between the contralateral joints, the film and the tube are centered midway between the two levels.

[1]Hickey, P.M.: Teleoroentgenography as an aid in orthopedic measurements, A.J.R. **11:**232-233, 1924.

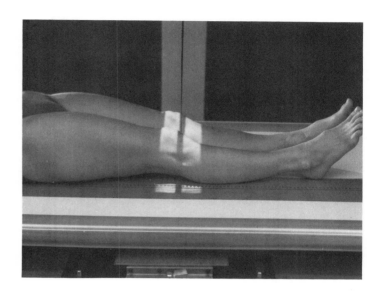

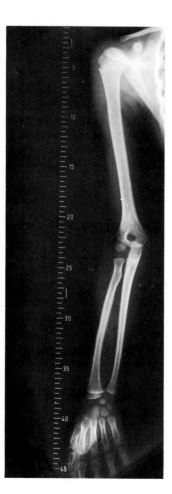

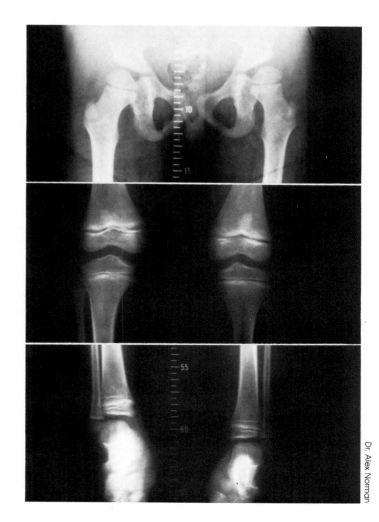

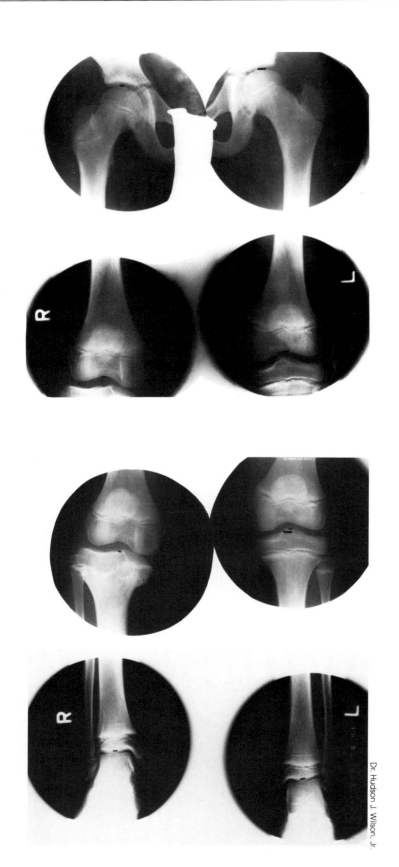

Dr. Hudson J. Wilson, Jr.

Spot scanography

Spot scanography was introduced by Gill[1] in 1944. This is the procedure wherein a closely collimated exposure is made over each joint, a restriction of the exposure field that considerably reduces radiation to the patient's body. All three joints of both extremities of the patient can be made on one film. A finely graduated metal ruler is placed under the extremity as pictured in the orthoroentgenogaphic method of lone bone measurment just described.

After the joint localization marks are made, the patient is positioned and immobilized and local gonad shielding is applied. The collimator is adjusted to limit the exposure field as much as possible. Alternately and successively centering to the localization marks, the right and left sides are exposed without moving the patient.

When the patient has low back pain, it may be necessary to determine whether the causative factor is faulty statics resulting from a difference in leg length and to determine the amount of corrective lift required to equalize the leg length. When the lengths are equalized, the leg measurements may be taken with the patient erect, as described. It is imperative that the patient does not move between any exposures.

[1]Gill, G.G.: A simple roentgenographic method for the measurement of bone growth; modification of Millwee's method of slit scanography, J. Bone Joint Surg. **26**:767-769, 1944.

7

Contrast arthrography

Arthrography (Gr. *arthron,* joint) is radiography of a joint or joints. *Pneumoarthrography, opaque arthrography,* and *double-contrast arthrography* are terms used to denote radiologic examinations of the soft tissue structures of joints (menisci, ligaments, articular cartilage, bursae) following the injection of a contrast agent or of two contrast agents into the capsular space. A gaseous medium is employed in pneumoarthrography, a water-soluble iodinated medium in opaque arthrography, and a combination of both in double-contrast arthrography. Although contrast studies may be made on any encapsuled joint, the knee is the most frequent site of investigation. Other joints sometimes examined by contrast arthrography are the shoulder, the hip, the elbow, the wrist, and the temporomandibular joints.

These examinations are usually performed with local anesthesia only. The injection is made under careful aseptic conditions, usually in a combination fluoroscopic-radiographic examining room, which should be carefully prepared in advance. The sterile items required, particularly the length and gauge of the needles, vary according to the part being examined. The sterile tray and the nonsterile items should be set up on a conveniently placed instrument cart or a small two-shelf table.

After aspirating any effusion, the physician injects the contrast agent or agents and manipulates the joint to ensure proper distribution of the contrast material. The examination is usually performed by fluoroscopy and spot films. Conventional radiographs may then be taken when special projections, such as an axial projection of the shoulder or an intercondyloid fossa projection of the knee, are desired.

Contrast arthrography of knee
VERTICAL RAY METHOD

Contrast arthrography of the knee by the vertical ray method requires the use of a stress device. The extremity is placed in the frame to widen or "open up" the side of the joint space under investigation. This widening, or spreading, of the intrastructural spaces permits better distribution of the contrast material around the meniscus.

After the contrast material is injected, the extremity is placed in the stress device. For the delineation of the medial side of the joint, for example, the stress device is placed just above the knee, and the lower leg is laterally stressed.

When contrast arthrograms are to be made by conventional radiography, the patient is turned to the prone position and the centering point for each side of the

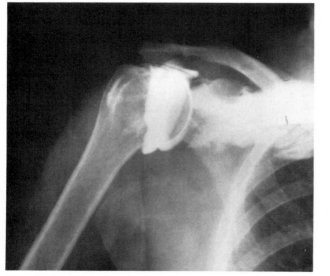

AP projection with arm in external rotation, showing normal filling of subscapular bursa and extension of contrast material into bicipital groove

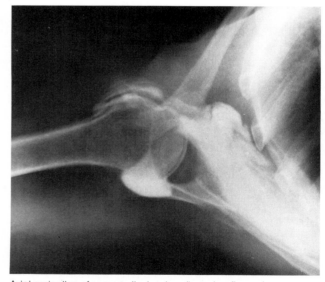

Axial projection of same patient as in adjacent radiograph

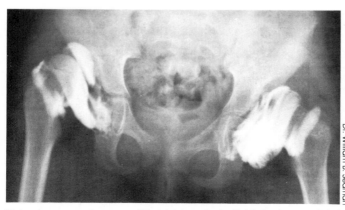
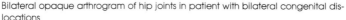

Dr. William B. Seaman

Bilateral opaque arthrogram of hip joints in patient with bilateral congenital dislocations

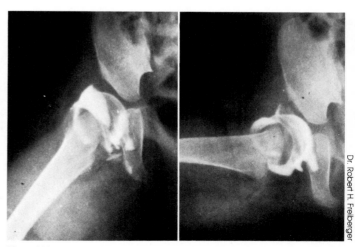

Dr. Robert H. Freiberger

AP and "frog" projections following contrast injection of a treated congenitally dislocated right hip

joint is fluroscopically localized. The mark ensures accurate centering for closely collimated studies of each side of the joint and permits multiple exposures to be made on one film. The projections taken of each side of the joint usually consist of a direct frontal projection and 20-degree right and left oblique projections. The oblique projections may be obtained by rotation of the leg or by central ray angulation. Following completion of these studies the frame is removed for a lateral and an intercondyloid fossa projection.

NOTE: Anderson and Maslin[1] recommended that tomography be utilized in knee arthrography, a technique that can frequently be used to advantage in other contrast-filled joint capsules.

[1]Anderson, P.W., and Maslin, P.: Tomography applied to knee arthrography, Radiology **110:**271-275, 1974.

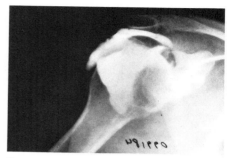

Opaque arthrogram of shoulder. Posterior dislocation with cuff tear. Subacromial bursa opacified.

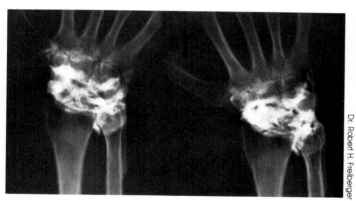

Opaque arthrogram of wrist. Rheumatoid arthritis.

Dr. Robert H. Freiberger

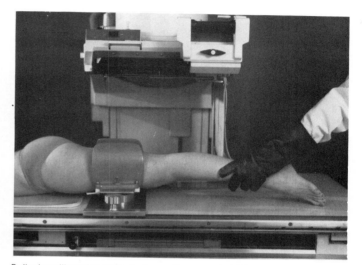

Patient positioned in stress device on fluoroscopic table

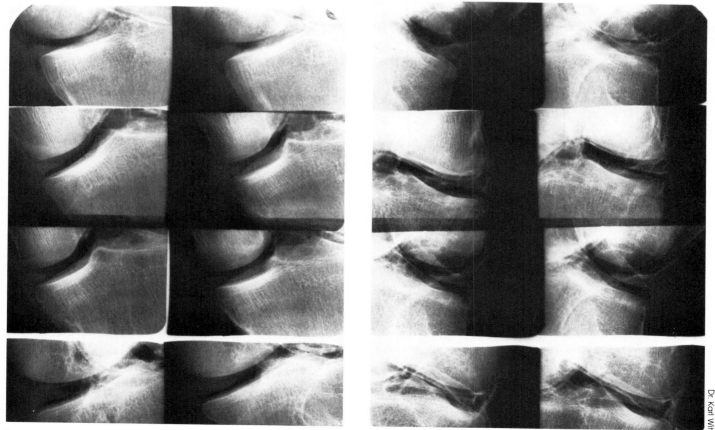

Pneumoarthrogram

Double-contrast arthrogram

Dr. Karl Witt

Double-contrast arthrography of knee
HORIZONTAL RAY METHOD

The horizontal ray method of performing double-contrast arthrography of the knee was first described by Andrén and Wehlin,[1] and later by Freiberger, Killoran, and Cardona.[2] It was found that by using horizontal ray projection and a comparatively small amount of each of the two contrast agents, improved double-contrast delineation of the knee joint structures could be obtained. This is because the excess of the heavy iodinated solution drains into the dependent part of the joint, leaving only the desired thin opaque coating on the gas-enveloped uppermost part, the part then under investigation.

Freiberger, Killovan, and Cardona[2] recommend that six projections be taken of each meniscus, these being consecutively exposed. The accessory equipment used for arthrography varies from institution to institution.

[1]Andrén, L., and Wehlin, L.: Double-contrast arthrography of knee with horizontal roentgen ray beam, Acta Orthop. Scand. **29**:307-314, 1960.
[2]Freiberger, R.H., and Killoran, P.J., and Cardona, G.: Arthrography of the knee by double contrast method, A.J.R. **97**:736-747, 1966.

Medial meniscus

1. The patient is adjusted in the semi-prone position that places the posterior aspect of the medial meniscus uppermost.
2. To widen the joint space the knee is manually stressed.
3. The central ray is directed along the line that is drawn on the medial side of the knee and centered to the meniscus.

With rotation toward the supine position, the leg is turned 30 degrees for each of the succeeding five exposures. The central ray is directed along the localization line. For the last three exposures the knee is adjusted to center the meniscus to the cassette.

Lateral meniscus

1. The patient is adjusted in the semi-prone position that places the posterior aspect of the lateral meniscus uppermost.
2. To widen the joint space the knee is manually stressed.

As for the medial meniscus, six projections may be made on one film. With movement toward the supine position, the leg is rotated 30 degrees for each of the consecutive exposures, from the initial prone oblique position to the supine oblique position. The central ray angulation is adjusted as required to direct it along the localization line.

NOTE: For the demonstration of the cruciate ligaments after filming of the menisci,[1] the patient is asked to stand and then to sit with his knee flexed 90 degrees over the side of the radiographic table. A firm cotton pillow is then adjusted under the knee so that some forward pressure is applied to the leg. With the patient holding a grid cassette in position, a closely collimated and slightly overexposed lateral projection is taken.

[1]Mittler, S., Freiberger, R.H., and Harrison-Stubbs, M.: A method of improving cruciate ligament visualization in double-contrast arthrography, Radiology **102**:441-442, 1972.

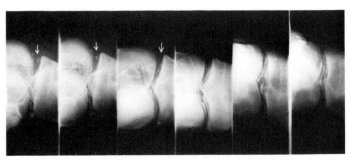

Medial meniscus. Tear in posterior half. Note irregular streaks of positive contrast material within meniscal wedge (arrows).

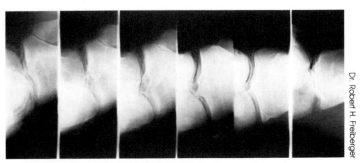

Dr. Robert H. Freiberger

Normal lateral meniscus on same patient as in above radiograph

8

Pelvis and upper femora

ANATOMY

The pelvis serves as a base for the trunk and as a girdle for the attachment of the lower extremities. The pelvic girdle is formed by the two hipbones in front and at the sides and by the sacrum and coccyx behind. The pubes of the hipbones articulate with each other anteriorly at the midline of the body, forming a joint called the symphysis pubis. The ilia articulate with the sacrum posteriorly, and these joints are called the sacroiliac joints. The pubic symphysis and the sacroiliac joints are amphiarthroses, which allow only a little movement.

HIP

The hipbone, also called the os coxae and os innominatum, consists of three parts—the ilium, the pubis, and the ischium. All three bones enter into the formation of the acetabulum, the cup-shaped socket that receives the head of the femur, where they are separated by cartilage in youth but become fused into one bone in adulthood.

Ilium. The ilium consists of a body and a broad, curved, winglike portion called the ala. The body of the ilium forms the upper portion of the acetabulum. The ala projects superiorly from the body to form the prominence of the hip. The ala has three margins, or borders—anterior, posterior, and superior. The anterior and posterior borders each present two prominent projections, which are separated from each other by a notch. These projections

are the superior and inferior spines, respectively. The superior margin extends from the anterior to the posterior superior iliac spines and is called the crest of the ilium. The medial surface of the ala is divided into anterior and posterior portions. The anterior portion is called the iliac fossa and is separated from the body of the bone by a smooth, arc-shaped ridge, the arcuate line, which forms a part of the circumference of the pelvic brim. The arcuate line passes obliquely inferiorly and medially to its junction with the pubis, where there is a slight, rounded elevation called the iliopectineal eminence. The lower part of the posterior portion of the ala presents a large facet, the auricular suface, for articulation with the sacrum.

Pubis. The pubic bone consists of a body and two rami—the superior, or ascending, ramus, and the inferior, or descending, ramus. The body of the pubis forms the lower anterior portion of the acetabulum. (The flattened portion of the pubis at the midline was formerly called the body of the bone.) The superior ramus projects inferiorly and medially from the acetabulum to the midline of the body. Here the bone curves inferiorly and then posteriorly and laterally to join the ischium. The lower prong is termed the inferior ramus. The upper surface of the superior ramus presents a ridge, the pectin, or pectineal line, which is continuous with the arcuate line of the ilium.

Ischium. The ischium, like the pubis, consists of a body and two rami. The body of the ischium forms the lower posterior portion of the acetabulum. Its superior ramus projects posteriorly and inferiorly from the acetabulum to an expanded portion called the ischial tuberosity. The inferior ramus projects anteriorly and medially from the tuberosity to its junction with the inferior ramus of the pubis. By this posterior union the rami of the pubis and the ischium enclose the obturator foramen. At the upper posterior border of the superior ramus is a prominent projection called the ischial spine.

The greater sciatic notch begins just below the posterior inferior iliac spine and extends to the ischial spine. The lesser sciatic notch lies between the ischial spine and the ischial tuberosity.

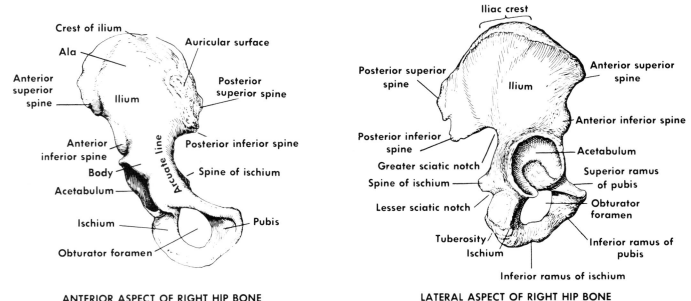

ANTERIOR ASPECT OF RIGHT HIP BONE   **LATERAL ASPECT OF RIGHT HIP BONE**

FEMUR

The proximal end of the femur consists of a head, a neck, and two large processes termed the greater and lesser trochanters. The head is smooth and rounded and is received into the acetabular cavity of the hip. It is connected to the shaft by a pyramid-shaped neck. The neck is constricted near the head but expands to a broad base at the shaft of the bone. The neck projects medially, superiorly, and anteriorly from the shaft. The trochanters are situated at the junction of the shaft and the base of the neck, the greater trochanter at the upper lateral part of the shaft and the lesser trochanter at the posterior medial part. The prominent ridge extending between the trochanters at the base of the neck on the posterior surface of the shaft is called the intertrochanteric crest. The less prominent ridge connecting the trochanters anteriorly is called the intertrochanteric line.

The upper portion of the greater trochanter projects above the neck and curves slightly posteriorly and medially. The most prominent point of the lateral surface of the greater trochanter is always in direct line with the upper border of the neck of the femur. The angulation of the neck of the femur varies considerably with age, sex, and stature. In the adult of average form the neck projects anteriorly from the shaft at an angle of approximately 15 to 20 degrees and superiorly at an angle of approximately 120 to 130 degrees to the long axis of the shaft. In youth the latter angle is wider; that is, the neck is more vertical in position. The angle is narrower—the neck is more horizontal in position—in wide pelves.

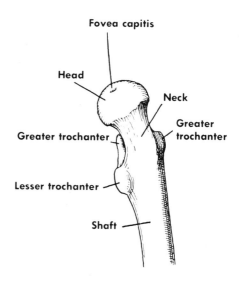

MEDIAL ASPECT OF UPPER END OF FEMUR

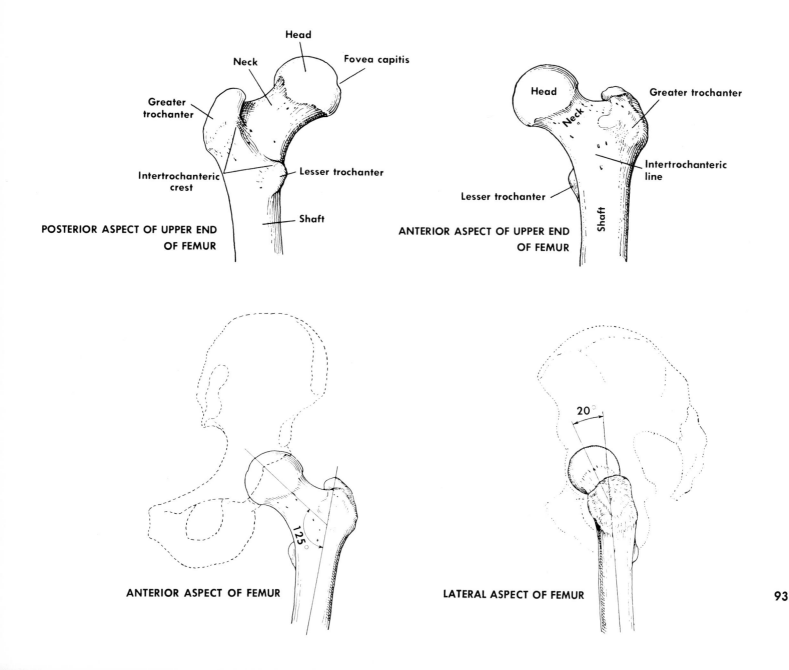

POSTERIOR ASPECT OF UPPER END OF FEMUR

ANTERIOR ASPECT OF UPPER END OF FEMUR

ANTERIOR ASPECT OF FEMUR

LATERAL ASPECT OF FEMUR

HIP JOINT

The articulation between the acetabulum and the head of the femur is a diarthrosis of the ball-and-socket type, which permits free movement in all directions. The knee and ankle joints are hinge joints, so that the wide range of movements of the lower extremity depends on the ball-and-socket joint of the hip. Because the knee and ankle joints are hinge joints, inversion and eversion of the foot cause rotation of the entire extremity and, if carried far enough, of the pelvis. This makes the position of the feet important in radiography of the hip and pelvis; they must be immobilized in the correct position to avoid rotation resulting in distortion of the upper end of the femur.

The two palpable bony points of localization for the hip joint are the anterior superior iliac spine and the superior margin of the pubic symphysis. The midpoint of a line drawn between these two points will lie directly above the center of the dome of the acetabular cavity. A line drawn at right angles to the midpoint of the first line will lie parallel with the long axis of the femoral neck of an average adult in the anatomic position.

For accurate localization of the femoral neck in atypical subjects, or when the extremity is not in the anatomic position, (1) draw a line between the anterior superior iliac spine and the upper margin of the pubic symphysis, and (2) draw a line from a point 1 inch inferior to the greater trochanter to the midpoint of the previously marked line. The femoral head will lie in the same plane as this line (see diagram).

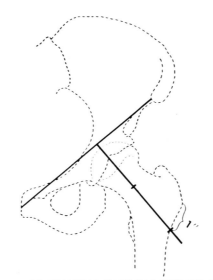

**SCHEMATIC DRAWING SHOWING METHOD OF
LOCALIZING LONG AXIS OF FEMORAL NECK**

PELVIC GIRDLE

The female pelvis is lighter in structure than the male pelvis. It is broader and shallower, and the inlet is larger and more rounded. The sacrum is wider, it curves more sharply posteriorly, and the sacral promontory is flatter. The width and depth of the pelvis vary with stature and with sex.

The pelvis is divided into two portions by an oblique plane that extends from the upper anterior margin of the sacrum to the upper margin of the symphysis pubis. The boundary line of this plane is called the brim of the pelvis. The region above the brim is called the greater or false pelvis, and the region below the brim is called the lesser or true pelvis.

The brim forms the superior strait, or inlet, of the true pelvis and is measured in three directions in pelvimetry. Its antero-posterior, or conjugate, diameter is measured from the upper anterior margin of

the sacrum to the upper margin of the symphysis pubis; its transverse diameter, across the widest region; and its oblique diameter, from the iliopectineal eminence of one side to the sacroiliac joint of the opposite side. The inferior strait, or outlet, of the true pelvis is measured from the tip of the coccyx to the lower margin of the pubic symphysis in the anteroposterior direction and between the ischial tuberosities in the transverse direction. The region between the inlet and the outlet is called the pelvic cavity.

When the body is in the erect or seated position, the pelvic brim forms an angle of approximately 60 degrees to the transverse plane. This angle varies with other body positions, the degree and direction of the variation depending on the lumbar and sacral curves.

The bony landmarks used in radiography of the pelvis and hips are the iliac

crests, the anterior superior iliac spines, the symphysis pubis, the greater trochanters of the femora, the ischial tuberosities, and the tip of the coccyx. Most of these points are easily palpable even in hyper-sthenic subjects. However, because of the heavy muscles immediately above the iliac crest, care must be exercised in locating this structure to avoid centering too high. It is advisable to have the patient inhale deeply, and, while the muscles are relaxed during exhalation, palpate for the highest point of the iliac crest.

The highest point of the greater trochanter, which can be palpated immediately below the depression in the soft tissues of the lateral surface of the hip, is in the same transverse plane as the midpoint of the hip joint and the coccyx. The most prominent point of the greater trochanter is in the same transverse plane as the symphysis pubis.

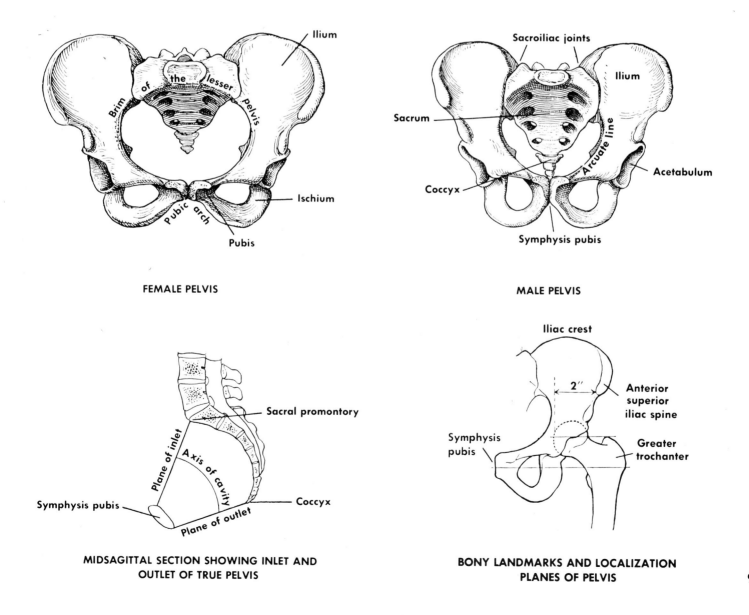

FEMALE PELVIS

MALE PELVIS

MIDSAGITTAL SECTION SHOWING INLET AND OUTLET OF TRUE PELVIS

BONY LANDMARKS AND LOCALIZATION PLANES OF PELVIS

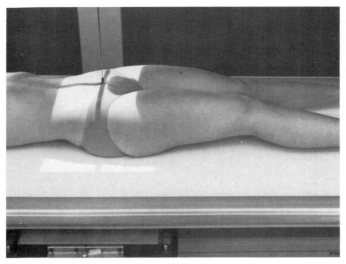

AP projection of pelvis with gonad (shadow) shield

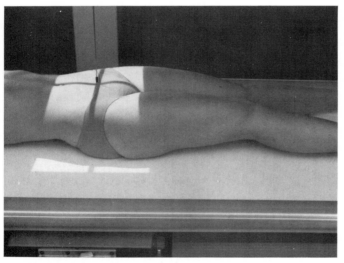

AP projection of pelvis without gonad shield

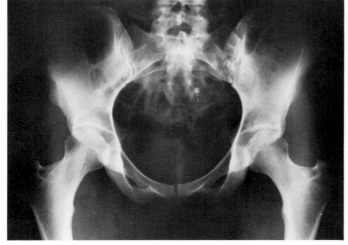

Feet correctly placed

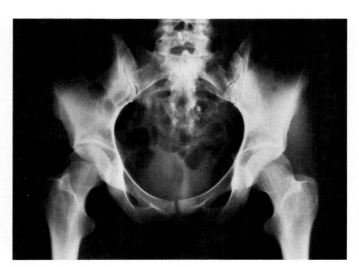

Feet incorrectly placed

Pelvis and upper femora
AP PROJECTION

For all examinations of the pelvis and the upper femora the use of gonad shielding should be considered, according to the criteria outlined in Chapters 1 and 4.

Film: $14'' \times 17''$ crosswise.

Position of patient

Place the patient on the table in the supine position.

Position of part

Center the midsagittal plane of the body to the midline of the table and adjust it in a true AP position. Adjust the shoulders to lie in the same transverse plane, flex the elbows, and rest the hands on the upper chest. Invert the feet about 15 degrees to overcome the anteversion of the femoral necks and thus place their long axes parallel with the plane of the film. Note the appearance of the femoral head, femoral neck, and trochanters in the two radiographs below. (Because the ankle and knee joints are hinge joints, inversion of the foot rotates the entire extremity medially. Inversion of the foot is performed by grasping the heel and turning the foot medially until the position of the longitudinal axis of the heel indicates that the desired degree of extremity rotation has been obtained.) Immobilize with a sandbag across the ankles.

Measure the distance from the anterior superior iliac spine to the tabletop on each side to be sure that there is no rotation of the pelvis. If a soft tissue abnormality (swelling or atrophy) is causing rotation of the pelvis, elevate one side on a radioparent pad to overcome the rotation.

With the cassette in the Bucky tray, center at the level of the soft tissue depression just above the greater trochanter. This centering will include the entire pelvic girdle and the upper fourth of the femora on pelves of average size and shape.

If the pelvis is deep, palpate for the crest of the ilium and adjust the position of the film so that its upper border will project 1 to 1½ inches above the crest of the ilium.

Instruct the patient to suspend respiration for the exposure.

Central ray

Direct the central ray perpendicularly to the midpoint of the film.

Structures shown

An AP projection of the pelvic girdle and of the head, neck, trochanters, and upper third or fourth of the shaft of the femora is presented.

Congenital dislocation of the hip

Martz and Taylor[1] recommend two AP projections of the pelvis for the demonstration of the relationship of the femoral head to the acetabulum in patients with congenital dislocation of the hip. The first projection is made with the central ray directed perpendicularly to the symphysis pubis to detect any lateral or superior displacement of the femoral head. The second projection is made with the central ray directed to the symphysis pubis at a cephalic angulation of 45 degrees. This angulation will cast the shadow of an anteriorly displaced femoral head above that of the acetabulum and the shadow of a posteriorly displaced head below that of the acetabulum.

[1]Martz, C.D., and Taylor, C.C.: The 45-degree angle roentgenographic study of the pelvis in congenital dislocation of the hip, J. Bone Joint Surg. **36-A:**528-532, 1954.

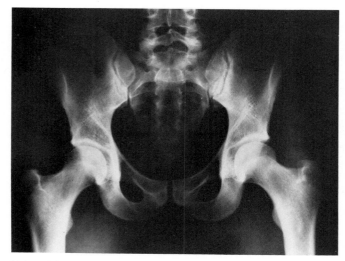

Male pelvis

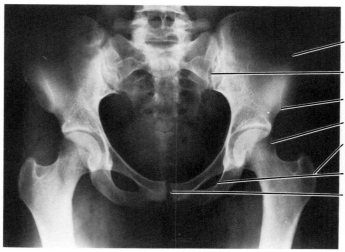

Female pelvis

Anterior superior iliac spine
Sacroiliac articulation
Anterior inferior iliac spine
Femoral head
Greater trochanter
Obturator foramen
Pubic symphysis

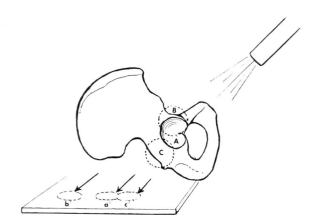

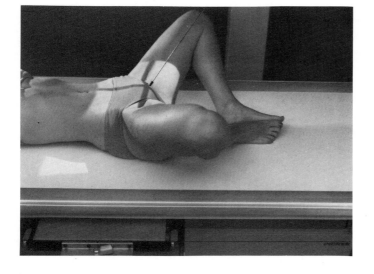

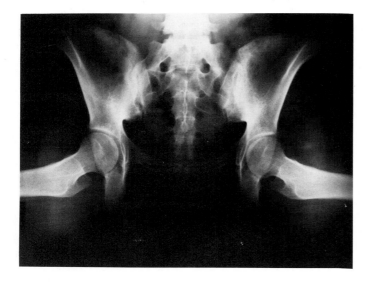

Femoral necks
AP AXIAL PROJECTIONS
CLEAVES METHOD

Film: 14″ × 17″ crosswise.

Position of patient

Place the patient in the supine position. Center the midsagittal plane of the body to the midline of the table. Adjust the shoulders to lie in the same transverse plane, flex the elbows, and rest the hands on the upper chest.

Position of part

Adjust the pelivs in a true AP position. A compression band may be placed well above the hip joints so that it will not interfere with their flexion.

1. Have the patient flex his hips and knees and draw his feet up as much as possible, that is, enough to place the femora in a near vertical position if the affected side will permit. Instruct the patient to hold this position, which is relatively comfortable, while you adjust the tube and cassette.

2. Angle the tube to direct the central ray to be parallel with the long axes of the femoral shafts, and center to the symphysis pubis.

3. With the cassette in the Bucky tray, adjust its position so that the midpoint of the film will coincide with the central ray.

4. Abduct the thighs and have the patient turn his feet inward to brace the soles against each other for support. Center the feet to the midline of the table. Check the position of the thighs, being careful to abduct them to the same degree. If possible, abduct the thighs approximately 40 degrees from the vertical to place the long axis of the femoral necks parallel with the plane of the film.

This position is adapted for a *unilateral examination* by adjusting the body position to center the anterior superior iliac spine of the affected side to the midline of the table. Have the patient flex the hip and knee of the affected side and draw the foot up to the opposite knee. After adjusting the central ray angulation and the position of the cassette tray, have the patient brace the sole of the foot against the opposite knee and lean the thigh laterally approximately 40 degrees.

Structures shown

This method demonstrates an axial projection of the femoral heads, necks, and trochanteric areas projected onto one film for comparison.

This projection is popularly known as the "frog" position.

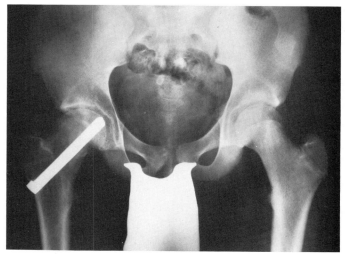

AP

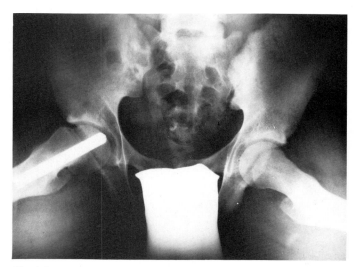

AP axial

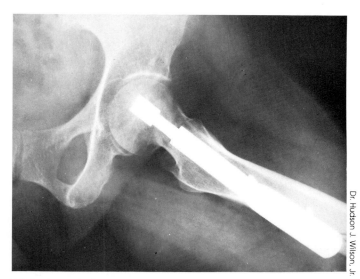

Unilateral examination

Dr. Hudson J. Wilson, Jr.

Pelvis and upper femora
LATERAL PROJECTION

Film: 14″ × 17″ lengthwise.

Position of patient

The patient may be examined in the recumbent or the erect position. If the recumbent position is used, the thighs should be extended enough to prevent the femora from obscuring the shadow of the pubic arch.

Position of part

Recumbent position. When the patient can be placed in the lateral position, center the midaxillary plane of the body to the midline of the table. Place a support under the lower thorax and adjust it to place the vertebral column to be parallel with the tabletop. If the vertebral column is allowed to sag, it will rotate the pelvis in the longitudinal plane.

Adjust the pelvis in a true lateral position, with the anterior superior iliac spines lying in the same vertical plane.

Berkebile, Fischer, and Albrecht[1] recommend a cross-table lateral projection of the pelvis for the demonstration of the gull-wing sign in cases of fracture disloca-

[1]Berkebile, R.D., Fischer, D.L., and Albrecht, L.F.: The gull-wing sign: value of the lateral view of the pelvis in fracture dislocation of the acetabular rim and posterior dislocation of the femoral head, Radiology **84**:937-939, 1965.

tion of the acetabular rim and posterior dislocation of the femoral head.

Erect position. Place the patient in the lateral position before a vertical grid device and center the midaxillary plane of the body to the midline of the grid. Have the patient stand straight, with the weight of the body equally distributed on the feet. Adjust the position of the body so the midsagittal plane is parallel with the plane of the film.

If the extremities are of unequal length, place a support of suitable height under the foot of the short side. Have the patient grasp the side of the stand for support.

Centering point

With the cassette in the Bucky tray, center at the level of the soft tissue depression just above the greater trochanter.

Central ray

Direct the central ray perpendicularly to the midpoint of the film.

Structures shown

A lateral projection of the lumbosacral junction, the sacrum and coccyx, and the superimposed hipbones and upper femora is demonstrated.

If the position is exact, the acetabular shadows will be perfectly superimposed. The larger circle of the fossa farther from the film will be equidistant from the smaller circle of the fossa nearer the film throughout their circumference.

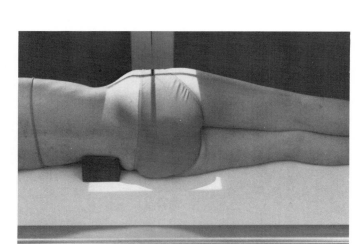

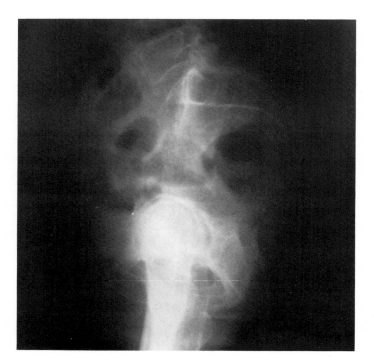

Pelvis and hip joints
AXIAL PROJECTION
CHASSARD-LAPINÉ METHOD

Chassard and Lapiné[1] devised this method for the purpose of measuring the transverse, or biischial, diameter in pelvimetry. It is being used by some to determine the relationship of the femoral head to the acetabulum and by others for the demonstration of the opacified rectosigmoid.

Film: 14″ × 17″ crosswise.

Position of patient

Seat the patient well back on the side or end of the table so that the posterior surface of the knees is in contact with the edge of the table.

Position of part

Center the longitudinal axis of the film to the midsagittal plane of the body, or, if the patient is seated on the end of the table, center the midsagittal plane of the body to the midline of the table. A bench or other suitable support may be placed under the feet.

[1]Chassard and Lapiné: Étude radiographique de l'arcade pubienne chez la femme enceinte; une nouvelle méthode d'appréciation du diamètre bi-ischiatique, J. Radiol. Electrol. **7:**113-124, 1923.

To prevent the thighs from limiting flexion of the body too greatly, have the patient abduct them as far as the end of the table permits. The patient is then instructed to lean directly forward until the symphysis pubis is in close contact with the table; the vertical axis of the pelvis will be tilted forward approximately 45 degrees. The average patient can achieve this degree of flexion without strain.

Have the patient grasp his ankles to aid in maintaining the position. Respiration is suspended for the exposure.

The exposure factors required for this projection are approximately the same as those required for a lateral projection of the pelvis.

Central ray

Direct the central ray perpendicularly through the lumbosacral region at the level of the greater trochanters.

When flexion of the body is restricted, direct the central ray anteriorly, perpendicular to the coronal plane of the symphysis pubis.

Structures shown

An axial projection of the pelvis is shown, demonstrating the relationship between the femoral heads and the acetabula, the pelvic bones, and any opacified structure within the pelvis.

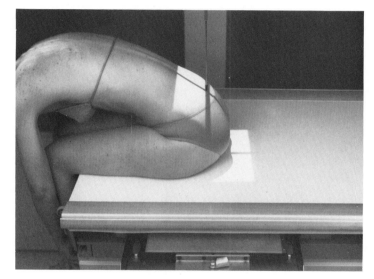

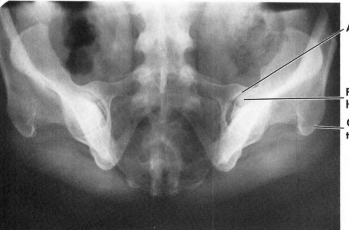

Acetabulum

Femoral head

Greater trochanter

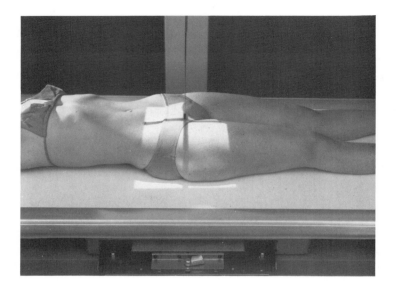

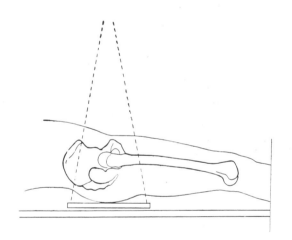

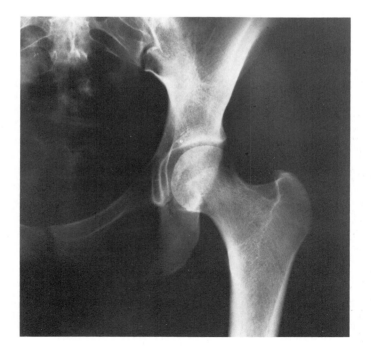

Hip

AP PROJECTION

Film: $10'' \times 12''$ lengthwise.

Position of patient

Place the patient in the supine position.

Position of part

Center the sagittal plane passing 2 inches medial to the anterior superior iliac spine to the midline of the table, and adjust the body in a true AP position. Place the arms in a comfortable position. Adjust the shoulders to lie in the same transverse plane.

Unless contraindicated or otherwise instructed, invert the feet approximately 15 degrees to overcome the anteversion of the femoral neck and thereby place its long axis parallel with the plane of the film.

With the cassette in the Bucky tray, center at the level of the highest point of the greater trochanter.

Central ray

Direct the central ray perpendicularly to the midpoint of the film.

Structures shown

An AP projection of the hip demonstrates the head, neck, trochanters, and upper third of the shaft of the femur.

In the initial examination of a hip lesion, whether traumatic or pathologic in origin, the AP projection is usually made on a film large enough to include the entire pelvic girdle and upper femora. Progress studies may be restricted to the affected side.

NOTE: Trauma patients who have sustained severe injury are not usually transferred to the radiographic table but are radiographed on the stretcher or bed. After the localization point has been established and marked, one assistant should be stationed on each side of the stretcher to grasp the sheet and lift the pelvis just enough for the placement of the cassette, while a third person supports the injured extremity. Any necessary manipulation of the extremity must be made by a physician.

Femoral neck
SUPEROINFERIOR PROJECTION
LEONARD-GEORGE METHOD

Film: $8'' \times 10''$ with a curved cassette.

Position of patient

With the patient in the supine position, the pelvis may be elevated on a small, firm pillow or folded sheets enough to place the greater trochanters 4 inches above the tabletop to center the hip to the vertically placed cassette. Support the affected extremity at hip level on pillows or sandbags.

Position of part

Flex the hip and knee of the unaffected side, if they are not immobilized, and abduct the thigh enough to accommodate the position of the curved cassette.

The affected extremity is usually in abduction in a cast or a splint. If not, and it is possible, abduct the leg enough for accurate placement of the curved cassette in the groin.

Place the cassette in the vertical position well up between the thighs and center it to the crease of the groin of the affected side. With the leg in abduction, this center point will be perpendicular to the femoral neck.

If the extremity can be safely moved, grasp the heel and invert the foot about 15 or 20 degrees to overcome the anteversion of the femoral neck and thus place its long axis parallel with the horizontal and its lateral aspect perpendicular to the plane of the film.

Central ray

Direct the central ray inferiorly and medially perpendicular to the long axis of the femoral neck. It enters the lateral surface of the hip just above the soft tissue depression.

Structures shown

This method demonstrates the head, neck, and trochanteric area of the femur. Because of the convexity of the cassette, the femoral head and the trochanteric areas are somewhat elongated.

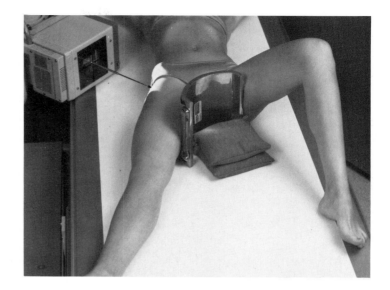

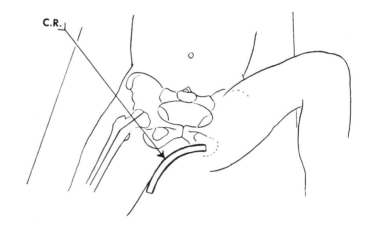

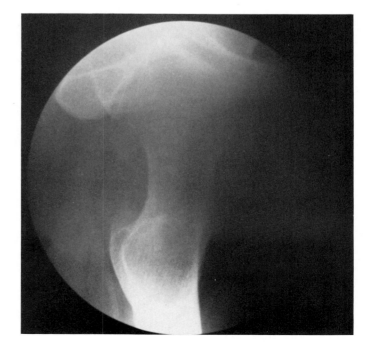

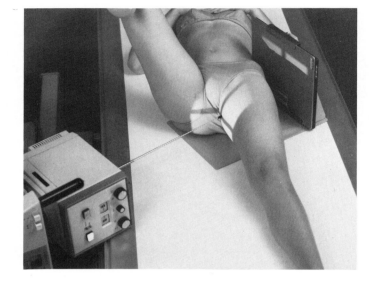

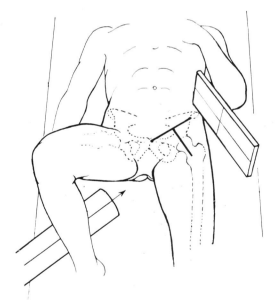

AXIOLATERAL PROJECTION
DANELIUS-MILLER MODIFICATION OF LORENZ[1] METHOD

Film: $8'' \times 10''$ lengthwise.

Position of patient

Adjust the patient in the supine position. When examining a subject who is thin or is lying on a soft bed, elevate the pelvis on a firm pillow or folded sheets enough to center the most prominent point of the greater trochanter to the film. The support must not extend beyond the lateral suface of the body; otherwise it will interfere with the placement of the cassette. Support the affected extremity at hip level on sandbags or firm pillows.

Localization point

To localize the long axis of the femoral neck, first draw a line between the anterior superior iliac spine and the upper border of the symphysis pubis and mark its center point. Palpate for the most prominent lateral projection of the greater trochanter and mark a point 1 inch distal to it. A line drawn between these two points will parallel the long axis of the femoral neck regardless of the position of the extremity.

Position of part

Flex the knee and hip of the unaffected side and adjust the extremity in a position that will not interfere with the projection of the central ray. If possible, rest the leg on a suitable support, with the thigh in a vertical position. Adjust the pelvis in a true AP position.

Grasp the heel and invert the foot of the affected side about 15 or 20 degrees if not contraindicated. The manipulation of patients with unhealed fractures should be done by a physician.

[1]Lorenz: Die röntgenographische Darstellung des subskapularen Raumes und des Schenkelhalses im Querschnitt, Fortschr. Roentgenstr. **25**:342-343, 1917-1918.

Position of film

Place the cassette in the vertical position with its upper border in contact with the lateral surface of the body at or just above the level of the crest of the ilium. Angle the lower border away from the body until the cassette is exactly parallel with the long axis of the femoral neck. The cassette is supported in position with sandbags or a vertical cassette holder. Be careful to place the grid so that the lead strips will be in the horizontal position.

Central ray

Direct the central ray perpendicularly to the long axis of the femoral neck, and center it about 2½ inches below the point of intersection of the localization lines.

Structures shown

This projection of the proximal femur demonstrates the head, neck, and trochanters of the femur.

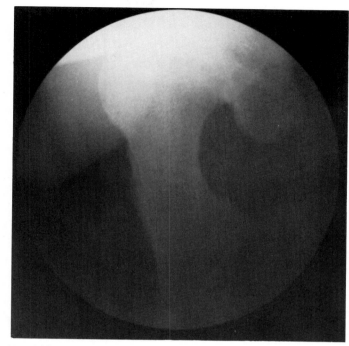

Nongrid film

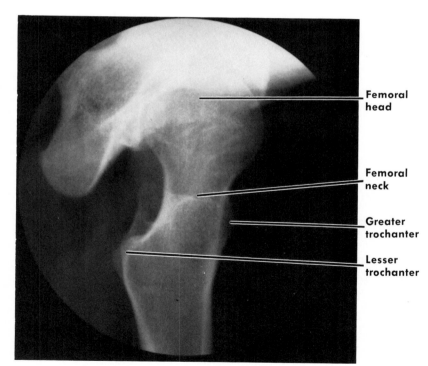

Stationary grid film

Femoral head

Femoral neck

Greater trochanter

Lesser trochanter

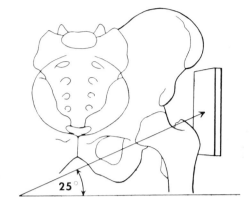

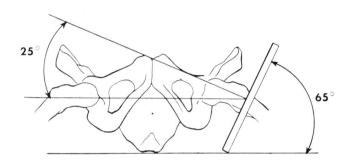

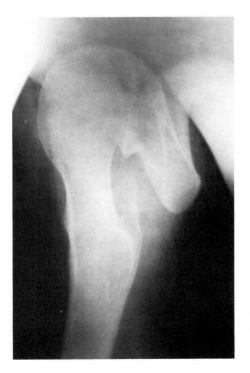

MEDIOLATERAL PROJECTION
JOHNSON METHOD[1]

The Johnson method of obtaining an axiolateral projection of the femoral neck is employed when the opposite femur cannot be adjusted for one of the two preceding positions.

Film: 8″ × 10″ placed lengthwise in a vertical position.

Position of part

When necessary, elevate the pelvis on folded sheets or a firm pillow to place the greater trochanters about 6 inches above the tabletop (2 inches above the center line of the film). This elevation is to allow for the laterodorsal angle of the central ray. Support the extremities at hip level on pillows or sandbags. Adjust the body in a true AP position.

Place the cassette in the vertical position along the lateral surface of the hip and center the transverse line of the cassette to the greater trochanter, which should be approximately 2 inches above the longitudinal line. Tilt the cassette backward 25 degrees from the vertical and support it in position.

Central ray

The central ray is directed to the greater trochanter at a double angle—25 degrees cephalad plus 25 degrees posteriorly. It enters at about the midsagittal plane of the thigh.

Structures shown

An axiolateral projection of the head, neck, and trochanteric region of the femur is shown.

[1]Johnson, C.R.: A new method for roentgenographic examination of the upper end of the femur, J. Bone Joint Surg. **30:**859-866, 1932.

Hip
AXIOLATERAL PROJECTION
FRIEDMAN METHOD

Film: 10″ × 12″ lengthwise.

Position of patient

Have the patient lie in the lateral recumbent position on the affected side. Center the midaxillary plane of the body to the midline of the table.

Position of part

Extend the affected extremity and adjust it in a true lateral position. Roll the upper side gently posteriorly approximately 10 degrees, and place a support under the knee to support it at hip level. The affected femur will not change position if it is properly immobilized; the pelvis will rotate from the femoral head.

With the cassette in the Bucky tray, adjust its position so that the midpoint of the film will coincide with the central ray.

Central ray

Direct the central ray to the femoral neck at an angle of 35 degrees cephalad.

Kisch[1] recommends that the central ray

[1]Kisch, E.: Eine neue Methode für röntgenologische Darstellung des Hüftgelenks in frontaler Ebene, Fortschr. Roentgenstr. **27**:309, 1920.

be angled 15 or 20 degrees cephalad for this projection.

Structures shown

This method presents an axiolateral projection of the head, neck, trochanters, and upper shaft of the femur.

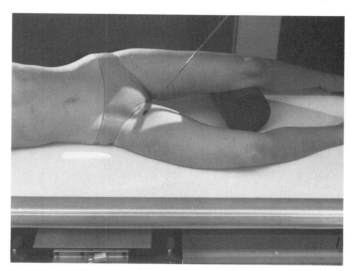

Angulation of 35 degrees

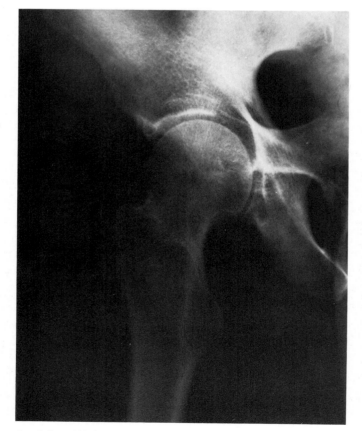

Angulation of 20 degrees

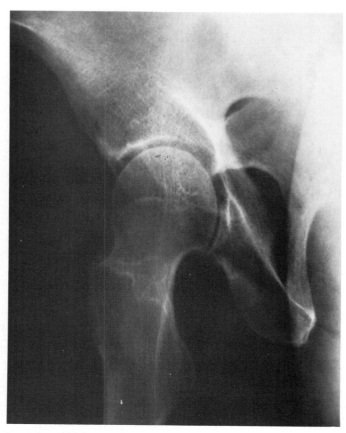

Angulation of 35 degrees

Hip joint
LATERAL PROJECTION
LAUENSTEIN AND HICKEY METHODS

The Lauenstein and Hickey methods are used to demonstrate the hip joint and the relationship of the femoral head to the acetabulum. Because of the danger of fragment displacement or injury, this body position is not used in the presence of an unhealed fracture or a destructive disease.

Film: 10″ × 12″ crosswise.

Position of patient

Following the AP projection have the patient turn toward the affected side to a near lateral position.

Position of part

Adjust the body and center the affected hip to the midline of the table. Ask the patient to flex the dependent knee and draw the thigh up to a near right-angle position. Extend the opposite thigh and support it at hip level. Adjust the position of the pelvis so that the upper side is rotated posteriorly enough to prevent its superimposition on the affected hip.

Position the Bucky tray so that the midpoint of the film will coincide with the central ray.

Central ray

Direct the central ray through the hip joint, which is located at a point midway between the anterior superior iliac spine and the pubic symphysis, (1) perpendicularly for the Lauenstein method and (2) at a cephalic angle of 20 to 25 degrees for the Hickey method.

Structures shown

A lateral projection of the hip is demonstrated, showing the acetabulum, the upper end of the femur, and the relationship of the femoral head to the acetabulum.

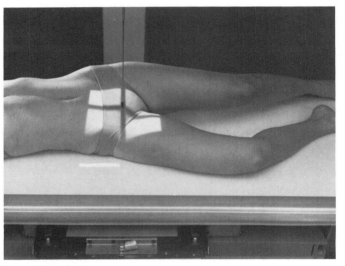

Lauenstein method

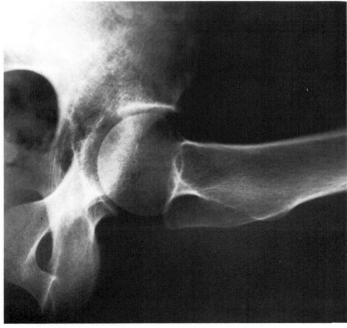

Lauenstein projection

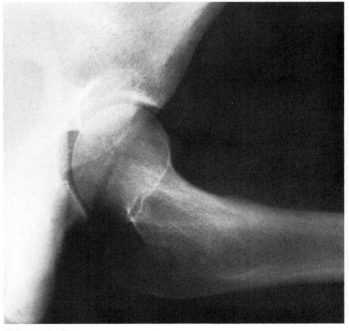

Hickey projection

Hip

PA OBLIQUE PROJECTION (RAO AND LAO)

HSIEH METHOD

Film: 10″ × 12″ lengthwise.

Position of patient

Place the patient in the semiprone position and center the affected hip to the midline of the table.

Position of part

Elevate the unaffected side approximately 40 to 45 degrees and have the patient support himself on the flexed knee and forearm of the elevated side.

Adjust the position of the body to place the posterior surface of the dependent iliac bone over the midline of the table.

With the cassette in the Bucky tray, adjust its position so that the center of the film will lie at the level of the superior border of the greater trochanter.

Central ray

Direct the central ray perpendicularly to the midpoint of the film. It should pass between the posterior surface of the iliac blade and the dislocated femoral head.

Structures shown

This method shows an oblique projection of the ilium, the hip joint, and the upper end of the femur. Hsieh[1] recommends this position for demonstrating posterior dislocations of the femoral head in other than acute fracture dislocations.

[1]Hsieh, C.K.: Posterior dislocation of the hip, Radiology 27:450-455, 1936.

NOTE: Urist[1] has recommended an AP oblique position for the demonstration of the posterior rim of the acetabulum in acute fracture-dislocation injuries of the hip. The patient is adjusted from the supine position for this projection. Elevate the injured hip 60 degrees to place the posterior rim of the acetabulum in profile, and adjust the body to center the sagittal plane passing through the anterior superior iliac spine to the midline of the table. Center the cassette at the level of the upper border of the greater trochanter. Direct the central ray perpendicularly to the midpoint of the film.

[1]Urist, M.R.: Fracture-dislocation of the hip joint, J. Bone Joint Surg. **30-A:**699-727, 1948.

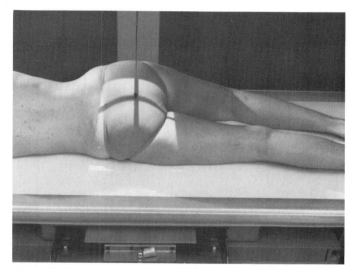

Hsieh method

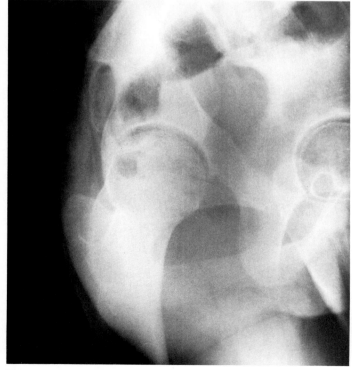

Urist projection

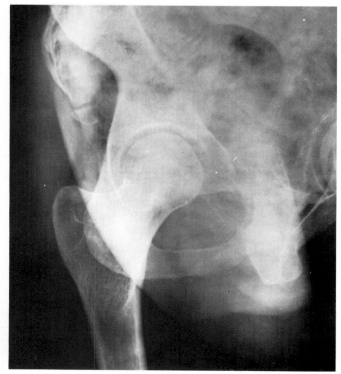

Hsieh projection

POSTEROLATERAL PROJECTION
LILIENFELD METHOD

The Lilienfeld method should not be used with patients who have an acute hip injury because of the danger of fragment displacement.

Film: 10″ × 12″ lengthwise.

Position of patient

Have the patient lie in the lateral recumbent position on the affected side.

Position of part

Center the midaxillary plane of the body to the midline of the table. Fully extend the affected thigh, adjust it in a true lateral position, and immobilize it with sandbags.

Have the patient grasp the side of the table to aid in stabilizing the position. Roll the upper side gently forward approximately 15 degrees, or just enough to separate the two sides of the pelvis, and support the extremity at hip level on sandbags. If the affected side is well immobilized and the upper side is gently rolled forward, it will not change position; the pelvis will rotate from the femoral head.

With the cassette in the Bucky tray, adjust its position so that the center point of the film will lie at the level of the greater trochanter.

Central ray

Direct the central ray perpendicularly to the midpoint of the film.

Structures shown

A posterolateral projection of the ilium, the acetabulum, and the upper end of the femur is demonstrated.

NOTE: The Lilienfeld position is not used with patients who have an acute hip injury because of the danger of fragment displacement. These patients can be comfortably, safely, and satisfactorily examined in the position described by Colonna.[1] The patient is positioned for this projection in approximately the manner described for the Lilienfeld position, except that he is placed *on the unaffected side* and adjusted to center the uppermost hip to the midline of the table. Colonna recommends that the uppermost side, the affected side, be rotated about 17 degrees forward from the true lateral position. He states that this degree of rotation separates the shadows of the hip joints and gives the optimum projection of the slope of the acetabular roof and the depth of the socket.

[1]Colonna, P.C.: A diagnostic roentgen view of the acetabulum, Surg. Clin. North Am. **33**:1565-1569, 1953.

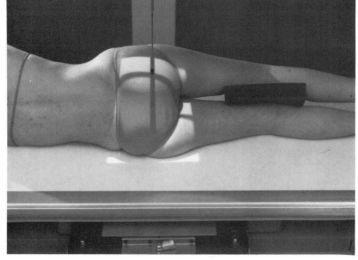

Lilienfeld method

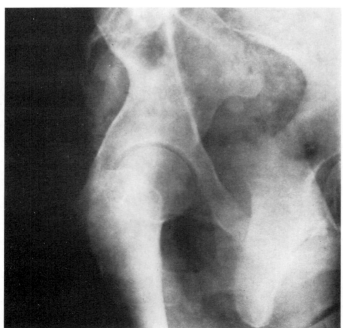

Lilienfeld projection

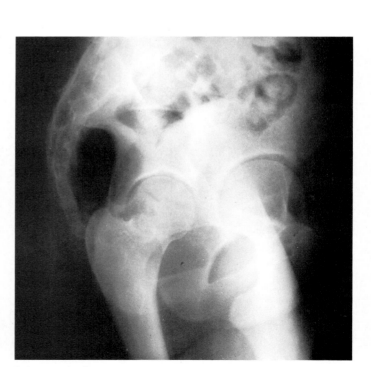

Colonna projection

Acetabulum
PA OBLIQUE PROJECTION (RAO AND LAO)
TEUFEL METHOD

Film: 8″ × 10″ lengthwise.

Position of patient

Have the patient lie in a semiprone position on the affected side, and have him support himself on the forearm and flexed knee of the elevated side.

Position of part

Align the body and center the hip being examined to the midline of the table. Adjust the elevation of the unaffected side so that the anterior surface of the body forms a 38-degree angle from the table.

With the cassette in the Bucky tray, adjust its position so that the midpoint of the film coincides with the central ray.

Central ray

Direct the central ray through the acetabulum at an angle of 12 degrees cephalad. The central ray enters the body at the inferior level of the coccyx and approximately 2 inches lateral to the midsagittal plane toward the side being examined.

Structures shown

Teufel[1] has recommended this position for the demonstration of the fovea capitis and, particularly, the upper posterior wall of the acetabulum.

[1]Teufel, S.: Eine gezielte Aufsichtsaufnahme der Hüftgelenkspfanne, Roentgenpraxis **10**:398-402, 1938.

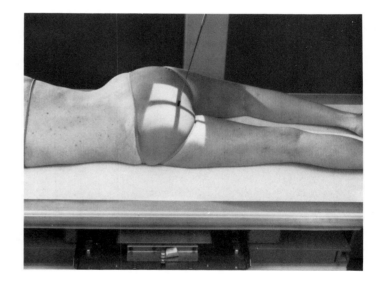

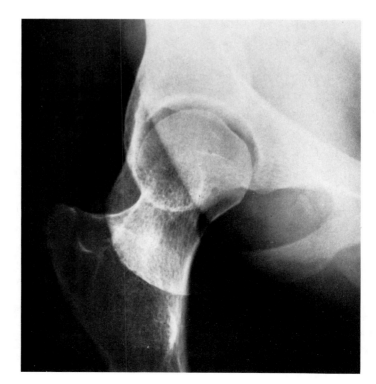

Acetabula

SUPEROINFERIOR PROJECTION

DUNLAP, SWANSON, AND PENNER METHOD

Film: 7″ × 17″ or 14″ × 17″ film, crosswise for bilateral projections of adults.

Close collimation is used to restrict the radiation to the adjacent half of the film.

Position of patient

The patient is placed in the seated-erect position on the side of the table.

Position of part

Ask the patient to move back far enough to place the posterior surface of his knees in contact with the edge of the table.

Center the midline of the longitudinal half of the cassette opposite to the side being examined to the midsagittal plane of the body. Mark the position of the grid so that it can be moved back to this position for the second exposure without disturbing the patient's position; then center the opposite half of the film to the midsagittal plane of the body for the first exposure.

Ask the patient to sit erect with his thighs together, and have him cross his arms over his chest so that they will be well away from the iliac crests. Instruct him to maintain the exact position when the x-ray tube is shifted for the second exposure. Respiration need not be suspended for the exposures.

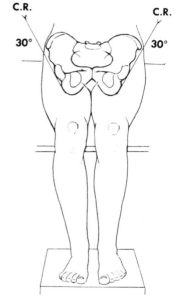

Central ray

Direct the central ray to the crest of the ilium at a medial angle of 30 degrees, first from one side and then from the other.

The originators[1] of this position have stated that the plane of the acetabulum forms an angle of 35 degrees with the sagittal plane in the average adult and 32 degrees in children, but they have found that a central ray angulation of 30 degrees results in the least superimposition of parts.

Structures shown

This method shows the acetabula in profile projected from a plane at right angles to the frontal projection and the relationship of the femoral heads to the acetabula. The femoral heads, necks, and trochanters are seen from a near frontal plane, because there is little change in the position of the femora between the supine and the seated positions.

[1]Dunlap, K., Swanson, A.B., and Penner, R.S.: Studies of the hip joint by means of lateral acetabular roentgenograms, J. Bone Joint Surg. **38-A:**1218-1230, 1956.

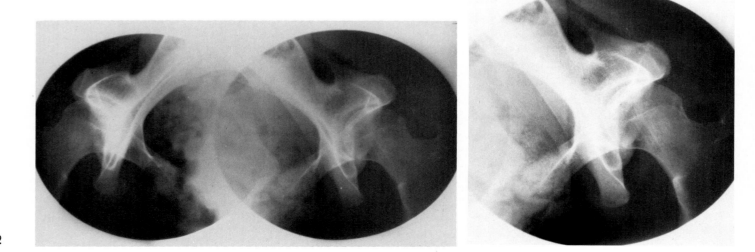

Anterior pelvic bones
AP AXIAL PROJECTION
TAYLOR METHOD

Film: $10'' \times 12''$ crosswise.

Position of patient

Place the patient in the supine position.

Position of part

Center the midsagittal plane of the body to the midline of the table and adjust it in a true AP position.

With the cassette in the Bucky tray, adjust its position so that the midpoint of the film will coincide with the central ray.

Central ray

Males. Direct the central ray approximately 25 degrees (20 to 35 degrees) cephalad and center to a point 2 inches distal to the upper border of the symphysis pubis.

Females. Direct the central ray approximately 40 degrees (30 to 45 degrees) cephalad and center to a point 2 inches distal to the upper border of the symphysis pubis.

The localization point may be established with sufficient accuracy from the most prominent lateral projection of the greater trochanter.

Structures shown

An inferosuperior projection of the pubic and ischial rami is presented, free of superimposition.

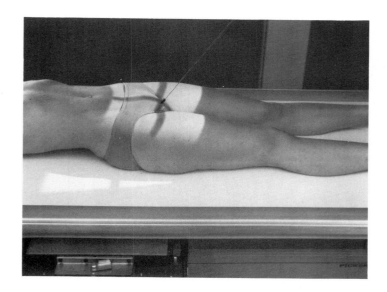

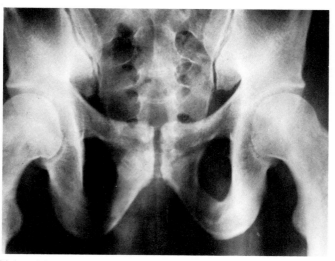

Male pelvis

Female pelvis

PA PROJECTION

Film: 8″ × 10″ crosswise.

Position of patient

Place the patient in the prone position and center the midsagittal plane of the body to the midline of the table.

Position of part

Adjust the body in a true PA position. With the cassette in the Bucky tray, center at the level of the greater trochanters; this will center the film to the symphysis pubis.

Central ray

Direct the central ray perpendicularly to the midpoint of the film.

Structures shown

A PA projection of the pubic and ischial bones is demonstrated, including the pubic symphysis and the obturator foramina.

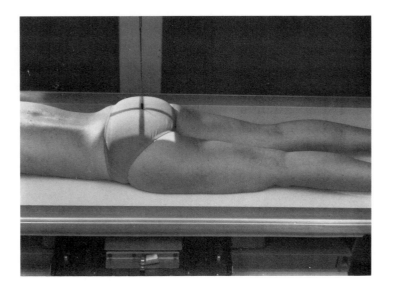

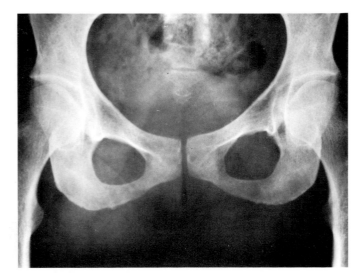

AP AXIAL PROJECTIONS
LILIENFELD METHOD

Film: 8″ × 10″ crosswise.

Position of patient

Place the patient on the radiographic table in a seated-erect position.

Position of part

Center the midsagittal plane of the body to the midline of the table. To relieve strain, flex the knees slightly and support them. If the travel of the cassette tray is great enough to permit centering near the end of the table, the patient will be more comfortable seated, so that his legs can hang over and his feet can rest on a suitable support.

Have the patient extend his arms for support, lean backward 45 or 50 degrees, and then arch his back to place the pubic arch in a vertical position.

With the cassette in the Bucky tray, center at the level of the greater trochanters.

Central ray

Direct the central ray perpendicularly to the midpoint of the film.

Structures shown

The radiograph demonstrates a superoinferior projection of the anterior pubic and ischial bones and the symphysis pubis.

STAUNIG METHOD

Film: 8″ × 10″ crosswise.

Position of patient

Place the patient in the prone position.

Position of part

Center the midsagittal plane of the body to the midline of the table. Adjust the body in a true PA position.

With the cassette in the Bucky tray, adjust its position so that the midpoint of the film will coincide with the central ray.

Central ray

With the central ray at an angle of 35 degrees cephalad, center to the symphysis pubis, which lies in the midsagittal plane at the level of the greater trochanters.

Structures shown

This method shows an inferosuperior projection of the pubic and ischial bones and of the symphysis pubis.

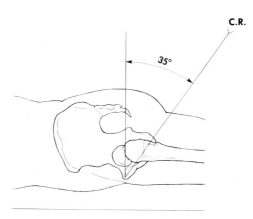

Staunig method

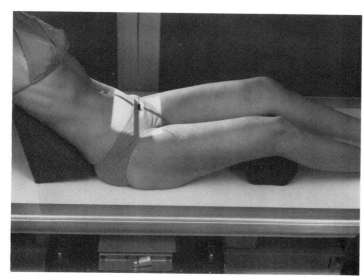

Lilienfeld method

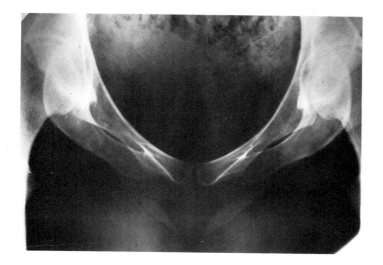

Ilium

AP AND PA OBLIQUE PROJECTIONS

Film: 10″ × 12″ lengthwise.

AP oblique position (RPO and LPO)

Place the patient in the supine position and center the sagittal plane passing through the hip joint of the affected side to the midline of the table. Elevate the unaffected side approximately 40 degrees to place the broad surface of the wing of the dependent ilium parallel with the plane of the film. Support the elevated shoulder, hip, and knee on sandbags. Adjust the position of the uppermost extremity to place the anterior superior iliac spines in the same transverse plane.

PA oblique position (RAO and LAO)

Place the patient in the prone position and center the sagittal plane passing through the hip joint of the affected side to the midline of the table. Elevate the unaffected side about 40 degrees to place the dependent ilium perpendicularly to the plane of the film. Have the patient rest on the forearm and flexed knee of the elevated side. Adjust the position of the uppermost thigh to place the anterior superior iliac spines in the same transverse plane.

Center the film at the level of the transverse plane passing midway between the anterior superior iliac spines and the upper border of the greater trochanters.

Central ray

Direct the central ray perpendicularly to the midpoint of the film.

Structures shown

The AP oblique projection shows an unobstructed image of the iliac wing and of the sciatic notches and a profile image of the acetabulum.

The PA oblique projection shows an oblique image of the ilium and of the upper end of the femur.

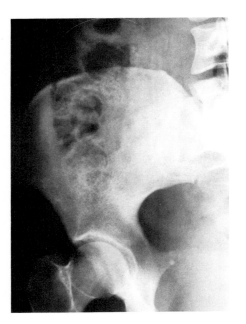

AP oblique

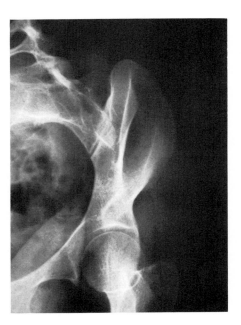

PA oblique

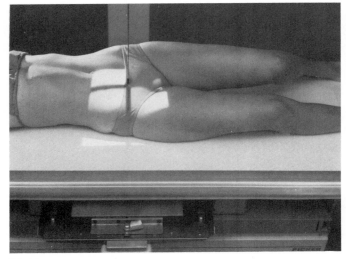

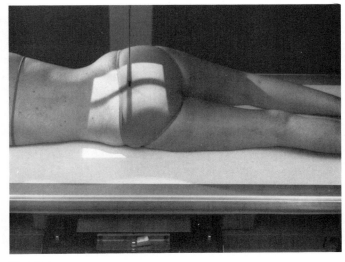

9

Upper extremity

ANATOMY

For purposes of study, anatomists divide the bones of the upper extremities into four main groups: the hand, the forearm, the arm, and the shoulder girdle. The upper end of the arm and the shoulder girdle are discussed in Chapter 10.

HAND

The hand consists of 27 bones, which are subdivided into three groups: the phalanges, or bones of the fingers; the metacarpals, or bones of the palm; and the carpals, or bones of the wrist.

Fingers. The fingers are numbered and named; however, the description by number is the more correct terminology. Beginning at the lateral side, the numbers and names are the first finger, or thumb; the second, or index, finger; the third, or middle, finger; the fourth, or ring, finger; and the fifth, or small, finger. There are 14 phalanges in the fingers—two in the thumb and three in each of the other fingers. The phalanges of the first finger are described as first and second or as proximal and distal. Those of the other fingers are described as first, second, and third or as proximal, middle, and distal. The phalanges consist of a cylindrical shaft and two articular ends and are slightly concave anteriorly. The distal phalanges are small and flattened and have a roughened rim around their distal anterior end, which gives them a spatular appearance. The interphalangeal articulations are diarthrodial joints of the hinge type, having only forward and backward movement.

Palm. There are five metacarpals, corresponding in position to the palm of the hand. The metacarpals are simply numbered one to five, beginning at the lateral, or thumb, side of the hand. The metacarpals consist of a body, or shaft, and two articular ends. They are cylindrical in shape and are slightly concave anteriorly. They articulate with the phalanges at their distal ends and with the carpus at their proximal ends.

With the exception of the thumb, the metacarpophalangeal articulations are diarthrodial joints of the condyloid type, having the movements of flexion, extension, abduction, adduction, and circumduction. In addition to these movements the thumb has axial rotation, which places it in the saddle joint classification.

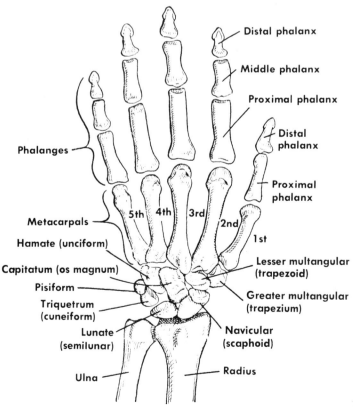

POSTERIOR ASPECT OF HAND AND WRIST

WRIST

The wrist has eight carpal bones. They are fitted closely together and arranged in two transverse rows. With one exception, each of these bones has two names, both in common usage. The names of those in the proximal row, beginning at the lateral, or thumb, side, are the navicular, or scaphoid; the lunate, or semilunar; the triquetral, or cuneiform (also called the triangular); and the pisiform. In the distal row, beginning at the lateral side, are the greater multangular, or trapezium; the lesser multangular, or trapezoid; the capitatum, or os magnum (also called the capitate); and the hamate, or unciform. The carpals are composed largely of cancellous tissue with an outer layer of compact bony tissue. They are classified as short bones. The carpals articulate with each other, with the metacarpals, and with the radius of the forearm.

In the carpometacarpal articulations the first metacarpal and the greater multangular form a saddle type of joint, which has great freedom of movement, whereas the articulations between the second, third, fourth, and fifth metacarpals and the lesser multangular, capitatum, and hamate form gliding joints of limited movement. The midcarpal articulations allow free flexion and extension and slight rotation. The radiocarpal articulation, which is considered the wrist joint proper, is a diarthrodial joint of the condyloid type, which has all movements except rotation.

The dorsal surface of the articulated carpals is convex. The palmar surface is concave from side to side, and the groove formed by the concavity is called the carpal sulcus (also carpal canal and carpal tunnel).

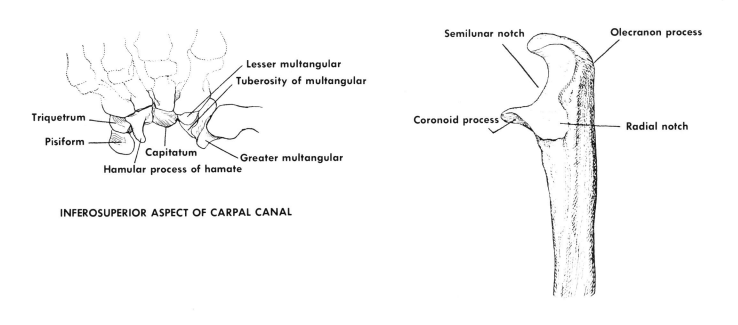

INFEROSUPERIOR ASPECT OF CARPAL CANAL

RADIAL ASPECT OF UPPER END OF ULNA

FOREARM

The forearm has two bones—the radius and the ulna. Like other long bones, the radius and ulna each consists of a shaft and two articular extremities. The ulna lies on the medial side of the forearm parallel with the radius, which lies on the lateral, or thumb, side.

Ulna. The shaft, or body, of the ulna is long and slender and tapers downward. Its upper extremity is large and presents two beaklike processes and two concave depressions. The upper process, the olecranon, is curved forward and slightly downward and forms the proximal part of the semilunar notch. The lower, or coronoid, process projects forward from the anterior surface of the shaft to form the lower part of the semilunar notch. The coronoid process is triangular in shape and curves slightly upward.

The semilunar notch, which is formed by the smooth, concave surfaces of the olecranon and coronoid processes, articulates with the trochlea of the humerus by a hinge joint. On the lateral side of the coronoid process there is a depression, the radial notch, for articulation with the disklike head of the radius.

The lower end of the ulna has a rounded process on its lateral side, termed the head of the ulna, which articulates with the lower end of the radius. On its posterior medial side is a slender conical projection called the styloid process. The head of the ulna is separated from the wrist joint by an articular disk.

Radius. The proximal end of the radius is small and presents a flat, disklike head above a constricted area called the neck. Just below the neck, on the medial side of the shaft, is a roughened process called

the radial tuberosity. The lower end of the radius is broad and flattened and has a conical projection on its lateral surface called the styloid process.

The head of the radius articulates with the capitellum of the humerus above and with the radial notch of the ulna at the side. The lower end of the radius articulates with the carpus below and with the head of the ulna at the median side. Both the superior and inferior radioulnar articulations are diarthrodial joints of the pivot type. The movements of supination and pronation of the forearm and hand are largely the result of the combined rotary action of these two joints. In the act of pronation the radius turns medially and crosses over the ulna at its upper third, while the ulna makes a slight counterrotation, which obliques the humerus by rotating it medially.

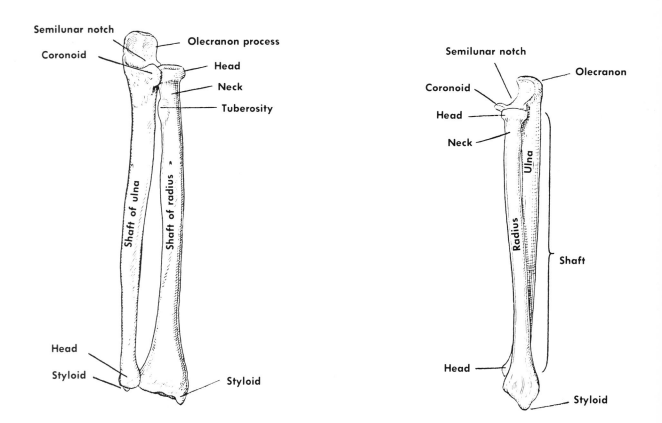

ANTERIOR ASPECT OF RADIUS AND ULNA

LATERAL ASPECT OF RADIUS AND ULNA

ARM

The arm has one bone, the humerus, which consists of a shaft, or body, and two articular extremities. The shaft is long and cylindrical in shape. The upper part of the humerus is considered with the shoulder girdle in Chapter 10. The lower part is broad and flattened and presents numerous processes and depressions. It has medial and lateral condyles and medial and lateral epicondyles. On its inferior surface are two smooth elevations for articulation with the bones of the forearm, the trochlea on the medial side for articulation with the ulna, and the capitellum on the lateral side for articulation with the flattened head of the radius.

On the anterior surface, just above the trochlea, is a shallow depression called the coronoid fossa for the reception of the coronoid process when the elbow is flexed. Immediately behind the coronoid fossa, on the posterior surface, is the olecranon fossa, which is a deep depression for the accommodation of the olecranon process when the elbow is extended.

The articulation between the humerus and the ulna is a hinge type of joint, allowing forward and backward movement only. The elbow joint proper includes the superior radioulnar articulation as well as the articulations between the humerus and the radius and ulna. The three joints are enclosed in a common capsule.

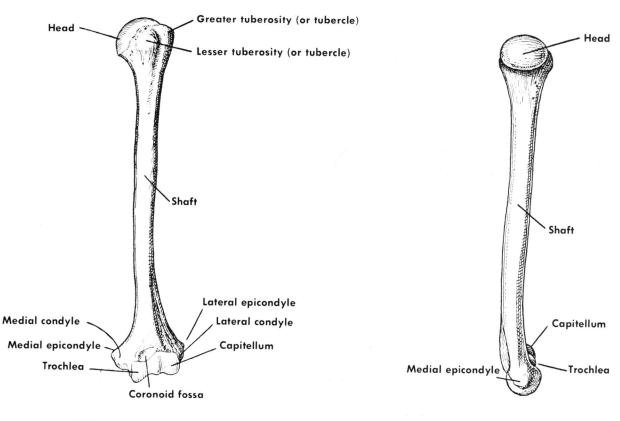

ANTERIOR ASPECT OF HUMERUS

MEDIAL ASPECT OF HUMERUS

When radiographing the upper extremity, seat the patient at the side or the end of the table in such a way that it will not be necessary for him to assume a strained or uncomfortable position. Place the cassette at a location and angle that will allow the patient to be positioned most comfortably. Since the degree of immobilization is limited, particularly of the hand and fingers, it is important that the patient be comfortable so that he can relax and cooperate in maintaining the position.

The central ray, unless otherwise specified, is directed at right angles to the midpoint of the film. The joint spaces of the extremities are narrow. Accurate centering is essential to avoid obscuring them. When a bilateral examination is requested of the hands and/or wrists, *each side should be correctly, separately positioned*. This positioning is for the purpose of preventing rotation distortion, particularly of the joint spaces, as happens when both sides are placed on the film for simultaneous projection.

The gonad area should be shielded from scattered radiation with a sheet of lead-impregnated rubber placed as shown in the adjacent photograph.

✱Hand
PA PROJECTION

Film: 8″ × 10″ for hand of average size.

Position of part

Have the patient rest his forearm on the table and place his hand on the cassette with the palmar surface down. Center the film to the metacarpophalangeal joints and adjust it so that the long axis of the film is parallel with the long axis of the hand and forearm. Spread the fingers only slightly.

Ask the patient to relax his hand to avoid motion. Involuntary movement can be prevented with the use of adhesive tape or positioning sponges.

Central ray

Direct the central ray vertically to the third metacarpophalangeal joint.

Structures shown

A PA projection demonstrates the carpals, the metacarpals, and the phalanges (except of the thumb), the interarticulations of the hand, and the lower ends of the radius and ulna. This position also demonstrates an oblique projection of the first finger.

NOTE: When the metacarpophalangeal joints are the point of interest and the patient cannot extend his hand enough to place its palmar surface in contact with the cassette, reverse the position of the hand for an AP projection. This position is also used for the metacarpals when, because of injury, a pathologic condition, or dressings, the hand cannot be extended.

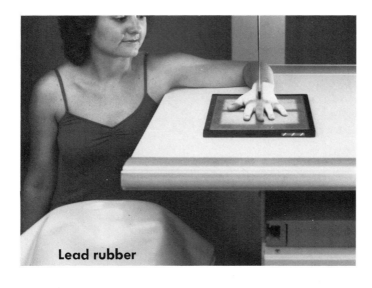

Lead rubber

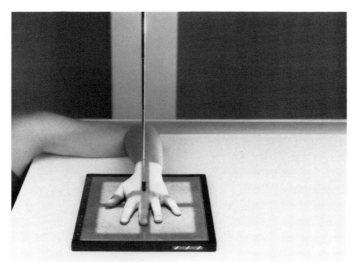

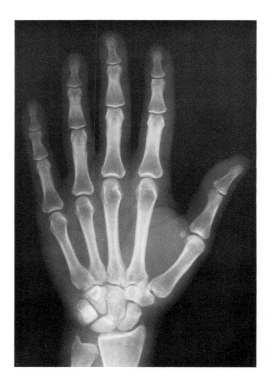

LATERAL IN FLEXION

Film: 8″ × 10″ lengthwise.

Position of part

Ask the patient to rest his forearm on the table and to place his hand on the film with the ulnar aspect down. Center the cassette to the metacarpophalangeal joints and adjust it so that its midline is parallel with the long axis of the hand and forearm.

With the patient relaxing his fingers so that the natural arch of the hand is maintained, arrange them so that they are perfectly superimposed. Have the patient hold his thumb parallel with the film. If he is unable to do so, immobilize it with tape or a sponge.

Central ray

Direct the central ray perpendicularly to the metacarpophalangeal joints.

Structures shown

A lateral projection of the bony structures and soft tissues of the hand in their normally flexed position is presented.

This projection is used to demonstrate anterior or posterior displacement in fractures of the metacarpals. The radiographic technique should be properly adjusted so

that the outline of each bone is clearly seen through the superimposed shadows of the other metacarpals.

NOTE: Fiolle[1,2] was the first to describe a small bony growth occurring on the dorsal surface of the third metacarpocarpal joint. He termed the condition "carpe bossu," or carpal boss, and found that it could be demonstrated to best advantage in a lateral projection with the wrist in palmar flexion.

[1]Fiolle, J.: Le "carpe bossu," Bull. Soc. Chir. Paris **57:**1687, 1931.
[2]Fiolle, J., and Ailland: Nouvelle observation de "carpe bossu," Bull. Soc. Chir. Paris **58:**187-188, 1932.

LAT - 2-5 Fingers straight
Thumb Right Angle
Ulna side close to film

CR.- perp. 2ⁿᵈ mcp. jt.

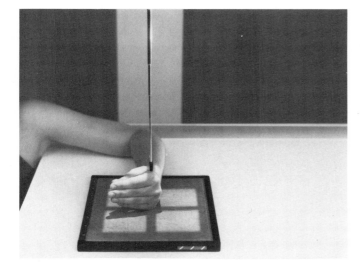

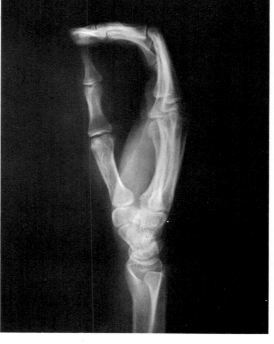

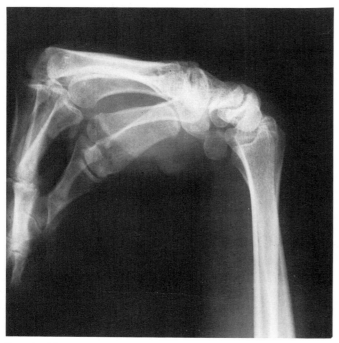

Normal wrist

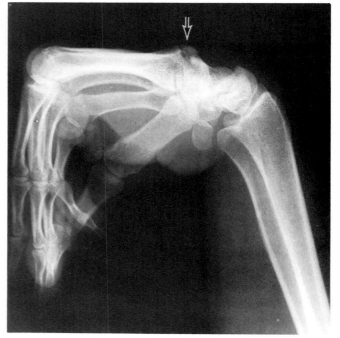

Carpal boss *(arrow)*

✳ LATERAL IN EXTENSION

Film: 8″ × 10″ for hand of average size.

Position of part

Have the patient completely extend his fingers with the thumb at right angles to the palm and his hand on the cassette, with the radial or the ulnar aspect down, as indicated. If the elbow is elevated, support it in position with sandbags.

Center the cassette to the metacarpophalangeal joints and adjust it so that the midline is parallel with the long axis of the hand and forearm. If the hand is resting on the ulnar surface, immobilization of the thumb may be necessary.

Central ray

Direct the central ray perpendicularly to the metacarpophalangeal joints.

Structures shown

This position shows a lateral projection of the hand in extension. This is the customary position for the localization of foreign bodies. The exposure technique will depend on the nature of the foreign body.

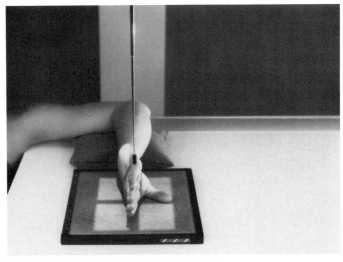

Radial surface to film

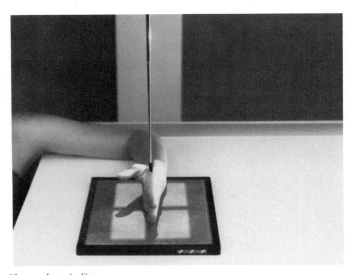

Ulnar surface to film

2-5 Finger straight
Thumb Right angle L
Ulna side close to film

CR - perp. 2ND mcp. Jt.

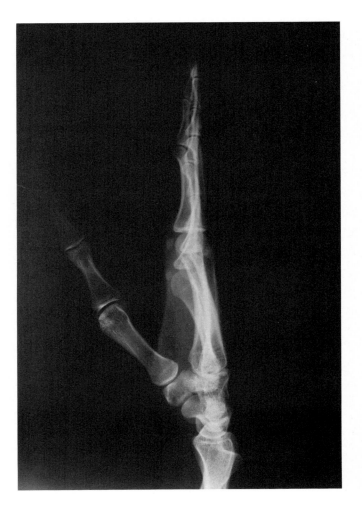

✳ PA OBLIQUE PROJECTION

Film: 8″ × 10″ lengthwise.

Position of part

Have the patient rest his forearm on the table and place his hand on the cassette in the lateral position, ulnar side down. From the lateral position, rotate the hand medially with the fingers slightly flexed so that their tips will touch the cassette. Center the film to the metacarpophalangeal joints and adjust it so that the midline is parallel with the long axis of the hand and forearm. Adjust the obliquity of the hand so that the metacarpophalangeal joints form an angle of approximately 45 degrees with the plane of the film.

If it is not possible to obtain the correct position with all fingertips resting on the cassette, elevate the index finger and thumb on a suitable radiolucent material.

When an oblique projection of the interphalangeal joints is desired, a foam wedge should be used to support the fingers in the intended position.

Central ray

Direct the central ray vertically to the third metacarpophalangeal joint.

Structures shown

An oblique projection of the bones and soft tissues of the hand is shown. This position is used largely in pathologic conditions or as a supplemental projection in the investigation of fractures.

*45° Rotation ulna side hand + wrist
Spread Fingers apart
CR - 3Rd mcp. Jt.*

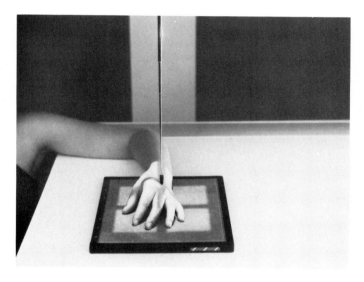

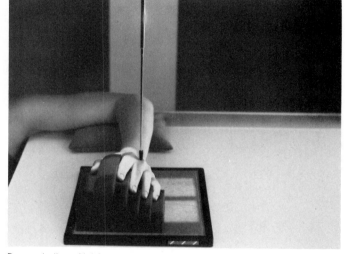

Demonstration of joint spaces

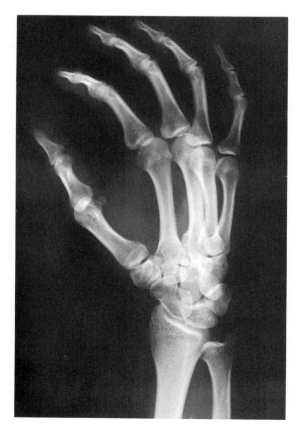

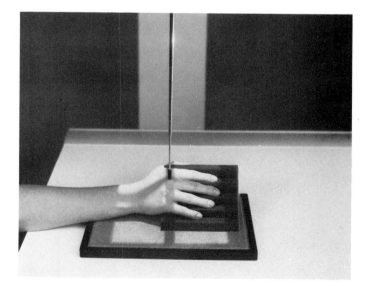

Fingers (second through fifth)
PA PROJECTIONS

Film: 8″ × 10″ crosswise for two projections on one film.

Position of part

When radiographing individual fingers (except the first), place the finger on the unmasked half of the cassette with the palmar surface down.

Separate the fingers slightly and center the finger being examined to the midline of the film, with its proximal interphalangeal joint over the center point of the film.

Central ray

Direct the central ray perpendicularly to the proximal interphalangeal jont.

NOTE: Fingers that cannot be extended can be examined in small sections with dental films. If a joint is in question, the projection should be an AP instead of a PA.

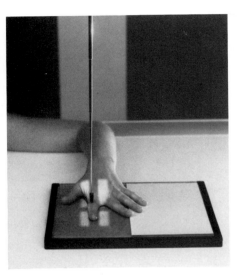

Second finger

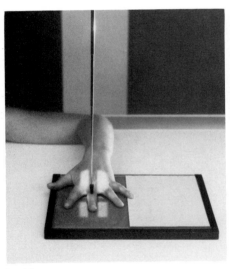

Third finger

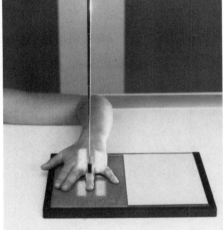

Fourth finger

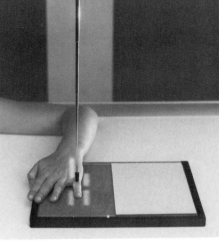

Fifth finger

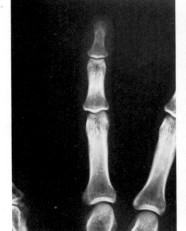

Second finger

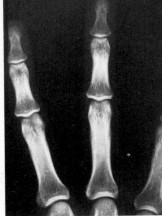

Third finger

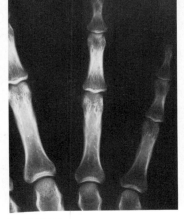

Fourth finger

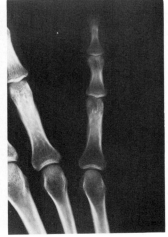

Fifth finger

LATERAL PROJECTION

Film: 8″ × 10″ crosswise for two projections on one film.

Position of part

Since lateral finger positions are difficult to hold, it is advisable to tell the patient how his finger is to be adjusted on the cassette. Demonstrate with your own finger, and then let the patient assume the position with his arm that will be most comfortable for him.

Ask the patient to extend the finger to be examined, close the rest of the fingers into a fist, and hold them in complete flexion with his thumb. When it is necessary to elevate the elbow to bring the finger into position, support it on sandbags or other suitable support.

With the finger to be examined extended and the other fingers folded into a fist, the patient's hand should rest (1) on the radial surface for the second or third finger or (2) on the ulnar surface for the fourth or fifth finger.

Before the final adjustment of the position of the finger, place the cassette so that the midline of its unmasked half is parallel with the long axis of the finger and center it to the proximal interphalangeal joint.

The second and fifth fingers rest directly on the cassette, but for accurate projection of the bones and joints the third and fourth fingers must be elevated to place their long axis parallel with the plane of the film.

Immobilize the extended finger by placing a strip of adhesive tape, a tongue depressor, or other support against its palmar surface. The patient can hold the support with his opposite hand. Finally, adjust the arterior or posterior rotation of the hand to obtain a true lateral position of the finger.

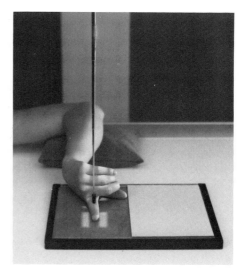

Second finger

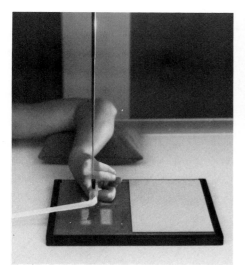

Third finger

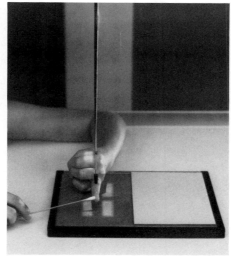

Fourth finger

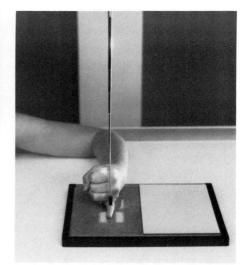

Fifth finger

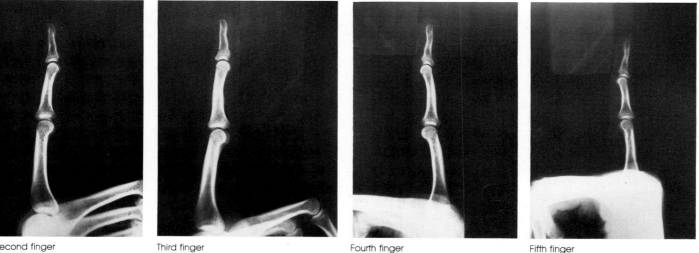

Second finger

Third finger

Fourth finger

Fifth finger

First finger (thumb)

FRONTAL, LATERAL, AND OBLIQUE
PROJECTIONS

Film: 8″ × 10″ crosswise for two projections on one film.

AP PROJECTION

To avoid motion or rotation it is advisable for the technologist to demonstrate the desired position with his own hand. The patient can then, by adjusting the position of his body on the chair, place his hand in the correct position with the least amount of strain on his arm. Place the cassette under the finger after the hand is in approximately the correct position. The patient will assume a more comfortable position if he is not asked to adjust his hand at a specific point.

Ask the patient to turn his hand to a position of extreme internal rotation. Have the patient hold the extended fingers back with tape or with his opposite hand and rest the thumb on the table. If the elbow is elevated, place a support under it and have the patient rest the opposite forearm against the table for support.

Place the cassette under the thumb and, with its midline parallel with the long axis of the finger, center to the metacarpophalangeal joint. Adjust the position of the hand to secure a true AP position of the thumb, being careful to have the fifth metacarpal back far enough to avoid superimposition.

PA PROJECTION

It is sometimes necessary to take the frontal projection of the first carpometacarpal joint and finger from the dorsal aspect. For this projection, place the hand in the lateral position, rest the elevated and abducted thumb on a radioparent support, and adjust the hand to place the dorsal surface of the finger parallel with the film. When the position requires that the wrist be elevated, support it on a small sandbag.

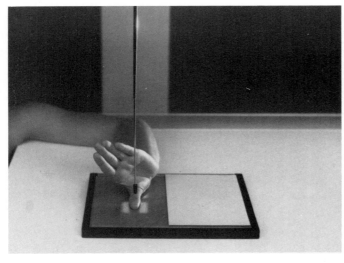

AP

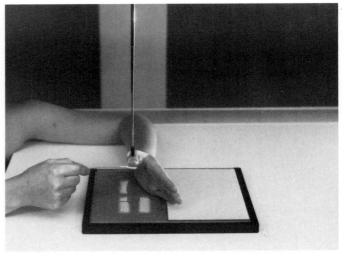

PA

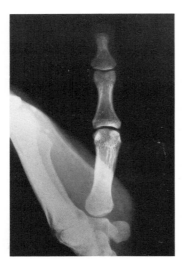

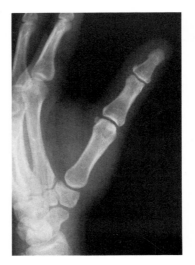

LATERAL PROJECTION

Have the patient place his hand in its natural arched position with the palmar surface down. Place the cassette so that its midline is parallel with the long axis of the finger and center it to the metacarpophalangeal joint. Adjust the arching of the hand until a true lateral position of the thumb is obtained.

OBLIQUE PROJECTION

With the thumb abducted, place the palmar surface of the hand in contact with the cassette. Align the longitudinal axis of the thumb with the long axis of the film. Direct the central ray perpendicular to the interphalangeal joint of the thumb.

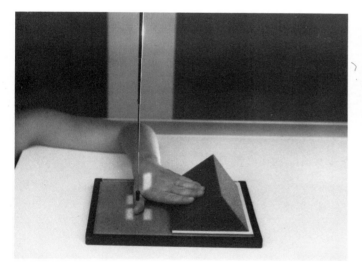

Lateral

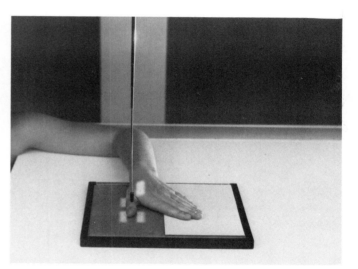

Oblique

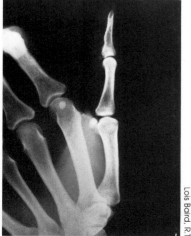

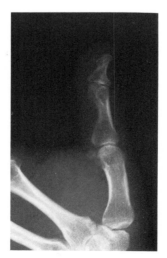

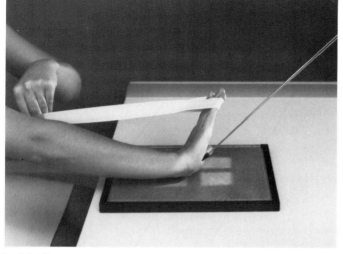

Radial shift

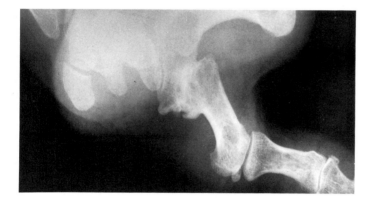

First carpometacarpal joint
AP PROJECTION

RADIAL SHIFT OF THE CARPAL CANAL POSITION

Burman,[1] who devised this projection, states that it gives a clearer projection of the first carpometacarpal joint than does the standard AP projection, which it may supplement when the wrist can be dorsiflexed.

Film: 8″ × 10″ crosswise.

Position of patient

Seat the patient at the end of the table in such a way that the forearm can be adjusted to lie approximately parallel with the long axis of the table.

Position of part

Hyperextend the hand and have the patient hold it in this position with his opposite hand or with a bandage looped around the fingers, and then rotate the hand to place the thumb in the horizontal position. Place the cassette under the wrist and finger and center it 1 inch proximal to the first carpometacarpal joint; the joint will be projected to the center of the film.

Central ray

Direct the central ray to a point about 1 inch distal to the first carpometacarpal joint at an angle of 45 degrees toward the elbow.

Structures shown

An AP projection showing the concavoconvex outline of the first carpometacarpal joint is demonstrated.

[1]Burman, M.: Anteroposterior projection of the carpometacarpal joint of the thumb by radial shift of the carpal tunnel view, J. Bone Joint Surg. **40-A:**1156-1157, 1958.

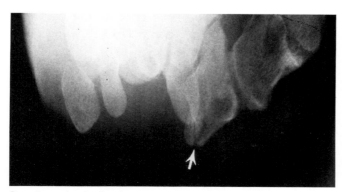

Carpal canal projection showing fracture of greater multangular

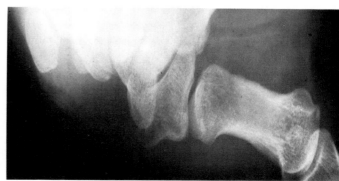

Radial shift projection on patient in adjacent radiograph

Wrist

PA AND AP PROJECTIONS

For examinations of the wrist, seat the patient low enough to place the axilla in contact with the table, or elevate the extremity to shoulder level on a suitable support. This is done for the purpose of placing the shoulder, elbow, and wrist joints in the same plane to permit right-angle rotation of the ulna and the radius for the lateral projection.

Film: 8″ × 10″ crosswise for two projections.

When it is difficult to determine the exact location of the carpus because of a swollen wrist, ask the patient to flex the wrist slightly, and then center to the point of flexion. When the wrist is in a cast or a splint, the exact point of centering can be determined by comparison with the opposite side.

PA PROJECTION

Position of part

Have the patient rest his forearm on the table. Place the cassette under the wrist and center to the carpus. Adjust the hand and forearm so they lie parallel with the long axis of the film. Arch the hand slightly at the metacarpophalangeal joints to place the wrist in close contact with the film.

When necessary, place a support under the fingers to immobilize them.

Central ray

Direct the central ray perpendicularly to the midcarpal area.

Structures shown

A PA projection of the carpals, the lower ends of the radius and ulna, and the upper ends of the metacarpals is shown.

The PA position gives a slightly oblique projection of the ulna. When this bone is the point of interest, the AP position should be used.

AP PROJECTION

Position of part

Have the patient rest his forearm on the table in the AP position. Place the cassette under the wrist and center to the carpals. Elevate the fingers on a suitable support to place the wrist in close contact with the cassette. Have the patient lean laterally to prevent rotation of the wrist.

Central ray

Direct the central ray perpendicularly to the midcarpal area.

Structures shown

The carpal interspaces are better demonstrated in this position, since, because of their oblique direction, they are more nearly parallel with the divergence of the x-ray beam.

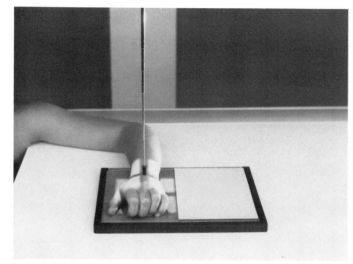

PA

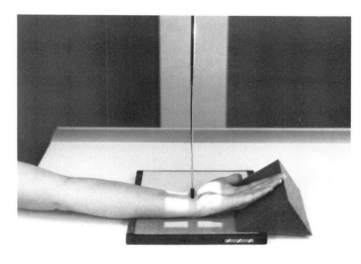

AP

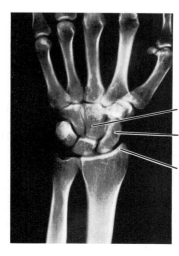

Capitate

Navicular

Radial styloid process

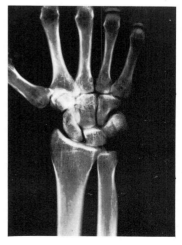

Film: $8'' \times 10''$ for two projections.

Position of part

Have the patient flex his elbow 90 degrees to rotate the ulna to the lateral position, and have him rest his *arm* and forearm on the table. Center the film to the carpals and adjust the forearm and hand so that the wrist is in a true lateral position.

Central ray

Direct the central ray perpendicularly to the wrist joint.

Structures shown

This position shows a lateral projection of the carpals, the upper ends of the metacarpals, and the lower ends of the radius and ulna.

NOTE: Burman et al.[1] suggest that the lateral projection of the navicular be made with the wrist in palmar flexion, because this action rotates the bone anteriorly into a dorsovolar position. They state, however, that this position is of value only when enough flexion is permitted.

[1]Burman, M.S., et al.: Fractures of the radial and ulnar axes, A.J.R. **51**:455-480, 1944.

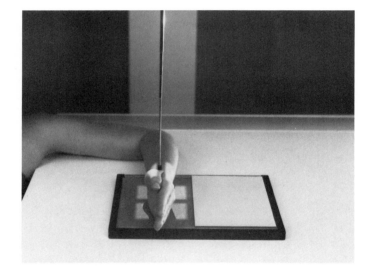

Ulnar surface to film

Navicular

Ulnar surface to film   Radial surface to film   Wrist in flexion

BENDING POSITIONS

Film: 8″ × 10″ for two projections.

Ulnar flexion
Position of part

Position the wrist and center the cassette for a PA projection. Next, with one hand cupped over the joint to hold it in position, move the elbow away from the patient's body, and then turn the hand outward until the wrist is in extreme ulnar flexion.

Central ray

Direct the central ray perpendicularly to the navicular; according to the direction of the fracture line, its clear delineation sometimes requires a central ray angulation of 10 to 15 degrees proximally or distally.

Structures shown

This position corrects the foreshortening of the navicular, which is obtained in the direct PA position, and opens the spaces between the adjacent carpals.

Radial flexion
Position of part

Position the wrist and center the cassette as for a PA projection. Cup one hand over the wrist joint to hold it in position and then move the elbow toward the patient's body and the hand medially until the wrist is in extreme radial flexion.

Central ray

Direct the central ray perpendicularly to the midcarpal area.

Structures shown

This position opens the interspaces between the carpals on the medial side of the wrist.

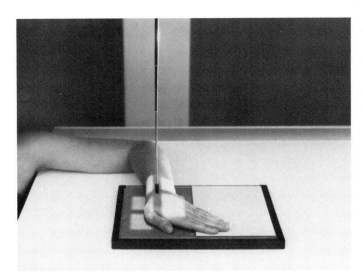

Ulnar flexion

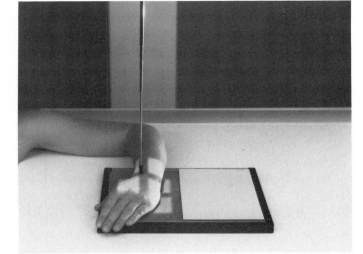

Radial flexion

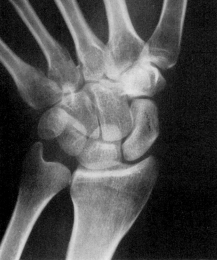

Ulnar flexion

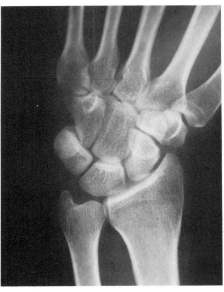

Radial flexion

AP AND PA OBLIQUE PROJECTIONS[1]

Film: 8″ × 10″ crosswise for two projections on one film.

A 45-degree foam wedge placed under the elevated side of the wrist permits exact positioning and ensures duplication in follow-up examinations.

AP OBLIQUE PROJECTION

Position of part

Have the patient rest his forearm on the table in the lateral position. Place the cassette under the wrist and center it at the dorsal surface of the carpus. Next rotate the wrist laterally until it forms an angle of approximately 45 degrees to the film.

[1]McBride, E.: Wrist joint injuries, a plea for greater accuracy in treatment, J. Okla. Med. Assoc. **19**:67-70, 1926.

Central ray

Direct the central ray perpendicularly to the midpoint of the film. It enters the anterior surface of the wrist midway between its medial and lateral borders.

Structures shown

This position separates the pisiform from the adjacent carpal bones. It also gives a more distinct projection of the triquetrum (cuneiform) and hamate (unciform).

PA OBLIQUE PROJECTION

Position of part

Place the wrist, resting on the ulnar surface, on the cassette. Adjust the cassette so that its center point is approximately 1½ inches anterior to the carpals; this will place it under the navicular when the wrist is rotated from the lateral position.

From the lateral position, rotate the wrist medially until it forms an angle of approximately 45 degrees with the plane of the film. Extend the wrist just slightly, and, if the fingers do not touch the table, support them on a sandbag. When the navicular is the point of interest, adjust the wrist in ulnar flexion. Place a sandbag across the forearm.

Central ray

Direct the central ray perpendicularly to the navicular. It enters just distal to the radius.

Structures shown

This position demonstrates the carpals on the lateral side of the wrist, particularly the navicular, which is stacked on itself in the direct PA projection.

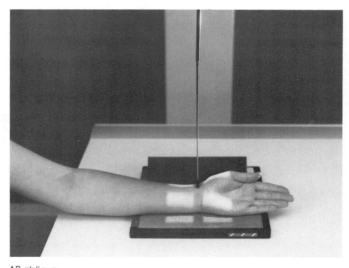

AP oblique

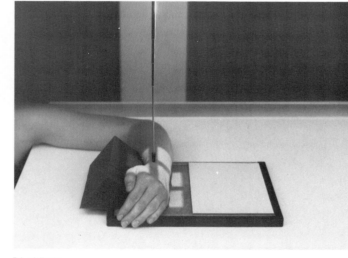

PA oblique

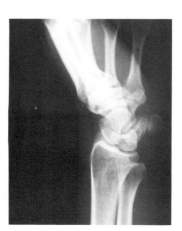

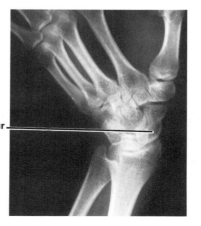

Navicular

NAVICULAR
STECHER METHOD

Film: 8″ × 10″.

Position of part

Place one end of the cassette on a support and adjust it so that it forms an angle inclined toward the elbow of 20 degrees to the horizontal.

Adjust the wrist on the cassette in the PA position and center the carpus approximately ½ inch above the midpoint of the cassette. Bridgman[1] suggests that the wrist be positioned in ulnar flexion for this projection.

[1]Bridgman, C.F.: Radiography of the carpal navicular bone, Med. Radiogr. Photogr. **25:**104-105, 1949.

Central ray

With the central ray perpendicular to the horizontal, direct it to the navicular.

Structures shown

The 20-degree angulation of the wrist places the navicular at the right angles to the central ray so that it is projected without self-superimposition.

Variations

1. Stecher[1] recommends the above method as being the preferable one; however, he says that a similar projection can be obtained by placing the film and wrist

[1]Stecher, W.R.: Roentgenography of the carpal navicular bone, A.J.R. **37:**704-705, 1937.

horizontally and directing the central ray 20 degrees toward the elbow.

For the demonstration of a fracture line that angles superoinferiorly these positions may be reversed; that is, the wrist may be angled inferiorly, or from the horizontal position the central ray may be angled toward the fingers.

2. A third method recommended by Stecher is to have the patient clench his fist. This tends to elevate the distal end of the navicular so that it will lie parallel with the film; it also tends to widen the fracture line. The wrist is positioned as for the PA projection, and no central ray angulation is used.

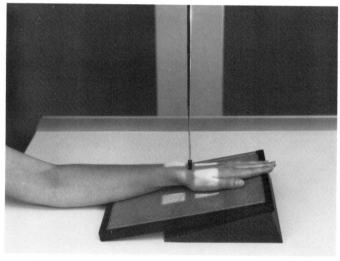

Angulation of part

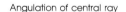

Angulation of central ray

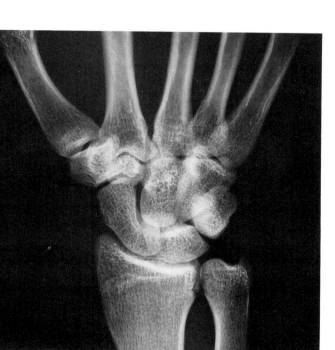

Carpal canal
TANGENTIAL PROJECTIONS
GAYNOR-HART METHOD

Film: 8″ × 10″ crosswise.

Inferosuperior projection
Position of patient

Seat the patient at the end of the table in such a way that the forearm can be adjusted to lie parallel with the long axis of the table.

Position of part

Hyperextend the wrist and center the cassette to the joint at the level of the radial styloid. Place a radioparent pad approximately ¾ inch thick under the lower forearm for support.

Adjust the position of the hand to place its long axis, as near as possible, vertically. To prevent superimposition of the shadows of the hamate and pisiform bones, rotate the hand slightly toward the radial side. Have the patient grasp the fingers with his opposite hand, or use a suitable device to hold the wrist in the extended position.

Central ray

Direct the central ray to the palm of the hand, to a point approximately 1 inch distal to the base of the fourth metacarpal, at an angle of 25 to 30 degrees to the long axis of the hand.

Structures shown

This projection of the carpal canal (sulcus carpi; carpal tunnel) shows the palmar aspect of the greater multangular, the tuberosity of the navicular, the lesser multangular, the capitate, the hamular process of the hamate, the triquetrum, and the entire pisiform.

Superoinferior projection

When the patient cannot assume or maintain the above position, a similar but not identical projection may be obtained by adjusting the wrist as shown in the photograph below. Have the patient dorsiflex his wrist as much as is tolerable and lean forward to place the carpal canal tangent to the film. The canal is easily palpable on the palmar aspect of the wrist as the concavity between the greater multangular laterally and the hamular hook and pisiform medially.

NOTE: Templeton and Zim[1] recommend a variation on this position wherein the forearm is placed at right angles to the film. The central ray is then directed through the carpal canal at an angle of 40 degrees toward the fingers.

[1]Templeton, A.W., and Zim, I.D.: The carpal tunnel view, Mo. Med. **61:**443-444, 1964.

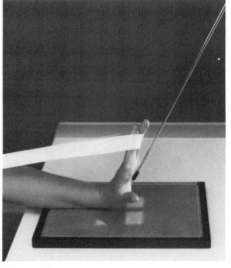

Inferosuperior

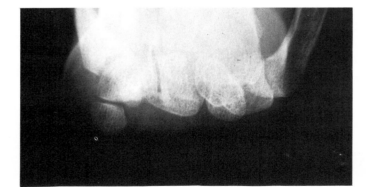

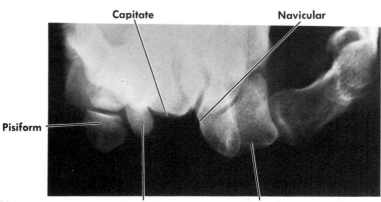

Capitate — Navicular

Pisiform —

Hamate — Greater multangular

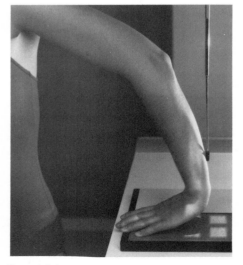

Superoinferior

Carpal bridge
TANGENTIAL PROJECTION

Film: $8'' \times 10''$ lengthwise.

Position of patient

The patient must be seated at the side of the table to permit the required manipulation of the x-ray tube.

Position of part

The originators[1] of this position recommend that the hand lie palm upward on the cassette, with the hand forming a right

[1]Lentino, W., et al.: The carpal bridge view. J. Bone Joint Surg. **39-A:**88-90, 1957.

angle to the forearm, as shown in the opposite photograph.

When the wrist is too painful to be adjusted in the above position, a similar but not identical projection can be obtained by elevating the forearm on sandbags or other suitable support and, with the wrist flexed to a right-angle position, placing the film in the vertical position, as shown in the photograph below.

Central ray

Direct the central ray to a point about $1\frac{1}{2}$ inches proximal to the wrist joint at a superoinferior angle of 45 degrees.

Structures shown

A tangential projection of the carpus is demonstrated. The originators recommend this projection for the demonstration of (1) fractures of the navicular, (2) lunate dislocations, (3) calcifications and foreign bodies in the dorsum of the wrist, and (4) chip fractures of the dorsal aspect of the carpal bones.

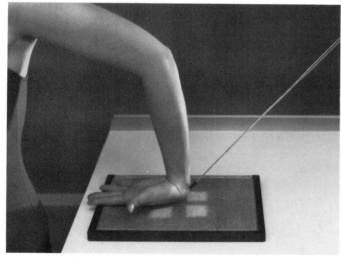

Original method

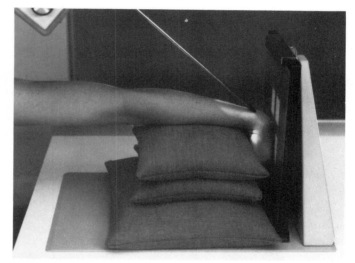

Modified method

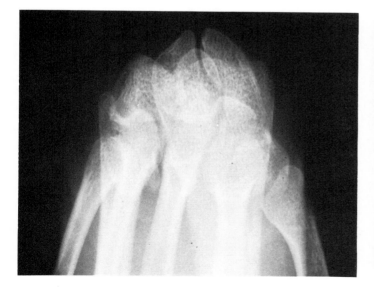

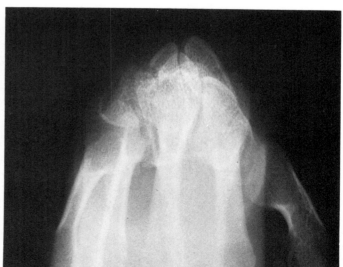

Forearm

AP AND LATERAL PROJECTIONS

Film

Select a film long enough to include the entire forearm from the olecranon process of the ulna to the styloid process of the radius. Take both projections of the forearm on one film by alternately covering one half with a lead mask.

AP PROJECTION

Position of patient

Seat the patient close to the table and low enough to place the entire extremity in the same plane.

Position of part

Supinate the hand, extend the elbow, and center the unmasked half of the cassette to the forearm. Have the patient lean laterally until the forearm is in a true AP position. Adjust the cassette so that its long axis is parallel with that of the forearm.

The hand *must be supinated*. Pronation of the hand crosses the radius over the ulna at its upper third and rotates the humerus medially, resulting in an oblique projection of the forearm.

LATERAL PROJECTION

Position of patient

The patient must be seated so that the shoulder joint and elbow will lie in the same plane to permit the ulna to rotate to the lateral position.

Position of part

Flex the elbow 90 degrees, place the unmasked half of the cassette under the forearm, parallel with its long axis, and center it. Adjust the extremity in a true lateral position. The thumb side of the hand *must be up*.

Central ray

Direct the central ray perpendicularly to the midpoint of the forearm.

Structures shown

AP and lateral projections of the forearm, the elbow joint, and the proximal row of carpal bones are demonstrated.

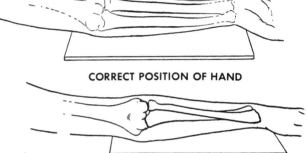

CORRECT POSITION OF HAND

INCORRECT POSITION OF HAND

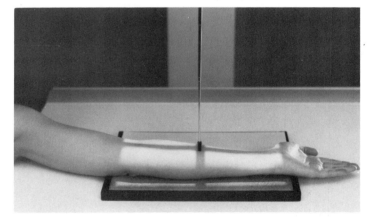

AP

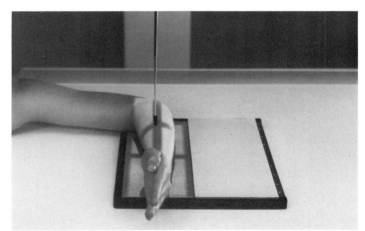

Lateral

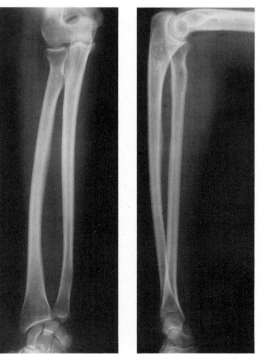

AP

Lateral

Elbow

AP AND OBLIQUE PROJECTIONS

Film: 8″ × 10″ lengthwise.

Position of patient

Seat the patient low enough to place the shoulder and elbow joints in the same plane.

AP PROJECTION

Position of part

Extend the elbow, supinate the hand, and center the cassette to the elbow joint. Have the patient lean laterally until the anterior surface of the elbow is parallel with the plane of the film. Adjust the cassette so that it is parallel with the long axis of the part.

The hand *must be supinated* to prevent rotation of the bones of the forearm.

Central ray

Direct the central ray perpendicularly to the elbow joint.

Structures shown

An AP projection of the elbow joint, the lower end of the arm, and the upper end of the forearm is presented.

MEDIAL OBLIQUE PROJECTION

Position of part

Extend the extremity as for the AP projection and center the midpoint of the cassette to the elbow joint.

Pronate the hand and adjust the elbow to place its anterior surface at an angle of 40 to 45 degrees. This degree of obliquity will usually clear the coronoid process of the radial head.

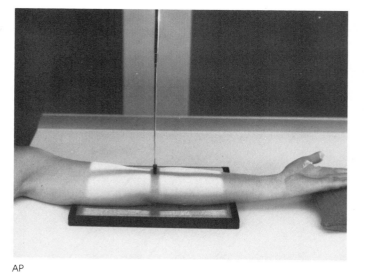

AP

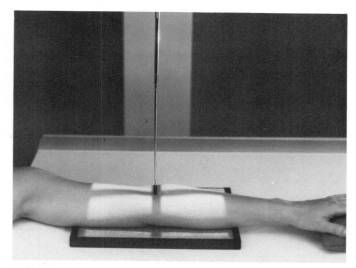

Medial oblique

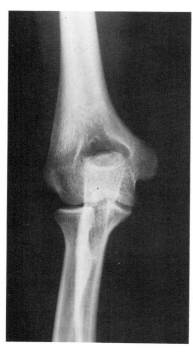

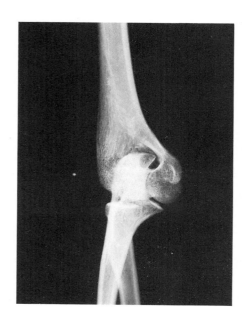

LATERAL OBLIQUE PROJECTION

Extend the extremity as for the AP projection and center the midpoint of the cassette to the elbow joint.

Rotate the hand laterally to place the posterior surface of the elbow at an angle of 40 degrees.

Central ray

Direct the central ray vertically to the midpoint of the film.

Structures shown

This projection shows an oblique image of the elbow with the coronoid process, projected free of superimposition.

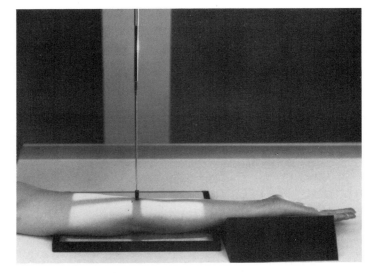

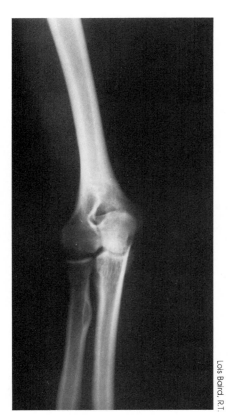

Lois Baird, R.T.

LATERAL PROJECTION

Film: 8″ × 10″ lengthwise.

Position of part

From the AP or oblique position, flex the elbow 90 degrees. Center the cassette to the joint and adjust it so that its long axis is parallel with the long axis of the forearm, as shown in the photograph and the lower radiograph. When it is desired to include more of the arm and forearm, adjust the cassette diagonally, as shown in the upper right radiograph.

To obtain a lateral projection of the elbow (1) the hand must be adjusted in the lateral position and (2) the humeral epicondyles must be perpendicular to the plane of the film.

Central ray

Direct the central ray perpendicularly to the elbow joint, regardless of its location on the film.

Structures shown

This position presents a lateral image of the elbow joint, the lower arm, and the upper forearm.

NOTE: When the soft structures about the elbow are in question, the joint should be flexed only 30 or 35 degrees as shown in the lower right radiograph.

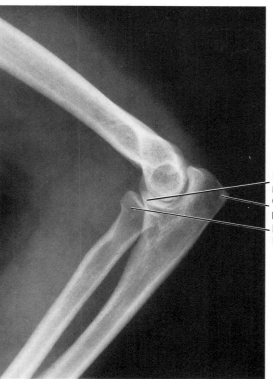

Coronoid process
Olecranon process
Radial head

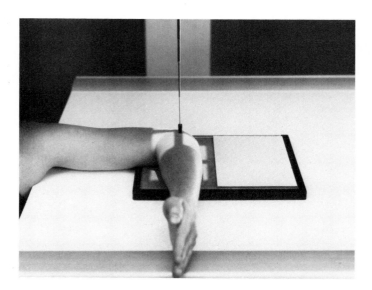

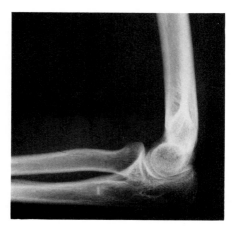

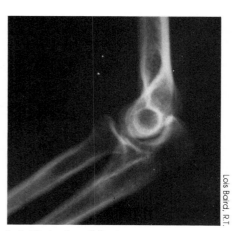

Partial flexion for soft tissue

Lois Baird, R.T.

AP PROJECTION
PARTIAL FLEXION

When the patient is unable to extend his elbow completely, the lateral position offers little difficulty, but it is necessary to make two AP exposures to avoid distortion. Both exposures can be made on one 8″ × 10″ film placed crosswise by alternately covering one half of the film with a lead mask.

Distal humerus

Seat the patient low enough to place the entire humerus in the same plane, and support the elevated forearm on a support. If possible, the hand should be supinated. Place the cassette under the elbow and center it to the condyloid area of the humerus.

Central ray

Direct the central ray to the midpoint of the film. Depending on the degree of flexion, it may be necessary to angle the central ray into the joint.

Proximal forearm

Seat the patient high enough to permit him to rest the dorsal surface of the forearm on the table. If this is not possible, elevate the extremity on a support, adjust it in the lateral position, place the cassette in the vertical position behind the upper end of the forearm, and direct the central ray horizontally.

Central ray

Direct the central ray perpendicularly to the long axis of the forearm and center to the elbow joint. Adjust the cassette so that the central ray will pass to its midpoint.

NOTE: Holly[1] has described an excellent method for obtaining the AP projection of the radial head. The patient is positioned as described above for the lower end of the humerus. Extend the elbow as much as possible and support the forearm. Holly states that the forearm should be supinated enough to place the transverse plane of the wrist at an angle of 30 degrees with the horizontal.

[1]Holly, E.W.: Radiography of the radial head, Med. Radiogr. Photogr. **32:**13-14, 1956.

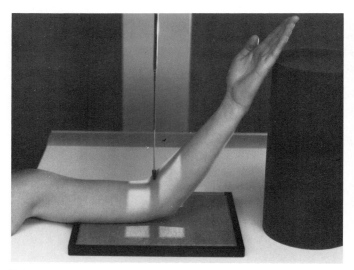

Distal humerus

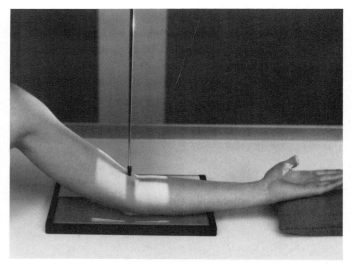

Joint and proximal radius and ulna

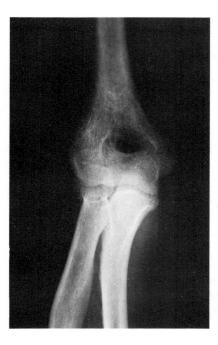

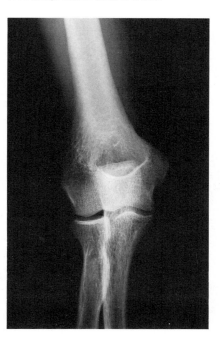

AXIAL PROJECTION
ACUTE FLEXION

Film: 8″ × 10″.

When fractures around the elbow are being treated in the Jones position (complete flexion), the lateral projection offers little difficulty, but the frontal projection must be made through the superimposed bones of the arm and forearm. The central ray should be directed perpendicularly to the humerus or to the radius and ulna, depending on the location of the fracture.

Distal humerus

The axial projection of the lower end of the arm is obtained by centering the cassette a little above the epicondyloid area of the humerus and directing the central ray perpendicularly to the film.

Adjust the arm or the tube and film so that there will be no rotation.

Proximal forearm

When the upper end of the forearm is in question, the tube should be angled so that the central ray will be perpendicular to the forearm. The cassette must be moved toward the shoulder so that the central ray will pass to its midpoint.

Structures shown

The outlines of the superimposed bones of the arm and forearm are shown in a frontal position. This position gives a very clear image of the olecranon process.

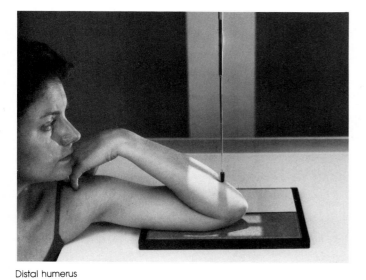

Distal humerus

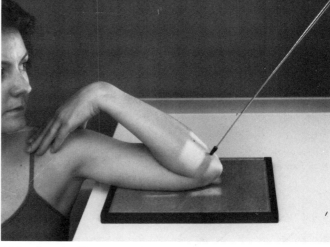

Joint and proximal forearm

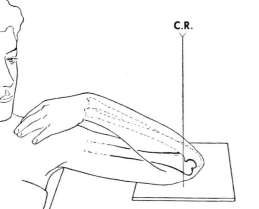

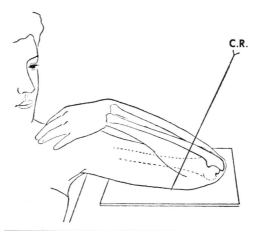

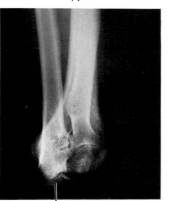

Olecranon
process

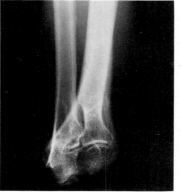

RADIAL HEAD

LATEROMEDIAL ROTATION

To demonstrate the entire circumference of the radial head free of superimposures, varying the position of the hand.

Film: 8″ × 10″ for four exposures on one film.

Place an 8″ × 10″ cassette in position and cover three fourths of the film area with sheet lead.

Position of patient

Seat the patient low enough to place the entire extremity in the same plane.

Position of part

Flex the elbow 90 degrees, center the joint to the unmasked fourth of the cassette tunnel, and position it for a lateral projection.

1. Make the first exposure with the hand supinated as much as is possible in this position.

2. Shift the film and make the second exposure with the hand in the lateral position, that is, with the thumb surface up.

3. Shift the film and make the third exposure with the hand pronated.

4. Shift the film and make the fourth exposure with the hand in extreme internal rotation, that is, resting on the thumb surface.

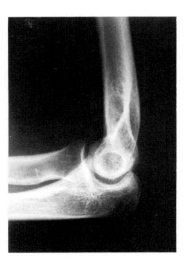

Hand supinated

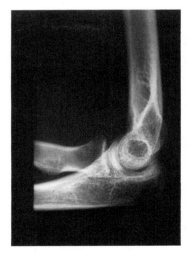

Hand lateral

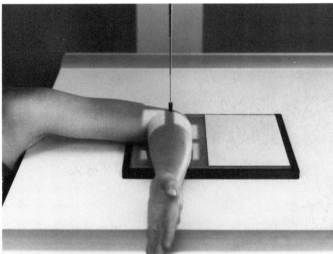

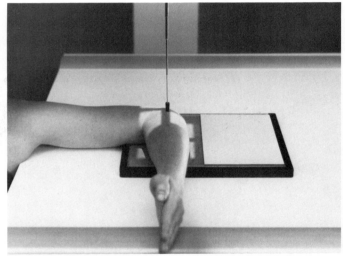

Central ray

Direct the central ray perpendicularly to the elbow joint.

NOTE: When the radial head is in question and it is not possible for the patient to rotate his forearm, the Schmitt[1] method of separating the radial head from the olecranon process can be employed.

The elbow is positioned as for an AP projection, and one radiograph is made with the central ray directed 45 degrees medially and one with it directed 45 degrees laterally.

[1]Schmitt, H.: Die röntgenologische Darstellung des Radius-köpfchens, Röntgenpraxis **11**:33-36, 1939.

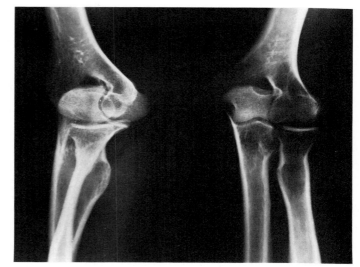

Angled projections

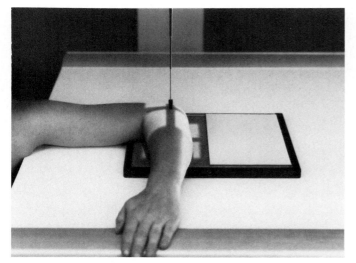

Hand pronated

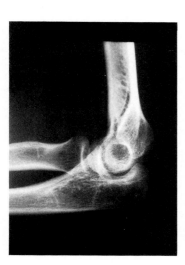

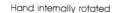

Hand internally rotated

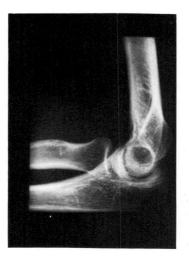

RADIAL HEAD
AXIAL PROJECTION

Film: $8'' \times 10''$.

Position of patient

Seat the patient low enough to place the shoulder joint and the elbow in the same plane.

Position of part

Center the humeral epicondyles to the midpoint of the film and flex the elbow so that the forearm forms an angle of 70 degrees to the horizontal. Rest the forearm against sandbags or other support.

1. Make the first exposure with the hand supinated.

2. Change the cassette and make the second exposure with the hand pronated.

Because the thick brachioradialis muscle is drawn over the head of the radius when the hand is pronated, it may be necessary to increase the radiographic technique for the second position.

Central ray

Direct the central ray perpendicularly to the head of the radius.

Structures shown

These two projections demonstrate the entire articular surface of the radial head free of bony superimposition.

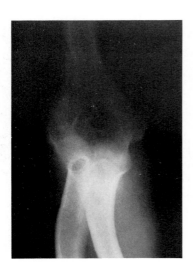

Hand supinated

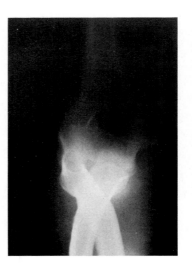

Hand pronated

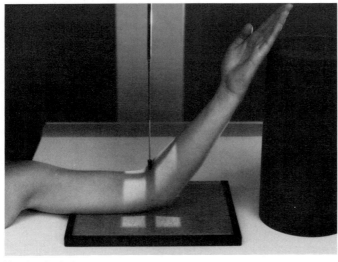

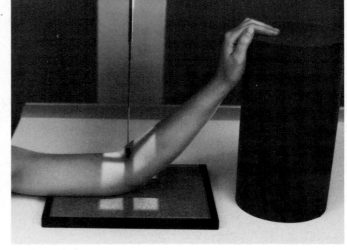

Distal humerus and olecranon process
AXIAL PROJECTIONS[1,2]

Film: 8″ × 10″ for two projections on one film.

Position of patient

For an axial projection of the distal end of the humerus, seat the patient high enough to enable him to rest his forearm on the table with the arm in the vertical position. The patient may be seated somewhat lower for an examination of the olecranon process. He must, for either region, be seated so that the forearm can be adjusted to be parallel to the long axis of the table.

[1]Laquerrière and Pierquin: De la nécessité d'employer une technique radiographique spéciale pour obtenir certains détails squelettiques, J. Radiol. Electrol. 3:145-148, 1918.
[2]Veihweger, G.: Zum Problem der Deutung der knochernen Gebilde distal des Epikondylus medialis humeri, Fortschr. Roentgenstr. 86:643-652, 1957.

Position of part

Ask the patient to rest his forearm on the table, and then adjust it so that its long axis is parallel with the table. Adjust the degree of flexion of the elbow to place the arm at the angle to be used. Center the cassette between the epicondyles, a little anterior to this level when central ray angulation is to be used.

Distal humerus
Position of part

Adjust the patient's arm in a near vertical position (10 to 15 degrees) so that there is no anterior or posterior leaning. Supinate the hand to prevent rotation of the humerus and ulna, and have the patient immobilize it with his opposite hand.

Central ray

Direct the central ray perpendicularly to the ulnar sulcus, a point just medial to the olecranon process.

Structures shown

This projection demonstrates the epicondyles, the trochlea, the ulnar sulcus (the groove between the medial epicondyle and the trochlea), and the olecranon fossa. It is used in radiohumeral bursitis (tennis elbow) for the detection of otherwise obscured calcifications located in the ulnar sulcus.

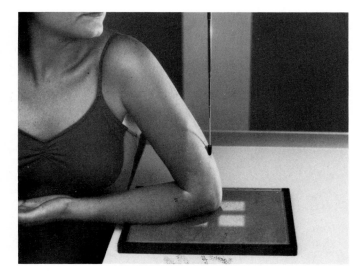

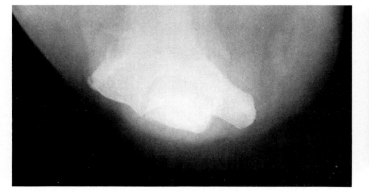

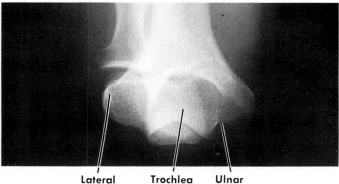

Lateral condyle　　Trochlea　　Ulnar sulcus

OLECRANON PROCESS
Position of part

For an axial projection of the olecranon process, adjust the arm at an angle of 45 to 50 degrees, so that there is no anterior or posterior leaning. Supinate the hand to place the ulna in the AP position, and have the patient immobilize it with his opposite hand.

Central ray and structures shown

Direct the central ray to the olecranon process (1) perpendicularly for the demonstration of the dorsum of the process and (2) at an anterior angle of 20 degrees for the demonstration of the curved extremity and articular margin of the process.

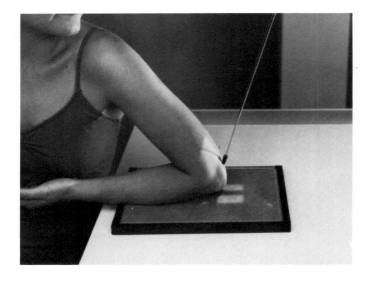

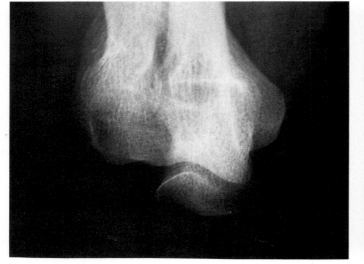

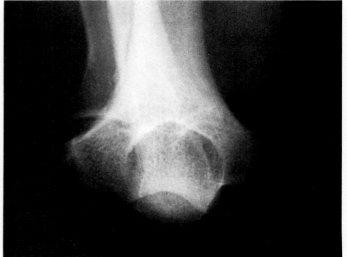

Angulation of 20 degrees

Angulation of 0 degrees

Humerus

AP AND LATERAL PROJECTIONS
ERECT POSITIONS

Shoulder and arm abnormalities, whether traumatic or pathologic in origin, are extremely painful. For this reason an erect position, either standing or seated, should be used whenever possible. By rotating the patient's body as required, the arm can be positioned quickly and accurately with minimum discomfort to the patient and, in the presence of fracture, with no danger of fragment displacement.

Film

The film selected should be long enough to include the humerus from its head to its condyles inclusively. An 11″ × 14″ film is adequate for most adults when the arm can be abducted enough for diagonal placement on the film.

Position of patient

Place the patient in the general position, adjust the height of the cassette to place the upper margin of the film about 1½ inches above the head of the humerus, and then adjust the tube to direct the central ray perpendicularly to the midpoint of the film.

The accompanying photographs illustrate the body position used for AP and lateral projections of the freely movable arm. The body position, whether oblique or facing toward or away from the film, is unimportant as long as true frontal and lateral projections of the arm are obtained.

Position of part

Locate the epicondyles and, while holding them between the thumb and index fingers of one hand, adjust the position of the arm or have the patient turn slowly until the desired position is reached. *A coronal plane passing through the epicondyles will be parallel with the plane of the film for the frontal (AP or PA) projection and at right angles to it for the lateral projection.*

Structures shown

These positions demonstrate AP and lateral projections of the entire length of the humerus, the accuracy of the positions being shown by the epicondyles.

NOTE: Radiographs of the humerus and shoulder may be taken with or without a grid. The size of the patient and the preference of the technologist and physician are the factors often considered in reaching a decision. Most medical facilities establish a policy for the routine procedures, and, whether the policy is to use a grid or to employ a nongrid technique, the positioning of the body part remains the same.

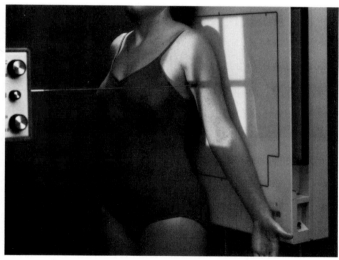

AP

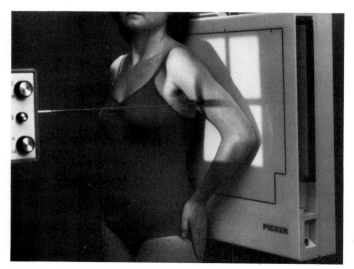

Lateral

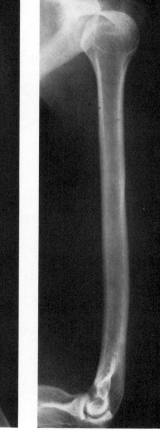

AP   Lateral

Dr. Edward M. Winant

AP AND LATERAL PROJECTIONS
RECUMBENT POSITION

Film

The cassette size selected should be long enough to include the bone from its head to its condyles inclusively.

AP projection

With the patient in the supine position, adjust the cassette to include the entire length of the humerus. Elevate the opposite shoulder on a sandbag to place the affected arm in contact with the cassette, or elevate the arm and cassette on sandbags. Supinate the hand and adjust the extremity to place the epicondyles parallel with the plane of the film.

Lateral projection

Abduct the arm somewhat and place the cassette under it. Flex the elbow, rotate the forearm medially enough to place the epicondyles perpendicular to the plane of the film, and rest the hand against the patient's side. Adjust the position of the cassette to include the entire length of the humerus.

Lateral position

When it is necessary to position the patient in the lateral decubitus position, place the cassette close to the axilla and center the arm to its midline. Flex the elbow, turn the thumb surface of the hand up, and rest it on a suitable support.

Adjust the position of the body to place the lateral surface of the arm perpendicular to the central ray.

Respiration is suspended for these exposures.

Central ray

Direct the central ray perpendicularly to the midpoint of the film.

Structures shown

AP and lateral projections of the lower portion or of the entire humerus are presented, depending on the size of the cassette.

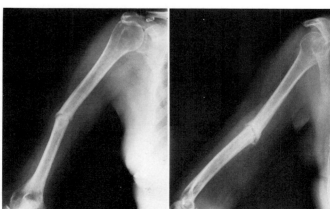

AP

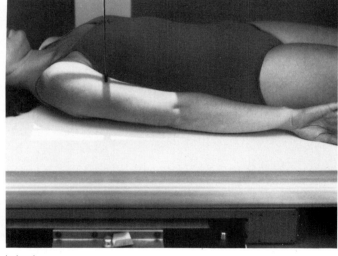

Lateral

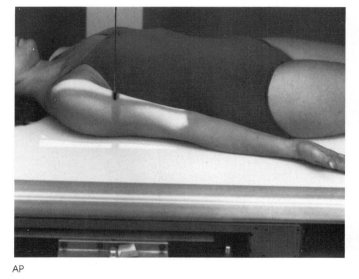

AP   Lateral

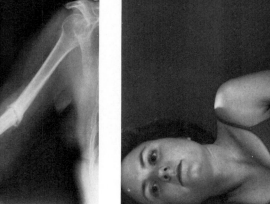

Lateral decubitus

Proximal humerus
TRANSTHORACIC LATERAL PROJECTION
LAWRENCE METHOD[1]

The Lawrence method is used when the arm cannot be abducted for an axial projection.

Film: 8″ × 10″ or 10″ × 12″ lengthwise.

Position of patient

Although this projection can be carried out with the patient in the supine or the erect position, the erect position facilitates accurate adjustment of the shoulder.

Position of part

Seat or stand the patient in the lateral position before a vertical grid device. Have the patient raise the uninjured arm, rest the forearm on his head, and elevate the shoulder as much as possible. The elevation of the uninjured shoulder will give the desired depression of the injured side, thus separating the shoulders to prevent superimposition. Center the cassette to the region of the surgical neck of the affected humerus.

While holding the humeral epicondyles between the thumb and forefinger of one hand, adjust the rotation of the patient's body to project the humerus between the vertebral column and the sternum. *The epicondyles should be perpendicular to the plane of the film.*

Instruct the patient to hold his breath at full inspiration when ready to make the exposure. Having the lungs full of air improves the contrast and also decreases the exposure necessary to penetrate the body.

When the patient is able to hold his breath for 5 or 6 seconds, lung detail may be blurred considerably by the action of the heart. When this is possible, maintain the usual mAs factor but convert to a low mA–long exposure time combination.

If the patient can be sufficiently well immobilized to prevent voluntary motion, breathing motion can be utilized. In this case, instruct the patient and have him practice slow, deep breathing. An exposure time of 7 to 10 seconds will give excellent results.

[1]Lawrence, W.S.: A method of obtaining an accurate lateral roentgenogram of the shoulder joint, A.J.R. **5:**193-194, 1918.

Central ray

Direct the central ray perpendicularly to the midpoint of the film.

Structures shown

A lateral projection of the upper half or two thirds of the humerus is shown, projected through the thorax. Although the definition may be poor, the outline of the humerus is clearly shown.

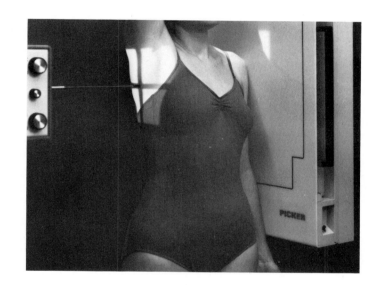

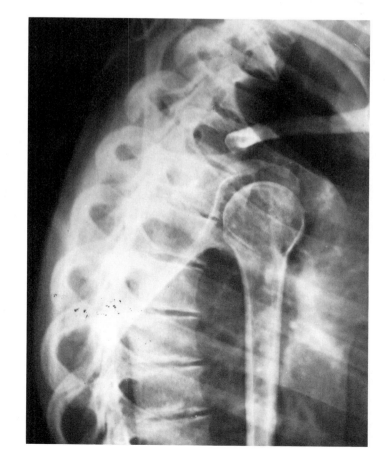

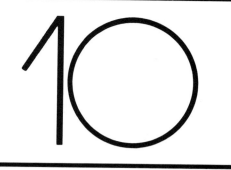

Shoulder girdle

ANATOMY

The shoulder girdle is formed by the clavicles and scapulae and serves to connect the upper extremities to the trunk. Although the alignment of these four bones is considered a girdle, it is incomplete both in front and behind. The girdle is completed in front by the sternum, which articulates with the medial ends of the clavicles, but the scapulae are widely separated in the back. Because the upper extremity of the humerus is included in the shoulder joint, it seems logical to consider its anatomy with that of the shoulder.

CLAVICLE

The clavicle is classified as a long bone, has a body, or shaft, and two articular extremities. It lies in an obliquely transverse plane just above the first rib, forming the anterior part of the shoulder girdle. Its lateral extremity articulates with the acromion process of the scapula, and its medial extremity with the upper segment of the sternum. The clavicle serves as a fulcrum for the movements of the arm and is doubly curved for strength. The curvature is more acute in the male than in the female.

The acromioclavicular articulation is a diarthrodial joint, permitting both gliding and rotary movements. The sternoclavicular articulation, which is the only bony union between the upper extremity and the trunk, is a diarthrodial joint adapted to circumduction, elevation, depression, and forward and backward movements of the clavicle. The clavicle carries the scapula with it through any movement.

SCAPULA

The scapula is classified as a flat bone. It forms the posterior part of the shoulder girdle. It is triangular in shape and has two surfaces, three borders, and three angles. It lies on the upper posterior thorax between the second and seventh ribs, with its vertebral border parallel with the vertebral column. The body of the bone is arched from above inferiorly for greater strength, and its surfaces serve for the attachment of numerous muscles.

The anterior, or costal, surface of the scapula is slightly concave and almost entirely filled by the subscapularis muscle, which arises from it. The serratus anterior muscle attaches to the vertebral border of the costal surface from the medial to the inferior angles.

The posterior, or dorsal, surface is divided into two portions by a prominent spinous process. The spine arises at the upper third of the vertebral border from a smooth, triangular area and runs obliquely

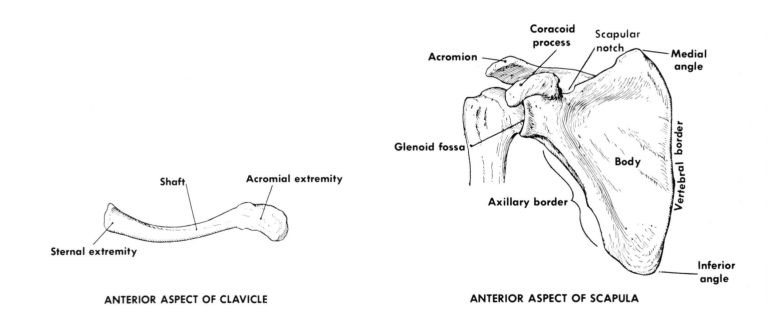

ANTERIOR ASPECT OF CLAVICLE

ANTERIOR ASPECT OF SCAPULA

upward to end in a flattened triangular projection called the acromion. The area above the spine is called the supraspinatus fossa and gives origin to the supraspinatus muscle. The infraspinatus muscle arises from the portion below the spine, which is called the infraspinatus fossa. The teres minor muscle arises from the upper two thirds of the axillary border of the dorsal surface, and the teres major from the lower third and from the inferior angle. The dorsal surface of the vertebral border affords attachment of the levator scapulae, the rhomboideus major, and the rhomboideus minor muscles.

The superior border extends from the medial angle to the coracoid process and presents a deep depression, the scapular notch, at its lateral end. The vertebral border extends from the medial to the inferior angles. The axillary border extends from the glenoid fossa to the inferior angle.

The medial angle is formed by the junction of the superior and vertebral borders. The inferior angle is formed by the junction of the vertebral and axillary borders. The lateral angle, the thickest part of the scapula, ends in a shallow, oval depression called the glenoid fossa. The glenoid fossa articulates with the head of the humerus. The constricted region around the glenoid fossa is called the neck of the scapula. The coracoid process arises from a thick base that extends from the scapular notch to the upper part of the neck of the scapula. It projects first anteriorly and medially and then curves on itself to project laterally. The coracoid process can be palpated just below and slightly medial to the acromioclavicular articulation.

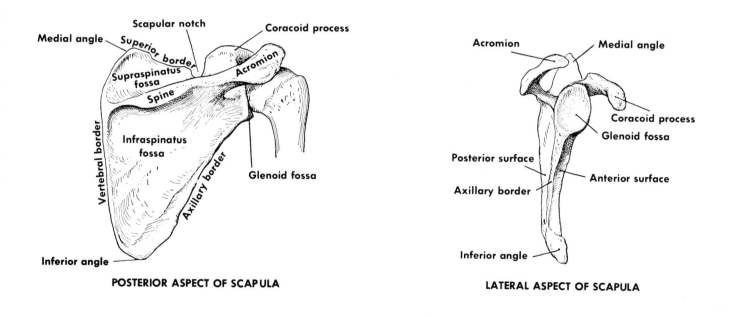

POSTERIOR ASPECT OF SCAPULA

LATERAL ASPECT OF SCAPULA

HUMERUS

The proximal end of the humerus consists of a head, an anatomic neck, two prominent processes termed the greater and lesser tuberosities, or tubercles, and a surgical neck. The head is large, smooth, and rounded and lies in an oblique plane on the upper medial side of the humerus. It articulates with the glenoid fossa of the scapula. Just below the head, lying in the same oblique plane, is the narrow constricted area called the anatomic neck. The constriction of the shaft just below the tuberosities is called the surgical neck.

The lesser tuberosity is situated on the anterior surface of the bone immediately below the anatomic neck. The tendon of the subscapularis is inserted at the lesser tuberosity. The greater tuberosity is located on the lateral surface of the bone just below the anatomic neck and is separated from the lesser tuberosity by a deep depression called the bicipital, or intertubercular, groove. The upper surface of the greater tuberosity slopes posteriorly at an angle of approximately 25 degrees and presents three flattened impressions for muscle insertions. The anterior impression is the highest of the three and affords attachment to the tendon of the supraspinatus. The middle impression is the point of insertion of the infraspinatus muscle. The tendon of the upper fibers of the teres minor is inserted at the posterior impression; its lower fibers are inserted into the shaft of the bone immediately below this point.

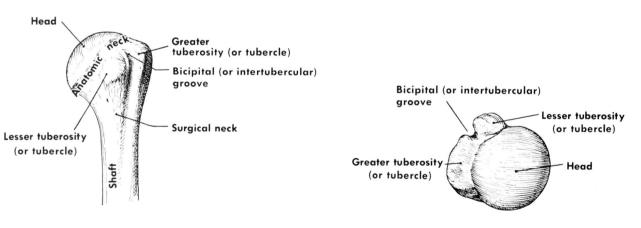

ANTERIOR ASPECT OF UPPER END OF HUMERUS

SUPERIOR ASPECT OF HUMERUS

SHOULDER JOINT

The articulation between the glenoid fossa and the head of the humerus forms a diarthrodial joint of the ball-and-socket type, which allows movement in all directions. Although many muscles connect with, support, and enter into the function of the shoulder joint, technologists are chiefly concerned with the insertion points of the short rotators. The insertion points of these muscles—the subscapularis, the supraspinatus, the infraspinatus, and the teres minor—have already been stated.

An articular capsule completely encloses the shoulder joint. The tendon of the long head of the biceps muscle, which arises from the upper margin of the glenoid fossa, passes through the capsule of the shoulder joint, arches over the head of the humerus, and descends through the bicipital groove. The short head of the biceps arises from the coracoid process and, with the long head of the muscle, is inserted at the radial tuberosity. Because it is connected with both the shoulder and the elbow joints, the biceps synchronizes their action.

Important bursae are located under the deltoid (between it and the capsule), under the tendon of the subscapularis, and in the bicipital groove under the tendon of the long head of the biceps.

The interaction of movement between the wrist joint and the elbow and shoulder joints makes the position of the hand important in the radiography of these parts. Any rotation of the hand also rotates these joints. The best approach to the study of the mechanics of joint and muscle action is to perform all the movements ascribed to each joint and carefully note the reaction in remote parts.

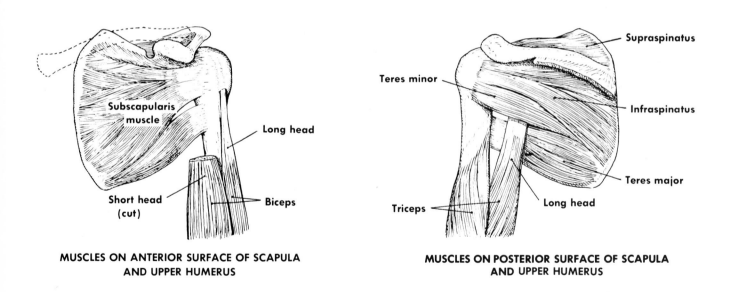

MUSCLES ON ANTERIOR SURFACE OF SCAPULA AND UPPER HUMERUS

MUSCLES ON POSTERIOR SURFACE OF SCAPULA AND UPPER HUMERUS

RADIOGRAPHY

Shoulder
AP PROJECTIONS

Film: 10″ × 12″ crosswise or lengthwise, according to the area to be included.

Position of patient

The patient may be examined in the erect or the supine position. It must be recalled, however, that shoulder and arm lesions, whether traumatic or pathologic in origin, are extremely sensitive to movement and to pressure. For this reason the erect position should be used whenever possible so that the patient's body position can be adjusted to require little or no manipulation of the arm.

Position of part

Adjust the position of the cassette and the patient's body to center the film to the coracoid process. To overcome the curve of the back and the resultant obliquity of the shoulder structures, rotate the patient enough to place the blade of the scapula parallel with the plane of the film. When the patient is in the supine position support the elevated shoulder and hip on sandbags. When the patient is in this basic body position, locate the epicondyles, and, while holding them between the thumb and index fingers of one hand, adjust the arm as follows:

1. Ask the patient to turn the palm of his hand forward. Abduct the arm slightly and adjust it so that the coronal plane of the epicondyles is parallel with the plane of the film. When the patient is erect, the arm may be immobilized by having him rest the hand against an IV standard or the back of a chair. This adjustment of the arm, referred to as the *external rotation position,* places the shoulder in the true AP, or anatomic, position. The external rotation position is used to demonstrate the bony and soft structures of the shoulder and upper humerus in their anatomic position. It shows the glenohumeral joint relationship and the region of the subacromial bursa and gives a profile projection of the greater tuberosity of the humerus, the site of the insertion of the supraspinatus tendon.

2. Ask the patient to rest the palm of his hand against his thigh. This position of the arm rolls the head of the humerus into a *neutral position,* placing the epicondyles at an angle of about 45 degrees to the plane of the film. The resultant projection shows the posterior part of the supraspinatus insertion site, sometimes profiling small calcific deposits not otherwise visualized.

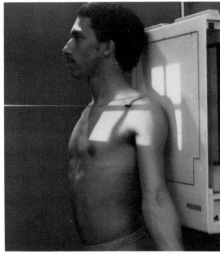

External rotation

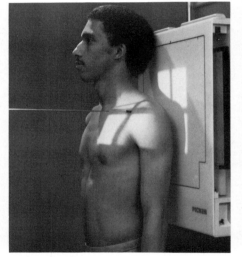

Neutral rotation

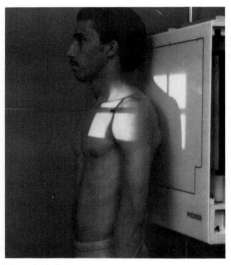

Internal rotation

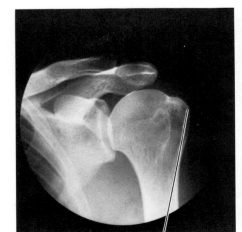

Greater
tuberosity

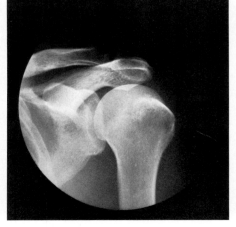

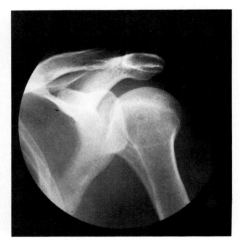

3. Ask the patient to flex his elbow somewhat, rotate the arm internally, and rest the back of the hand on his hip. Adjust the arm to place the coronal plane of the epicondyles perpendicular to the plane of the film. (When the shoulder is too painful for adequate internal rotation of the arm, the patient may turn somewhat away from the film, but, if the part-film distance becomes too great, he should be turned for adjustment from the PA position.) This adjustment of the arm, referred to as the *internal rotation position,* rolls the humerus into the true lateral position. The internal rotation position demonstrates the region of the subdeltoid bursa and, when the arm can be abducted enough to clear the lesser tuberosity of the head of the scapula, a profile projection of the site of the insertion of the subscapularis tendon.

Central ray

Direct the central ray perpendicularly to the coracoid process.

Infraspinatus insertion. With the patient's arm in the AP position (external rotation), direct the central ray to the coracoid process at an angle of 25 degrees caudad. The resultant projection profiles the second impression on the greater tuberosity, the site of insertion of the infraspinatus tendon, and also opens up the subacromial space.

Subacromial space. Berens and Lockie[1] recommend an AP projection, with the central ray directed to the coracoid process at an angle of 15 degrees caudad to open the subacromial space and thus to demonstrate ossification of the coracoac-

[1]Berens, D.L., and Lockie, L.M.: Ossification of the coracoacromial ligament, Radiology **74:**802-805, 1960.

romial ligament or other lesions of the subacromial space. They state that ossification of the coracoacromial ligament shows as a tongue of bone projecting from the anteroinferior aspect of the acromion process.

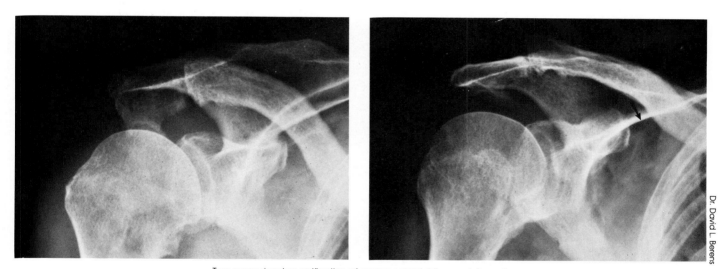

Two cases showing ossification of coracoacromial ligament *(arrow)*

Dr. David L. Berens

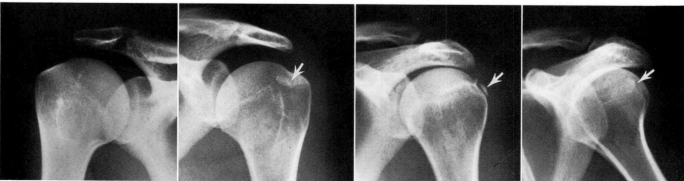

Caudal angulation of 25 degrees   External rotation   Neutral rotation   Internal rotation

Calcareous peritendinitis *(arrows)*

Dr. Hudson J. Wilson, Jr.

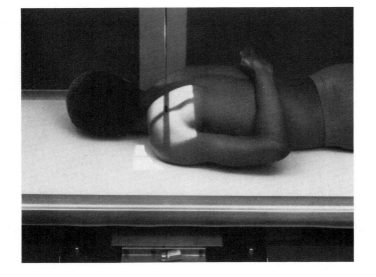

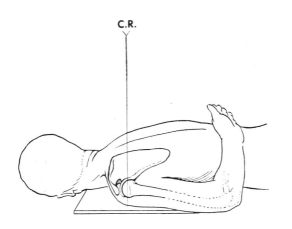

C.R.

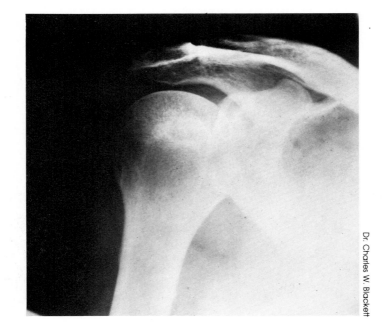

Dr. Charles W. Blackett

TERES MINOR INSERTION
BLACKETT-HEALY METHOD

Film: 8″ × 10″ crosswise.

Position of patient

Adjust the patient in the prone position, his arms along the sides of the body and his head resting on the cheek of the affected side. Place a long sandbag under the ankles for the patient's comfort.

Position of part

Place the cassette under the shoulder and center it to a point about 1 inch distal to the coracoid process. Turn the arm to a position of extreme internal rotation and, if possible, flex the elbow and place the hand on the patient's back.

Respiration is suspended at the end of exhalation for a more uniform density.

Central ray

Direct the central ray perpendicularly to the head of the humerus.

Structures shown

This position rotates the head of the humerus so that the third impression of the greater tuberosity is brought anteriorly, giving a tangential projection of the insertion of the teres minor at the outer edge of the bone just below the articular surface of the head.

NOTE: Blackett[1] states that the teres minor insertion can be demonstrated with the patient in the AP position by turning the arm to a position of extreme internal rotation.

[1]Blackett, C.W.: Personal communication.

SUBSCAPULARIS INSERTION
BLACKETT-HEALY METHOD

Film: 8″ × 10″ or 10″ × 12″ crosswise.

Position of patient

Place the patient in the supine position, his arms resting along the sides of the body.

Position of part

Align the body so that the affected shoulder joint is centered to the midline of the table.

The opposite shoulder may be elevated approximately 15 degrees and supported with a sandbag. Abduct the affected arm to the long axis of the body, flex the elbow, and rotate the arm internally by pronating the hand.

Place one sandbag under the hand and another on top, if necessary for immobilization. Respiration is suspended at the end of exhalation.

Central ray

Direct the central ray perpendicularly to the shoulder joint.

Structures shown

This method presents a tangential projection of the insertion of the subscapularis at the lesser tuberosity. On the radiograph the lesser tuberosity presents itself along the inferior margin of the humerus.

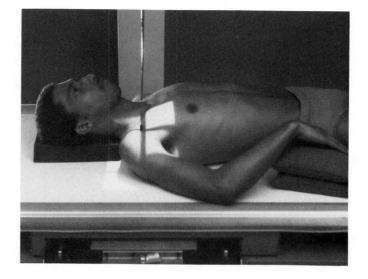

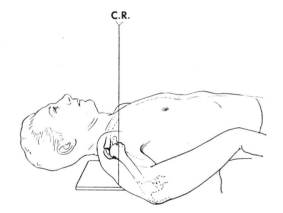

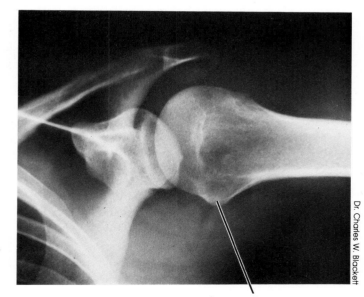

Lesser tuberosity

Dr. Charles W. Blackett

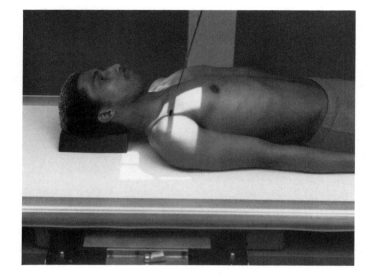

CORACOID PROCESS
AP AXIAL PROJECTION

Film: $8'' \times 10''$ or $10'' \times 12''$ cross-wise.

Position of patient

Place the patient in the supine position, his arms along the sides of the body.

Position of part

Adjust the position of the body and center the affected coracoid process to the midline of the grid. Position the cassette so that the midpoint of the film will coincide with the central ray.

Adjust the shoulders to lie in the same transverse plane. Abduct the arm of the affected side slightly, and supinate the hand and immobilize it with a sandbag across the palm. Respiration is suspended at the end of exhalation for a more uniform density.

Central ray

Direct the central ray to the coracoid process at an angle of 15 to 30 degrees cephalad. The degree of angulation depends on the shape of the patient's back; round-shouldered patients will require a greater angulation than those who have a straight back.

Structures shown

A slightly inferosuperior projection of the carocoid process is shown, projected free of self-superimposition. Because the coracoid is curved on itself, it casts a small, oval shadow in the direct AP projection of the shoulder. The scapular notch is also clearly demonstrated in this projection.

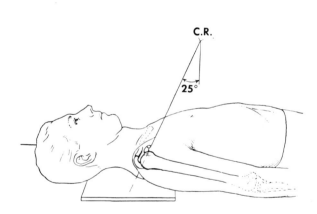

C.R.

25°

Coracoid process

Scapular notch

GLENOID FOSSA
GRASHEY METHOD

Film: 8″ × 10″ or 10″ × 12″ cross-wise.

Position of patient

Although this projection can be made with the patient in the supine or the erect position, the erect position is more comfortable for the patient and facilitates accurate adjustment of the part.

Position of part

Center the cassette to the shoulder joint. Rotate the body approximately 45 degrees toward the affected side. If the patient is in the supine position, support the elevated shoulder and hip on sandbags.

Adjust the degree of rotation to place the scapula parallel with the plane of the film and the head of the humerus in contact with it. Abduct the arm slightly in internal rotation.

Respiration is suspended at the end of exhalation for a more uniform density.

Central ray

Direct the central ray perpendicularly to a point 2 inches medial and 2 inches distal to the upper outer border of the shoulder.

Structures shown

The joint space between the humeral head and the glenoid fossa is shown. This projection shows the glenoid fossa in profile.

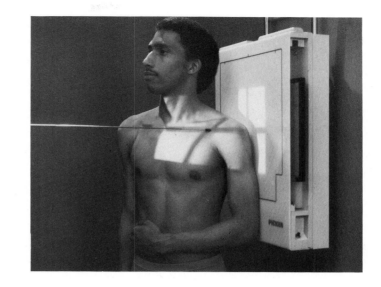

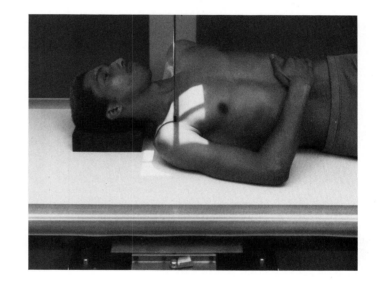

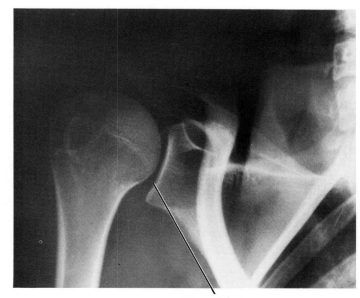

Glenoid fossa

Bicipital groove
TANGENTIAL PROJECTION
FISK METHOD[1]

Film: 8″ × 10″.

Position of patient

The patient is asked to stand facing the end of the table. When necessary, this position can be easily adapted to the seated position. When this is done, a local gonad shield should be applied.

[1]Fisk, C.: Adaptation of the technique for radiography of the bicipital groove, Radiol. Technol. **37:**47-50, 1965.

Position of part

Ask the patient to flex his elbow, lean forward, and rest his forearm on the table with the hand supinated.

Place the cassette on the forearm, with its longitudinal midline parallel with the long axis of the forearm, and ask the patient to close his fingers over the end of the cassette. Adjust a sandbag under the hand and wrist to place the cassette in the horizontal position.

Have the patient lean forward or backward as required to place the humerus at an angle of 10 to 15 degrees, open anteriorly from the vertical. Palpate and mark the location of the biciptal groove; it is the easily palpable depression between the greater and lesser tuberosities.

Central ray

Direct the central ray perpendicularly through the previously marked bicipital groove.

Structures shown

This method shows an axial projection of the acromioclavicular joint as well as of the bicipital groove. The bicipital groove is often superimposed but not obscured by the acromion process.

Inferosuperior projection

If the x-ray tube can be lowered enough for an *inferosuperior projection,* the patient may be examined in the erect position. The arm may be retracted, or the patient may be asked to lean forward 10 to 15 degrees to place the bicipital groove in a tangential position. The palm of the hand is rested against the thigh. After localizing and marking the bicipital groove, place an 8″ × 10″ cassette on the shoulder and ask the patient to hold it in position with his opposite hand. The central ray is directed vertically through the bicipital groove.

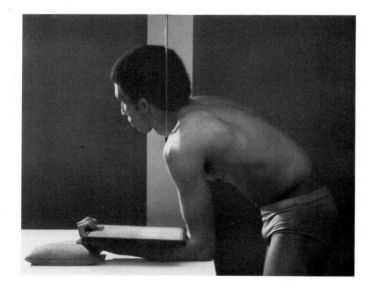

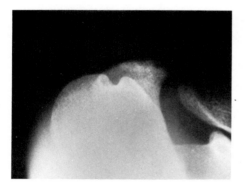

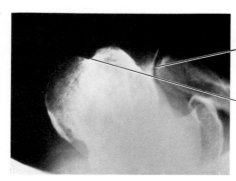

Acromioclavicular joint

Bicipital groove

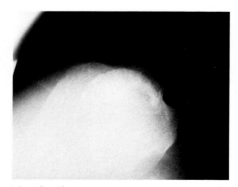

Inferosuperior

Shoulder
ROLLED-FILM AXIAL PROJECTION
CLEAVES METHOD

Cleaves[1] devised this method of obtaining an axial projection of the shoulder joint for use with patients who cannot or should not abduct the arm enough for one of the routine axial projections.

Film

This projection requires that an 8″ × 10″ film be enclosed in a lightproof envelope and gently curved around a small tube approximately 2 inches in diameter. A tube smaller than this will cause too much distortion on the radiograph, and a tube that is too large will be difficult to place high in the axilla.

To reduce radiation exposure to the patient the envelope used to enclose the film may include a pair of flexible intensifying screens. The loaded envelope is curved around the tube and secured at each end. If screens are used, extreme care must be used to avoid damaging them when loading and unloading.

Position of patient

The patient is seated laterally at the end of the table. When necessary, this projection can be adapted to the supine position.

Position of part

Place the film roll as high in the axilla as possible and adjust it so that it is horizontal.

Central ray

Direct the central ray perpendicularly to the shoulder, at a point 1 cm posterior to the acromioclavicular joint.

Variations. Direct the central ray to the acromioclavicular articulation (1) at a 5-degree medial angulation to demonstrate the lesser tuberosity and the bicipital groove and (2) at a 5-degree lateral angulation to demonstrate the coracoid process.

Structures shown

An axial projection is demonstrated, showing the glenohumeral joint, the greater and lesser tuberosities, the bicipital groove, and the coracoid process.

[1]Cleaves, E.N.: A new film holder for roentgen examination of the shoulder, A.J.R. **45**:288-290, 1941.

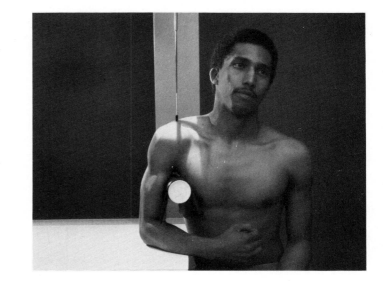

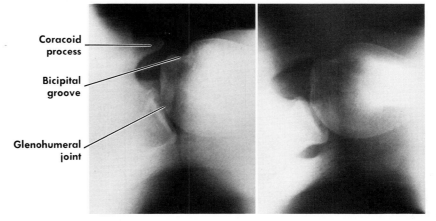

Coracoid process

Bicipital groove

Glenohumeral joint

Angulation of 0 degrees

Medial angulation of 5 degrees

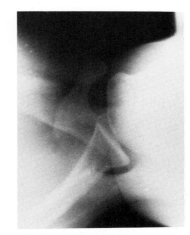

Lateral angulation of 5 degrees

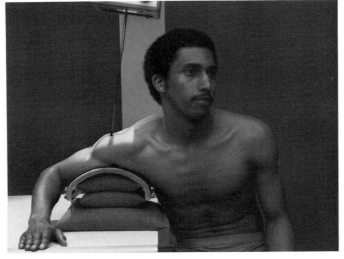

Curved cassette

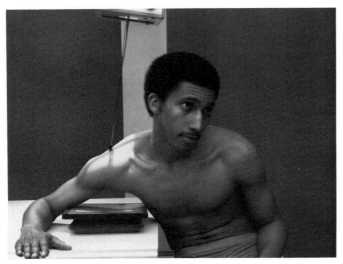

Cassette

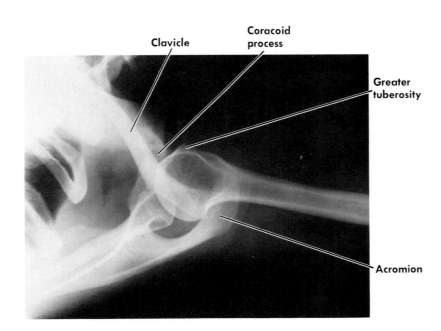

Clavicle

Coracoid process

Greater tuberosity

Acromion

Shoulder joint
AXIAL PROJECTION

The patient's ability to abduct his arm to a near right angle to the long axis of his body and the advisability of his doing so should be verified before this position is undertaken.

Film: 8″ × 10″ film placed lengthwise for accurate centering to the shoulder joint.

A curved cassette may be used for this position.

Position of patient

Seat the patient at the end of the table with the shoulder centered to the midline of the table. The patient should be seated on a stool or chair high enough to enable him to extend the affected shoulder well over the cassette.

Position of part

Place the cassette near the end of the table and parallel with its long axis.

Ask the patient to hold the hand of the affected side and raise the arm to a position as near as possible at right angles to the long axis of his body. Have him then lean laterally over the cassette until the shoulder joint is over the midpoint of the film and bring the elbow to rest on the table. Flex the patient's elbow 90 degrees, and place the hand in the neutral position. To obtain a direct lateral projection of the head of the humerus, adjust any anterior or posterior leaning of the body to place the humeral epicondyles in the vertical position.

Respiration is suspended for the exposure.

Central ray

Have the patient bend his head toward the unaffected shoulder. Direct the central ray to the shoulder joint at an angle of 5 to 15 degrees toward the elbow.

Structures shown

A superoinferior projection shows the joint relationship of the upper end of the humerus and the glenoid fossa. The acromioclavicular articulation, the outer portion of the coracoid process, and the points of insertion of the subscapularis and the teres minor are well demonstrated. Depending on the flexibility of the patient, a greater or lesser portion of the medial structures is shown.

INFEROSUPERIOR AXIAL PROJECTION
LAWRENCE METHOD

When abduction is limited, inferosuperior projections of the shoulder may be more easily obtained with the patient in the seated position. If necessary, a mobile x-ray unit may be helpful.

Film: 8″ × 10″ placed in the vertical position above the shoulder.

Position of patient

With the patient in the supine position, elevate the head and shoulders about 3 or 4 inches.

Position of part

As nearly as possible, abduct the arm of the affected side at right angles to the long axis of the body. While keeping the arm in external rotation, adjust the forearm and hand in a comfortable position, grasping a vertical support or extended on sandbags or a firm pillow.

Have the patient turn his head away from the side being examined. Place the cassette on edge above the shoulder and as close as possible to the neck. Support the cassette in position with sandbags.

Respiration is suspended for the exposure.

Central ray

Direct the central ray horizontally through the axilla to the region of the acromioclavicular articulation. The degree of medial angulation of the central ray depends on the degree of abduction of the arm.

Structures shown

An inferosuperior projection shows the glenohumeral joint, the lateral portion of the coracoid process, and the acromioclavicular articulation. The insertion site of the subscapularis tendon on the anterior border of the head of the humerus and the point of insertion of the teres minor tendon on the posterior border of the humeral head are also shown.

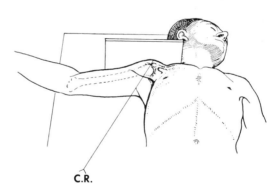

C.R.

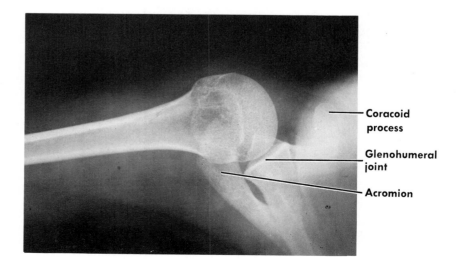

Coracoid process

Glenohumeral joint

Acromion

AXIAL PROJECTION

Film: 8″ × 10″ crosswise.

Position of patient

The patient may be in the erect or supine position.

Position of part

Center the glenohumeral joint of the affected shoulder to the midline of the grid.

Central ray

Direct the central ray through the shoulder at a cephalic angle of 35 degrees.

Structures shown

This axial projection shows the relationship of the head of the humerus to the glenoid fossa useful in diagnosing cases of posterior dislocation.

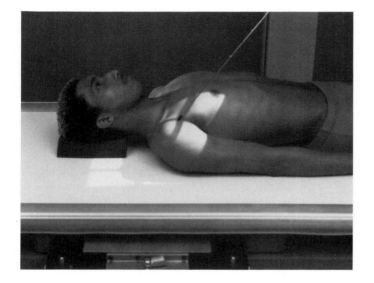

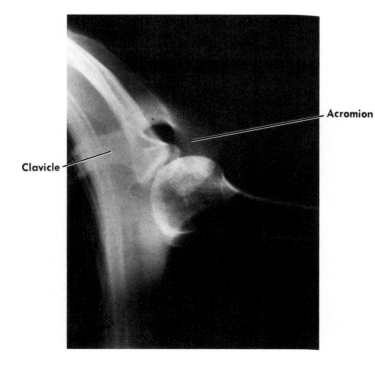

Acromion

Clavicle

Glenohumeral joint
AP AXIAL PROJECTION

The AP axial position is used to demonstrate the relationship of the head of the humerus to the glenoid fossa when the arm cannot be abducted, usually in cases of posterior dislocation. This condition is demonstrated when the shadow of the head of the humerus is cast distal to the shadow of the glenoid fossa.

This position is also used to obtain an axial projection of the clavicle and of the scapular spine. For this purpose and to obtain less distortion the cassette is adjusted at an angle of 45 degrees to place the film perpendicularly to the central ray.

Film: 8″ × 10″ lengthwise behind the shoulder.

Position of patient

The patient is seated with his back toward, and resting against, the end of the table.

Position of part

Ask the patient to sit erect. Since most of the patients for whom this position is used have a dislocation, provide whatever support is needed for the forearm, but make no attempt to change the position of the arm.

Place the cassette on the table and center it in line with the glenohumeral joint. When necessary, support the cassette on sandbags or angle sponges to elevate it to the middorsal area.

Central ray

Direct the central ray to the region of the coracoid process at a caudal angle of 40 to 45 degrees.

Structures shown

The relationship of the head of the humerus to the glenoid fossa is demonstrated. Depending on the size of the exposure field, an axial image of the clavicle and the spine of the scapula is also shown.

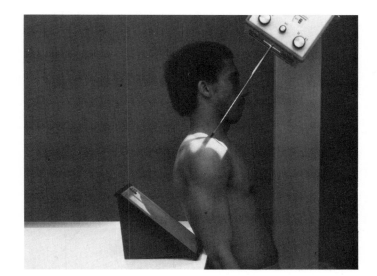

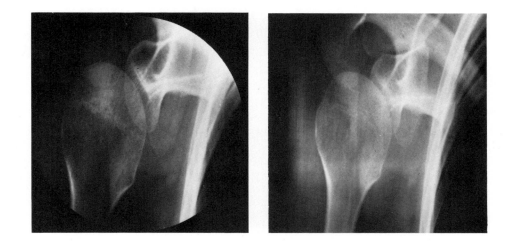

Acromioclavicular articulations

BILATERAL AP AND PA PROJECTIONS

PEARSON METHOD

Film: 7″ × 17″ or two 8″ × 10″ films, as needed to fit the patient.

Position of patient

Because a dislocation, partial or complete, of the acromioclavicular joint tends to reduce itself in the recumbent position, the demonstration of this condition requires the erect position. This projection must therefore be made with the patient in the erect position, seated or standing, if the condition of the patient permits.

Position of part

Place the patient in the AP or the PA position before a vertical grid device, and adjust the height of the cassette so that the midpoint of the cassette will lie at the level of the acromioclavicular joints. Center the midsagittal plane of the body to the midline of the grid. The weight of the body must be equally distributed on the feet to avoid rotation.

With the arms hanging by the sides, adjust the shoulders to lie in the same transverse plane. It is important that the arms hang unsupported, and, if possible, the patient should hold sandbags of equal weight in each hand.

Central ray

Direct the central ray perpendicularly to the midline of the body at the level of the acromioclavicular joints.

Structures shown

A bilateral frontal projection of the acromioclavicular joints is presented. This position is used to demonstrate dislocation, separation, and function of the joints.

AP AND LATERAL PROJECTIONS

ALEXANDER METHODS

Alexander[1] suggested that these positions be used in cases of suspected acromioclavicular subluxation or dislocation.

Film: 8″ × 10″ lengthwise.

Position of patient

The patient is placed in the erect position, either standing or seated.

[1]Alexander, O.M.: Radiography of the acromioclavicular articulation, Med. Radiogr. Photogr. **30:**34-39, 1954.

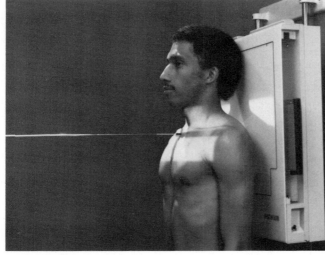

Bilateral AP examination

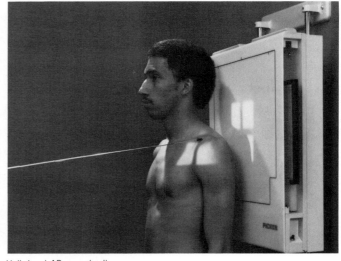

Unilateral AP examination

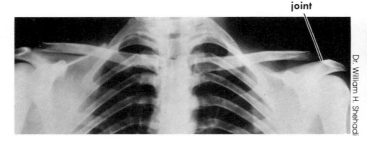

Acromioclavicular joint

Dr. William H. Shehadi

Separated acromioclavicular joint

Normal and abnormal acromioclavicular joints on same patient

Dr. Ramsay Spillman

AP PROJECTION

Position of part

Have the patient place his back against the vertical grid device, and ask him to sit or stand erect. Center the affected shoulder to the grid. Adjust the height of the cassette so that the midpoint of the film is at the level of the acromioclavicular joint. Adjust the patient's position to center the coracoid process to the film.

Central ray

Direct the central ray to the coracoid process at a cephalic angle of 15 degrees. This angulation projects the shadow of the acromioclavicular joint above that of the acromion.

LATERAL PROJECTION

Position of part

Turn the patient to the PA position with the hand of the affected side placed well up under the opposite axilla. Rotate the unaffected side 30 to 35 degrees away from the film, and adjust the patient's position to center the acromioclavicular joint to the midline of the grid.

Just before making the exposure, have the patient lean the affected shoulder against the cassette stand with the arm pulled firmly across the chest. Placing the arm across the chest draws the scapula laterally and forward. The slight obliquity of the chest and the pressure against the glenohumeral joint further rotate the scapula laterally and anteriorly. The scapula and the acromioclavicular joint are thus placed in the lateral position.

Central ray

Direct the central ray through the coracoid process at an angle of 15 degrees caudad.

Structures shown

The AP and lateral projections demonstrate the acromioclavicular joint and the relationship of the bones of the shoulder.

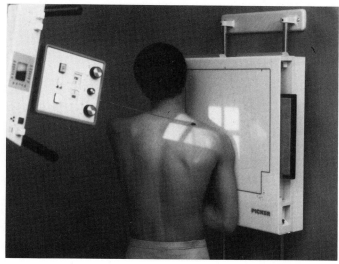

Lateral

Lateral projections of normal and abnormal acromioclavicular joints on same patient

Clavicle

PA AND PA AXIAL PROJECTIONS

PA PROJECTION

Film: 10″ × 12″ crosswise.

Position of patient

The patient may be placed in the prone or the erect position. However, if the clavicle is being examined for a fracture or a destructive disease and if the patient cannot be placed in the erect position, the AP position is used to obviate the possibility of fragment displacement or additional injury.

Position of part

Adjust the body to center the clavicle to the midline of the table or vertical grid device. Place the arms along the sides of the body, and adjust the shoulders to lie in the same transverse plane. Center the cassette to a point midway between the midsagittal plane of the body and the outer border of the shoulder at the level of the coracoid process.

Respiration is suspended at the end of exhalation for a more uniform density.

Central ray

Direct the central ray perpendicularly to the midpoint of the film.

Structures shown

This method demonstrates a frontal projection of the clavicle. The detail is better when the radiograph is taken in the PA direction because of the decreased part-film distance.

PA AXIAL PROJECTION

The patient is positioned similar to that for the PA projection described above. Direct the central ray to the supraclavicular fossa at an angle of 25 to 30 degrees caudad. The angulation of the central ray is reversed when the patient is in the supine position.

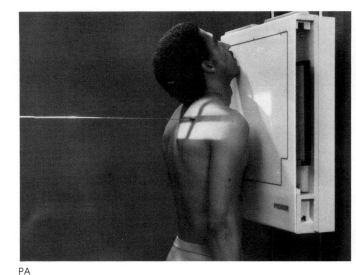

PA

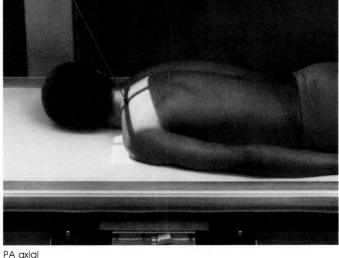

PA axial

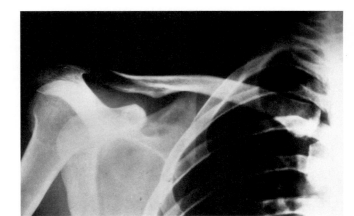

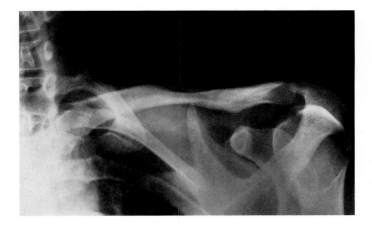

TANGENTIAL PROJECTION

The tangential projection is similar to the axial projection described on the previous page. However, the increased angulation of the central ray required for this tangential approach places the central ray nearly parallel with the rib cage. The clavicle is thus projected free of the chest wall.

Film: 8″ × 10″.

Position of patient

With the patient in the supine position, place the arms along the sides of the body.

Position of part

Depress the shoulder, if possible, to place the clavicle in a transverse plane. Have the patient turn his head away from the side being examined. Place the cassette on edge at the top of the shoulder and support it in position. The cassette should be as close to the neck as possible. Respiration is suspended for the exposure.

Central ray

Angle the tube so that the central ray will pass between the clavicle and the chest wall, perpendicular to the plane of the film.

If the medial third of the clavicle is in question, it is also necessary to angle the central ray laterally; from 15 to 25 degrees is usually sufficient.

Structures shown

An inferosuperior image of the clavicle is demonstrated, projected free of superimposed shadows.

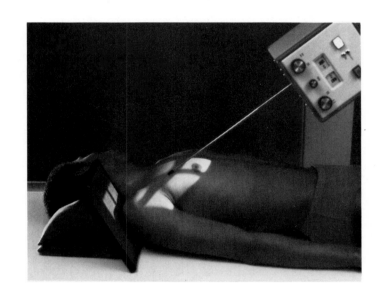

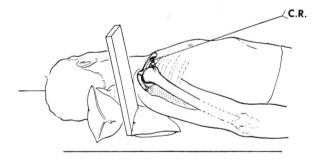

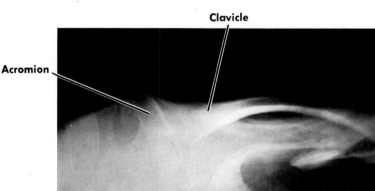

TANGENTIAL PROJECTION
TARRANT METHOD

The Tarrant method[1] is particularly useful with patients who have multiple injuries or who, for some other reason, cannot assume the lordotic position.

Film: $10'' \times 12''$ crosswise.

Position of patient

The patient is examined in the sitting position.

Position of part

Adjust a sheet of leaded rubber over the gonad area. A folded pillow or blankets may be placed on the patients lap to support the horizontally placed cassette. Center the cassette to the affected shoulder, and have the patient hold the cassette in position. Ask the patient to lean slightly forward.

Central ray

Direct the central ray anteriorly to the calvicle. It should pass perpendicularly to the coronal plane of the clavicle.

Because of the considerable part-film distance a long SID should be used to reduce magnification.

Structures shown

By this method the clavicle is projected above the thoracic cage.

[1]Tarrant, R.M.: The axial view of the clavicle, Xray Techn. **21:**358-359, 1950.

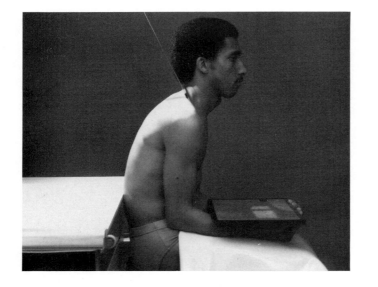

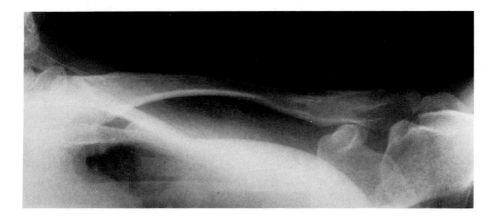

AP AXIAL PROJECTION

An axial projection of the clavicle can be obtained with far less discomfort to the patient when he can be adjusted from the erect position. This is particularly true of young patients who assume the lordotic position with ease.

Film: 10″ × 12″ for adults.

Position of patient

Place the patient in the AP position, standing or seated, approximately 1 foot away from the cassette stand.

Position of part

Adjust the patient's position to center the affected shoulder to the vertical grid device. Assist the patient in assuming the lordotic position, and center the cassette to the clavicle. Estimate the required angulation of the central ray, and then have the patient reassume the erect position while the tube is being adjusted for position, ask him to place his arms in a comfortable position. The technologist should place one hand against the patient's lumbar region to give the patient support and then have him lean backward in a position of extreme lordosis and rest his neck and shoulder against the vertical grid device. The neck will be in extreme flexion.

Respiration is suspended at the end of full inhalation to further elevate and angle the clavicle.

Central ray

Direct the central ray into the inferior border of the clavicle at right angles to its coronal plane.

Structures shown

An exact axial projection of the clavicle is obtained when the anterior and posterior ends of the first rib are seen to be exactly superimposed.

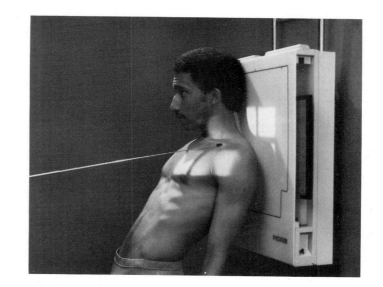

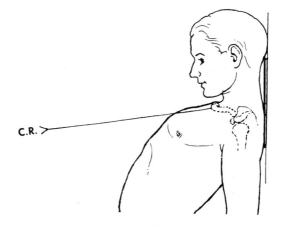

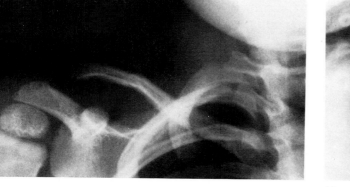

PA

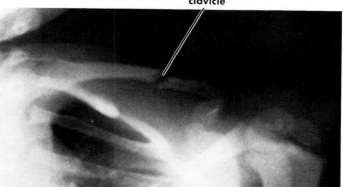

Fractured clavicle

AP axial projection on same patient as in adjacent radiograph, 3 years of age

RIGHT-ANGLE PROJECTIONS
QUESADA METHOD

Film: 10″ × 12″ crosswise for each exposure.

Position of patient

Place the patient in the prone position and adjust the body to center the clavicle to the midline of the table.

Position of part

With the patient's clavicle centered to the midline of the table, place the arms along the sides of the body, and adjust the shoulders to lie in the same transverse plane. Rest the head on the cheek of the affected side. Adjust the cassette so that the center point of the film will coincide with the central ray.

To obtain better delineation of the clavicle, instruct the patient to hold his breath at the end of inhalation.

Central ray

1. Direct the central ray to the midpoint of the clavicle at an angle of 45 degrees caudad.

2. Change the cassette; direct the central ray 45 degrees cephalad, and center to the midpoint of the clavicle.

Structures shown

Quesada[1] recommends that this method of obtaining exact right-angle projections of the clavicle be used as a preoperative procedure for patients with a comminuted fracture.

[1]Quesada, F.: Technique for the roentgen diagnosis of fractures of the clavicle, Surg. Gynecol. Obstet. **42:**424-428, 1926.

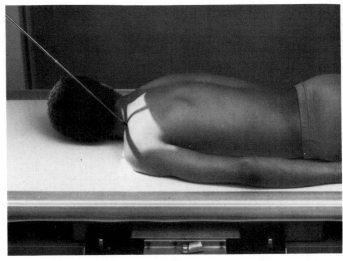

Caudal angulation of 45 degrees

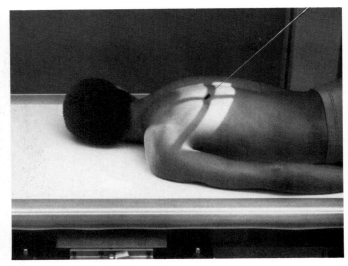

Cephalic angulation of 45 degrees

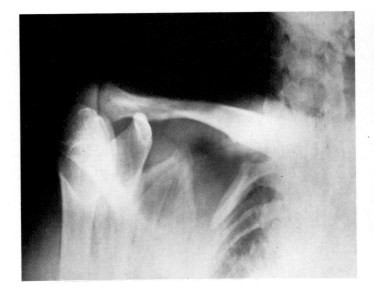

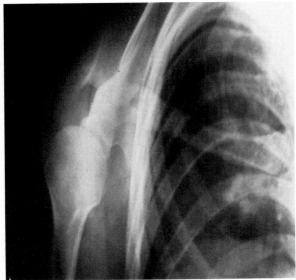

Scapula
AP PROJECTION

Film: $10'' \times 12''$ lengthwise.

Position of patient

The patient may be placed in the erect or the supine position, the erect position being preferred if the shoulder is tender.

Position of part

Adjust the body and center the affected scapula to the midline of the grid. Abduct the arm to a right angle to the body to draw the scapula laterally; then flex the elbow and support the hand in a comfortable position. Do not rotate the body toward the affected side for this projection, because the resultant obliquity would offset the effect of drawing the scapula laterally.

This projection of the scapula should be made during quiet breathing to obliterate lung detail.

Central ray

Direct the central ray prependicularly to the midscapular area.

Structures shown

An AP projection of the scapula is demonstrated with the lateral portion of its body free of superimposition.

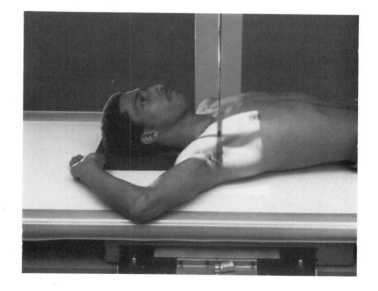

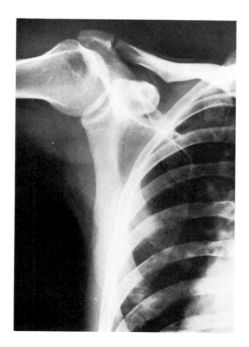

PA OBLIQUE PROJECTIONS
LORENZ AND LILIENFELD METHODS

Film: 10″ × 12″ lengthwise.

Position of the patient

The patient may be placed in the erect or the lateral recumbent position. When the shoulder is painful, the erect position should be used if possible.

Position of part

With the patient in the lateral position, erect or recumbent, align the body and center the scapula to the midline of the Bucky diaphragm. Adjust the arm according to the projection desired.

1. For the Lorenz method, adjust the arm at a right angle to the long axis of the body, flex the elbow, and rest the hand against the patient's head. Rotate the body slightly forward, and have the patient grasp the side of the table or the stand for support.

2. For the Lilienfeld method, extend the arm of the affected side obliquely upward, and have the patient rest the hand on his head. Rotate the body slightly forward and have the patient grasp the side of the table or the stand for support.

For either method, grasp the axillary and vertebral borders of the scapula between the thumb and index fingers of one hand, and adjust the rotation of the body so that the scapula will be projected free of the rib cage.

Central ray

With the central ray perpendicular to the plane of the film, direct it between the chest wall and the midarea of the protruding scapula.

Structures shown

An oblique projection of the scapula is shown, the degree of obliquity depending on the position of the arm. Compare the delineation of the different parts of the bone in the two oblique studies shown.

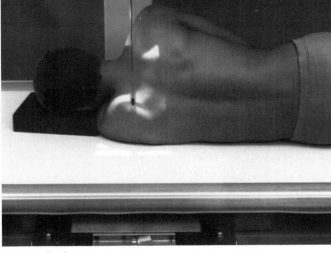

Lorenz method

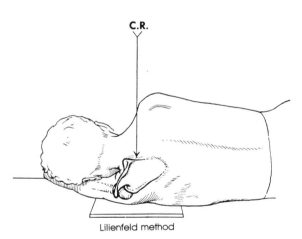

Lilienfeld method

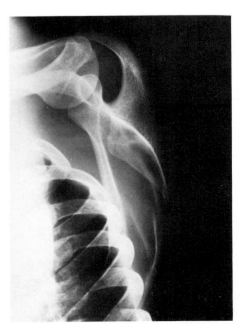

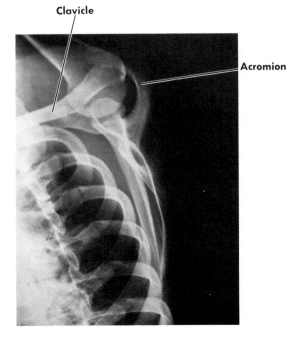

Clavicle

Acromion

LATERAL PROJECTIONS

Film: $10'' \times 12''$ lengthwise.

Position of patient

The patient is placed in the erect position, standing or seated, facing a vertical grid device.

When a patient cannot be placed in the erect position, a lateral projection of the scapula can be obtained by adjusting the degree of body rotation and the placement of the arm from the prone or the supine position.

Position of part

Adjust the patient in an oblique position, with the affected scapula centered to the grid. The arm is placed according to the area of the scapula to be demonstrated.

1. For the delineation of the body of the scapula, the elbow is flexed and the hand placed on the anterior or posterior chest at a level that will prevent the shadow of the humerus from overlapping that of the scapula. Marzujian[1] suggests that the arm may be adjusted across the upper chest by grasping the opposite shoulder.

2. For the demonstration of the acromion and coracoid processes, ask the patient to extend the arm upward and rest the forearm on his head.

3. For the demonstration of the glenohumeral joint, to prove or disprove posterior dislocation, McLaughlin[2] recommends that the arm hang beside the body and be adjusted to have it superimposed by the wing of the scapula.

After the placement of the arm for any one of the above projections, grasp the axillary and vertebral borders of the scapula between the thumb and index fingers of one hand, and adjust the body rotation to place the wing of the scapula perpendicular to the plane of the film.

Central ray

Direct the central ray horizontally to the medial border of the protruding scapula.

[1]Mazujian, M.: Lateral profile view of the scapula, Xray Techn. **25**:24-25, 1953.
[2]McLaughlin, H.L.: Posterior dislocation of the shoulder, J. Bone Joint Surg. **34-A**:584-590, 1952.

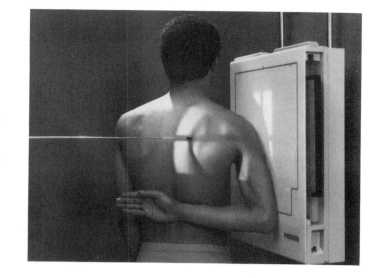

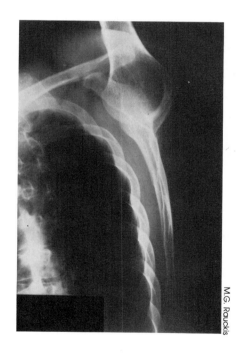

M.G. Rauckis

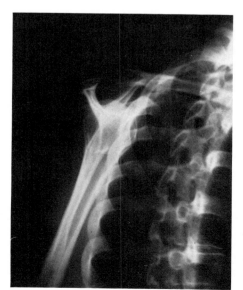

Scapula and arm superimposed

AP OBLIQUE PROJECTIONS

Film: $10'' \times 12''$ lengthwise.

Position of patient

The patient may be examined in the supine or the erect position, although the erect position should be used when the shoulder is painful.

Position of part

Have the patient in the AP position, supine or erect. Align the body and center the affected scapula to the midline of the grid.

1. For an AP oblique projection, ask the patient to extend his arm superiorly, flex the elbow, and place the supinated hand under his head. Have him turn away from the affected side enough to oblique the shoulder slightly.

2. For an oblique lateral projection, ask the patient to extend his arm and rest the flexed elbow on his forehead. Rotate the body away from the affected side. Grasp the axillary and vertebral borders of the scapula between the thumb and index fingers of one hand, and adjust the rotation of the body to project the scapula free of the rib cage.

3. For a direct lateral projection, draw the arm across the chest and adjust the body rotation to place the scapula perpendicular to the plane of the film.

Central ray

Direct the central ray perpendicularly to the lateral border of the rib cage at the midscapular area.

Structures shown

An oblique (or a lateral) image of the scapula is presented, projected free or nearly free of rib superimposition. Compare the delineation of the different parts of the bone in the two projections shown.

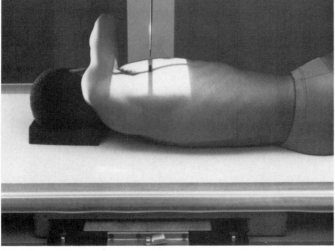

AP oblique

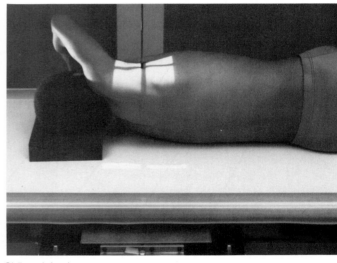

Oblique lateral

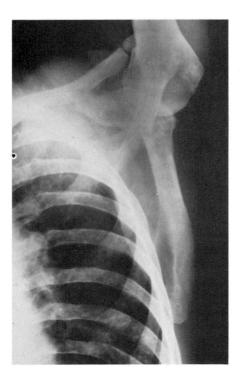

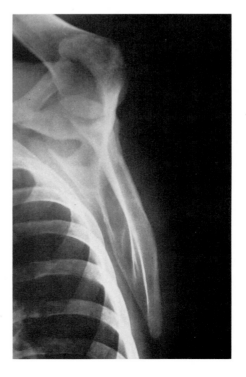

Scapular spine
TANGENTIAL PROJECTION
LAQUERRIERE-PIERQUIN METHOD

Film: 8″ × 10″ crosswise.

Position of patient

As described by the originators[1] the patient is placed in the supine position.

Position of part

Center the shoulder to the midline of the table. Adjust the patient's rotation to place the wing of the scapula in a horizontal position. When this requires that the opposite shoulder be elevated, support it on sandbags or radioparent sponges. The head should be turned away from the affected shoulder enough to prevent superimposition.

Funke[2] found that in the examination of flat-chested patients, clavicular superimposition can be prevented by inserting a 15-degree radioparent wedge under the shoulder to angle it caudally.

Central ray

The central ray is directed through the posterosuperior region of the shoulder at an angle of 45 degrees caudad. A 35-degree angulation suffices for obese and round-shouldered subjects.

After the adjustment of the x-ray tube, position the cassette so that it is centered to the central ray.

Structures shown

The spine of the scapula is projected in profile and free of bony superimposition except for the outer end of the clavicle.

NOTE: When the shoulder is too painful to tolerate the pressure of the supine position, the tangential projection of the spine of the scapula can be equally well obtained with the patient in the prone position[3] or the erect position as on the following page.

[1] Laquerrière and Pierquin: De la nécessité d'employer une technique radiographique spéciale pour obtenir certains détails squelettiques, J. Radiol. Electr. **3**:145-148, 1918.
[2] Funke, T.: Tangential view of the scapular spine, Med. Radiogr. Photogr. **34**:41-43, 1958.
[3] Voorhis, M.W.: The spine of the scapula, Du Pont X-ray News, no. 42.

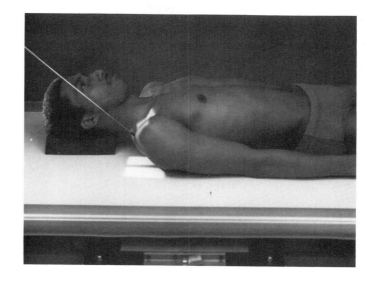

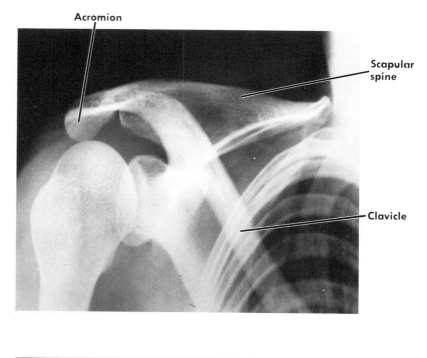

Acromion

Scapular spine

Clavicle

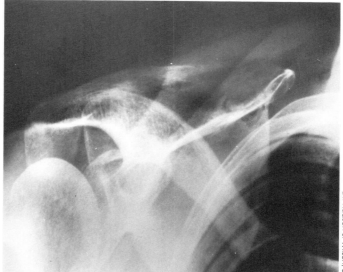

Dr. Hudson J. Wilson, Jr.

TANGENTIAL PROJECTION

Film: $8'' \times 10''$ crosswise.

Prone position
Position of part

Place the patient in the prone position, and center the shoulder to the midline of the table. Place the arms along the sides of his body, and adjust the shoulders to lie in the same transverse plane. Care must be taken to prevent lateral rotation of the scapula. Have the patient rest his head on the chin or the cheek of the affected side. Supinate the hand of the affected side. A radioparent wedge may be adjusted under the side of the shoulder and upper arm to place the scapula in the horizontal position.

Central ray

The central ray is directed through the scapular spine at an angle of 45 degrees cephalad. It exits at the anterosuperior aspect of the shoulder.

Erect position (seated)

A long SID is recommended because of the increased part-film distance.

Position of part

Seat the patient with his back toward and resting against the end of the table. Place the cassette on the table, center it in line with the shoulder, and adjust it on supports to place it at an angle of 45 degrees.

Central ray

Direct the central ray through the anterosuperior aspect of the shoulder at a posteroinferior angle of 45 degrees. The central ray should be perpendicular to the plane of the film.

Structures shown

The tangential projection presents the scapular spine in profile and free of superimposition of the scapular body.

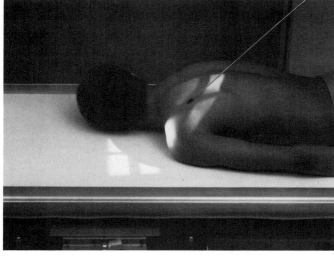

Prone

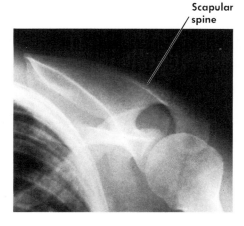

Seated

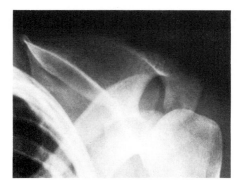

Scapular spine

Bony thorax

Sternum

Ribs

ANATOMY

The bony thorax is formed by the sternum, the 12 pairs of ribs, and the 12 thoracic vertebrae. It is more or less conical in shape, being narrower above than below. Its width is greater than its depth, and it is longer in back than in front.

STERNUM

The sternum, or breastbone, is directed anteriorly and inferiorly in the midsagittal plane of the anterior thorax. It is a narrow, flat bone about 6 inches long and consists of three parts—the manubrium, the gladiolus, or body, and the xiphoid, or ensiform, cartilage. The sternum supports the clavicles at the upper manubrial angles and affords attachment to the costal cartilages of the first seven pairs of ribs at its lateral borders.

The manubrium, which is the upper part of the sternum, is quadrilateral in shape and is the broadest part of the sternum. It has a depression on its upper border termed the manubrial or jugular notch. On each side of the manubrial notch the bone slants laterally and posteriorly and bears an articular surface for the reception of the sternal end of the clavicle. On its lateral borders, immediately below the articular notches for the clavicles, are shallow depressions for the attachment of the cartilages of the first pair of ribs. The manubrial notch is easily palpable, and in the thorax of average form it lies anterior to the interspace between the second and third thoracic vertebrae when the body is erect.

The gladiolus, or body, which is the longest part of the sternum, is joined to the manubrium at an obtuse angle, called the sternal angle, at the level of the junction of the second costal cartilage. Both the manubrium and the gladiolus contribute to the attachment of the second costal cartilage. The succeeding five pairs of costal cartilages are attached to the lateral borders of the gladiolus. The sternal angle is palpable and, in the normally formed thorax, lies anterior to the interspace between the fourth and fifth thoracic vertebrae when the body is erect.

The xiphoid process, which forms the distal part of the sternum, is variable in shape. It is a cartilaginous structure in early life but ossifies, at least in part, in later life. The xiphoid often deviates from the midsagittal plane of the body.

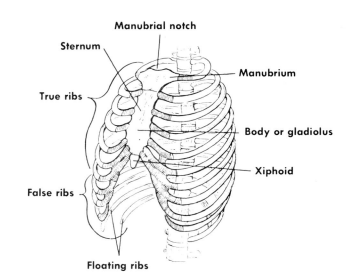

ANTEROLATERAL ASPECT OF BONY THORAX

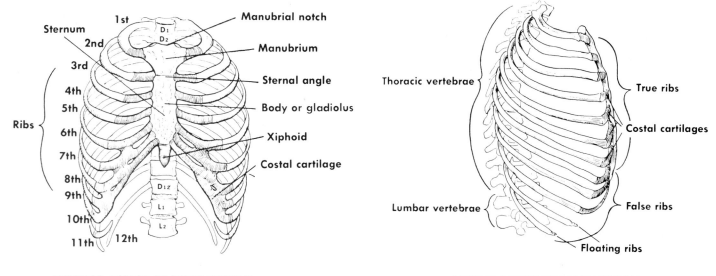

ANTERIOR ASPECT OF BONY THORAX

LATERAL ASPECT OF BONY THORAX

STERNOCLAVICULAR JOINTS

The sternoclavicular joints, which are the only points of articulation between the upper extremities and the trunk, are diarthroses that permit limited movement in almost all directions. These joints are formed by the articulation between the sternal ends of the clavicles and the clavicular notches of the manubrium. A circular disk of fibrocartilage is interposed in each joint between the articular ends of the bones, and the joints are enclosed in articular capsules.

RIBS

The 12 pairs of ribs are simply numbered from the neck inferiorly. With the exception of the last two pairs, in which the cartilage is absent, each rib consists of a long, slender, arched bone and a costal cartilage. The ribs are attached posteriorly to the bodies of the thoracic vertebrae. The first, tenth, eleventh, and twelfth ribs each articulates with one vertebral body, and the others articulate with two bodies. Anteriorly the cartilages of the first seven pairs of ribs are attached directly to the sternum and are called true, or vertebrosternal, ribs. The succeeding three pairs of ribs are attached cartilage to superjacent cartilage and are called false, or vertebrochondral, ribs. The last two pairs have no anterior attachment and are called floating, or vertebral, ribs. The term *false rib* is applied to both the vertebrochondral and the floating ribs.

The ribs are situated in an oblique plane slanting anteriorly and inferiorly so that their anterior ends lie from 3 to 5 inches below the level of their vertebral ends. The degree of obliquity gradually increases from the first to the ninth rib and then decreases to the twelfth rib. The spaces between the ribs are referred to as the intercostal spaces. The ribs vary in breadth and length. From the first rib, which is the shortest and broadest, the breadth gradually decreases to the twelfth rib, which is the narrowest rib. The length increases from the first to the seventh and then gradually decreases to the twelfth rib.

A typical rib consists of (1) a head that articulates with the vertebral bodies, forming the costovertebral articulations, (2) a flattened neck, (3) a tubercle that articulates with the transverse process of a thoracic vertebra, forming the costotransverse articulations, except in the eleventh and twelfth ribs, and (4) a shaft. From the point of articulation with the vertebral body, the rib projects obliquely posteriorly to the point of articulation with the transverse process. Then it turns laterally to the angle of the shaft, where the bone arches anteriorly, medially, and inferiorly in an oblique plane.

The heads of the ribs are closely bound to the vertebral bodies, and only slight gliding movement is permitted. These articulations are called costovertebral joints. The articulations between the necks and tubercles of the ribs and the transverse processes of the vertebrae, the costotransverse joints, permit only slight superior and inferior movements of the first six pairs. Greater freedom of movement is permitted in the succeeding four pairs. With the exception of the first pair, which are rigidly attached to the sternum, the sternocostal articulations permit gliding movements.

Respiratory excursion

The normal oblique position of the ribs changes very little during quiet respiratory movements; however, the degree of obliquity is decreased with deep inhalation and is increased with deep exhalation. The first pair of ribs, which are rigidly attached to the manubrium, rotate at their vertebral ends and move with the sternum as one structure during respiratory movements.

On deep inhalation the anterior ends of the ribs are carried anteriorly, superiorly, and laterally, while their necks are rotated inferiorly. On deep exhalation the anterior ends are carried inferiorly, posteriorly, and medially, while the necks are rotated superiorly. The last two pairs of ribs are depressed and held in position by the action of the diaphragm when the anterior ends of the upper ribs are elevated during respiration.

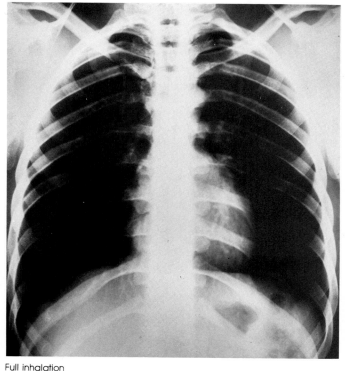

Full inhalation

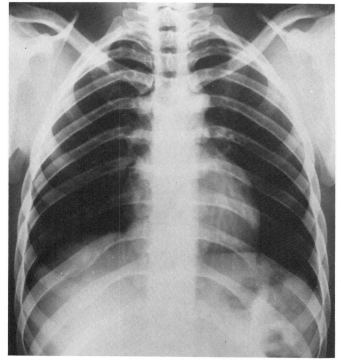

Full exhalation

Diaphragm

The ribs situated above the diaphragm are examined through the air-filled lungs, whereas those situated below the diaphragm must be examined through the upper abdomen. Because of the difference in penetration required for the two regions, the position and respiratory excursion of the diaphragm plays a large part in radiography of the ribs.

The position of the diaphragm varies with bodily habitus, being at a higher level in hypersthenic subjects and at a lower level in hyposthenic subjects. In the subject of average size and shape the right side of the diaphragm arches posteriorly from the level of about the sixth or seventh costal cartilage to the level of the ninth or tenth thoracic vertebra when the body is in the erect position. The left side of the diaphragm will lie at a slightly lower level. Because of the oblique position of both the ribs and the diaphragm, several pairs of ribs lie partially above and partially below the diaphragm.

The position of the diaphragm changes considerably with the position of the body, being at its lowest level when the body is erect and at its highest level when the body is supine. For this reason it is desirable to place the patient in the erect position when examining the ribs above the diaphragm and in a recumbent position when examining the ribs below the diaphragm. When the body is in a lateral recumbent position, the diaphragm lies in an oblique plane, the side against the table being higher in position than the upper half.

The respiratory excursion of the diaphragm averages about 1½ inches between deep inhalation and deep exhalation. The excursion will be less in hypersthenic subjects and more in hyposthenic subjects. Deeper inhalation or exhalation, and therefore greater depression or elevation of the diaphragm, is achieved on the second respiratory movement than is achieved on the first. This point should be utilized when examining the ribs that lie at the diaphragmatic level.

When the body is placed in the supine position, the anterior ends of the ribs are displaced superiorly, laterally, and posteriorly. For this reason the anterior ends of the ribs are less sharply visualized when the patient is radiographed in the supine position.

Body position

Although it is desirable in rib examinations to take advantage of the effect that body position has on the position of the diaphragm, the effect is not of sufficient importance to justify subjecting a patient to a painful change in position from the erect to the recumbent or vice versa. Rib injuries, minor as well as extensive, are painful, and even slight movement frequently causes the patient considerable distress. Therefore unless the change can be effected with a tilt table, patients with recent injury should be examined in the position in which they arrive in the department. The ambulatory patient can be positioned for recumbent projections with a minimum of discomfort by bringing the tilt table to the vertical position for each position change. With the patient standing on the footboard, he can be comfortably adjusted and then lowered to the horizontal position.

Casualty patients

The first and usually the only requirement in the initial radiographic examination of the casualty patient who has sustained severe trauma to the rib cage is to take frontal (PA or AP) and lateral projections of the chest. These projections are made not only to demonstrate the site and extent of rib injury but also to investigate the possibility of injury to the underlying structures by depressed rib fractures. The patient is examined in the position in which he arrives, usually recumbent on a stretcher. This body position necessitates a decubitus projection to demonstrate the presence of fluid and/or air levels.

Less seriously injured patients sometimes arrive after adhesive strapping has been applied around the lower thorax to restrict rib movement and thus to make breathing less painful. Fractures having appreciable fragment separation or displacement are readily detected through smooth, recently applied strapping. Nondisplaced transverse fractures frequently are not demonstrated radiographically before the appearance of callus formation, even without strapping. Failure to demonstrate small fissure fractures of this type is not of major clinical importance, since surgical intervention is seldom required.

It is desirable to radiograph ribs before the application of adhesive strapping, but no patient needs to be subjected to the discomfort of having freshly applied strapping removed, since no fracture of clinical significance will be missed as a result of its presence. It is, however, necessary to remove old, wrinkled strapping for progress examinations. Fortunately the patient will have recovered enough after an interval of 2 or 3 weeks to tolerate the removal without too much discomfort.

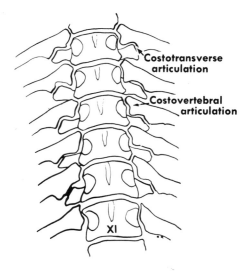

Sternum

The position of the sternum with respect to the denser thoracic structures, both bony and soft, makes it one of the more difficult organs to radiograph satisfactorily. Few problems are involved in obtaining a lateral projection, but, because of the location of the sternum directly anterior to the thoracic spine, a direct frontal projection contains little useful diagnostic information without the aid of tomography. To separate the shadows cast by the vertebrae and the sternum, it is necessary to rotate the body from the PA position or to angle the central ray medially. The exact degree of angulation required depends on the depth of the chest, deep chests requiring less angulation than shallow chests.

Although angulation of the body or of the central ray clears the sternum of the vertebral shadow, it superimposes the shadows of the posterior ribs and the lung markings. If the sternum is projected to the left of the thoracic vertebrae, it is also overshadowed by the heart and other mediastinal structures. The superimposition of the homogeneous density of the heart shadow can be used to advantage, as will be seen by comparing the radiographs on p. 188.

The pulmonary markings, particularly of elderly persons and of heavy smokers, can cast confusing shadows over the sternum, unless the motion of shallow breathing is used to eliminate them. If motion is desired, the exposure time should be long enough to cover several phases of shallow respiration. The milliamperage must be relatively low to achieve the desired milliampere-seconds.

If the female patient has large, pendulous breasts, they should be drawn to the sides and held in position with a wide bandage to prevent their shadows from overlapping the sternum and to obtain closer proximity of the sternum to the cassette. This is particularly important in the lateral projection, in which the breast shadows can obscure the lower portion of the sternum.

NOTE: In the early years of radiography a technique was often used in which the cone was removed from the radiographic tube and the x-ray tube then placed in contact with the patient's spine. This technique greatly magnified the spine and posterior ribs, which aided in the demonstration of the sternum. This technique is no longer employed because of the extremely high radiation dose received by the patient when such a short radiographic tube–part distance is used.

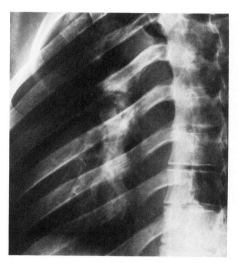

Suspended respiration

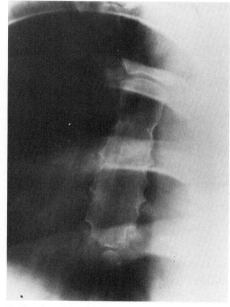

Shallow breathing during exposure

Sternum

RIGHT PA OBLIQUE PROJECTION (RAO)

Film: 10″ × 12″ lengthwise.

Position of patient

With the patient in the prone position, adjust him for a right PA oblique projection (RAO) to utilize the heart shadow. Have the patient support himself on the forearm and the flexed knee.

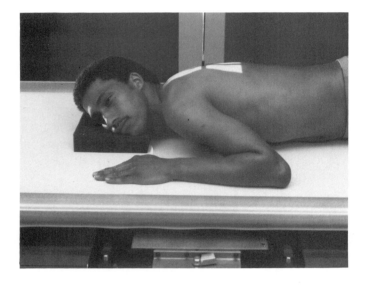

Position of part

Align the patient's body so that the long axis of the sternum is centered to the midline of the table. Adjust the elevation of the left shoulder and hip so that the thorax is rotated just enough to prevent superimposition of the vertebral and sternal shadows. The required degree of rotation can be estimated with sufficient accuracy by placing one hand on the patient's sternum and the other hand directly above it on his thoracic vertebrae to act as guides while adjusting the position.

Center the cassette to the midsternal area.

When breathing motion is to be utilized, instruct the patient to take slow, shallow breaths during the exposure.

When a short exposure time is to be used, instruct the patient to hold his breath at the end of exhalation to obtain a more uniform density.

Central ray

Direct the central ray perpendicularly to the midpoint of the film.

Structures shown

This method shows a slightly oblique PA projection of the sternum. The detail demonstrated depends largely on the technical procedure employed. If breathing motion is utilized, the pulmonary markings will be obliterated.

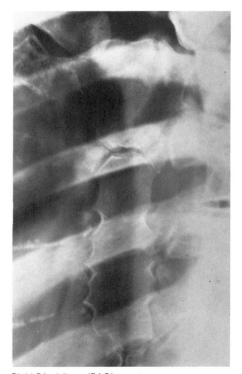

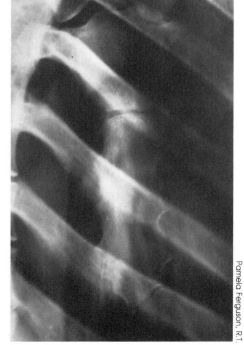

Pamela Ferguson, R.T.

Right PA oblique (RAO)   Left PA oblique (LAO)

LATERAL PROJECTION
ERECT POSITION

Film: $10'' \times 12''$ lengthwise.

Position of patient

Place the patient in a lateral position, either seated or standing, before a vertical grid device.

Position of part

Have the patient sit or stand straight, and adjust the height of the film so that its upper border is 1½ inches above the manubrial notch.

Rotate the shoulders posteriorly, and have the patient lock his hands behind his back. Center the sternum to the midline of the grid. Being careful to keep the mid-sagittal plane of the body vertical, place the patient close enough to the grid so that he can rest his shoulder firmly against it. Adjust the patient so that the broad surface of the sternum is perpendicular to the plane of the film.

The breasts of female patients should be drawn to the sides and held in position with a wide bandage so that their shadows will not obscure the lower portion of the sternum.

Respiration is suspended at the end of deep inhalation to obtain sharper contrast between the posterior surface of the sternum and the adjacent structures.

For a direct lateral projection of the sternoclavicular region only, center a vertically placed $8'' \times 10''$ cassette at the level of the manubrial notch.

Central ray

Direct the central ray horizontally to the midpoint of the film.

Structures shown

A lateral projection of the entire length of the sternum is demonstrated, showing the superimposed sternoclavicular joints and medial ends of the clavicles.

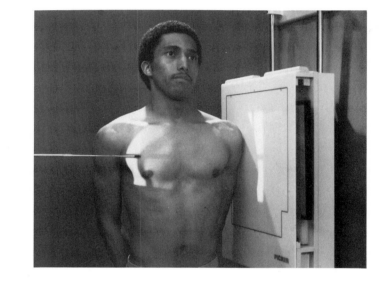

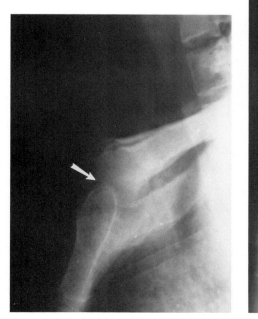

Sternoclavicular joint *(arrow)*

Sternum

LATERAL PROJECTION
RECUMBENT POSITION

Film: 10″ × 12″ lengthwise.

Position of patient

Place the patient in the lateral recumbent position, and center the long axis of the sternum to the midline of the table.

Position of part

Flex the patient's hips and knees to a comfortable position. Extend the arms over the head to prevent their shadows from overlapping that of the sternum. Rest the patient's head on the dependent arm or a pillow.

If necessary, place a support under the lower thoracic region to position the long axis of the sternum horizontally. Adjust the rotation of the body so that the broad surface of the sternum is perpendicular to the plane of the film.

A compression band may be applied across the hips for immobilization. Respiration is suspended at the end of deep inhalation to obtain shorter-scale contrast between the posterior surface of the sternum and the adjacent structures.

Center the cassette to the midsternal area.

Central ray

Direct the central ray perpendicularly to the plane of the film.

Structures shown

The lateral aspect of the entire length of the sternum is shown. In cases of severe injury the patient can be examined in the supine position by cross-table or horizontal ray projection. In this case a grid-front cassette or a stationary grid should be used as shown.

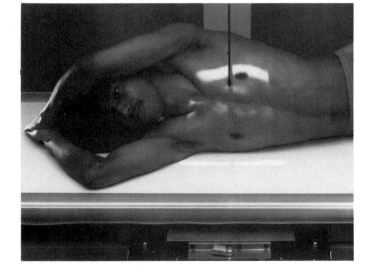

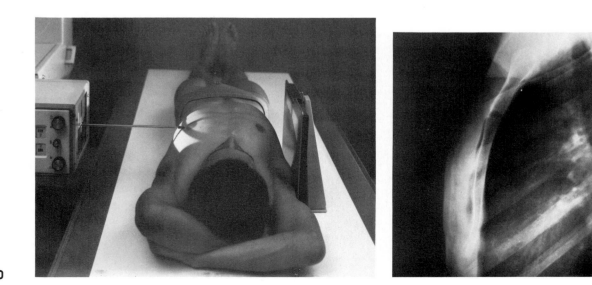

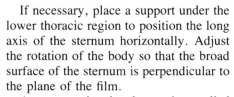

Sternoclavicular articulations

PA PROJECTION

Film: 8″ × 10″ crosswise.

Position of patient

Place the patient in the prone position, and center the midsagittal plane of the body to the midline of the table. The same procedure can be adapted for use with the patient who is standing or seated erect.

Position of part

Center the cassette at the level of the spinous process of the third thoracic vertebra, which lies posterior to the manubrial notch. Place the arms along the sides of the body with the palms facing upward, and adjust the shoulders to lie in the same transverse plane.

1. For a bilateral examination, rest the patient's head on the chin and adjust it so that the midsagittal plane is vertical.

2. For a unilateral examination, ask the patient to turn his head to face the affected side and then to rest his head on his cheek. The rotation of the head rotates the spine slightly away from the side being examined and thus gives better visualization of the lateral portion of the manubrium.

Respiration is suspended at the end of exhalation to obtain a more uniform density.

Central ray

Direct the central ray perpendicularly to the midpoint of the film.

Structures shown

This method presents a PA projection of the sternoclavicular joints and of the medial portions of the clavicles.

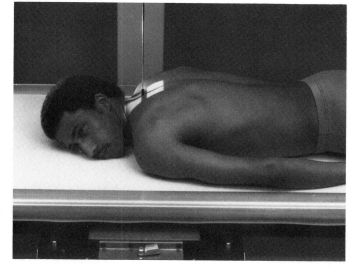

Unilateral examination

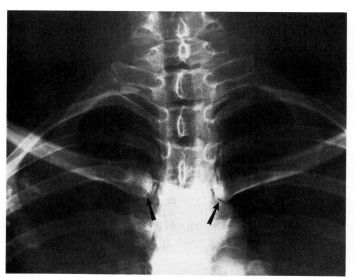

Bilateral

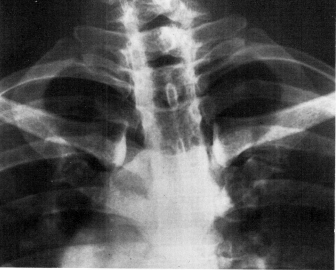

Unilateral

PA OBLIQUE PROJECTIONS (RAO AND LAO)

Film: 8″ × 10″ crosswise.

Body rotation method
Position of patient

The patient may be placed in a prone or in a seated-erect position.

Position of part

Keeping the affected side adjacent to the film, oblique the patient enough to project the vertebral shadow well behind that of the sternoclavicular joint, and then adjust his position to center the joint to the midline of the grid device. Adjust the shoulders to lie in the same transverse plane. Center the cassette at the level of the sternoclavicular joint.

Central ray

Direct the central ray perpendicularly to the midpoint of the film.

Central ray angulation method
Position of patient

Place the patient in the prone position. Adjust the cassette directly under his upper chest, and center the film to the affected sternoclavicular joint. A nongrid technique must be used to avoid grid cut-off because of the cross-table angulation.

Position of part

Extend the arms along the sides of the body with the palms of the hands facing upward, and adjust the shoulders to lie in the same transverse plane. Ask the patient to rest his head on his chin or to rotate the chin to the side.

Central ray

From the side being examined the central ray is directed to the midpoint of the film at an angle of 15 degrees toward the midsagittal plane of the body.

A small angle is satisfactory in examinations of the sternoclavicular articulations, because there is only a slight AP overlapping of the vertebrae and these joints.

Structures shown

A slightly oblique projection of the sternoclavicular joint is demonstrated by either method. Because the joint is closer to the plane of the film, less distortion is obtained with the central ray angulation method than with the body rotation method.

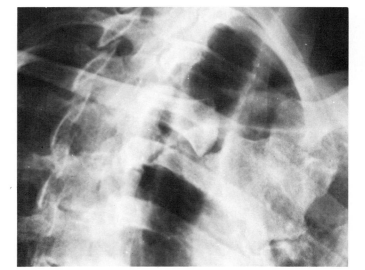

Body rotation

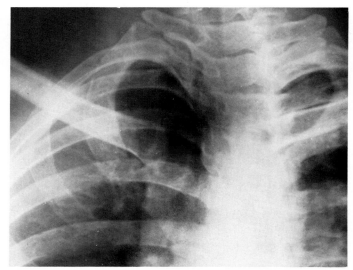

Central ray angulation

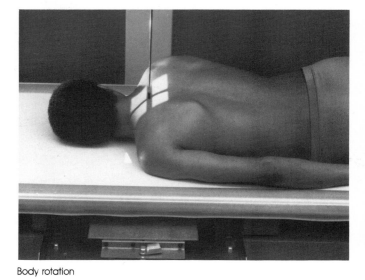

LATERAL PROJECTION
KURZBAUER METHOD[1]

Film: 8″ × 10″ lengthwise.

Position of patient

The patient lies in the lateral recumbent position on the side being examined, with the sternoclavicular region centered to the midline of the table. Flex the patient's hips and knees to a comfortable position.

Position of part

Have the patient fully extend the dependent arm and grasp the end of the table for support. Make any necessary adjustment

[1]Kurzbauer, R.: The lateral projection in the roentgenography of the sternoclavicular articulation, A.J.R. **56**:104-105, 1946.

to center the sternoclavicular articulation to the midline of the table. Place the uppermost arm along the side of the body, and have the patient grasp the dorsal surface of his hip to hold the shoulder in a depressed position. The extension of the dependent shoulder, coupled with the depression of the uppermost shoulder, prevents the superimposition of the shadows of the articulations.

Adjust the thorax to place the anterior surface of the manubrium perpendicular to the plane of the film.

Adjust the position of the cassette so that its midpoint will coincide with the central ray.

Respiration is suspended at the end of full inhalation.

Central ray

Direct the central ray through the lowermost sternoclavicular articulation at an angle of 15 degrees caudad.

Structures shown

This method presents an unobstructed lateral projection of the sternoclavicular articulation adjacent to the film.

Although the best result is obtained with the patient in the recumbent position, a comparable radiograph can be obtained with the erect position when the shoulder is too tender for pressure.

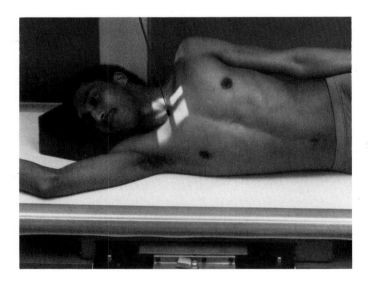

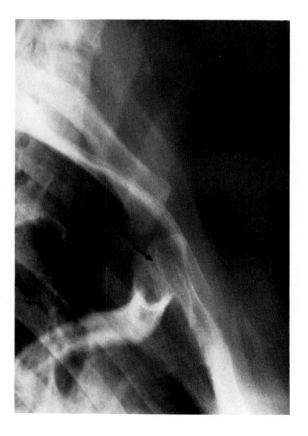

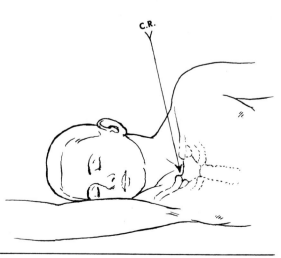

Ribs

In radiography of the ribs, unless the affected area is definitely localized near one end of the thorax, where the first or the last rib will be included on a smaller film, a 14″ × 17″ radiograph should be taken to identify the rib or ribs involved and to establish the extent of the suspected trauma or pathologic condition.

After localizing the lesion determine (1) the position required to place the affected rib region parallel with the plane of the film and (2) whether the projection should be made from above or below the diaphragm.

The anterior portions of the ribs, usually referred to simply as the anterior ribs, are often examined in the PA position. The posterior portions of the ribs, or more simply the posterior ribs, are examined in the AP position if the SID is less than 36 inches. The posterior ribs are well shown in the PA position if the SID is 36 inches or more.

The axillary portions of the ribs are best shown in an oblique position. Because the lateral position results in superimposition of the two sides, it is usually used only in the investigation of fluid and/or air levels.

When the ribs that are overshadowed by the heart are involved, the body must be rotated to project the ribs free of the heart shadow, or the radiographic exposure must be increased to compensate for the density of the heart. While the anterior and posterior ends are superimposed, the left ribs are cleared of the heart shadow in the left PA oblique position or the right AP oblique position. These two positions place the right-sided ribs parallel with the plane of the film and are reversed to obtain comparable projections of the left-sided ribs.

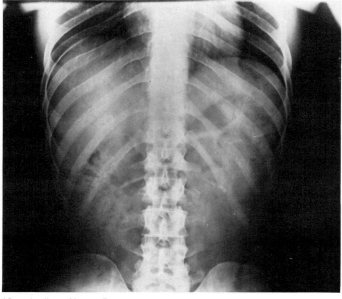

AP projection of lower ribs

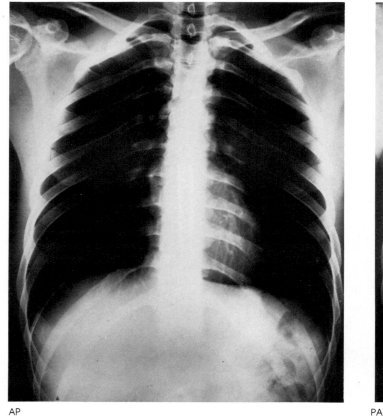

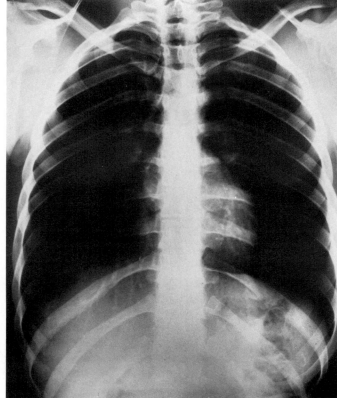

AP

PA

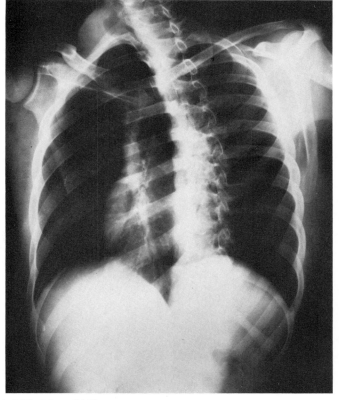

Left PA oblique (LAO)

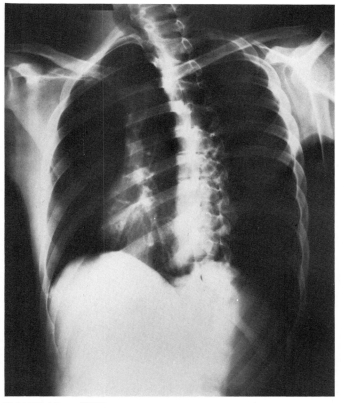

Right AP oblique (RPO)

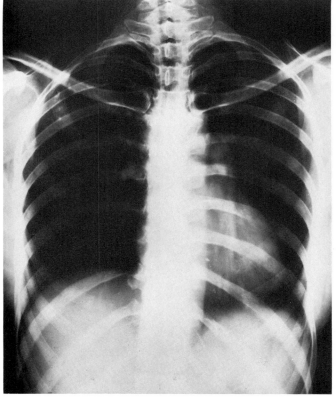

Quiet breathing

Suspended respiration

Upper anterior ribs
PA PROJECTION

Film: 14″ × 17″ lengthwise.

Position of patient

Place the patient for a PA projection, either erect or recumbent. Because the diaphragm descends to its lowest level in the erect position, the standing or the seated-erect position should be used for projections of the upper ribs when the patient's condition permits.

Position of part

Center the midsagittal plane of the body to the midline of the grid. Adjust the position of the cassette so that it projects approximately 1½ inches above the upper border of the shoulders.

Rest the patient's hands against his hips with the palms turned outward to rotate the scapulae away from the rib cage. Adjust the shoulders to lie in the same transverse plane. If the patient is supine, rest the head on the chin and adjust the midsagittal plane so that it is vertical.

Respiration is suspended at the end of full inhalation to depress the diaphragm as much as possible.

Central ray

With the central ray perpendicular to the plane of the film, center (1) to the midpoint of the film for the upper ribs or (2) approximately 5 inches proximal to the midpoint of the film for the seventh, eighth, and ninth ribs. In the latter case, high centering aids in projecting the shadow of the diaphragm below that of the affected rib.

Structures shown

A PA projection demonstrates the ribs above the diaphragm.

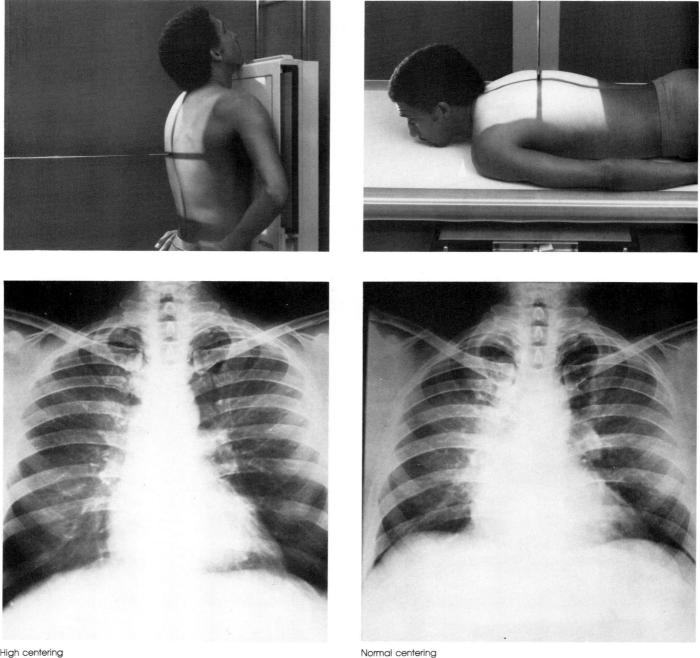

High centering

Normal centering

Posterior ribs
AP PROJECTION

Film: 14″ × 17″ lengthwise.

Position of patient

Place the patient in the AP position, either erect or recumbent. When the patient's condition permits, the erect position should be used for ribs above the diaphragm and the supine position for ribs below the diaphragm.

Position of part

Center the midsagittal plane of the body to the midline of the grid.

Ribs above diaphragm. Place the cassette lengthwise and center at the level of the sixth thoracic vertebra; the cassette will project about 1½ inches above the upper border of the shoulders.

Rest the patient's hands, palms outward, against the hips. Adjust the shoulders to lie in the same transverse plane, and rotate them forward to draw the scapulae away from the rib cage. The angle of the ribs can be decreased somewhat by having the patient extend his arms to the vertical position, the hands being supported on or under the head.

Have the patient suspend respiration at the end of full inhalation to depress the diaphragm.

Ribs below diaphragm. Place the cassette crosswise and center it at the level of the twelfth thoracic vertebra. The cassette will project approximately 1½ inches below the crests of the ilia.

Adjust the shoulders to lie in the same transverse plane, and place the arms in a comfortable position.

Respiration is suspended at the end of full exhalation for the purpose of elevating the diaphragm.

Central ray

With the central ray perpendicular to the plane of the film, center to the midpoint of the cassette.

Structures shown

An AP projection shows the posterior ribs above or below the diaphragm, according to the region examined.

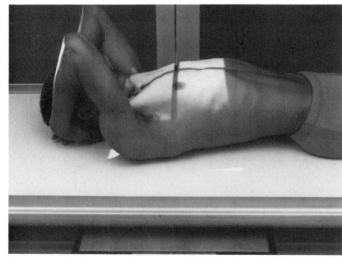

Ribs above diaphragm

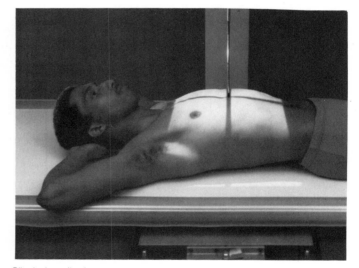

Ribs below diaphragm

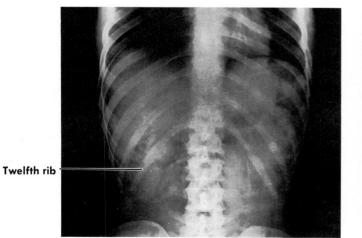

Twelfth rib

Full inhalation

Full exhalation

Axillary portion of ribs
AP OBLIQUE PROJECTION (RPO OR LPO)

Film: 14″ × 17″ lengthwise.

Position of patient

The patient may be examined in the erect or the recumbent position. Unless contraindicated by the patient's condition, the erect position is preferable for ribs above the diaphragm and the recumbent position for ribs below the diaphragm.

Position of part

From the AP position, rotate the body to an angle of approximately 45 degrees, the affected side toward the film. Center a plane midway between the midsagittal plane and the lateral surface of the body to the midline of the grid. If the patient is in the recumbent position, support the elevated hip.

Abduct the arm of the affected side and elevate it to carry the scapula away from the rib cage. Rest the hand on the patient's head if he is in the erect position, or place it under or above the head if he is in the recumbent position. The opposite extremity should be abducted with the hand on the hip.

Center the cassette at the level of the sixth thoracic vertebra for ribs above the diaphragm and at the level of the twelfth thoracic vertebra for ribs below the diaphragm. The cassette, placed lengthwise, may be centered midway between these points for a scout projection.

Breathing instructions

Respiration is suspended at the end of deep exhalation for ribs below the diaphragm and at the end of full inhalation for ribs above the diaphragm.

Central ray

With the central ray directed perpendicularly to the plane of the film, center to the midpoint of the cassette.

Structures shown

In this projection the axillary portion of the ribs are projected free of self-superimposition.

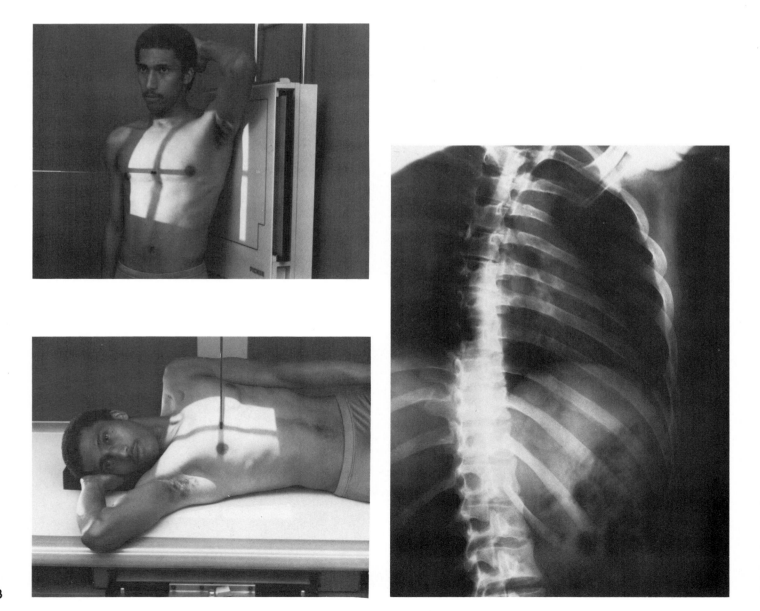

PA OBLIQUE PROJECTIONS
(RAO AND LAO)

Film: 14″ × 17″ lengthwise.

Position of patient

The patient may be examined in the erect or the recumbent position. Unless contraindicated by the patient's condition, the erect position should be used for ribs above the diaphragm, and the recumbent position for ribs below the diaphragm.

Position of part

From the PA position, rotate the body to an angle of approximately 45 degrees, with the affected side away from the cassette. If the patient is in the recumbent position, have him rest on the forearm and the flexed knee of the elevated side. Align the body so that a longitudinal plane midway between the midsagittal plane and the lateral surface of the body is centered to the midline of the grid.

Center the film at the level of the sixth thoracic vertebra for ribs above the diaphragm, at the level of the tenth thoracic vertebra for ribs below the diaphragm, or, placed lengthwise, midway between these points for a scout projection.

Breathing instructions

Respiration is suspended at the end of full exhalation for ribs above the diaphragm and at the end of full inhalation for ribs above the diaphragm.

Central ray

With the central ray perpendicular to the plane of the film, center to the midpoint of the cassette.

Structures shown

This projection demonstrates the axillary portion of the ribs, free of bony superimposition.

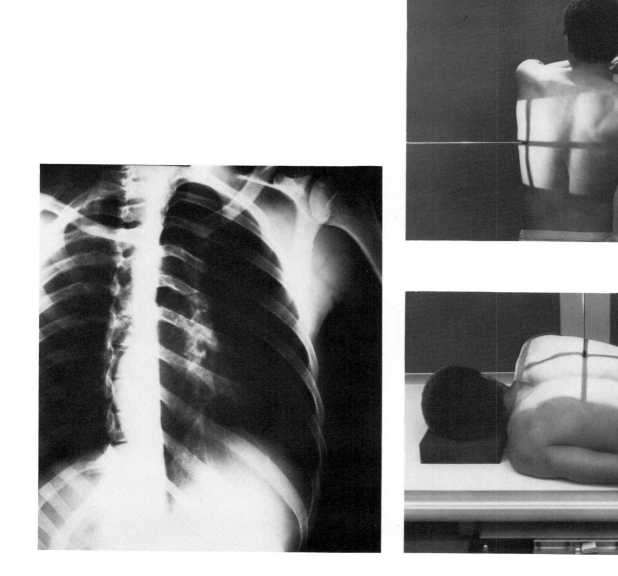

Costal joints
AP AXIAL PROJECTION
WILLIAMS METHOD

Williams[1] recommends this position for the demonstration of the costal joints in cases of rheumatoid spondylitis.

Film: $11'' \times 14''$ lengthwise.

Position of patient

Place the patient in the supine position. Let the head rest directly on the table to avoid accentuating the dorsal kyphosis.

Position of part

Adjust the body in a true AP position, with its midsagittal plane centered to the

[1]Williams, A. J.: Personal communication.

midline of the table. If the patient has an accentuated dorsal kyphosis, extend the arms over the head; otherwise the arms may be placed along the sides of the body. Adjust the shoulders to lie in the same transverse plane.

With the cassette in the Bucky tray, adjust its position so that the midpoint of the film will coincide with the central ray. The film will project approximately 4 inches beyond the upper border of the shoulders.

Compression may be applied across the thorax. Respiration is suspended at the end of full inhalation because the lung markings are less prominent at this phase of breathing.

Central ray

Direct the central ray through the sixth thoracic vertebra at an average angle of 20 degrees cephalad. Increase the central ray angulation slightly (5 to 10 degrees) when examining patients who have an accentuated dorsal kyphosis.

Structures shown

The costovertebral and costotransverse joints are demonstrated.

NOTE: Williams[1] states that in large-boned subjects it may be necessary to examine the two sides separately to demonstrate the costovertebral joints. This is done by alternately rotating the body approximately 10 degrees medially.

Hohmann and Gasteiger[2] state that in their studies of the costal joints (costovertebral and costotransverse) they have found that the central ray must usually be angled 30 degrees cephalad on the average patient. They increase the central ray angulation to 35 to 40 degrees when accentuated kyphosis is present, and in cases of severe curvature of the spine they also elevate the pelvis on a suitable support. For localized studies the central ray may be centered to T4 for the upper area and to T8 for the lower area.

These investigators have found a caudal angulation of the central ray, with the patient supine, helpful in differentiating osteoarthritis from degenerative changes of the ligamentum tuberculi costae.

They have further found that the lower costotransverse joints are best demonstrated in an oblique position wherein the patient is alternately rotated 20 degrees from the supine position. The joints of the elevated side are delineated.

[1]Williams, A.J.: Personal communication.
[2]Hohmann, D., and Gasteiger, W.: Roentgen diagnosis of the costovertebral joints, Fortschr. Roentgenstr. **112**:783-789, 1970. (In German.) Abstract: Radiology **98**:481, 1971.

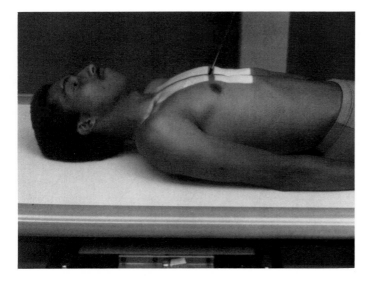

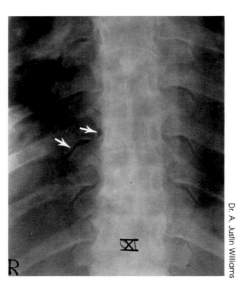

Dr. A. Justin Williams

12

Vertebral column

VERTEBRAL COLUMN

The vertebral column, which forms the central axis of the skeleton, is situated in the midsagittal plane of the posterior part of the trunk. It encloses and protects the spinal cord and acts as a support for the trunk. It supports the skull above and affords attachment for the ribs laterally, through which it supports the upper extremities. The column is supported by the hipbones at the sacroiliac joints, which through the hip joints transmit the weight of the trunk to the lower extremities. The column is composed of small segments of bone with disks of fibrocartilage interposed between their bodies to act as cushions; the whole is held together by ligaments and is so jointed and so curved that it has considerable flexibility and resilience.

In early life the vertebral column normally consists of 33 small, irregular bones called vertebrae. The vertebrae are divided into five groups and named according to the regions they occupy. The upper seven vertebrae occupy the region of the neck and are termed cervical vertebrae; the succeeding twelve bones lie in the dorsal portion of the thorax and are called the thoracic vertebrae. The five vertebrae occupying the region of the loin, or lumbus, are termed lumbar vertebrae; the following five are termed sacral vertebrae; and the vertebrae in the terminal group, which vary from three to five in number, are called the coccygeal vertebrae. The 24 segments in the upper three regions remain distinct throughout life and are termed the true, or movable, vertebrae. The segments in the two lower regions are called false, or fixed, vertebrae because of the change they undergo in the adult. The sacral segments always fuse into one bone termed the sacrum, whereas the coccygeal segments, referred to as the coccyx, have a tendency to fuse into one bone.

Viewed from the side the vertebral column presents four AP curves that arch anteriorly and posteriorly from the midaxillary line of the body. These curves are called cervical, thoracic, lumbar, and pelvic curves, for the regions they occupy. The cervical and lumbar curves are convex forward and are called lordotic curves. The thoracic and pelvic curves are concave forward and are called kyphotic curves. The upper curves merge smoothly, but the lumbar and pelvic curves are joined at an obtuse angle, the lumbosacral, or sacrovertebral, angle, which varies in different subjects. The thoracic and pelvic curves are called primary curves, because they are present at birth. The cervical and lumbar curves are called secondary, or compensatory, curves, because they are developed after birth. The cervical curve, which is the least pronounced of the curves, develops when the child begins to hold his head up at about 3 or 4 months of age and when he begins to sit alone at about 8 or 9 months of age. The lumbar curve develops when the child begins to walk at about 1 to 1½ years of age. The lumbar and pelvic curves are more pronounced in female subjects, causing a more acute angle at the lumbosacral junction.

Viewed from the front the vertebral column is seen to vary in width in the several regions. Generally the width gradually increases from the second cervical vertebra to the upper part of the sacrum, from which level it decreases sharply. There is sometimes a slight lateral curvature in the upper thoracic region. The convexity of this curve is to the right in right-handed persons and to the left in left-handed persons; for this reason it is believed to be the result of muscle action and to be influenced by occupation.

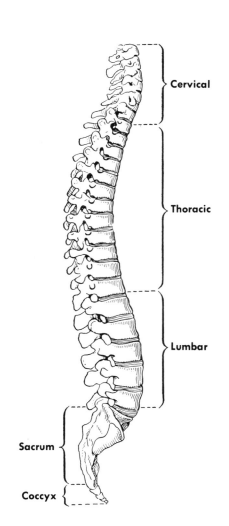

LATERAL ASPECT OF VERTEBRAL COLUMN

Viewed from the back the laminae and the projecting transverse and spinous processes are seen to form a deep depression on each side of the spinous processes. These bilateral depressions are called the *vertebral grooves,* and they contain the deep muscles of the back. The vertebral grooves are deeper in the thoracic region because of the sharp curve of the attached ribs.

The vertebral articulations consist of two types of joints: (1) amphiarthrodial joints, which are between the bodies of the vertebrae and permit only slight movement to individual vertebrae and (2) diarthrodial joints, which are between the vertebral arches and permit gliding movements. The movements permitted in the vertebral column by the combined action of the joints are flexion, extension, lateral, and rotary.

Typical vertebra. A typical vertebra is composed of two main parts—an anterior mass of bone called the body and a posterior, ringlike portion called the vertebral arch. The body and the vertebral arch enclose a space called the vertebral foramen. In the articulated column the vertebral foramina form the spinal, or neural, canal.

The body of the vertebra is composed largely of cancellous tissue covered by a layer of compact tissue. It is approximately cylindrical in shape. From above inferiorly its posterior surface is flattened, and its anterior and lateral surfaces are concave. The superior and inferior surfaces of the bodies are flattened and are covered by a plate of articular cartilage. In the articulated column the bodies are separated by cartilaginous disks that consist of a central mass of soft, pulpy, semigelatinous material called the nucleus pulposus, surrounded by an outer, firm portion called the annulus fibrosus.

The vertebral arch is formed by two pedicles and two laminae that support four articular processes, two transverse processes, and one spinous process. The pedicles are short, thick processes that project posteriorly, one from each side, from the upper lateral part of the posterior surface of the body. The upper and lower surfaces of the pedicles, or roots, are concave. These concavities are called vertebral notches, and by articulation with the vertebrae above and below the notches form intervertebral foramina for the transmission of the spinal nerves and blood vessels. The laminae are broad and flat and are directed posteriorly and medially from the pedicles.

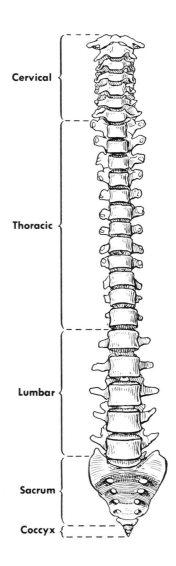

ANTERIOR ASPECT OF VERTEBRAL COLUMN

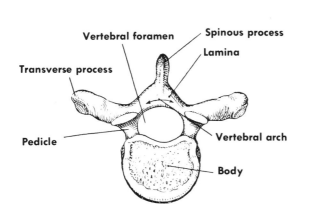

SUPERIOR ASPECT OF TYPICAL VERTEBRA

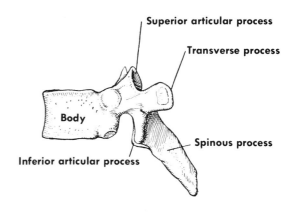

LATERAL ASPECT OF TYPICAL VERTEBRA

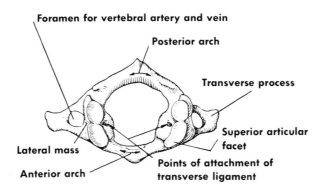

SUPERIOR ASPECT OF ATLAS

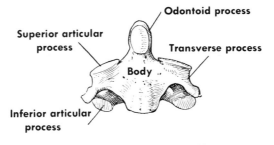

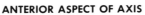

ANTERIOR ASPECT OF AXIS

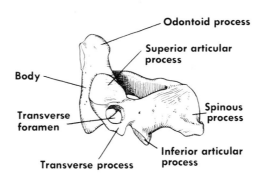

LATERAL ASPECT OF AXIS

The four articular processes (apophyses), two superior and two inferior, arise from the junction of the pedicles and laminae to articulate with the superjacent and subjacent vertebrae. Each superior apophysis presents an articular facet on its posterior surface, whereas the inferior processes present facets on their anterior surface. The planes of the facets vary in direction in the different regions and often in the same vertebra. The articulations between the vertebral arches are referred to as apophysial joints to distinguish them from the articulations between the bodies of the vertebrae.

The transverse processes project laterally and slightly posteriorly from the junction of the pedicles and laminae. The spinous process projects posteriorly and inferiorly from the junction of the laminae in the posterior midline.

The movable vertebrae, with the exception of the first and second cervical, are similar in general structure; however, each group has certain distinguishing characteristics that must be considered in radiography of the vertebral column.

CERVICAL VERTEBRAE

The *atlas,* the first cervical vertebra, is a ringlike structure having no body and no spinous process. It consists of an anterior arch, a posterior arch, two lateral masses, and two transverse processes. The anterior and posterior arches extend between the lateral masses, and the ring formed by them is divided into anterior and posterior portions by a ligament called the transverse atlantal ligament. The anterior portion of the ring receives the odontoid process of the axis, and the posterior portion transmits the proximal spinal cord.

The transverse processes are longer than those of the other cervical vertebrae, and they project laterally and slightly inferiorly from the lateral masses. Each lateral mass bears a superior and an inferior articular facet. The superior facets lie in a transverse plane, are large and deeply concave, and are shaped for the reception of the condyles of the occipital bone of the cranium. The articulations between the atlas and the occipital bone are diarthroses and are called the occipitocervical, or occipitoatlantal, articulations. The inferior facets are directed laterally and slightly inferiorly to articulate with the axis.

The *axis,* the second cervical vertebra, has a strong conical process arising from the upper surface of its body, which is called the odontoid process, or the *dens.* The odontoid is received into the anterior portion of the atlantal ring to act as a pivot or body for the atlas. At each side of the odontoid on the upper surface of the body are the superior articular facets, which are adapted to the inferior facets of the atlas. This pair of joints differs in both position and direction from the other cervical apophysial joints. The inferior articular processes of the axis have the same direction as those of the succeeding cervical vertebrae. The laminae of the axis are broad and thick. The spinous process is long and is horizontal in position.

The seventh cervical vertebra, which is termed the *vertebra prominens,* has a long, prominent spinous process that projects almost horizontally posteriorly. The spinous process of the vertebra prominens is easily palpable at the base of the neck posteriorly. It is convenient to use this process as a guide in localizing other vertebrae.

The *typical cervical* vertebrae have small, transversely oblong bodies that have slightly prolonged anteroinferior borders, resulting in an anteroposterior overlapping of the bodies in the articulated column.

The transverse processes of the cervical vertebrae arise partially from the side of the body and partially from the vertebral arch, are short and wide, are perforated by the transverse foramen for the transmission of the vertebral artery and vein, and present a deep concavity on their upper surfaces for the passage of the spinal nerves.

The pedicles project laterally and posteriorly from the body, and their superior and inferior vertebral notches are nearly equal in depth. The laminae are narrow and thin. The spinous processes are short, have bifid tips, and are directed posteriorly and slightly inferiorly. Their palpable tips lie at the level of the interspace below the body of the vertebra from which they spring.

The superior and inferior articular processes are situated behind the transverse process, where, arising at the junction of the pedicle and the lamina, they form a short column of bone that is usually referred to as the articular pillar. The superior and inferior articulating surfaces of the pillars are directed obliquely posteriorly and inferiorly so that the apophysial joints are not radiographically demonstrable in conventional frontal plane projections. The apophysial joints of the lower six cervical vertebrae are situated at right angles to the midsagittal plane of the body so that they are clearly demonstrated in a true lateral projection.

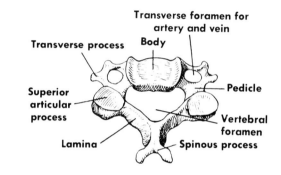

SUPERIOR ASPECT OF TYPICAL CERVICAL VERTEBRA

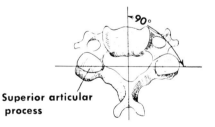

DIRECTION OF CERVICAL APOPHYSIAL JOINTS

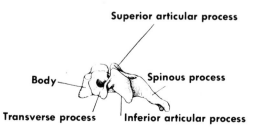

LATERAL ASPECT OF TYPICAL CERVICAL VERTEBRA

The *intervertebral foramina* of the cervical region lie at an angle of 45 degrees, open anteriorly to the midsagittal plane of the body and at an angle of approximately 15 degrees, open inferiorly, to the transverse plane of the body. Accurate radiographic demonstration of these foramina requires a longitudinal angulation of the central ray as well as medial rotation of the patient or a medial angulation of the central ray.

THORACIC VERTEBRAE

The bodies of the thoracic segments increase in size from above inferiorly and vary in form from those resembling the cervical bodies in the upper part of the region to those resembling the lumbar bodies in the lower part of the region. The bodies of the typical thoracic vertebrae, from the third to the ninth, are approximately triangular in form. The thoracic bodies are deeper behind than in front, and their posterior surface is concave from side to side. On each side of the bodies, at both the upper and lower posterior borders, are demifacets that form, with the demifacet of the superjacent and subjacent vertebrae, the articular surfaces for the heads of the ribs. The body of the first thoracic vertebra presents a whole facet above for the first rib and a demifacet below; the tenth, eleventh, and twelfth bodies present whole facets above and none below. The articulations between the ribs and the vertebral bodies are called costovertebral joints.

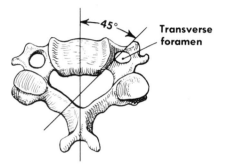

DIRECTION OF CERVICAL INTERVERTEBRAL FORAMINA

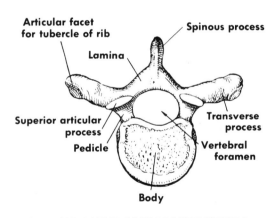

SUPERIOR ASPECT OF THORACIC VERTEBRA

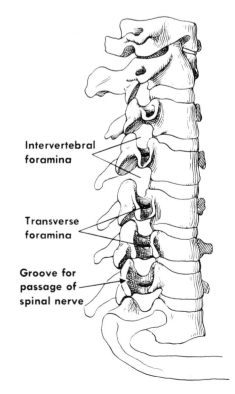

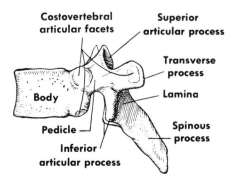

LATERAL ASPECT OF THORACIC VERTEBRA

ANTEROLATERAL ASPECT OF CERVICAL VERTEBRAE SHOWING INTERVERTEBRAL AND TRANSVERSE FORAMINA

The transverse processes of the thoracic vertebrae project obliquely laterally and posteriorly. With the exception of the eleventh and twelfth pairs, each process has, on the anterior surface of its extremity, a small concave facet for articulation with the tubercle of a rib. The articulations between the ribs and the transverse processes of the thoracic vertebrae are termed the costotransverse joints. The laminae are broad and thick and overlap the subjacent lamina. The spinous processes are long. From the fifth to the ninth vertebrae they project sharply inferiorly and overlap each other but are less vertical in direction above and below this region. The palpable tips of the spinous processes of the fifth to the ninth vertebrae correspond in position with the body of the subjacent vertebra. The upper and lower processes correspond in position with the interspace below the body from which they spring.

The *apophysial joints* of the thoracic region, except the inferior processes of the twelfth vertebra, angle forward approximately 15 to 20 degrees to form an angle of 70 to 75 degrees, open forward, to the midsaggital plane of the body. For the radiographic demonstration of the apophysial joints of the thoracic region, the body must be rotated 15 to 20 degrees from the lateral position, using anterior rotation to demonstrate the joints nearer the film and posterior rotation to demonstrate those farther from the film.

The *intervertebral foramina* of the thoracic region are perpendicular to the midsagittal plane of the body. They are clearly demonstrated radiographically in a true lateral position. The arms must be raised enough to elevate the ribs, which otherwise cross the intervertebral foramina.

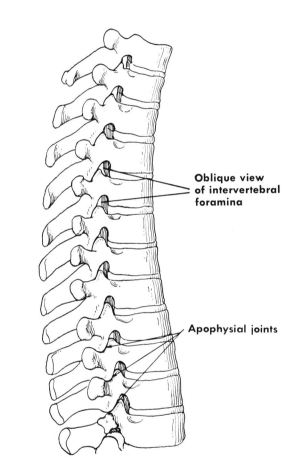

Oblique view of intervertebral foramina

Apophysial joints

POSTEROLATERAL ASPECT OF THORACIC VERTEBRAE SHOWING APOPHYSIAL JOINTS

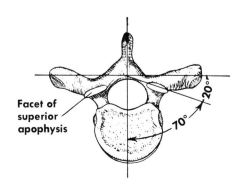

Facet of superior apophysis

DIRECTION OF THORACIC APOPHYSIAL JOINTS

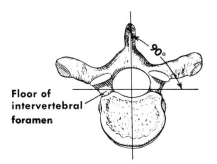

Floor of intervertebral foramen

DIRECTION OF THORACIC INTERVERTEBRAL FORAMINA

LUMBAR VERTEBRAE

The lumbar segments have large, bean-shaped bodies that increase in size from above inferiorly. They are deeper in front than behind, and their superior and inferior surfaces are flattened or slightly concave. The lumbar body, at its posterior surface, is flattened from above inferiorly and is transversely concave. Its anterior and lateral surfaces are concave from above inferiorly.

The transverse processes are smaller than those of the thoracic region. The upper three pairs are directed almost exactly laterally, whereas the lower two pairs are inclined slightly superiorly. The spinous processes are large, thick, and blunt and project almost horizontally posteriorly; their palpable tips correspond in position with the interspace below the vertebra from which they spring.

The body of the fifth lumbar segment is considerably deeper in front than behind, which gives it a wedge shape that adapts it for articulation with the sacrum. The articular disk of this joint is also more wedge shaped than are those in the interspaces above. The spinous process of the fifth lumbar vertebra is smaller and shorter and the transverse processes are much thicker than are those of the upper lumbar vertebrae.

The *apophysial joints* of the lumbar region are inclined posteriorly from the coronal plane, forming an angle, open posteriorly, of 30 to 50 degrees to the midsaggital plane of the body. These joints can be demonstrated radiographically by rotating the body from the AP or the PA position.

The *intervertebral foramina* of the lumbar region are situated at right angles to the midsagittal plane of the body, except the fifth, which turns slightly anteriorly. The upper four pairs of foramina are demonstrated in a true lateral position; the last pair requires a slight obliquity of the body.

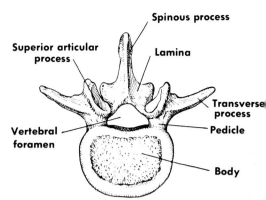

SUPERIOR ASPECT OF LUMBAR VERTEBRA

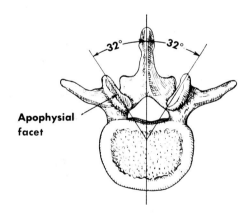

LATERAL ASPECT OF LUMBAR VERTEBRA

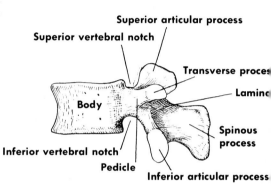

DIRECTION OF LUMBAR APOPHYSIAL JOINTS

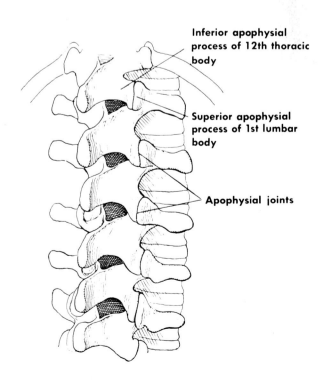

POSTEROLATERAL ASPECT OF LUMBAR VERTEBRAE SHOWING APOPHYSIAL JOINTS

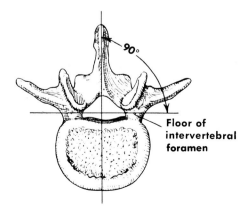

DIRECTION OF LUMBAR INTERVERTEBRAL FORAMINA

SACRUM AND COCCYX

The *sacrum* is formed by the fusion of the five sacral segments into a curved, triangular bone. The sacrum is wedged between the iliac bones of the hips, its broad base directed obliquely superiorly and anteriorly, and its apex directed posteriorly and inferiorly. Although there is a considerable variation in the size and in the degree of curvature of the sacrum in different subjects, the bone is normally longer, narrower, more evenly curved, and more vertical in position in male than in female subjects. The female sacrum is more acutely curved on itself, the greatest curvature being in the lower half of the bone, and it lies in a more oblique plane, which results in a sharper angle at the junction of the lumbar and pelvic curves.

The upper portion of the first sacral segment remains distinct and resembles the vertebrae of the lumbar region. The superior surface of the body of the sacrum corresponds in size and shape to the inferior surface of the last lumbar segment, with which it articulates to form the sacrovertebral, or lumbosacral, junction. The concavities on the upper surface of the pedicles of the first sacral segment, with the corresponding concavities on the lower surface of the pedicles of the last lumbar segment, form the last pair of intervertebral foramina. The superior articular processes of the first sacral segment articulate with the inferior articular processes of the last lumbar vertebra to form the last pair of apophysial joints.

The body of the sacrum has a prominent ridge at its upper anterior margin that is termed the sacral promontory. Directly behind the body is the sacral canal, the

continuation of the spinal canal, which is contained within the bone and transmits the sacral nerves. The anterior and posterior walls of the sacral canal are each perforated by four pairs of foramina for the passage of the sacral nerves and blood vessels.

On each side of the sacral body is a large, winglike lateral mass, or *ala*. At the upper anterior part of the lateral surface of each ala is a large articular process, the auricular surface, for articulation with similarly shaped processes on the iliac bones of the hips. The articulations between the sacrum and the ilia, the sacroiliac joints, slant obliquely posteriorly and medially at an angle of 25 to 30 degrees, open anteriorly to the midsagittal plane of the body. These joints are amphiarthroses by classification.

The inferior surface of the apex of the sacrum has an oval facet for articulation with the coccyx and two processes, the sacral cornua, which project inferiorly from the posterolateral aspect of the last sacral segment to join the cornua of the coccyx.

The *coccyx* is composed of three to five (usually four) rudimentary vertebrae that have a tendency to fuse into one bone in the adult. The coccyx diminishes in size from its base inferiorly to its apex. From its articulation with the sacrum it curves inferiorly and anteriorly, often deviating from the midsagittal plane of the body. Two processes, the coccygeal cornua, project superiorly from the posterolateral aspect of the first coccygeal segment to join the sacral cornua.

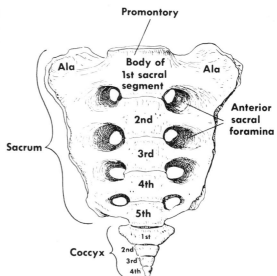

ANTERIOR ASPECT OF SACRUM AND COCCYX

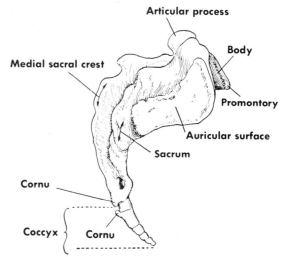

LATERAL ASPECT OF SACRUM AND COCCYX

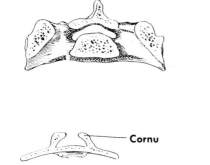

TRANSVERSE SECTIONS OF SACRUM

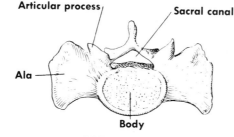

BASE OF SACRUM

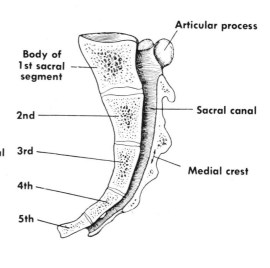

SAGITTAL SECTION OF SACRUM

209

RADIOGRAPHY

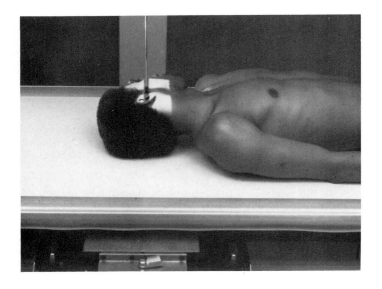

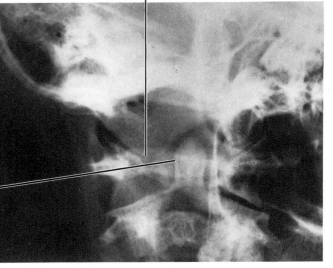

Occipitoatlantal articulation

Odontoid process

Occipitocervical articulations
AP OBLIQUE PROJECTION

Film: $8'' \times 10''$.

Position of patient

Place the patient in the supine position. Center the midsagittal plane of the body to the midline of the table, and adjust the shoulders to lie in the same transverse plane.

Position of part

Place the cassette in the Bucky tray and adjust the patient's head so that the midpoint of the cassette is 1 inch lateral to the midsagittal plane of the head at the level of the external auditory meatuses.

Rotate the head away from the side being examined. Adjust the flexion of the head to place the infraorbitomeatal line perpendicular to the film. Respiration is suspended for the exposure.

Central ray

Direct the central ray perpendicularly to the midpoint of the film. It enters 1 inch anteriorly to the external auditory meatus and emerges at the occipitoatlantal articulation.

Structures shown

A slightly oblique AP projection of the occipitoatlantal articulation is presented, the joint being projected between the orbit and the vertical ramus of the mandible. Both sides are examined for comparison.

The odontoid process of the axis is also well demonstrated in this projection so that it can be used for this purpose when a patient cannot be adjusted in the open-mouth position.

NOTE: Buetti[1] recommends a position for the occipitocervical articulations wherein the head is turned 45 to 50 degrees to one side, and with the mouth wide open the chin is drawn down as much as the open mouth will allow. The central ray is then directed vertically through the open mouth to the dependent mastoid tip.

[1]Buetti, C.: Zur Darstellung der Atlanto-epistropheal-Gelenke bzw. der Procc. transversi atlantis und epistrophei, Radiol. Clin. **20:**168-172, 1951.

BILATERAL PA PROJECTION

Film: 8″ × 10″ crosswise.

Position of patient

With the patient in the prone position, center the midsagittal plane of the body to the midline of the table. If the patient is thin, place a small, firm pillow under the chest to relieve strain in holding the position. Flex the patient's elbows, place the arms in a comfortable position, and adjust the shoulders to lie in the same transverse plane.

Position of part

Rest the patient's head on his forehead and nose and adjust it so that the midsagittal plane is perpendicular to the midline of the table.

Adjust the flexion of the head to place the orbitomeatal line perpendicular to the plane of the film; center the film at or slightly below the level of the infraorbital margins. Respiration is suspended for the exposure.

Central ray

Direct the central ray perpendicularly to the midpoint of the film. It enters the back of the neck at the level of the infraorbital margins.

Structures shown

This method demonstrates a PA projection of the occipitocervical joints projected through the antra.

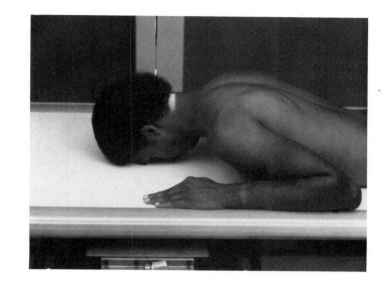

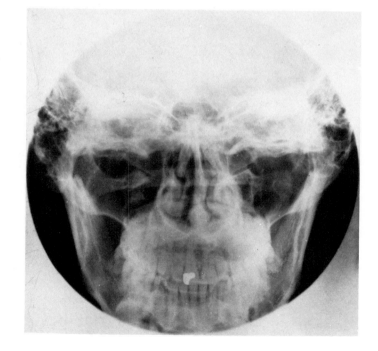

Atlas and axis (open mouth)

AP PROJECTION

The open-mouth method was described by Albers-Schönberg[1] in 1910 and by George[2] in 1919.

Film: 8″ × 10″.

Position of patient

With the patient in the supine position, center the midsagittal plane of the body to the midline of the table. Place the patient's arms along the sides of his body, and adjust the shoulders to lie in the same transverse plane.

[1]Albers-Schönberg, H.E.: Die Röntgentechnik, ed. 3, Hamburg, 1910, Gräfe & Sillem.
[2]George, A.W.: Method for more accurate study of injuries to the atlas and axis, Boston Med. Surg. J. **181**:395-398, 1919.

Position of part

Place the cassette in the Bucky tray and center it at the level of the second cervical segment. Adjust the patient's head so that the midsagittal plane is perpendicular to the plane of the table.

Set the exposure, and move the x-ray tube into position so that any minor change can be made quickly after the final adjustment of the patient's head. This position is not easy to hold; however, the patient is usually able to cooperate fully, unless he is kept in the final, strained position too long.

Have the patient open his mouth as wide as possible, and then adjust the head so that a line from the lower edge of the upper incisors to the tip of the mastoid process is perpendicular to the film.

Instruct the patient to keep his mouth wide open and to softly phonate "ah" during the exposure. This will affix the tongue in the floor of the mouth so that its shadow will not be projected on that of the atlas and axis and will prevent movement of the mandible.

Central ray

Direct the central ray perpendicularly to the midpoint of the open mouth.

Structures shown

This method presents an AP projection of the atlas and axis through the open mouth.

If the patient has a deep head or a long mandible, the entire atlas will not be demonstrated. When the exactly superimposed shadows of the inferior margins of the upper teeth and the base of the skull are in line with those of the tips of the mastoid processes, the position cannot be improved.

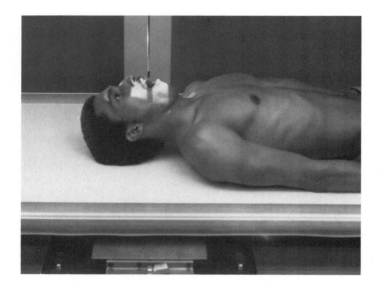

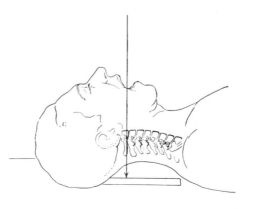

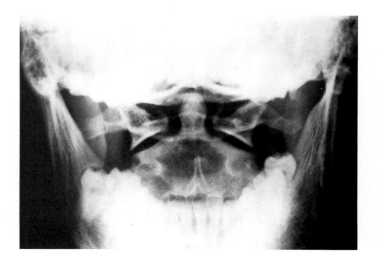

Odontoid process
AP PROJECTION
FUCHS METHOD

Film: 8″ × 10″ crosswise.

Position of patient

With the patient in the supine position, center the midsagittal plane of the body to the midline of the table. Place the arms along the sides of the body, and adjust the shoulders to lie in the same transverse plane.

Position of part

Place the cassette in the Bucky tray and center it to the level of the tips of the mastoid processes. Extend the chin until the tip of the chin and the tip of the mastoid process are vertical. Adjust the head so that the midsagittal plane is perpendicular to the plane of the table. Respiration is suspended for the exposure.

Central ray

Direct the central ray perpendicularly to the midpoint of the film; it enters the neck just distal to the tip of the chin.

Structures shown

An AP projection of the odontoid process is shown, lying within the shadow of the foramen magnum.

Fuchs[1] has recommended this position for the demonstration of the dens when its upper half is not clearly shown in the open-mouth position. This position must not be attempted if there is a fracture or degenerative disease of the upper cervical region. Patients suspected of having such a condition should be examined by tomography.

[1]Fuchs, A.W.: Cervical vertebrae (part 1), Radiogr. Clin. Photogr. **16**:2-17, 1940.

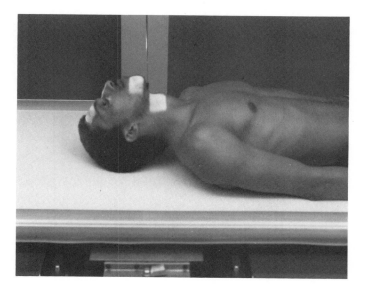

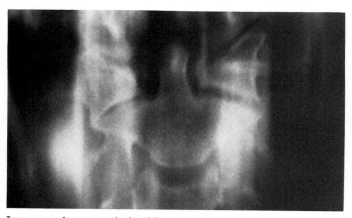

Tomogram of upper cervical vertebrae

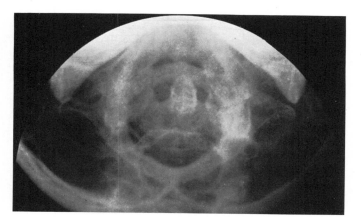

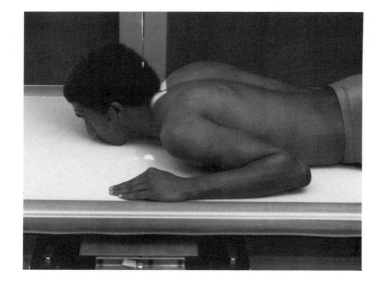

Atlas and odontoid process
PA PROJECTION
JUDD METHOD

Film: 8″ × 10″ crosswise.

Position of patient

With the patient in the prone position, center the midsagittal plane of the body to the midline of the table. Flex the patient's elbows, place the arms in a comfortable position, and adjust the shoulders to lie in the same transverse plane.

Position of part

Have the patient extend his chin and rest it on the table. Place the cassette in the Bucky tray and adjust it so that the midpoint is centered to the throat at the level of the upper margin of the thyroid cartilage.

Adjust the head so that the tip of the nose is about 1 inch from the tabletop and so that the midsagittal plane is perpendicular to the table. Respiration is suspended for the exposure.

Central ray

Direct the central ray perpendicularly to the midpoint of the film. It enters the occiput just posterior to the mastoid tips.

Structures shown

An AP projection of the odontoid process is shown, as seen through the foramen magnum.

The technologist should not attempt this position with a patient who has an unhealed fracture nor with a patient who has a degenerative disease of the upper cervical region.

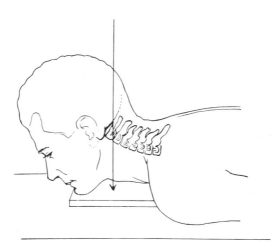

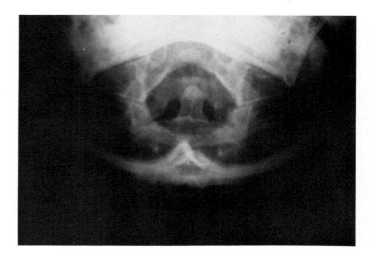

Odontoid process
AP OBLIQUE PROJECTION
KASABACH METHOD

Film: 8″ × 10″.

Position of patient

With the patient in the supine position, center the midsagittal plane of the body to the midline of the table. Place the arms along the sides of the body, and adjust the shoulders to lie in the same transverse plane.

Position of part

Place the cassette in the Bucky tray and center it to the midsagittal plane at the level of the mastoid tip.

Rotate the head approximately 40 to 45 degrees away from the side being examined and adjust the head so that the infraorbitomeatal line is perpendicular to the plane of the table. Respiration is suspended for the exposure.

For right-angle projections of the odontoid make one exposure with the head turned to the right and one with it turned to the left.

Central ray

With the central ray angled 10 to 15 degrees caudad, center to a point midway between the outer canthus and the external auditory meatus.

Structures shown

An oblique projection of the odontoid process is shown, which Kasabach[1] has recommended for use in conjunction with the AP and lateral projections.

The head of a patient who has a possible fracture or degenerative disease must not be rotated. Kasabach[1] has recommended that the entire body, rather than only the head, be rotated.

NOTE: Herrmann and Stender[2] have described a position for the demonstration of the occipitoatlantal-odontoid relationship, wherein the head is adjusted as for the Kasabach method. The central ray is then directed vertically midway between the mastoid processes at the level of the occipitocervical joints.

[1]Kasabach, H.H.: A roentgenographic method for the study of the second cervical vertebra, A.J.R. **42**:782-785, 1939.

[2]Herrmann, E., and Stender, H.: Ein einfache Aufnahmetechnik zur Darstellung der Dens axis, Fortsenr. Roentgenstr. **96**:115-119, 1962.

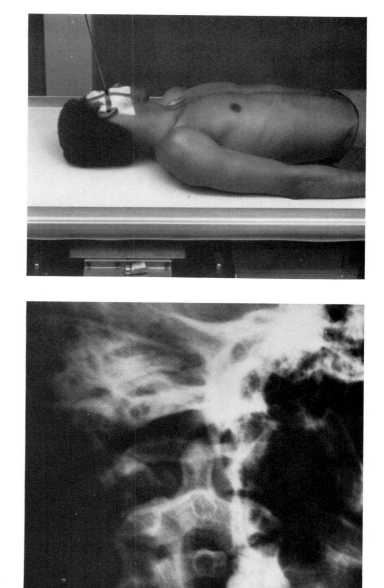

Atlas and axis
LATERAL PROJECTION

Film: 8″ × 10″.

Position of patient

With the patient supine, adjust the body in a true AP position. Place the arms along the sides of the body, and adjust the shoulders to lie in the same transverse plane.

Position of part

With the cassette in the vertical position and in contact with the upper neck, center at the level of the atlantoaxial articulation (1 inch distal to the tip of the mastoid process). Adjust the cassette so that it is parallel with the midsagittal plane of the neck and then support it in position.

Extend the chin slightly so that the shadow of the mandibular rami will not overlap that of the spine. Adjust the head so that the midsagittal plane is perpendicular to the table. Respiration is suspended for the exposure.

Central ray

Direct the central ray horizontally to a point 1 inch distal to the adjacent mastoid tip.

Structures shown

A lateral projection of the atlas and axis is demonstrated. The occipitocervical articulations are also demonstrated. Because of the short part-film distance, better detail is obtained with this method than with the customary method of performing the lateral examination of the cervical vertebrae. A grid and close collimation should be used to minimize secondary radiation.

Pancoast, Pendergrass, and Schaeffer[1] recommend that the head be rotated slightly to prevent superimposition of the laminae of the atlas. They recommend a slight transverse tilt of the head for the demonstration of the arches of the atlas.

NOTE: Smith and Abel[2] describe a method for the demonstration of the laminae and articular processes of the upper cervical vertebrae. They slightly extend the patient's head, and the mouth is opened wide. The central ray is directed 35 degrees caudad and centered to the third cervical vertebra. The exposure is made with the head passively rotated 10 degrees to the side, thus removing the mandible from the overlying areas of interest.

[1]Pancoast, H.K., Pendergrass, E.P., and Schaeffer, J.P.: The head and neck in roentgen diagnosis, Springfield, Ill., 1940, Charles C Thomas, Publisher.
[2]Smith, G., and Abel, M.: Visualization of the posterolateral elements of the upper cervical vertebrae in the anteroposterior projection, Radiology 115:219-220, 1975.

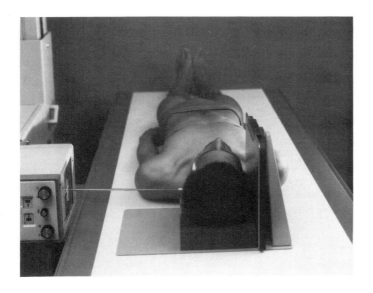

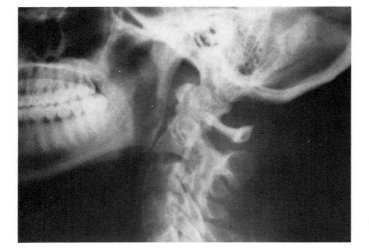

Lower cervical vertebrae
AP PROJECTION

Film: 8″ × 10″ lengthwise.

Position of patient

The patient is placed in the AP position, either recumbent or erect.

Position of part

Center the midsagittal plane of the patient's body to the midline of the table or vertical grid device. Adjust the shoulders to lie in the same transverse plane to prevent rotation.

Extend the head enough to place the occlusal plane and the mastoid tips in the same transverse plane to prevent superim-

position of the mandible and the midcervical vertebrae.

Adjust the position of the cassette so that the center of the cassette will coincide with the central ray.

Central ray

Direct the central ray through the fourth cervical body at an angle of 15 to 20 degrees cephalad. It enters at or slightly inferior to the most prominent point of the thyroid cartilage.

Structures shown

This projection shows the lower five cervical bodies and the upper two or three thoracic bodies, the interpediculate spaces, the superimposed transverse and articular processes, and the intervertebral disk spaces.

This position is also used to demonstrate the presence or absence of cervical ribs.

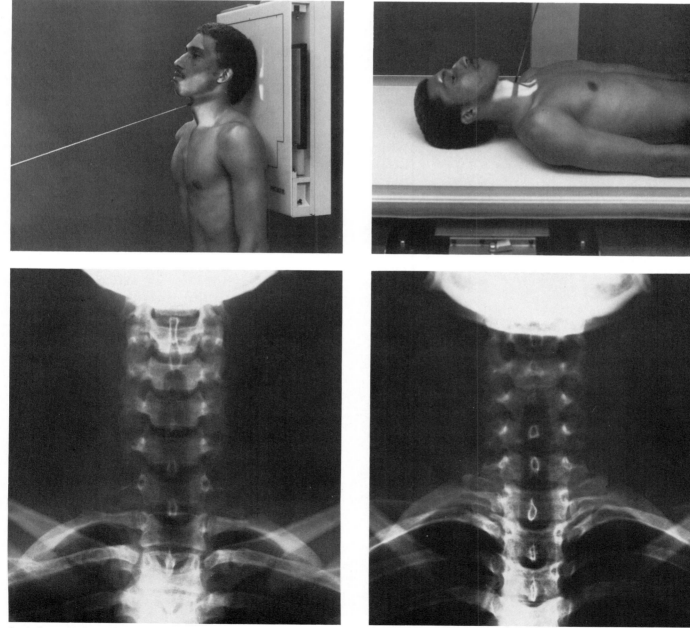

Cephalic angulation of 20 degrees

Angulation of 0 degrees; same patient as in adjacent radiograph

217

Cervical vertebrae
LATERAL PROJECTIONS
Grandy method[1]

Film: 8″ × 10″ lengthwise.

Position of patient

Place the patient in a lateral position, either seated or standing, before a vertical grid device. Have him sit or stand straight, and adjust the height of the cassette so that it is centered at the level of the fourth cervical segment.

Position of part

Center the coronal plane that passes through the tips of the mastoid processes

[1]Grandy, C.C.: A new method for making radiographs of the cervical vertebrae in the lateral position, Radiology 4:128-129, 1925.

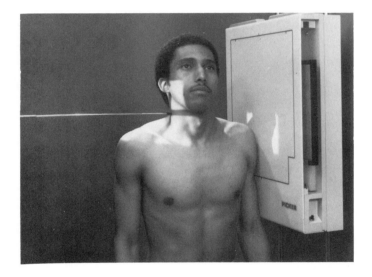

to the midline of the film. Move the patient close enough to the stand to permit him to rest the adjacent shoulder against it for support.

Rotate the shoulders anteriorly or posteriorly, according to the natural kyphosis of the back: if the subject is round shouldered, rotate them anteriorly; otherwise, rotate them posteriorly. Adjust the shoulders to lie in the same transverse plane, depress them as much as possible, and immobilize them by having the patient hold one small sandbag in each hand. The sandbags should be of equal weight. Another method that is sometimes more suitable is to place a long strip of gauze bandage under the patient's feet, or, if he is seated, under the rungs of the stool, and

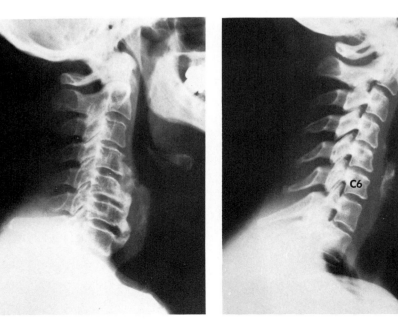

have him grasp one end of the gauze in each hand and pull. This will allow the shoulders to be depressed, according to the needs of the patient.

Adjust the body in a true lateral position, with the long axis of the cervical vertebrae parallel with the plane of the film. Elevate the chin slightly to prevent superimposition of the mandibular rami and the spine, and, with the midsagittal plane of the head vertical, ask the patient to look steadily at one spot on the wall to aid in maintaining the position of his head. The fraction of a second needed for the exposure time of this projection makes elaborate immobilization measures unnecessary in a majority of cases.

Respiration is suspended at the end of full exhalation to obtain maximum depression of the shoulders.

Central ray

Direct the central ray horizontally to the midpoint of the film.

Taylor[1] recommends centering at the level of the external auditory meatuses for the purpose of projecting the magnified shadow of the shoulder remote from the film below those of the lower cervical segments.

Because of the great part-film distance, an S.I.D. of at least 60 inches should be used to obtain the finest detail possible.

Structures shown

This method presents a lateral projection of the cervical bodies and their interspaces, the articular pillars, the lower five articular facets, and the spinous processes. Depending on how well the shoulders can be depressed, the seventh cervical vertebra and sometimes the upper one or two thoracic vertebrae can also be seen.

NOTE: This method of obtaining the lateral projection of the cervical spine was described by Grandy[2] in 1925. Before that time the patient was examined in the recumbent position, with the cassette in contact with the neck.

[1]Taylor, H.K.:Personal communication.
[2]Grandy, C.C.: A new method for making radiographs of the cervical vertebrae in the lateral position, Radiology 4:128-129, 1925.

Flexion-extension studies

As for the neutral lateral projection of the cervical vertebrae, the patient is adjusted in an exact lateral position and instructed to sit or stand erect.

While keeping the midsagittal plane of his head and neck parallel with the plane of the film:

1. Ask the patient to drop his head forward and then to draw his chin as close as possible to his chest to place the cervical vertebrae in a position of extreme flexion for the first exposure.

2. Ask the patient to elevate his chin as much as possible to place the cervical vertebrae in a position of extreme extension for the second exposure.

Functional studies of the cervical vertebrae in the lateral position are made for the purpose of demonstrating normal ante-roposterior movement or, as a result of trauma or disease, an absence of movement. The spinous processes are elevated and widely separated in the flexion position and are depressed in close approximation in the extension position.

NOTE: Ott et al.[1] recommend, in addition to the routine projections, tomography in the neutral lateral position and in the hyperflexed lateral position for the demonstration of luxation of the atlantoaxial joint in cases of rheumatoid arthritis.

[1]Ott, H., et al.: Radiologic examination of the cervical spine in rheumatoid arthritis, Schweiz. Med. Wochenschr. 100:1726-1730. (In German.) Abstract: Radiology 100:233, 1971.

Spinous processes

The demonstration of the cervicothoracic spinous processes is frequently requested for patients who have sustained an injury of a direct or a whiplash type. When the patient has reasonably flexible shoulders, he can be adjusted in a direct lateral position, as described below. When, because of pain or bodily habitus, the patient cannot be so positioned, the spinous processes can be demonstrated quite satisfactorily with the AP oblique apophysial joint position, described on pp. 233 and 234.

Seat the patient in a lateral position before a vertical grid device. Center the cassette and the central ray at the level of the second or third thoracic vertebra. Rotate the shoulders well anteriorly and inferiorly, and have the patient hold them in position by grasping his knees or by crossing his forearms and grasping his upper arms. Readjust the body position to center the cervicothoracic vertebrae to the midline of the grid. Instruct the patient to drop his head forward and pull his chin down as much as possible to elevate the spinous processes into a position of prominence. Respiration is suspended for the exposure.

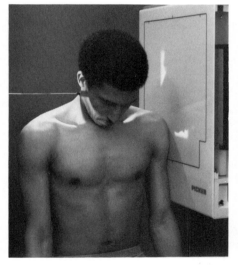
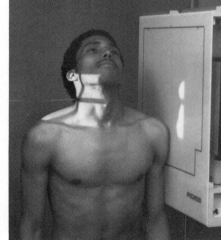

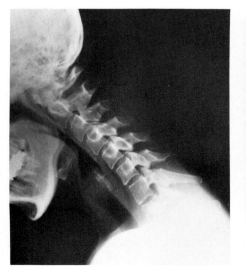

Flexion

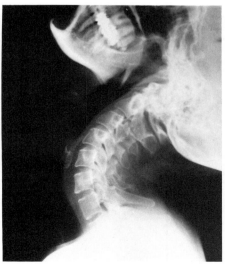

Extension

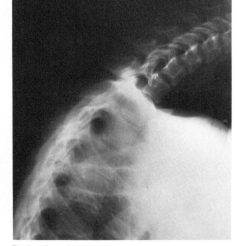

Flexion for spinous processes

Cervical intervertebral foramina

PA OBLIQUE AXIAL PROJECTION (RAO AND LAO)

Oblique projections for the demonstration of the cervical intervertebral foramina were first described by Barsóny and Koppenstein.[1,2]

Film: 8″ × 10″ lengthwise.

Position of patient

The patient is placed in the PA position. For the patient's comfort and to facilitate accurate adjustment of the part, the standing or seated erect position is preferable for oblique studies of the cervical spine.

[1]Barsóny, T., and Koppenstein, E.: Eine neue Method zur Röntgenuntersuchung der Halswirbelsäule, Fortschr. Roentgenstr. **35**:593-594, 1926.
[2]Barsóny, T., and Koppenstein, E.: Beitrag zur Aufnahmetechnik der Halswirbelsäule; Darstellung der Foramina intervertebralia, Röntgenpraxis **1**:245-249, 1929.

Position of part

Keeping one shoulder adjacent to the film (both sides are examined for comparison), rotate the patient's *entire body* to approximately the 45-degree angle required to place the foramina parallel with the film, and then center the cervical spine to the midline of the vertical grid device or table. The foramina *closest* to the cassette are demonstrated.

To allow for the caudal angulation of the central ray the cassette is centered at the level of the fifth cervical segment (1 inch distal to the most prominent point of the thyroid cartilage).

Erect position. Ask the patient to sit or stand straight without strain and, with the arm hanging free, to rest the adjacent shoulder against the grid device. Adjust the degree of body rotation with the use of a protractor.

With the midsagittal plane of the head coextensive with that of the spine, elevate the chin slightly to prevent superimposition of the shadows of the mandibular rami and the foramina. If preferred, the head may be turned slightly, but care must be exercised to avoid rotation of the upper cervical segments.

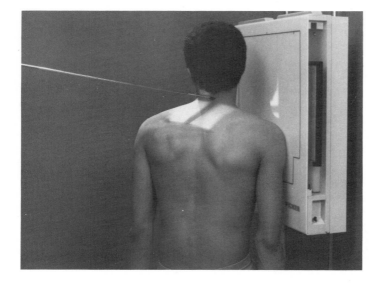

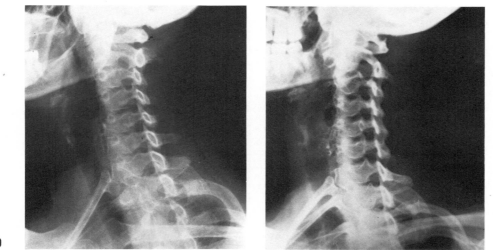

Semiprone position. With the patient's body at an angle of 45 degrees and the cervical spine centered to the midline of the table, have the patient support himself on the forearm and flexed knee of the elevated side. Adjust a suitable support under the head to place the long axis of the cervical column parallel with the film. Check and adjust the degree of body rotation.

Adjust the position of the patient's head so that the midsagittal plane is coextensive with that of the spine, and extend the head just enough to prevent superimposition of the shadows of the mandibular rami and the intervertebral foramina.

Central ray

Direct the central ray to the fourth cervical vertebra at an angle of 15 to 20 degrees caudad so that it will coincide with the angle of the foramina.

Structures shown

This method demonstrates the intervertebral foramina and pedicles closest to the film and an oblique projection of the bodies and other parts of the cervical column.

Oblique flexion-extension projections

Boylston[1] has suggested functional studies of the cervical vertebrae in the oblique position for the demonstration of fractures of the articular processes and of obscure dislocations and subluxations. The manipulation of the patient's head must be performed by a physician when an acute injury has been sustained.

The patient is placed in a direct PA position with his shoulders held firmly against the grid device. The head is carefully rotated maximally to one side and kept so, while the neck is flexed for the first exposure and extended for the second exposure. Both sides are examined for comparison.

[1]Boylston, B.F.: Oblique roentgenographic views of the cervical spine in flexion and extension; an aid in the diagnosis of cervical subluxations and obscure dislocations, J. Bone Joint Surg. **39-A:**1302-1309, 1957.

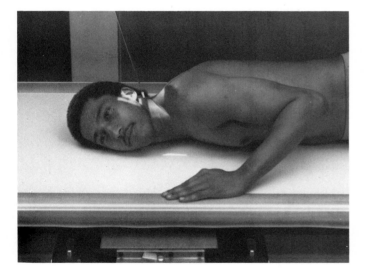

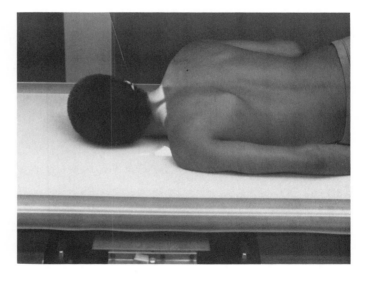

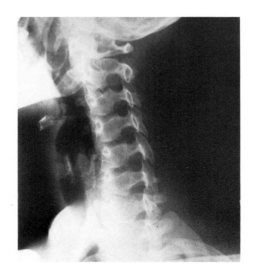

AP OBLIQUE AXIAL PROJECTION (RPO AND LPO)

Film: 8″ × 10″ lengthwise.

Position of patient

The patient is placed in the AP position. The erect position, standing or seated, is preferable for the patient's comfort and for greater ease of adjustment.

Position of part

Adjust the body at a 45-degree angle to obtain a profile of the foramina, and center the cervical spine to the midline of the cassette.

To compensate for the cranial angulation of the central ray, center the cassette to the third cervical body (1 inch proximal to the most prominent point of the thyroid cartilage).

Erect position. Ask the patient to sit or stand straight without strain and to rest the adjacent shoulder firmly against the vertical film holder for support. Check and adjust the degree of body rotation with a protractor. Being careful not to rotate the cervical spine, turn the head away from the side being examined (the side remote from the film) just enough to prevent superimposition of the shadows of the mandibular rami and the foramina.

Semisupine position. With the patient's body rotated approximately 45 degrees and the cervical spine centered to the midline of the table, place suitable supports under the lower thorax and the elevated hip. Place a support under the head and adjust it so the the cervical column is horizontal.

Using a protractor, check and adjust the 45-degree body rotation. Turn the head just enough to prevent superimposition of the shadows of the mandibular rami and the foramina, being careful to avoid rotation of the cervical spine.

Central ray

Direct the central ray to the fourth cervical vertebra at an angle of 15 to 20 degrees cephalad so that the beam coincides with the angle of the foramina.

Structures shown

The angulation of the central ray demonstrates the intervertebral foramina and pedicles farthest from the film and an oblique projection of the bodies and other parts of the cervical vertebrae.

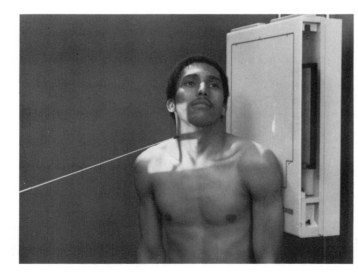

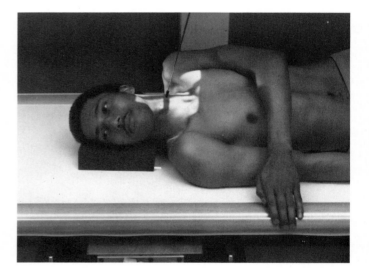

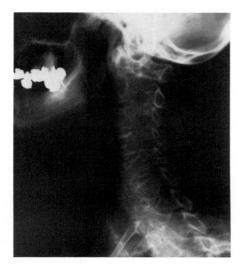

Cervical vertebrae
AP PROJECTION
OTTONELLO METHOD

With the Ottonello method, the mandibular shadow is blurred, if not obliterated, by utilizing an even chewing motion of the mandible during the exposure. The head must be rigidly immobilized to prevent movement of the vertebrae. The exposure time must be long enough to cover several complete excursions of the mandible.

Film: 8″ × 10″ lengthwise.

Position of patient

With the patient in the supine position, center the midsagittal plane of the body to the midline of the table. Place the arms along the sides of the body, and adjust the shoulders to lie in the same transverse plane. Place a long sandbag under the ankles for the patient's comfort.

Position of part

Adjust the head so that the midsagittal plane is perpendicular to the table. Elevate the chin enough to place the edges of the upper incisors and the mastoid tips in the same transverse plane. Immobilize the head, and have the patient practice opening and closing his mouth until he can move the mandible smoothly without striking the teeth together.

With the cassette in the Bucky tray, center it at the level of the fourth cervical vertebra.

Central ray

Direct the central ray perpendicularly to the midpoint of the film.

Structures shown

An AP projection of the entire cervical column is shown with the shadow of the mandible being blurred if not obliterated.

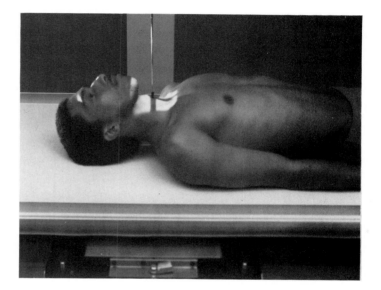

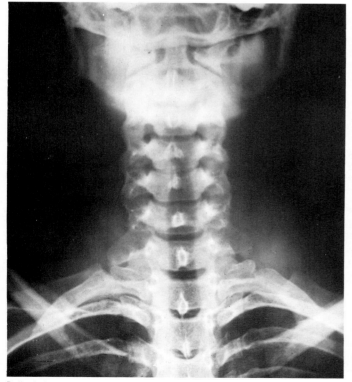

Patient chewing motion

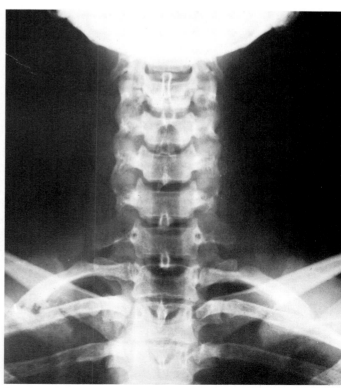

Conventional

Cervical and upper thoracic vertebrae
VERTEBRAL ARCH PROJECTIONS[1,2]

The vertebral arch projections, sometimes referred to as *pillar* or *lateral mass* projections, are employed for the demonstration of the posterior elements of the cervical and upper three or four thoracic vertebrae, the articular processes and their facets, the laminae, and the spinous processes. The central ray angulations employed project the vertebral arch elements free of the shadows of the anteriorly situated vertebral bodies and transverse processes so that when the central ray angu-

[1]Dorland, P., and Frémont, J.: Aspect radiologique normal du rachis postérieur cervicodorsal (vue postérieure ascendante), Semaine Hop. PP.1457-1464, 1957.

[2]Dorland, P., et al.: Techniques d'examen radiologique de l'arc postérieur des vertebres cervicodorsales, J. Radiol. Electrol. 39:509-519, 1958.

lation is correct the resultant film resembles a hemisection of the vertebrae. In addition to frontal plane delineation of the articular pillars and facets, these projections are especially useful for the demonstration of the cerviothoracic spinous processes in patients with a whiplash injury.[1]

Film: 8″ × 10″ or 10″ × 12″ lengthwise.

AP axial projection
Position of patient

The patient is adjusted in the supine position, with the midsagittal plane of the body centered to the midline of the table.

[1]Abel, M.S.: Moderately severe whiplash injuries of the cervical spine and their roentgenologic diagnosis, Clin. Orthop. 12:189-208, 1958.

Depress his shoulders and adjust them to lie in the same transverse plane; if necessary, place a long strip of bandage around the patient's feet, and with his knees slightly flexed, have him grasp the ends of the bandage and then extend his knees to depress the shoulders.

Position of part

With the midsagittal plane of the head perpendicular to the table, *hyperextend* the head; the success of this axial projection depends on the hyperextension. When the patient cannot tolerate hyperextension without undue discomfort, use an oblique projection.

Adjust the position of the cassette so that the upper edge of the film is at the level of the external auditory meatuses.

Central ray

Direct the central ray to the seventh cervical vertebra at an average angle of 25 (20 to 30) degrees caudad. It enters the neck in the region of the thyroid cartilage.

The degree of the central ray angulation is determined by the cervical lordosis. The aim is to have the central ray coincide with the plane of the articular facets, so that a greater angle is required when the cervical curve is accentuated and a lesser angle is required when the curve is diminished. To reduce an accentuated cervical curve and thus place the third to seventh cervical vertebrae in the same plane as the first to fourth thoracic vertebrae, the originators[1] have suggested that a radioparent wedge be placed under the neck and shoulders, with the head extended somewhat over the edge of the wedge.

[1]Dorland, P., et al.: Techniques d'examen radiologique de l'arc postérieur des vertebres cervicodorsales, J. Radiol. Electrol. 39:509-519, 1958.

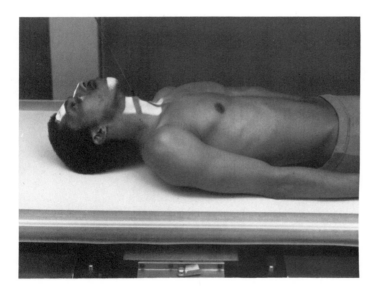

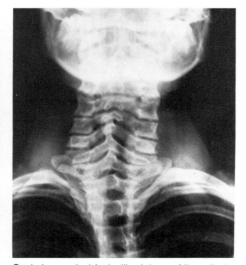

Head fully extended but central ray angulation inadequate

Central ray coincident with plateau of the articular facets

OBLIQUE AXIAL PROJECTIONS

AP oblique axial projection
Position of part

With the patient adjusted in the supine position, as for the direct AP projection, rotate the head 45 to 50 degrees toward the unaffected side. Examine both sides for comparison. A 45- to 50-degree rotation of the head usually demonstrates the articular facets of the second to seventh cervical vertebrae and of the first thoracic vertebra. A rotation of as much as 60 to 70 degrees is sometimes required for the demonstration of the facets of the sixth and seventh cervical vertebrae and of the first to fourth thoracic vertebrae.

Central ray

Direct the central ray to the seventh cervical vertebra at an average angle of 35 (30 to 40) degrees caudad.

PA oblique axial projection
Position of patient

Adjust the patient in the prone position, which seems to be more comfortable for injured patients than the supine position. Center the midsagittal plane of the body to the midline of the table. When the patient is thin, place a pillow under his chest to obviate accentuation of the cervical curve. Depress the shoulders and adjust them to lie in the same transverse plane.

Position of part

1. For a PA axial projection showing both sides on one film, rest the patient's head on his fully extended chin with the midsagittal plane of the head perpendicular to the table.

2. For a PA oblique axial projection, rest the patient's head on one cheek (both sides are examined for comparison), and adjust the head so that the midsagittal plane is at an angle of 45 degrees.

For the demonstration of the second to fifth cervical vertebrae, flex the head somewhat to reduce the cervical curve. For the fifth to seventh cervical vertebrae and the first to fourth thoracic vertebrae, adjust the head in moderate extension.

Position the cassette so that the distal edge of the film is at the level of the tip of the seventh cervical spinous process.

Central ray

Direct the central ray to the seventh cervical vertebra (1) at an average angle of 40 (35 to 45) degrees cephalad for the direct PA axial projection and (2) at an average angle of 35 (30 to 40) degrees cephalad for the PA oblique axial projections; it exits at the level of the mandibular symphysis.

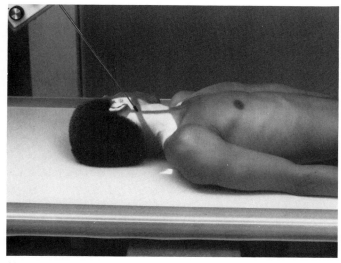

AP oblique axial

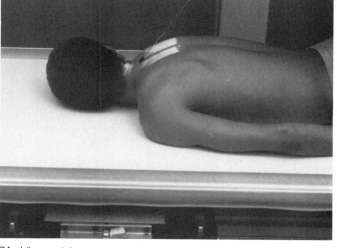

PA oblique axial

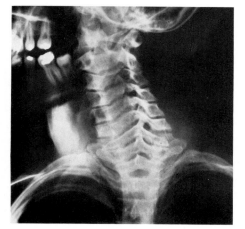

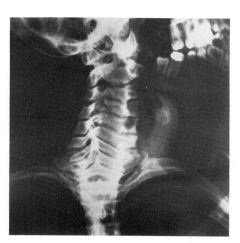

Cervical vertebrae
ADAPTATION OF POSITIONS TO THE SEVERELY INJURED PATIENT

When a patient who has sustained a severe injury of the cervical spine arrives by stretcher or bed, he should not be transferred to the radiographic table and he must not be rotated. To preclude the possibility of damaging the spinal cord by the sharp edge of a bone fragment or by a subluxated vertebra as a result of movement, any necessary manipulation of the patient's head must be performed by a physician.

If there is not a specially equipped emergency room, the initial examination is performed with a mobile unit or in an examining room that is large enough to accommodate the placement of a stretcher or bed where the x-ray tube can be brought into position for the required projections.

Grid-front cassettes or a stationary grid should be used for the AP and oblique projections.

Lateral projection

The lateral projection, taken by horizontal ray, presents no problem because it requires little or no adjustment of the patient's head and neck.

The cassette is placed in the vertical position, with its lower portion in contact with the lateral aspect of the shoulder, centered to the fourth cervical vertebra and then immobilized. The central ray is directed horizontally to the fourth cervical vertebra.

For the demonstration of the seventh cervical vertebra, the shoulders must be fully depressed. Depending on the patient's condition, this can be done by looping a long strip of bandage around his feet, and, with his knees slightly flexed, have him grasp the ends of the bandage and then extend his knees to pull the shoulders down if his condition permits. If not, an assistant can depress the shoulders by applying symmetrical traction on the arms. To prevent additional injury to the patient any body adjustments must be made only by qualified personnel.

NOTE: Although a grid is used in the lateral projection photographs, it need not be used because of the increased part-film distance. The increase in the part-film distance creates an air gap, which reduces the amount of scatter radiation reaching the film.

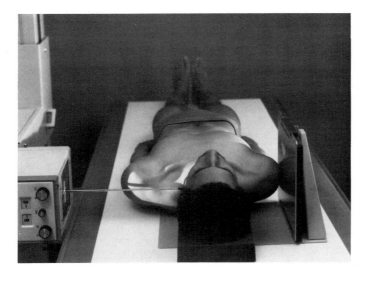

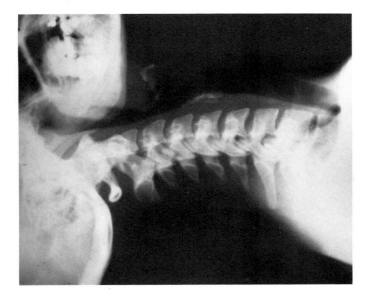

AP axial projections

For AP axial projections the patient's head must be held to prevent it from turning and lifted enough for the cassette to be slipped into position without appreciable movement of the patient's head and neck.

Two AP projections may be made: (1) a 15- to 20-degree cephalic angulation of the central ray for the demonstration of the vertebral bodies and their interspaces and (2) a 20- to 30-degree caudal angulation of the central ray for the demonstration of the posterior vertebral elements, the articular pillars and facets, the laminae, and the spinous processes. The latter study should be made on a 10″ × 12″ film to include the upper three or four thoracic vertebrae.

AP oblique axial projection

For the demonstration of the pedicles and the intervertebral foramina the cassette must be positioned near the side opposite the one being examined so that its midpoint will coincide with the 45-degree lateromedial angulation of the central ray.

Have the patient's head lifted slightly and, with the cassette held so that its midpoint is at the level of the third cervical body, gently slide it under the head just far enough to center it under the adjacent mastoid process. This centering places the midline of the film approximately 3 inches lateral to the midsagittal plane of the neck.

From the opposite side, the side being projected, the central ray is directed to the fourth cervical vertebra at an eccentric angle of 45 degrees medial and 15 to 20 degrees cephalad.

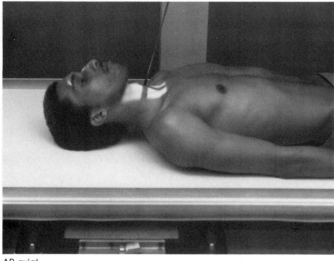

AP axial

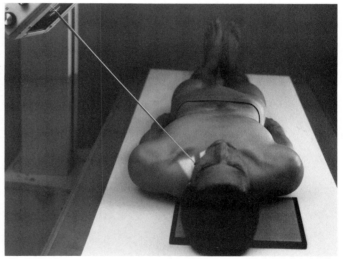

AP axial oblique

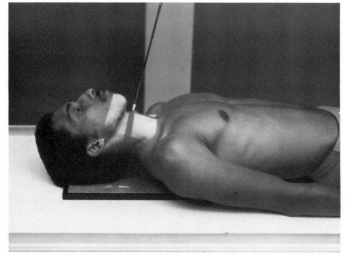

AP axial oblique

AP axial oblique

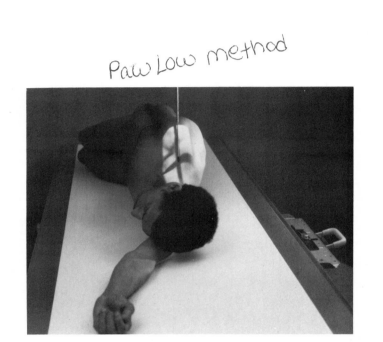

Paw Low method

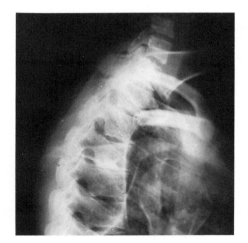

Cervicothoracic region
LATERAL PROJECTION
TWINING METHOD

Film: $10'' \times 12''$ lengthwise.

Position of patient

Place the patient in a lateral position, either seated or standing, before a vertical grid device. Have the patient sit or stand straight, and adjust the height of the cassette so that the film is centered at the level of the second thoracic vertebra.

Position of part

Center the midaxillary line of the body to the midline of the cassette. Elevate the arm that is adjacent to the stand to a vertical position, flex the elbow, and rest the forearm on the patient's head.

Rotate the shoulder posteriorly or anteriorly, according to what seems better for the individual patient; the opposite shoulder is rotated in the opposite direction. Move the patient close enough to the stand so that he can rest his shoulder firmly against it for support. Adjust the head so that the midsagittal plane is vertical.

Adjust the body in a true lateral position, with the midsagittal plane parallel with the plane of the film. Depress the shoulder that is remote from the film as much as possible, rotate it according to the placement of the opposite side, and immobilize it by having the patient hold a sandbag or an anchored strip of gauze. The goal is to have one shoulder rotated anteriorly and the other posteriorly just enough to prevent their superimposition on the shadow of the vertebrae. Respiration is suspended for the exposure.

Central ray

Direct the central ray to the midpoint of the film (1) perpendicularly if the shoulder is well depressed or (2) at a caudal angle of 5 degrees when the shoulder cannot be well depressed.

Structures shown

A lateral image of the lower cervical and upper thoracic vertebrae is shown, projected between the shadows of the shoulders.

LATERAL PROJECTION
PAWLOW METHOD

Film: 10″ × 12″ lengthwise.

Position of patient

Place the patient in a lateral recumbent position with his head elevated on sandbags or small, firm pillows.

Position of part

Center the midaxillary line of the body to the midline of the table. Extend the patient's dependent arm and adjust it to place the humeral head behind or in front of the vertebrae, the uppermost arm to be adjusted in the opposite direction. Adjust the support under the head, and place another support under the lower thorax so that the long axis of the cervicothoracic vertebrae is horizontal.

Depress the upper shoulder, adjust it to separate the shoulder shadows, and immobilize it by having the patient grasp the dorsal surface of his thigh. Adjust the body in an exact lateral position.

Center the cassette at the level of the second or third thoracic vertebra.

Central ray

Direct the central ray to the midpoint of the film at an angle of 3 to 5 degrees caudad.

Structures shown

A lateral projection of the cervicothoracic vertebrae is seen between the shadows of the shoulders.

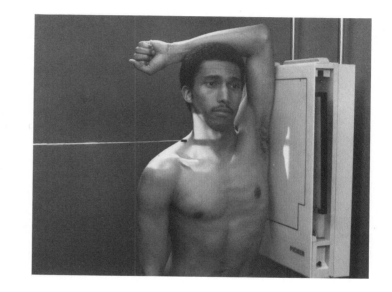

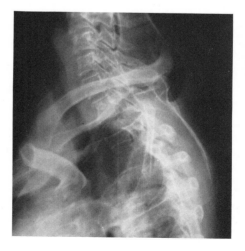

Twining method

Thoracic vertebrae

AP PROJECTION

Film: 14″ × 17″ lengthwise.

Position of patient

Place the patient in the AP position, either recumbent or erect. If the patient is supine, let the head rest directly on the table or on a thin pillow to avoid accentuating the dorsal kyphosis.

Position of part

Center the midsagittal plane of the body to the midline of the table or vertical grid device. Place the patient's arms along the sides of the body, and adjust the shoulders to lie in the same transverse plane.

If the supine position is being used, further reduce the dorsal kyphosis by flexing the hips and knees enough to place the back in contact with the table. Adjust the thighs in a vertical position, and immobi-

lize the feet with sandbags. If the extremities cannot be flexed, support the knees to relieve strain and invert the feet slightly.

When the erect position is used, have the patient stand so that his weight is equally distributed on the feet to prevent rotation of the vertebral column. If the lower extremities are of unequal length, place a support of correct height under the foot of the shorter side.

The patient may be allowed to take shallow breaths during the exposure unless his breathing is labored. In this case, respiration is suspended at the end of full exhalation to obtain a more uniform density.

Center the film at the level of the sixth thoracic vertebra. Depending on the stature of the patient, the anterior localization point will lie 3 to 4 inches distal to the manubrial notch; as a quick check, the

upper edge of the film should lie 1½ to 2 inches above the upper border of the shoulders.

Central ray

Direct the central ray perpendicularly to the midpoint of the film.

As suggested by Fuchs,[1] a more uniform density of the thoracic vertebrae will be obtained if the "heel effect" of the tube is utilized. This is done by positioning the tube so that its long axis coincides with the midsagittal plane of the body, with the anode over the head end of the body, that is, with the anode facing caudally. With the tube in this position, the greatest percentage of the beam of radiation is projected toward the thickest region of the thoracic vertebrae, that is, toward the vertebrae situated behind the sternum and mediastinal structures and toward those below the diaphragm. Compare the radiographs shown on this page.

Structures shown

This method demonstrates an AP projection of the thoracic bodies, their interpediculate spaces, and the surrounding structures.

The intervertebral spaces are not well demonstrated unless the SID is adjusted to the center of the radius of the thoracic curve to place the spaces parallel with the divergent rays. This is not desirable as a routine procedure, because it necessitates changing the SID for different patients and results in varying degrees of magnification. It should be employed only when an AP projection of the spaces is indicated and in conjunction with a radiograph made at the routine SID. A more practical method of demonstrating the disk spaces of a localized area is to angulate the central ray so that it is perpendicular to the long axis of the particular vertebral area. The degree of central ray angulation required can be estimated with reasonable accuracy by noting the angle of the dorsal curve at the area under investigation. Abnormal accentuation of the dorsal kyphosis requires that the patient be placed in the seated erect or decubitus position before a vertical grid device so that localized areas can be placed as nearly parallel with the film as possible.

[1]Fuchs, A.W.: Thoracic vertebrae, Radiogr. Clin. Photogr. **17:**2-13, 1941.

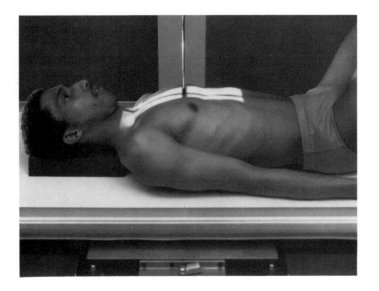

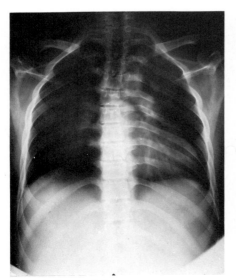

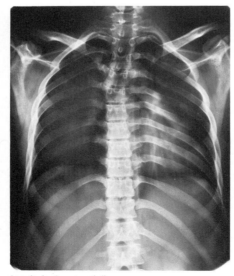

Anode facing cranially

Anode facing caudally

Lateral projection

Film: 14″ × 17″ lengthwise.

Position of patient

Place the patient in a lateral position, either recumbent or erect. If possible, the left lateral position should be used to place the heart closer to the film and thus minimize its shadow.

Oppenheimer[1] recommends the use of the orthostatic (erect) position to reproduce the physiologic conditions, and he says that the subject should be allowed to stand in a normal position—no attempt should be made to force him into an unwonted position, especially straightening of the vertebral column.

The patient should be dressed in an open-backed gown so that the vertebral column can be exposed for the adjustment of the position.

Recumbent position

Place a firm pillow under the patient's head to elevate the midsagittal plane to the level of the long axis of the vertebral column. Flex the hips and knees to a comfortable position. Center the midaxillary line of the body to the midline of the table. Elevate the lower knee to hip level and support it. With the knees exactly superimposed to prevent rotation of the pelvis, a small sandbag should be placed between them.

Adjust the arms at right angles to the long axis of the body to elevate the ribs enough to clear the intervertebral foramina. This placement of the arms gives a clear view of the vertebrae distal to the level of the glenohumeral joints. Drawing the arms forward or extending them to more than a right-angle position carries the scapulae forward where their shadows superimpose those of the upper thoracic vertebrae.

[1]Oppenheimer, A.: The apophyseal intervertebral articulations roentgenologically considered, Radiology **30:**724-740, 1938.

Unless central ray angulation is to be used, place a radioparent support under the lower thoracic region, and adjust the position of the support so that the long axis of the vertebral column is horizontal, as illustrated.

Stand with your eyes in the vertical plane that passes down the posterior surface of the patient's back, and adjust the body in a true lateral position.

When necessary, apply a compression band across the trochanteric area of the pelvis. This does not interfere with the alignment of the body, as does a band placed higher. Respiration is suspended at the end of exhalation unless the exposure is to be made during quiet breathing.

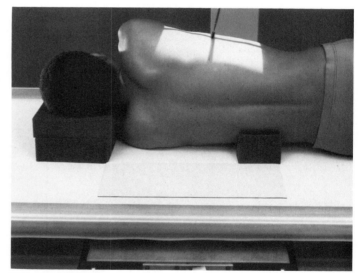

Support: straight spine

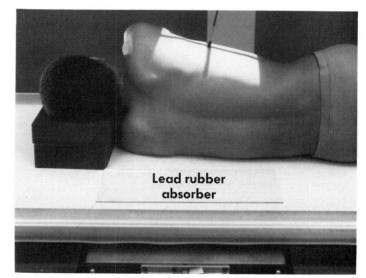

Nonsupport: curved spine

Erect position

Have the patient stand straight without strain, and adjust the height of the vertical grid device so that the midpoint of the film is at the level of the sixth thoracic vertebra. Center the midaxillary line of the body to the midline of the grid, and move the patient close enough to the grid to allow him to rest the adjacent shoulder firmly against the grid front for support.

The weight of the body must be equally distributed on the feet. If the extremities are of unequal length, place a support of correct height under the foot of the shorter side. Adjust the body so that the long axis of the vertebral column is parallel with the plane of the film.

To elevate the ribs, raise the arms to a position at right angles to the long axis of the body and support them in this position. An I.V. standard is very useful for this purpose. Place it in front of the patient, immobilize it with sandbags, and, placing one of the patient's hands on the other for correct alignment of the arms, have him grasp the standard at the correct height.

The support of the upper extremities usually furnishes sufficient immobilization.

Breathing. To obliterate, or at least diffuse, overlapping shadows of the vascular markings and ribs it is often desirable to make the exposure during quiet breathing.

Central ray

Direct the central ray perpendicularly to the midpoint of the film.

If the vertebral column is not elevated to a horizontal plane when the patient is in a recumbent position, the tube should be angled to direct the central ray perpendicular to the long axis of the thoracic column and then centered at the level of the sixth thoracic vertebra. An average angle of 10 degrees cephalad on female patients and, because of greater shoulder width, an average angle of 15 degrees on male patients are satisfactory for a majority of patients.

Structures shown

A lateral image of the thoracic bodies is demonstrated, showing their interspaces, the intervertebral foramina, and the lower spinous processes. Because of the overlapping shadows of the shoulders the upper three or four segments are not demonstrated in this position.

Improving radiographic quality

The quality of the radiograph can be improved if a sheet of leaded rubber is placed on the table behind the patient, as shown in the photographs. The lead will absorb the scatter radiation coming from the patient; scatter radiation serves only to decrease the quality of the radiograph. More important perhaps is that with automatic exposure control (AEC), the scatter radiation coming from the patient is often sufficient to prematurely terminate the exposure. The resultant radiograph may be too light because of the effect of the scatter radiation on the AEC device. For the same reason close collimation is necessary for lateral spine projections.

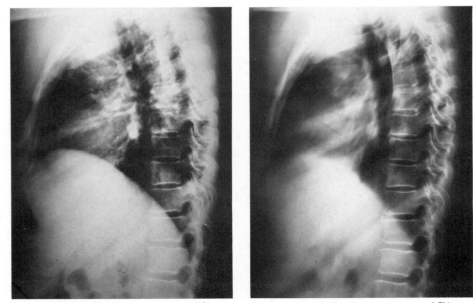

Suspended respiration for an exposure of ¾ second

Suspended respiration for an exposure of 7½ seconds on patient in adjacent radiograph

APOPHYSIAL ARTICULATIONS
OBLIQUE PROJECTIONS

The thoracic apophysial joints may be examined by anterior rotation of the body, as recommended by Oppenheimer,[1] or by posterior rotation of the body, as recommended by Fuchs.[2] The joints are well demonstrated with either position, those of the side nearer the film with anterior rotation and those of the side farther from the film with posterior rotation. Although the difference in part-film distance between the two positions is not great, the same method of rotation should be used bilaterally in each case.

Film: $14'' \times 17''$ lengthwise.

Erect position
Position of patient

Place the patient in a lateral position before a vertical grid device. Adjust the height of the grid to center the film to the sixth thoracic vertebra.

Position of part

Rotate the body slightly anteriorly or posteriorly so that the coronal plane forms an angle of 70 degrees from the plane of the film (the midsagittal plane forming an angle of 20 degrees with the film). Center the vertebral column to the midline of the grid, and have the patient rest the adjacent shoulder firmly against it for support.

Flex the elbow of the arm adjacent to the grid, and rest the hand on the hip. If the patient is rotated forward, have him grasp the side of the grid device for support; if he is rotated backward, place his hand on his hip. Adjust the shoulders to lie in the same transverse plane.

Have the patient stand straight to place the long axis of the vertebral column parallel with the film. The weight of the body must be equally distributed on the feet, and the head must not be turned laterally.

Having the shoulder rest against the vertical stand usually furnishes sufficient support. Respiration is suspended at the end of exhalation.

[1]Oppenheimer, A.: The apophyseal intervertebral articulations roentgenologically considered, Radiology **30:**724-740, 1938.
[2]Fuchs, A.W.: Thoracic vertebrae (part 2), Radiogr. Clin. Photogr. **17:**42-51, 1941.

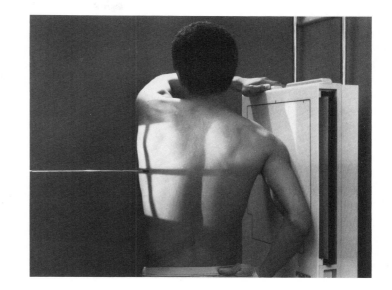

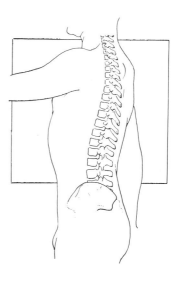

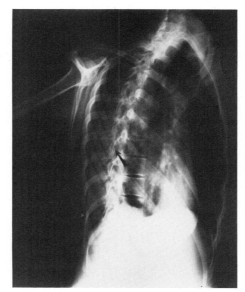

Forward rotation

Recumbent position
Position of patient

Place the patient in a lateral recumbent position. Elevate the head on a firm pillow so that its midsagittal plane is continuous with that of the vertebral column. Flex the patient's hips and knees to a comfortable position.

Position of part

For anterior rotation, place the dependent arm behind the back.

For posterior rotation, adjust the dependent arm at right angles to the long axis of the body, flex the elbow, and place the hand under or beside the head. After the body has been adjusted, draw the opposite arm posteriorly and support it.

Rotate the body slightly, either anteriorly or posteriorly as preferred, so that the coronal plane forms an angle of 70 degrees with the horizontal (20 degrees with the vertical). Center the vertebral column to the midline of the table; then check and adjust the body rotation.

A compression band may be applied across the hips, but care must be used not to change the position. Respiration is suspended for the exposure.

With the cassette in the Bucky tray, center at the level of the sixth thoracic vertebra.

Central ray

Direct the central ray perpendicularly to the midpoint of the film.

Structures shown

An oblique projection of the thoracic vertebrae is shown, demonstrating the apophysial articulations (arrow on radiograph). The number of joints shown depends on the dorsal curve. A greater degree of rotation from the lateral position is required to show the joints at the proximal and distal ends of the region on patients having an accentuated dorsal kyphosis. The inferior facets of the twelfth thoracic vertebra, having an inclination of about 45 degrees, are not shown in this position.

NOTE: The posterior rotation position gives an excellent demonstration of the cervicothoracic spinous processes and is used for this purpose when the patient cannot be satisfactorily positioned for a direct lateral projection.

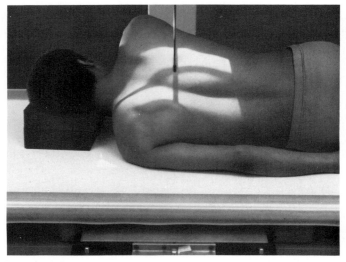

Forward rotation

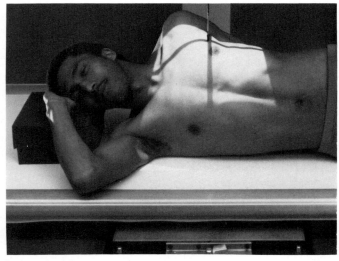

Backward rotation

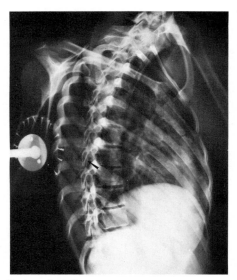

Backward rotation

Lumbar-lumbosacral vertebrae

AP AND PA PROJECTIONS

It is desirable to have the intestinal tract free of gas and fecal material for examinations of the bones lying within the abdominal and pelvic regions. The urinary bladder should be emptied just before the examination to eliminate the shadow cast by and the secondary radiation generated within the filled bladder. This is especially important in examinations of older men, in whom it is frequently possible to detect prostatic enlargement, as shown by urinary retention.

Film: 14″ × 17″ for general survey examinations.

Position of patient

The frontal projection of the lumbar-lumbosacral spine may be taken either AP or PA, with the patient recumbent or erect. Acute back disorders are excruciatingly painful. The technologist can spare the ambulatory patient much distress by radiographing him in the erect position whenever possible. When the patient cannot maintain the erect position without movement, he may be placed and positioned on the footboard of the elevated tilt table for each change in position and then returned to the horizontal position. This procedure takes a few minutes, but the patient is most appreciative.

Because the PA position presents the concave side of the lordotic curve to the x-ray tube, it places the intervertebral disk spaces at an angle closely paralleling the divergence of the beam of radiation. For this reason the PA position is sometimes used for erect studies of the lumbar-lumbosacral spine. The position does not increase the part-film distance, except with subjects who have a large abdomen. When used in the recumbent position it has the advantage of being more comfortable for the patient with a painful back and is especially more comfortable for the emaciated patient.

The AP position is generally used for recumbent examinations and, unfortunately, generally with the back fully arched by extension of the lower extremities. The extended position accentuates the lordotic curve, which in turn increases the angle between the vertebral bodies and the divergent rays, with resultant distortion of the bodies as well as poor delineation of the intervertebral disk spaces. The lordotic curve can be reduced and the intervertebral disk spaces clearly delineated in the AP direction simply by flexing the hips and knees enough to place the back in firm contact with the table.

Comparison of the films below shows that when the patient is correctly adjusted in the supine position there is little difference between the PA and AP projections. The only consideration left is the patient's comfort.

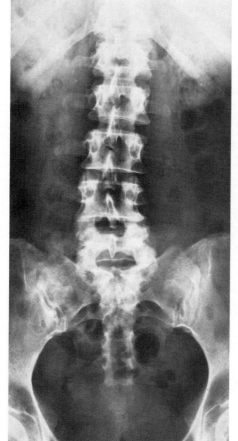

AP projection, the extremities extended

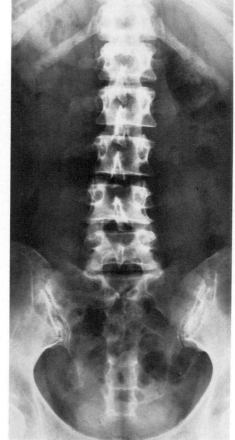

AP projection, the extremities flexed

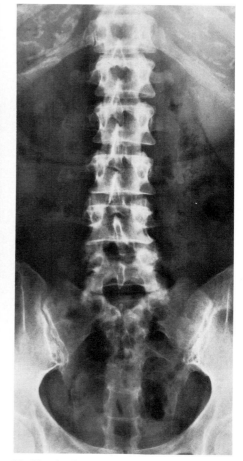

PA. All projections are of same patient.

Position of part

Supine position. Center the midsagittal plane of the body to the midline of the table. To prevent rotation of the spine, adjust the shoulders to lie in the same transverse plane, and adjust the head so that its midsagittal plane is coextensive with that of the spine. So that the forearms will not lie within the exposure field, flex the patient's elbows and place his hands on the upper chest. When a soft tissue abnormality (atrophy or swelling) is causing rotation of the pelvis, adjust a radioparent support under the lower side.

To delineate the intervertebral disk spaces it is necessary to adjust them at an angle closely paralleling that of the divergent beam of radiation. This adjustment requires that the lumbar lordosis be reduced by flexing the hips and knees enough to place the back in firm contact with the table. Have the patient lean his knees together for support.

When the knees cannot be flexed and the patient cannot be turned for a PA projection, place supports under the knees to relieve strain and invert the feet 15 to 20 degrees.

Prone position. Center the midsagittal plane of the body to the midline of the table. With elbows flexed, adjust the arms and forearms in a comfortable, bilaterally symmetrical position. Adjust the shoulders to lie in the same transverse plane, and have the patient rest his head on his chin to prevent rotation of the spine.

Film centering

Center the 14″ × 17″ film at the level of the iliac crests. Care must be used to palpate for the crest of the bone to avoid being misled by the contour of the heavy muscles and fatty tissue lying above it.

When two 10″ × 12″ films are used, center the first to the third lumbar body (at the level of the inferior midaxillary costal margin), and direct the central ray vertically. Center the second film to coincide with the cranially or caudally angulated central ray, which is directed through the lumbosacral joint.

Central ray

Direct the central ray vertically to the midpoint of the cassette for the general survey study.

Structures shown

The AP and PA projections demonstrate the lumbar bodies, the intervertebral disk spaces, the interpediculate spaces, the laminae, and the spinous and transverse processes. When the larger film is used, one or two of the lower thoracic vertebrae, the sacrum and coccyx, the pelvic bones, and the hip joints are included. Because of the angle at which the last lumbar segment joins the sacrum, the lumbosacral disk space is not well shown in direct frontal projections. The positions used for this purpose are described on the following pages.

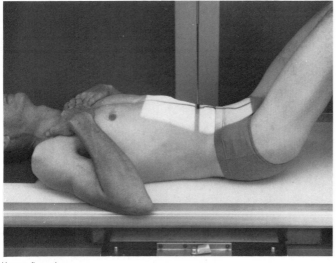

Knees flexed

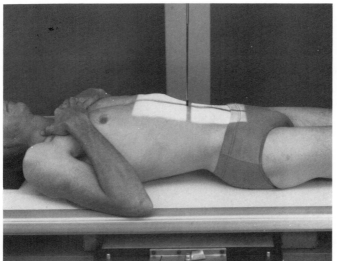

Knees extended

Lumbosacral junction and sacroiliac joints
AP AND PA AXIAL PROJECTIONS

Film: 8″ × 10″ or 10″ × 12″ lengthwise.

Position of patient

The axial projection, which is required for the demonstration of the lumbosacral and sacroiliac joints, is made with the patient in the same position as for, and usually immediately following, the AP or PA projection of the lumbar vertebrae.

If the patient was in the prone position for the PA projection, no change is required for the axial projection. If he is in the supine position, the lower extremities may be extended to remove them from the path of the cephalically angled central ray, or the thighs may be abducted and adjusted in the vertical position.

In each of these positions the central ray is directed through the lumbosacral junction. This joint is situated 1½ inches posterior to the midaxillary line at the intersection of the midsagittal plane and a transverse plane that passes midway between the iliac crests and the anterior superior iliac spines.

Supine extended position

With the patient supine and his lower extremities extended, direct the central ray through the lumbosacral joint at an average angle of 30 to 35 degrees cephalad.

An angulation of 30 degrees for the male patient and 35 degrees for the female patient is satisfactory in a majority of patients. By noting the contour of the lower back, unusual accentuation or diminution of the lumbosacral angle can be estimated and the central ray angulation varied accordingly.

Prone position

Lumbosacral joint. Direct the central ray through the joint to the midpoint of the cassette at an average angle of 35 degrees caudad. It enters the spinous process of the fourth lumbar segment.

Sacroiliac joints. Direct the central ray vertically and center at the level of the anterior superior iliac spines. It will enter about 2 inches distal to the spinous process of the fifth lumbar segment.

Meese[1] recommends the prone position for examinations of the sacroiliac joints since, their obliquity, it places them in a position more nearly parallel with the divergence of the beam of radiation.

[1]Meese, T.: Die dorso-ventrale Aufnahme der Sacroiliacalgelenke, Fortschr. Roentgenstr.**85**:601-603, 1956.

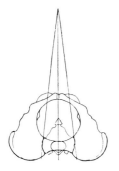

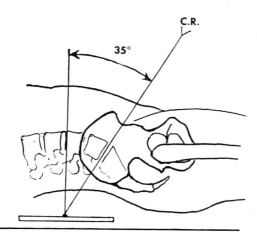

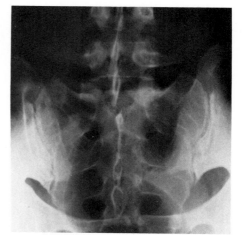

AP

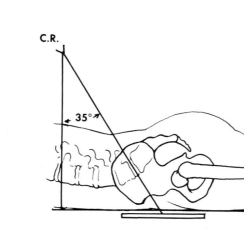

PA

Lumbar-lumbosacral vertebrae
LATERAL PROJECTIONS

Film: 14″ × 17″ for general survey examinations.

Position of patient

The body position (recumbent or erect) used for the frontal projection is maintained for the lateral projection.

It is desirable to have the patient dressed in an open-back gown so that the spine can be exposed for final adjustment of the position.

Recumbent position
Position of part

Ask the patient to turn onto the indicated side and to flex his hips and knees to a comfortable position. When examining a thin patient, adjust a suitable pad under the dependent hip to relieve pressure.

Center the midaxillary line of the body to the midline of the table. It must be remembered that no matter how large the patient, the long axis of the spine is situated in the midaxillary line.

Adjust the pillow to place the midsagittal plane of the head coextensive with that of the spine. With the patient's elbow flexed, adjust the dependent arm at right angles to his body.

To prevent rotation, exactly superimpose the knees, and place a small sandbag between the knees.

Unless central ray angulation is to be used, place a suitable radioparent support under the lower thorax and adjust it so that the long axis of the spine is horizontal. Recheck the position for rotation. Rotation can be detected and easily corrected by standing to look down the back while adjusting the position.

When using a large film, center at the level of the iliac crest. When using two 10″ × 12″ films, the first is centered at the level of the third lumbar segment. For the lumbosacral area, move the film to the level of the anterior superior iliac spines. The central ray is not moved from the midaxillary line of the body.

Central ray

After the spine has been adjusted in the horizontal position, direct the central ray perpendicularly to the midpoint of the film.

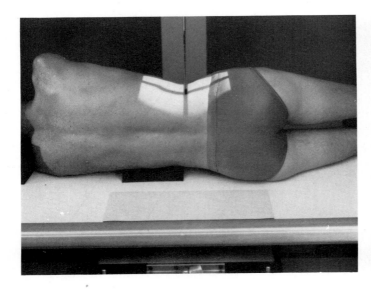

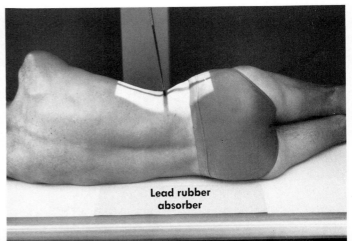

Lead rubber absorber

When the spine is not adjusted in the horizontal position, the central ray is directed perpendicularly to its long axis. The degree of central ray angulation depends on the angulation of the lumbar column, which depends on the breadth of the pelvis. An average caudal angle of 5 degrees for male patients and of 8 degrees for the female patients with a wide pelvis is satisfactory in a majority of cases.

Erect position
Position of part

From the position assumed for the PA projection, ask the patient to turn to the side and to center the midaxillary line of the body to the midline of the table. Immobilize the patient by placing a standard in front of him, while having him grasp it with both hands at shoulder height.

Care must be taken to see that the patient stands normally erect. Subjects who have severe low back pain tend to relieve the discomfort by tilting the pelvis anteriorly and superiorly. This movement reduces the lumbosacral angle and thus defeats the aim to demonstrate it in the orthostatic (erect) position. The weight of the body must be equally distributed on the feet.

Central ray

Direct the central ray horizontally to the midpoint of the film.

Structures shown

This shows a lateral projection of the lumbar bodies and their interspaces, the spinous processes, the lumbosacral junction, and the sacrum and coccyx. This projection gives a profile image of the upper four lumbar intervertebral foramina. The last lumbar intervertebral foramina (right and left) are not usually well visualized in this position because of their oblique direction. Oblique projections and the special Kovács position are used for these foramina.

Improving radiographic quality

The quality of the radiograph can be improved if a sheet of leaded rubber is placed on the table behind the patient, as shown in the photographs. The lead will absorb the scatter radiation coming from the patient; scatter radiation serves only to decrease the quality of the radiograph. More important perhaps is that with automatic exposure control (AEC), the scatter radiation coming from the patient is often sufficient to prematurely terminate the exposure. The resultant radiograph may be too light because of the effect of the scatter radiation on the AEC device. For the same reason close collimation is necessary for lateral spine projections.

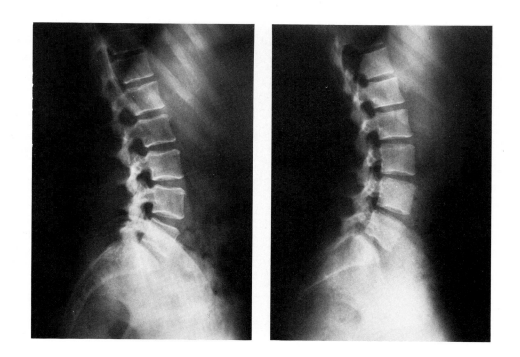

Lumbosacral junction
LOCALIZED LATERAL PROJECTION

Film: 8″ × 10″ lengthwise.

Position of patient

It is recommended that the lumbosacral region be examined in the recumbent position, because patients who have low back pain tend, when erect, to assume a protective position that reduces the lumbosacral angle. It is further recommended that questionable cases be checked with a lateral projection made in the erect position as well as in the usual recumbent position.

Position of part

To center the laterally positioned lumbosacral joint to the film, align the patient's body so that the coronal plane passing 1½ inches posterior to the midaxillary line is centered to the midline of the table or vertical grid device.

With the patient in the recumbent position, adjust the pillow to place the midsagittal plane of the head coextensive with that of the spine. With the patient's elbow flexed, adjust the dependent arm in a position at right angles to the body.

It is desirable to have the hips fully extended for this study. When this cannot be done extend them as much as possible, and support the dependent knee at hip level on sandbags. Place sandbags under and between the ankles and knees.

With the cassette in the Bucky tray, center the cassette at the level of the transverse plane that passes midway between the iliac crests and the anterior superior iliac spine.

Central ray

Direct the central ray perpendicularly to the midpoint of the cassette.

When the spine is not adjusted in the horizontal position, the central ray is angled caudally, 5 degrees for male patients and 8 degrees for female patients. It enters midway between the level of the iliac crest and anterior superior iliac spine.

Structures shown

A lateral projection of the lumbosacral joint, the lower one or two lumbar vertebrae, and the upper sacrum is demonstrated.

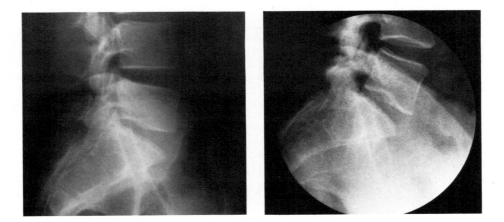

Last lumbar intervertebral foramina

PA OBLIQUE AXIAL PROJECTION
KOVÁCS METHOD[1]

Film: 8″ × 10″ lengthwise.

Position of patient

The patient is placed in the recumbent position and alternately turned onto the side being examined.

Position of part

Adjust the patient in the lateral position and align the body so that the coronal plane that passes 1½ inches posterior to the midaxillary line is centered to the midline of the table. Have the patient extend

[1]Kovács, A.: X-ray examination of the exit of the lowermost lumbar root, Radiol. Clin. **19:**6-13, 1950.

the uppermost arm and grasp the end of the table to aid in maintaining the thorax in the lateral position when the pelvis is rotated.

Keeping the patient's thorax exactly lateral, rotate the pelvis 30 degrees anteriorly from the lateral position. Place a sandbag support under the flexed uppermost knee to prevent too much rotation of the hips. Check and adjust the degree of rotation with a protractor.

Adjust the position of the cassette so that its midpoint will coincide with the central ray.

Central ray

Angle the tube to direct the central ray along a straight line extending from the superior edge of the uppermost iliac crest through the fifth lumbar segment to the inguinal region of the dependent side. According to the alignment of the spine, the central ray angulation will vary from 15 to 30 degrees caudad.

Structures shown

A profile image of the lowermost lumbar intervertebral foramen is demonstrated. Both sides are examined for comparison.

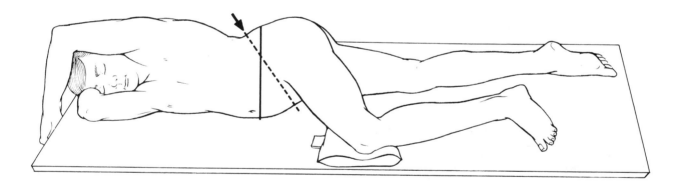

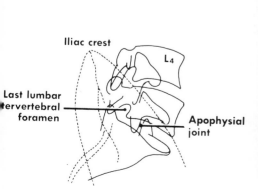

Kovács method

Direct lateral projection on same patient as in adjacent radiograph

Lumbar-lumbosacral apophysial joints
PA OBLIQUE PROJECTIONS (RAO AND LAO)

The articular facets of the lumbar vertebrae form an angle of 45 degrees and those between the last lumbar vertebra and the sacrum form an angle of 30 degrees to the midsagittal plane in a majority of patients. The angulation does vary, however, not only from patient to patient but from side to side in the same patient. Exact adjustment of the part on the first examination makes it possible to determine any necessary change in rotation for further studies.

Film: 14″ × 17″ lengthwise; 8″ × 10″ for the last apophysial joint.

Position of patient

The patient may be examined in the erect or the recumbent position. The recumbent position is generally used, because it facilitates immobilization.

Greater ease in positioning the patient and a resultant higher percentage of success in duplicating results make the semiprone position preferable to the semisupine position.

Position of part

Have the patient turn to a semiprone position and support himself on the forearm and flexed knee of the elevated side. Align the body to center the third lumbar vertebra of the elevated side to the midline of the table.

With the use of a protractor, check and, if necessary, adjust the degree of body rotation. It is adjusted at an angle of 45 degrees for the lumbar region and at an angle of 30 degrees from the horizontal for the lumbosacral apophysial joint. Center the film at the level of the third lumbar vertebra.

To demonstrate the last intervetebral foramen, position the patient as described above but center to the apophysial joint of the fifth lumbar vertebra.

Central ray

Direct the central ray perpendicularly to the midpoint of the film.

Structures shown

An oblique projection of the lumbar and/or the lumbosacral vertebrae is shown, demonstrating the articular facets of the side farther from the film. The articulation between the twelfth thoracic and first lumbar vertebrae, having the same direction as those in the lumbar region, is shown on the larger film.

The last intervertebral foramen is usually well shown in oblique projections.

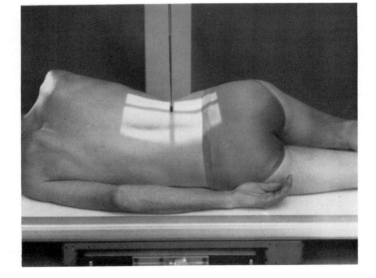

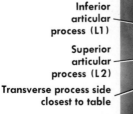

Inferior articular process (L1)

Superior articular process (L2)

Transverse process side closest to table

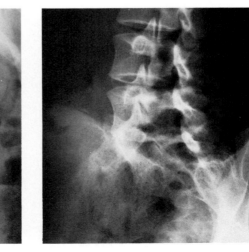

AP OBLIQUE PROJECTIONS (RPO AND LPO)

Film: 14" × 17" lengthwise; 8" × 10" for last apophysial joint.

Position of patient

Oblique projections are, when indicated, taken immediately following the frontal projection and in the same body position—recumbent or erect. The recumbent position is described because it is more frequently used, but the directions can be easily adapted to the erect position.

Position of part

Have the patient turn from the supine position to the approximate degree of obliquity to be used. Center the spine to the midline of the table. In the oblique position the lumbar spine overlies the longitudinal plane that passes along the dependent side 2 inches lateral to the spinous processes.

Ask the patient to place his arms in a comfortable position. Place suitable supports under the elevated shoulder, the hip, and the knee.

With the use of a protractor, check and adjust the degree of body rotation. It is adjusted at an angle of 45 degrees for the demonstration of the articular facets in the lumbar region and at an angle of 30 degrees from the horizontal plane for the demonstration of the lumbosacral facets.

Center the cassette at the level of the third lumbar segment for the lumbar region and at the level of the transverse plane passing midway between the iliac crests and the anterior superior iliac spines for the last apophysial joint.

Central ray

Direct the central ray perpendicularly to the midpoint of the film.

Structures shown

An oblique projection of the lumbar and/or the lumbosacral spine is shown, demonstrating the articular facets of the side *nearer* the film. Both sides are examined for comparison.

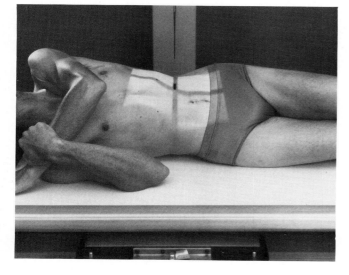 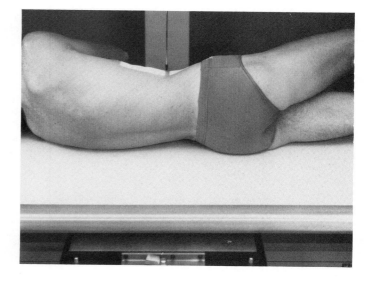

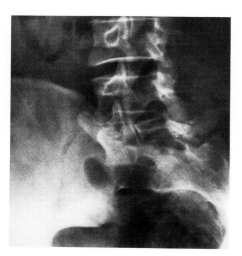 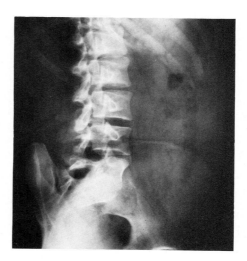

Lumbar intervertebral disks

WEIGHT-BEARING FLEXION AND EXTENSION STUDIES

DUNCAN-HOEN METHOD OF DETERMINING LEVEL OF DISK HERNIATION

Film: 14" × 17" lengthwise.

Position of patient

This examination is made with the patient in the standing position. Duncan and Hoen[1] recommend that the PA position be used, because in this direction the divergent rays are more nearly parallel with the intervertebral disk spaces.

With the patient standing before a vertical grid device, adjust the height of the

[1]Duncan, W., and Hoen, T.: A new approach to the diagnosis of herniation of the intervertebral disc, Surg. Gynecol. Obstet. **75:**257-267, 1942.

cassette so that its midpoint is at the level of the third lumbar vertebra. This centering will include several of the thoracic interspaces as well as all of the lumbar interspaces.

Position of part

Center the midsagittal plane of the patient's body to the midline of the vertical grid device, and adjust the body in a PA position. Let the arms hang unsupported by the sides.

One radiograph is made with right bending and one with left bending. Have the patient lean directly laterally as far as possible without rotation and without lifting his foot. The degree of leaning must not be forced, and the patient must not be supported in position.

Central ray

Direct the central ray to the midpoint of the film at an angle of 15 to 20 degrees caudad, or it may be directed perpendicular to the film.

Structures shown

Two PA projections of the lower thoracic and the lumbar regions are presented in lateral flexion for the demonstration of the mobility of the intervertebral joints. This method of examination is used in cases of disk protrusion to localize the involved joint as shown by limitation of motion at the site of the lesion.

Duncan and Hoen[1] also recommend that lateral projections be made with the patient in extreme flexion and in extreme extension to demonstrate mechanical obstruction of the posterior portion of the intervertebral joints. The method of positioning for these studies is shown in the accompanying drawings. Again, the degree of leaning must not be forced, and the patient must not be supported in position.

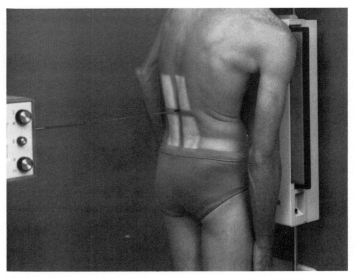

Right bending

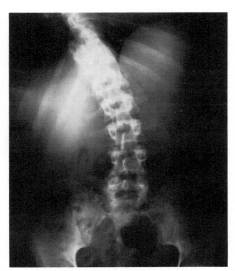

Lumbar intervertebral disk

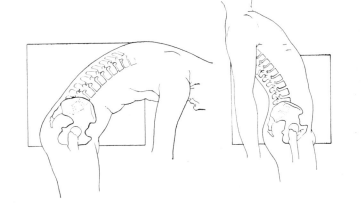

Sacroiliac joints
PA OBLIQUE PROJECTIONS (RAO AND LAO)

Film: 8″ × 10″ or 10″ × 12″ lengthwise.

Position of patient

Place the patient in a semiprone position, the side being examined adjacent to the table, and have him rest on the forearm and flexed knee of the elevated side. Place a small, firm pillow under the head.

Position of part

Adjust the rotation so the upper side is elevated about 25 degrees, and then align the body so a longitudinal line passing 1 inch medial to the dependent anterior superior iliac spine is centered to the midline of the table. Adjust the shoulders to lie in the same transverse plane. Place supports under the ankles and under the flexed knee. Adjust the position of the elevated thigh so that the anterior superior iliac spines lie in the same transverse plane.

Using a protractor to check the rotation, adjust the body so that it is obliqued 25 to 30 degrees from the prone position. Check the degree of rotation at several points along the anterior surface of the body.

The forearm and flexed knee usually furnish sufficient support for this position. Respiration is suspended for the exposure.

Adjust the position of the cassette so that its midpoint will coincide with the central ray.

Central ray

1. With the central ray perpendicular to the plane of the film, center at the level of the anterior superior iliac spines.

2. With the central ray at an angle of 20 to 25 degrees caudad, center at the level of the transverse plane passing 1½ inches distal to the fifth lumbar spinous process; it will exit at the level of the anterior superior iliac spine.

Structures shown

A profile image of the sacroiliac joint nearer the film is presented. Both sides are examined for comparison.

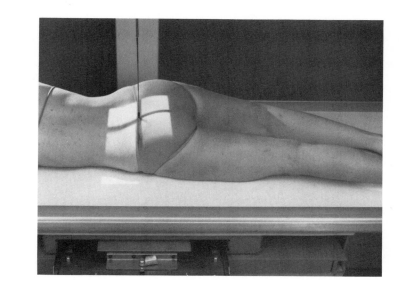

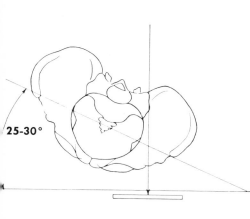

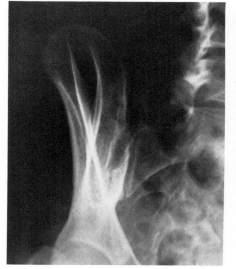

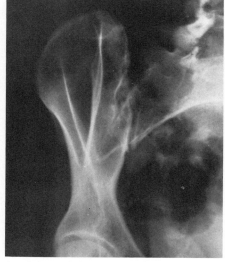

Angulation of 25 degrees   Angulation of 0 degrees

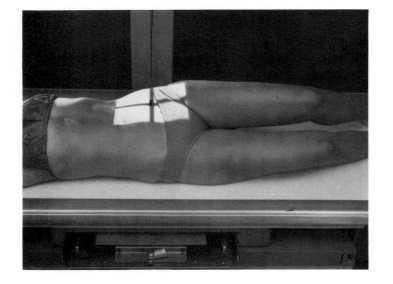

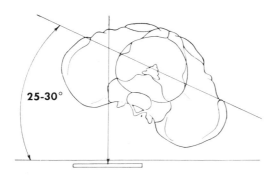

25-30°

AP OBLIQUE PROJECTIONS (RPO AND LPO)

Film: $8'' \times 10''$ or $10'' \times 12''$ lengthwise.

Position of patient

Place the patient in the supine position and elevate the head on a firm pillow.

Position of part

Elevate the side being examined approximately 25 degrees and support the shoulder, the lower thorax, and the upper thigh on sandbags. Align the body so that the sagittal plane passing 1 inch medial to the anterior superior iliac spine of the elevated side is centered to the midline of the table. Place the arms in a comfortable position, and adjust the shoulders to lie in the same transverse plane.

Adjust the position of the elevated thigh to place the anterior superior iliac spines in the same transverse plane. Place sandbag supports under the knee to elevate it to hip level if needed.

Using a protractor to check the position, adjust the degree of rotation so that the posterior surface of the body forms a 25- to 30-degree angle from the table. Check the rotation at several points along the back.

Respiration is suspended for the exposure. Adjust the position of the cassette so that its midpoint will coincide with the central ray.

Central ray

1. With the central ray directed perpendicularly, center at the level of the anterior superior iliac spines.

2. With the central ray at an angle of 20 to 25 degrees cephalad, center to a point 1½ inches distal to the level of the anterior superior iliac spines.

Structures shown

A profile projection of the sacroiliac joint farther from the film and an oblique projection of the adjacent structures are seen. Both sides are examined for comparison.

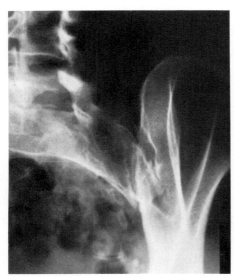

Angulation of 0 degrees

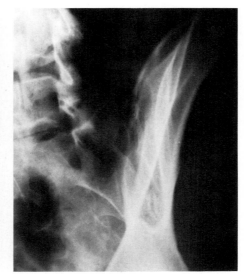

Angulation of 25 degrees

CHAMBERLAIN METHOD OF DEMONSTRATING ABNORMAL SACROILIAC MOTION

Chamberlain[1] recommends the following erect projection in cases of sacroiliac slip or relaxation:

1. A conventional lateral projection centered to the lumbosacral junction. Chamberlain[2] prefers to have this projection made with the patient erect.

2. Two PA projections of the pubic bones, with the patient in the erect position and with weight-bearing on the alternate legs to demonstrate symphysis reaction by a change in the normal relation of the pubic bones in cases of sacroiliac slip or relaxation.

This examination requires two blocks or box stools approximately 6 inches high, the blocks being alternately removed to allow one leg to hang free.

Film: 8″ × 10″ lengthwise for each exposure.

Position of patient

Place the patient in the PA position, standing on the two blocks, before a vertical grid device. Adjust the height of the grid, and center the film to the symphysis pubis.

Position of part

Center the midsagittal plane of the body to the midline of the grid, and adjust the body in a true PA position.

The patient may be allowed to grasp the sides of the device to steady himself, but he must not be allowed to aid in supporting his weight in this way. A compression band may be placed across the pelvis to immobilize the patient but not to aid in supporting the weight of the body. Respiration is suspended for the exposures.

[1] Chamberlain, W.E.: The symphysis pubis in the roentgen examination of the sacroiliac joint, A.J.R. **24:**621-625, 1930.

[2] Chamberlain, W.E.: Personal communication.

For the first exposure, remove one of the blocks so that one leg hangs free. The patient should be instructed to "let the leg hang like a dead weight," so that he will not overcome the desired effect through muscular resistance. For the second exposure, replace the first support and remove the opposite one. Chamberlain suggests that the identification marker be placed on the weight-bearing side.

Central ray

Direct the central ray horizontally to the midpoint of the film.

Structures shown

Two PA projections of the pubic bones are shown, demonstrating any abnormal motion of the sacroiliac joints as shown by a change in the normal relation of the pubic bones to each other when the body weight is borne on one leg.

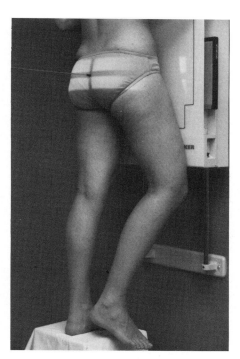

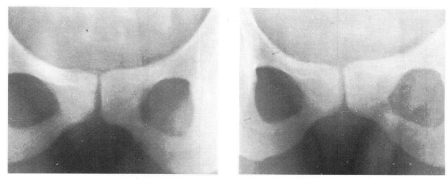

PA projection in a normal female patient

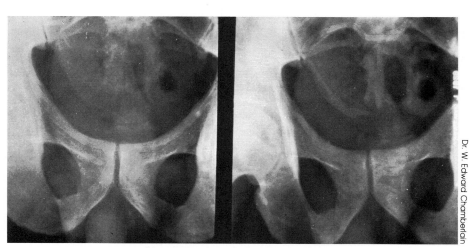

PA projection in a normal male patient

Sacrum and coccyx
AP AND PA PROJECTIONS

It is particularly desirable to have the colon free of gas and fecal material for examinations of the sacrum and coccyx. The urinary bladder should be emptied before the examination.

Film: $10'' \times 12''$ for sacrum; $8'' \times 10''$ for coccyx.

Position of patient

The patient is routinely adjusted in the supine position for the AP projection of the sacrum and coccyx to place the part as close as possible to the film. The prone position can be used without appreciable loss of detail and should be used with patients who have a painful injury or a destructive disease.

Position of part

With the patient either supine or prone, center the midsagittal plane of the body to the midline of the table. Have the patient flex the elbows and place the arms in a comfortable, bilaterally symmetrical position. Adjust the shoulders to lie in the same transverse plane.

When the pelvis is rotated by a soft tissue abnormality (swelling or atrophy), adjust a radioparent support under the low side. When the patient is supine, a support may be placed under the knees.

Position the cassette so that its midpoint will coincide with the central ray angulation.

Central ray

Sacrum. With the patient supine, direct the central ray 15 degrees cephalad. Center it to the midpoint of the transverse plane that passes midway between the pubic symphysis and the anterior superior iliac spines. With the patient prone, angle the central ray 15 degrees caudad and center it to the clearly visible sacral curve.

Coccyx. With the patient supine, angle the central ray 10 degrees caudad and center to a point about 2 inches superior to the pubic symphysis. With the patient prone, angle the central ray 10 degrees cephalad and center it to the easily palpable coccyx.

Structures shown

A true frontal projection of the sacrum or the coccyx is demonstrated, projected free of superimposition.

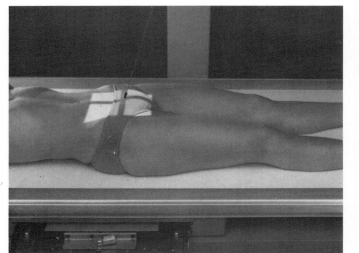

Central ray angulation for sacrum

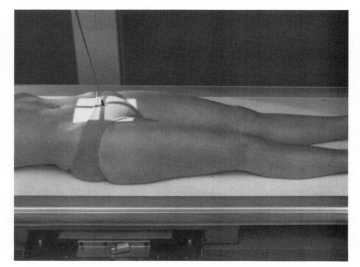

Central ray angulation for coccyx

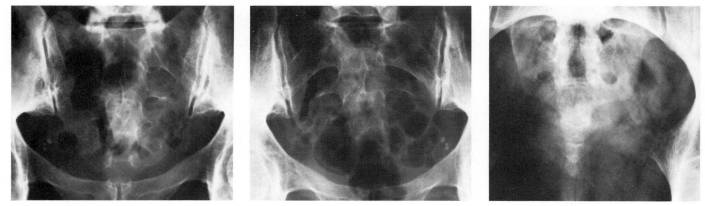

Supine projection of sacrum

Prone projection of sacrum

Supine projection of coccyx

LATERAL PROJECTIONS

Film: 10″ × 12″ for sacrum; 8″ × 10″ for coccyx.

Position of patient

Ask the patient to turn onto the indicated side and flex his hips and knees to a comfortable position.

Position of part

For the sacrum, align the body so that the coronal plane passing 3 inches posterior to the midaxillary line is centered to the midline of the table.

The coccyx lies approximately 5 inches posterior to the midaxillary line with its exact position depending on the pelvic curve. It can easily be palpated between the buttocks at the base of the spine, and the body can then be aligned to place the coccyx over the center line of the table.

Adjust the arms in a position at right angles to the body, and have the patient grasp the side of the table with the upper hand to aid in maintaining the position. Exactly superimpose the knees, and elevate the lower knee to hip level and support it on sandbags. Place sandbags under and between the ankles and between the knees.

Adjust a support under the body to place the long axis of the spine horizontal. Adjust the pelvis so that there is no rotation from the exact lateral position.

Position the film so that its midpoint is at the level of the anterior superior iliac spines for the sacrum or at the level of the center of the coccyx.

Central ray

Direct the central ray perpendicularly to the midpoint of the film.

Structures shown

This projection shows the lateral aspect of the sacrum and/or coccyx.

Improving radiographic quality

The quality of the radiograph can be improved if a sheet of leaded rubber is placed on the table behind the patient, as shown in the photographs. The lead will absorb the scatter radiation coming from the patient; scatter radiation serves only to decrease the quality of the radiograph. More important perhaps is that with automatic exposure control (AEC), the scatter radiation coming from the patient is often sufficient to prematurely terminate the exposure. The resultant radiograph may be too light because of the effect of the scatter radiation on the AEC device. For the same reason close collimation is necessary for lateral spine projections.

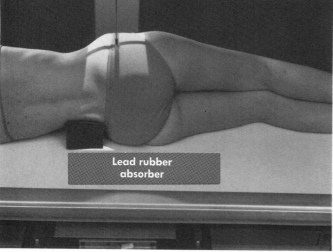

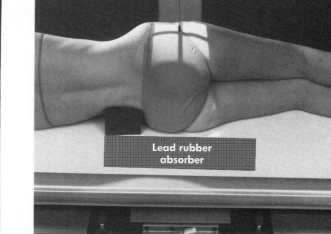

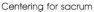
Centering for sacrum

Centering for coccyx

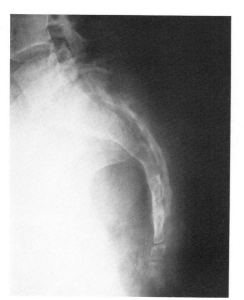

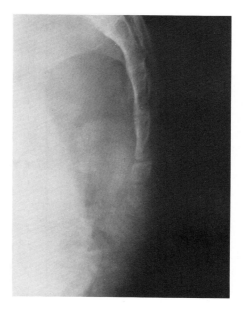

Sacral canal—sacroiliac joints
AXIAL PROJECTION
NÖLKE METHOD

Film: 8″ × 10″ or 10″ × 12″ crosswise.

Position of patient

In the examination of the sacral canal the patient is seated on the end of the table and is then flexed in different degrees for the several regions of the canal. The exact degree of flexion depends on the curvature of the sacrum.

Seat the patient far enough back on the table to center the midaxillary line of the body to the transverse axis of the Bucky tray. If the patient is too short to be comfortably seated so far back, the cassette can be shifted off center so that its midpoint will coincide with the region of the canal being projected. Support the feet on a chair or a stool.

Position of part

Adjust the position of the body so that the midsagittal plane is perpendicular to the midline of the table. Have the patient lean forward enough so that the upper, the middle, or the lower portion of the sacral canal is vertical, being careful not to let him lean laterally.

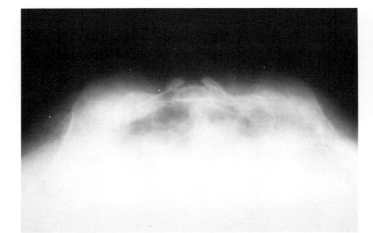

Slight flexion

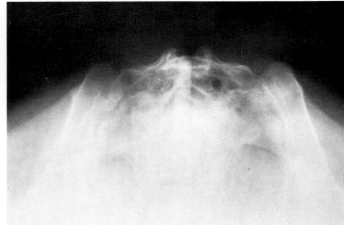

Moderate flexion

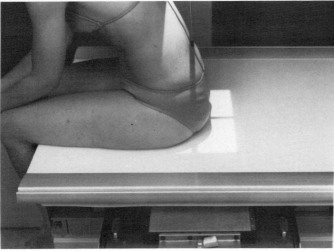

Have the patient grasp the sides of the table, or his legs or ankles, depending on the degree of leaning, to maintain the position. Respiration need not be suspended for the exposure unless the patient's breathing is labored.

With the cassette in the Bucky tray, center to the vertically placed portion of the sacrum.

Central ray

Direct the central ray perpendicularly to the midpoint of the film.

Structures shown

With the patient leaning forward in a position of acute flexion, as illustrated in the third photograph, the resultant radiograph shows the upper sacral canal projected into the angle formed by the ascending rami of the ischial bones just posterior to the pubic symphysis. The spinous process of the last lumbar segment is projected across the shadow of the canal.

With the patient leaning forward in a position of slight flexion, as illustrated in the first photograph, the resultant radiograph shows the lower sacral canal, the junction of the sacrum and the coccyx, and the last lumbar vertebra.

With the patient leaning forward in a position of moderate flexion, as illustrated in the second photograph, the resultant radiograph shows a cross section of the upper and lower sacral canal. The sacroiliac joints are also demonstrated in this position.

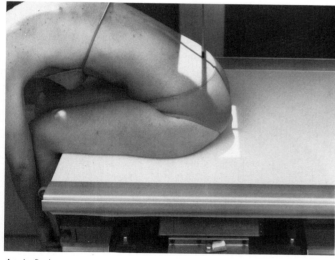

Acute flexion

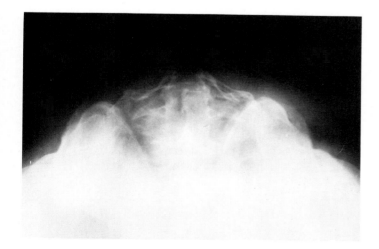

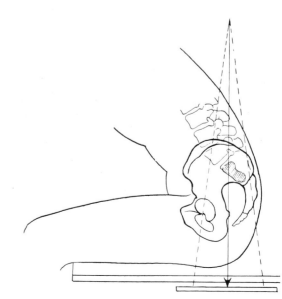

Scoliosis series

FERGUSON METHOD OF DISTINGUISHING DEFORMING CURVE FROM COMPENSATORY CURVE

Film: 14″ × 17″ placed lengthwise for each exposure.

Position of patient

Place the patient in the AP position, either seated or standing, before a vertical grid device. Have the patient sit or stand straight, and then adjust the height of the cassette to include about 1 inch of the iliac crests.

Position of part

For the first radiograph, the patient is adjusted in a normally seated or standing position to check the spinal curvature. Center the midsagittal plane of the body to the midline of the grid. Allow the arms to hang relaxed at the sides.

For the second radiograph, elevate the hip or foot of the convex side of the curve approximately 3 or 4 inches by placing a block, a book, or sandbags under the buttock or the foot. Ferguson[1] specifies that the elevation must be sufficient to make the patient expend some effort in maintaining the position.

The patient must not be supported in these positions. A compression band is not employed. Respiration is suspended for the exposures.

[1]Ferguson, A.B.: Roentgen diagnosis of the extremities and spine, New York, 1939, Harper & Row, Publishers.

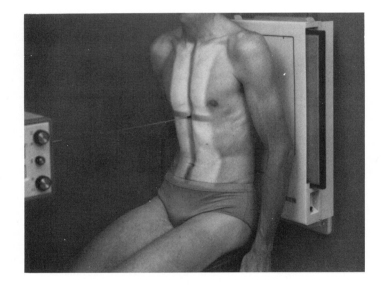

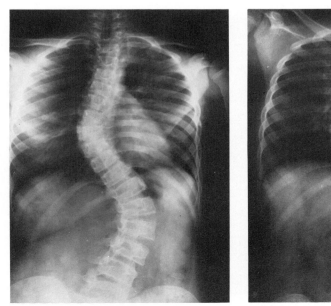

Standing   Supine

Dr. Lawson E. Miller, Jr.

Central ray

Direct the central ray horizontally to the midpoint of the film.

Structures shown

Two AP projections of the thoracic and lumbar vertebrae are shown, used for comparison to distinguish the deforming, or primary, curve from the compensatory curve in cases of scoliosis.

NOTE: Another widely used scoliosis series consists of four projections of the thoracic and lumbar spine: (1) a direct AP projection with the patient standing, (2) a direct AP projection with the patient supine, and (3) and (4) AP projections with alternate right and left flexion in the supine position. The right and left bending positions are described on the following page. For the scoliosis series, however, 14″ × 17″ films are used and are placed to include about 1 inch of the iliac crests.

Young, Oestreich, and Goldstein[1] have recently described their application of this scoliosis procedure in detail. They recommend the addition of a lateral projection made with the patient standing erect to show spondylolisthesis or to demonstrate exaggerated degrees of kyphosis or lordosis.

Kittleson and Lim[2] have described both the Ferguson and the Cobb methods of measurement of scoliosis.

[1]Young L.W., Oestreich, A.E., and Goldstein, L.A.: Roentgenology in scoliosis: contribution to evaluation and management, Radiology **97**:778-795, 1970.
[2]Kittleson, A.C., and Lim, L.W.: Measurement of scoliosis, A.J.R. **108**:775-777, 1970.

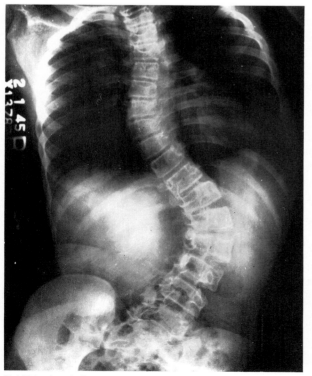

Right hip elevated

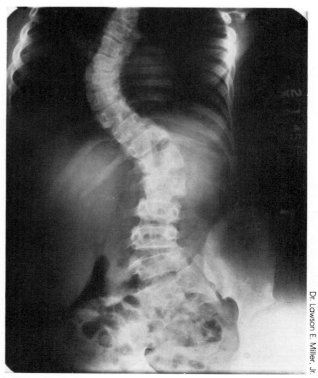

Left hip elevated

Dr. Lawson E. Miller, Jr.

Spinal fusion series

SUPINE RIGHT AND LEFT BENDING POSITIONS

Film: 10" × 12" or 14" × 17" placed lengthwise for each exposure.

Position of patient

Place the patient in the supine position, and center the midsagittal plane of the body to the midline of the table.

Position of part

The first radiograph is made with maximum right bending and the second with maximum left bending. To obtain equal bending force throughout the spine, cross the patient's leg on the side to be flexed over his opposite leg. Place one hand against the side of the lumbar region, draw the thighs laterally enough to place the dependent heel near the edge of the table, and immobilize with sandbags. Next, draw the shoulders directly lateral as far as is possible without rotating the pelvis.

After the patient is in position a compression band may be applied to prevent movement. Respiration is suspended for the exposure.

Center the cassette to the midarea of the region being examined.

Central ray

Direct the central ray perpendicularly to the midpoint of the film.

Structures shown

Two AP projections of the lumbar vertebrae, made in maximum right and left flexion, are presented. These studies are employed (1) in cases of early scoliosis to determine the presence of structural change by unequal bend to right and left, (2) to localize a herniated disk as shown by limitation of motion at the site of the lesion, and (3) to demonstrate whether there is motion in the area of a spinal fusion. The latter examination is usually performed after a period of 6 months following the fusion operation.

The density of the spinal fusion radiographs must be sufficient to demonstrate the degree of movement when they are superimposed.

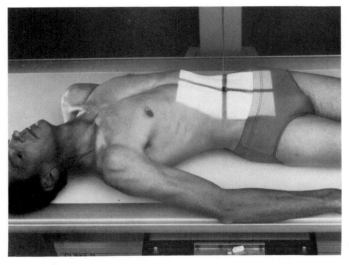

Right bending

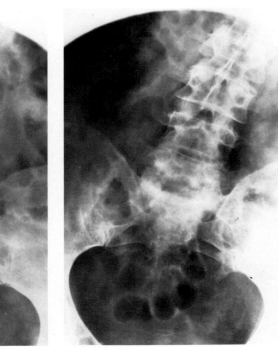

Right bending

Left bending

Dr. Lawson E. Miller, Jr.

LATERAL PROJECTION IN FLEXION AND EXTENSION

Film: 10" × 12" or 14" × 17" placed lengthwise for each exposure.

Position of patient

Adjust the patient in a lateral recumbent position. Center the coronal plane that lies approximately 2 inches posterior to the midaxillary line to the midline of the table.

Position of part

For the first radiograph, have the patient lean forward and draw his thighs up to flex the spine as much as possible.

For the second radiograph, have the patient lean backward and then extend his hips and thighs as much as possible. After the patient is in position a compression band may be applied across the pelvis to prevent movement.

Center the cassette at the level of the midarea of the region being examined.

Respiration is suspended for the exposures.

Central ray

Direct the central ray perpendicularly to the midpoint of the film.

Structures shown

These projections show two lateral images of the spine made in flexion and extension for the purpose of determining whether there is motion in the area of a spinal fusion or to localize a herniated disk as shown by limitation of motion at the site of the lesion.

The density of spinal fusion radiographs must be sufficient to demonstrate the degree of movement when they are superimposed.

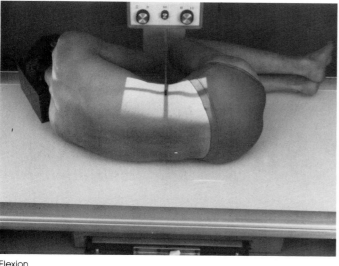

Flexion

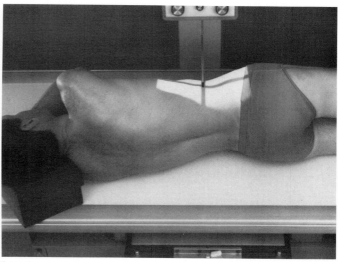

Extension

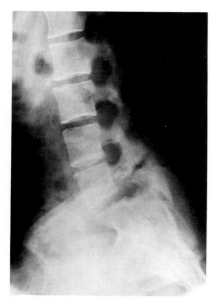

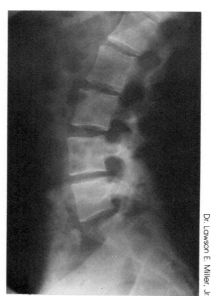

Dr. Lawson E. Miller, Jr.

13

Tomography

JEFFREY BOOKS

Since its inception in the 1890s, radiography has presented the problem of trying to record accurately three-dimensional body structures on two-dimensional films. This unavoidably results in the superimposition of structures, which often obscures important diagnostic information. One familiar method used to attempt to overcome this problem is the technique of right-angle projections. Over the years many other techniques have been developed that partially circumvent the problem of superimposition, such as multiple projections, stereoscopic projections, and subtraction techniques in angiography.

The partial or complete elimination of obscuring shadows by the effect of motion on shadow formation is a common technique used in radiography. This effect is frequently used with conventional projections. For example, in conjunction with a long exposure time, breathing motion is used to reduce rib and pulmonary shadows to a background blur on frontal projections of the sternum and on lateral projections of the thoracic spine.

Body-section radiography, or more appropriately tomography, is a term used to designate the radiographic technique with which most of the problems of superimposed images are overcome.

Tomography is the term used to designate the technique whereby a predetermined plane of the body is demonstrated in focus on the radiograph. Other body structures above or below the plane of interest are eliminated from the image or are rendered as a low-density blur caused by motion.

The origin of tomography cannot be attributed to any one particular person; in fact, tomography was developed by several different gifted men experimenting in different countries at about the same time without any knowledge of each other's work.

In 1921 one of the early pioneers in tomography, a French dermatologist, Dr. André-Edmund-Marie Bocage, described in an application for a patent many of the principles used in modern tomographic equipment. Many other early investigators made significant contributions to the field of tomography. Each of these pioneers applied a different name to his own particular device or process of body-section radiography. Bocage (1922) termed the result of his process *moving film roentgenograms;* the Italian, Vallebona (1930), chose the term *stratigraphy;* the Dutch physician, Ziedses des Plantes (1932), who made several significant contributions, called his process *planigraphy.* The term *tomography* came from the German investigator Grossman as does the *Grossman Principle,* which will be discussed later in this section. Tomography was invented in the United States in 1928 by Jean Kieffer, a radiologic technologist, who developed the special radiographic technique to demonstrate a form of tuberculosis that he had. His process was termed *laminagraphy* by another American, J. Robert Andrews, who assisted Kieffer in the construction of his first tomographic device, the *laminagraph.*[1]

A great deal of confusion arose over the multiplicity of names given to the general process of body-section radiography. To eliminate this confusion the International Commission of Radiological Units and Standards appointed a committee in 1962 to select a single term to represent all of the processes. *Tomography* is the term that they chose, and it is this term that is now recognized throughout the medical community as the single appropriate term for all forms of body-section radiography.[2]

[1]Littleton, J.T.: Tomography: physical principles and clinical application, Baltimore, 1976, The Williams & Wilkins Co., pp. 1-13.

[2]Vallebona, A., and Bistolfi, F.: Modern thin-section tomography, Springfield, Ill., 1973, Charles C Thomas, Publisher.

In tomography, as in conventional radiography, there are three basic requirements: an x-ray source, an object, and a recording medium (film). However, in tomography, to create an image of a single plane of tissue a fourth requirement must be met—synchronous movement of any two of the three essential elements during the x-ray exposure. This is usually achieved by moving the x-ray source and film in opposing directions about the stationary patient. The basic tomographic blurring principle is demonstrated in the diagram. At the beginning of the exposure the tube and film are at positions T_1 and F_1, respectively. During the exposure the tube and film travel in opposite directions, and their movements are terminated at the end of the exposure at positions T_2 and F_2. The focal plane is at the axis of rotation or the *fulcrum*. Structures at the same level of the focal plane remain in focus, while structures in other planes above and below this level are blurred from view. Tomography may be thought of as a process of controlled blurring. Note that the object located at point B is projected at the left side of the film at the beginning of the exposure. Now observe that at the end of the exposure the relative position of the projected object has now moved to the right of the film. Since this is not a static projection but a dynamic one, this structure is now nothing more than a blurred density on the film. An object at point A located at the level of the focal plane, however, is projected at the same place on the film throughout the entire exposure and therefore is not blurred but remains in focus.

Tomographic sections of different layers may be obtained by altering the level of the focal plane. This may be accomplished by one of two methods, depending on the principle utilized in the operation of the tomographic device. These two principles, the *planigraphic principle* and the *Grossman principle*, are the basis of all modern tomographic equipment. The Grossman principle utilizes a fixed fulcrum system in which the axis of rotation, or the fulcrum, remains at a fixed height. The focal plane level is changed by raising and lowering the tabletop and patient through this fixed point to the desired height. In contrast, the planigraphic principle utilizes an adjustable fulcrum system. The actual fulcrum or pivot point is raised or lowered to the height of the desired focal plane level, while the table and patient remain stationary at a fixed height.

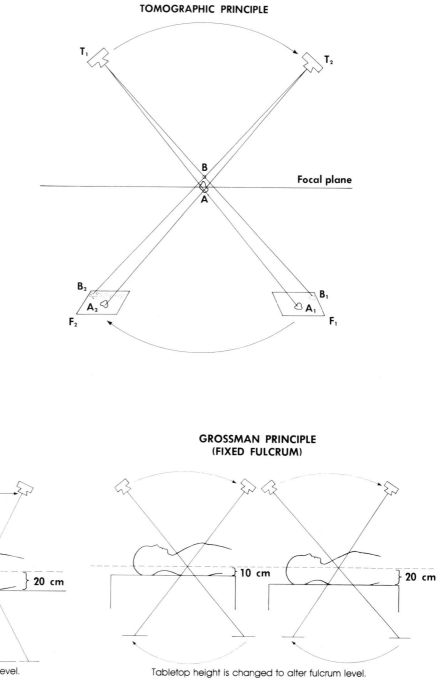

TOMOGRAPHIC PRINCIPLE

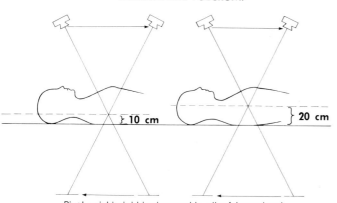

**PLANIGRAPHIC PRINCIPLE
(ADJUSTABLE FULCRUM)**

Pivot point height is changed to alter fulcrum level.

**GROSSMAN PRINCIPLE
(FIXED FULCRUM)**

Tabletop height is changed to alter fulcrum level.

The *exposure angle* is that angle of arc that is described by the movement of the tube and film during the tomographic exposure. The width of the focal plane or the plane of tissue that is in maximum focus is called the *section thickness*. The thickness of the tomographic section may be changed by altering the exposure angle. Tomograms using wide exposure angles will demonstrate thin sections; conversely, smaller exposure angles will demonstrate comparatively thicker sections.

The range of focal plane thickness produced by wide-angle tomography is approximately from 1 to 5 mm, and that with narrow-angle tomography, or zonography, is from slightly less than 1 cm to about 2.5 cm. *Zonography,* or the tomographic technique used to demonstrate relatively thick sections or zones of tissue, was first described by Zeidses des Plantes, who recommended it for examining sections of the cranium and the spinal column. Zonography is now used for a number of other regions and is particular-

ly useful in tomographic examinations of the abdominal structures.

There is no sharp line of focal plane demarcation, but the degree to which definition decreases with distance from the focal plane is dependent on the width of the angle described by the tube motion. This depends on the width of the angle described by the tube. Wide angles of the tube movement provide excellent blurring of structures close to the focal plane, as well as of those remote from it. Narrow angles of tube movement provide excellent blurring of structures remote from the focal plane but only moderate to slight blurring of structures close to the focal zone.

Although visibility of the objective area is greatly enhanced by the partial or complete elimination of obscuring shadows, the appearance of the tomogram is quite different from that of a conventional radiograph. The customary sharp definition and clear contrast are diminished, and the contours of all but the thinnest objects are absent. The contrast is reduced because of the blurring action diffusing elements in other planes over the focal plane image. The formation of the tomographic image is a cumulative process. The shadows of structures in the plane of focus accumulate on the film as the area traversed by the beam of radiation swings over the arc. The images are not sharp, since the radiation traversed structures from many angles, outlining clearly only those boundaries to which it is momentarily tangential in its passage.

Zonograms are comparable in appearance to conventional radiographs, because (1) the cuts are thick enough to show structural contours, (2) the narrow arc described by the tube directs the radiation at only slightly oblique angles, so that it projects structural contours more nearly true to shape, and (3) because of less blurring, contrast and detail are superior to those of the tomograms. However, this is not to say that there is more diagnostic information in a zonogram than in a wide-angle tomogram; each has its definite place in tomography. The choice between using a wide or narrow exposure angle primarily depends on the thickness of the structure or structures to be tomographed and their proximity to other structures outside the focal plane.

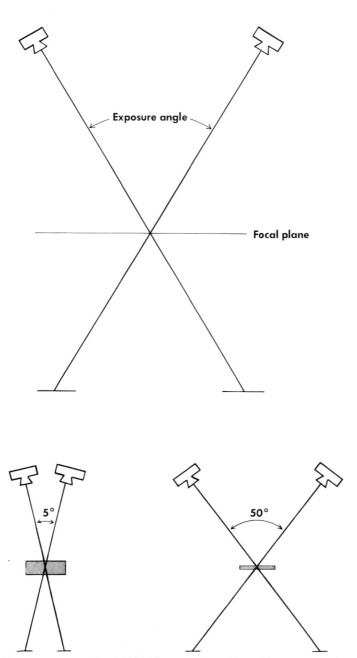

Narrow exposure angles yield thick tomographic sections; wide exposure angles yield thin tomographic sections.

BLURRING MOTIONS

Modern tomographic equipment offers a variety of different blurring patterns. These blurring motions fall under two separate categories: *unidirectional*, or *linear*, and *pluridirectional*, or *complex*, *motions*, which include circular, elliptical, hypocycloidal, and spiral motions. A basic understanding of the characteristics of these blurring patterns is necessary for understanding their advantages as well as their limitations.

Linear motion

The basic tomographic blurring pattern is the undirectional, or linear, motion. The blurring action of linear motion is provided by elongation of structures outside of the focal plane so that they become indistinguishable linear streaks or blurs over the focal plane image. Maximum blurring occurs to those elements of structures outside the focal plane that are oriented perpendicularly to the relative motion of the tube. In linear tomography therefore elements of structures oriented parallel to the motion of the tube are incompletely blurred and form false shadows over the focal plane image. This results in an inaccurate representation of the focal plane because of the summation of the focal plane image and images of some structures outside the plane of focus. This characteristic is demonstrated in the following tomogram of a test object.

The test object consists of two wire patterns: pattern A, is located at the level of the focal plane; pattern B is 5 mm away from the level of the focal plane and therefore exhibits the effects of the blurring motion used.

The best blurring occurs to those elements of the patterns that are perpendicular to the tube movement, and the least occurs to those parallel. In linear tomography it is important to orient those structures to be blurred at right angles to the tube movement. For example, in tomography of the chest the tube movement is oriented perpendicularly to the ribs for maximum blurring of those structures.

A more efficient blurring motion would be one in which all of the elements of an object would be perpendicular to the movement of the tube at some time during the exposure. This is the principle of the second type of blurring motion, the multidirectional, or pluridirectional, motion.

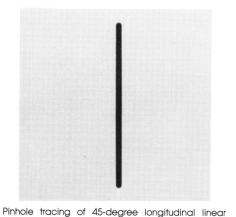

Pinhole tracing of 45-degree longitudinal linear motion

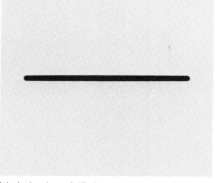

Pinhole tracing of 45-degree transverse linear motion

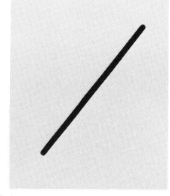

Pinhole tracing of 45-degree oblique linear motion

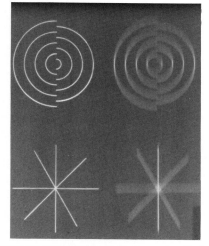

Tomogram of test object at 45-degree longitudinal linear motion. Left pattern is at level of focal plane. Right pattern is 5 mm above level of focal plane. With linear motion the best blurring occurs to elements of test object oriented perpendicular to movement of tube and the least blurring to elements oriented parallel.

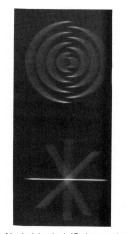

Tomogram of test object at 45-degree transverse linear motion

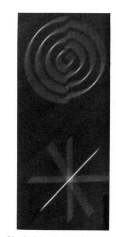

Tomogram of test object at 45-degree oblique linear motion

Circular motion

The basic pluridirectional motion is the circular pattern. The circular motion does not blur by mere elongation but by evenly diffusing the densities of those structures outside the focal plane over the focal plane image. Tomograms using a circular or any other complex motion therefore exhibit more even but less contrast than do linear tomograms with their characteristic linear streaking. Note that all elements of the test pattern are equally blurred regardless of their orientation. The circular motion maintains a constant radius and angle throughout the exposure, which results in a sharp cutoff margin of the blurred structures. This in turn may result in the formation of phantom images superimposed over the focal plane image.

The phenomenon of phantom images occurs more often in circular tomography using small angles as in circular zonography. The phantom images are created by the fusion of the margins of the blurred shadows of structures slightly outside the focal plane or by annular shadows of dense structures again slightly outside the focal plane.

These phantom images are usually less dense and distinct than the actual focal plane images. They can be identified as such on successive tomograms as the real structure or structures come into focus.

The characteristics of wide-angle circular tomography are identical to small-angle circular tomography, with one exception. The wider angle results in greater displacement of the blurred shadows, reducing the possibility of phantom image formation.

Elliptical motion

The elliptical motion, having both linear and circular aspects to the pattern, exhibits blurring characteristics of both. It requires the same perpendicular orientation as the linear motion and exhibits similar phantom shadow characteristics to the circular motion. Although it is a more efficient blurring motion than the simple linear motion, the quality of blur is much less than the circular motion or the more complex motions, *hypocycloidal* and *spiral motion*.

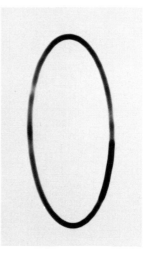

A

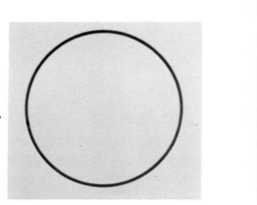

A

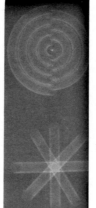

B

Circular motion of 45 degrees. **A,** Pinhole tracing. **B,** Tomogram of test object demonstrating annular shadow formation and fusion of marginal blur pattern characteristics of circular motion.

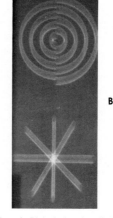

B

Elliptical motion. **A,** Pinhole tracing. **B,** Tomogram of test object demonstrating characteristics of both linear and circular motions.

Hypocycloidal motion

The hypocycloidal motion offers excellent displacement of the marginal blur pattern, nearly eliminating the possibility of phantom image formation. It provides excellent blurring of structures both close to and remote from the focal plane and has a focal plane thickness of slightly less than 1 mm.

Spiral motion

Tomographic equipment capable of producing a spiral motion is usually designed for a three-spired motion or a five-spired motion. The spiral motion, although different in pattern from the hypocycloidal motion, also offers excellent displacement of the marginal blur pattern, exceptional resolving power, and an extremely thin section thickness of less than 1 mm.

These excellent blurring characteristics make both the hypocycloidal and spiral motion useful in examinations of any area of the body, and they are especially useful in tomographic examinations of the skull, where structures are very small and compact and require greater separation of tissue planes.

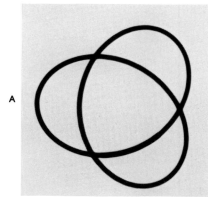

A

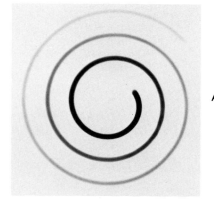

A

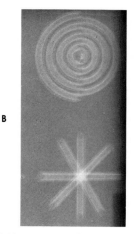

B

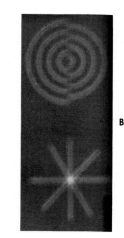

B

Hypocycloidal motion. **A,** Pinhole tracing. **B,** Tomogram of test object demonstrating excellent blurring characteristics.

Trispiral motion. **A,** Pinhole tracing. **B,** Tomogram of test object demonstrating excellent blurring characteristics.

FACTORS AFFECTING TOMOGRAPHIC IMAGE

"The difference between a high quality tomogram and a poor one is very slight; hence, it is extremely important that attention be given to all the parameters which contribute to the focal plane image."[1] The factors that affect the tomographic image can be divided into two categories: (1) patient variables and (2) equipment variables.

Patient variables

As in conventional radiography, proper positioning of the patient and centering of the central ray are of critical importance. Another and equally important factor that must be considered in tomography is the selection of the proper focal plane level. The part must be adequately immobilized, because any motion will add unwanted blur to the focal plane image. Object size and the relative density of structures will affect density and contrast of the image.

Equipment variables

The tomographic principle utilized will affect several different properties of the image, with magnification being affected the most. Tomographic machines utilizing the fixed fulcrum principle will maintain a constant magnification factor at any focal plane level, because the distance between the focal plane and the film remains the same at any level. Conversely, with the adjustable fulcrum system, the focal plane–film distance changes as the fulcrum height is varied, resulting in different magnification of the focal plane image at different fulcrum heights. This magnification is, however, at most working levels, less than the fixed rate of magnification of the fixed fulcrum machines.

[1] Littleton, J.T.: Tomography: physical principles and clinical application, Baltimore, 1976, The Williams & Wilkins Co., p. 33.

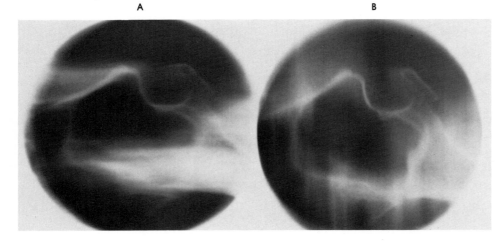

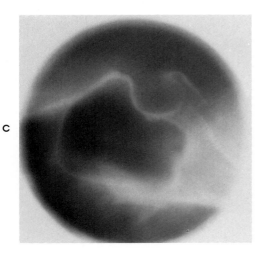

Tomograms of sella turcica in lateral projection through midplane. **A,** Transverse linear motion. **B,** Longitudinal transverse motion. **C,** Trispiral motion demonstrating the sella turcica much more clearly and without parasitic linear streaking that is found in **A** or **B.**

The degree to which structures outside the focal plane are blurred is a function of the geometry of the blurring pattern and the angle of the tomographic arc. The more complex the blurring pattern is, the greater the effacement will be of those structures outside the focal plane. Wide exposure angles provide greater blurring of structures close to the focal plane as well as those that are remote. The exposure angle also determines the thickness of the focal plane image. As previously mentioned, the wider the exposure angle, the thinner the section thickness will be, and, conversely, the narrower the exposure angle, the thicker the section thickness.

Each blurring pattern requires a specific amount of time to complete its motion. Therefore the exposure time must be of sufficient length to allow completion of the motion before terminating the exposure. Linear motions generally take less time to complete than do the more complex pluridirectional movements. The exposure time is the other half of the mAs formula, but, since there are restrictions for certain exposure times for each different pattern, the mA and kV must be altered to change the density. Since contrast levels are inherently low in tomography, high mAs and relatively low kV techniques are used in most examinations to enhance the contrast between structures.

Collimating to the smallest possible field size also improves the contrast of the image.

The focal spot size will affect the detail of the focal plane image. In areas in which great detail is required, such as the skull, cervical spine, and extremities, the smallest available focal spot should be used. Extreme care must be taken not to exceed the recommended tube limits or cooling rate.

Tomographic machines must provide synchronous, vibration-free movement of the tube and film, because any mechanical instability may transmit unwanted motion and blur to the focal plane image. For this reason, the exposure is started after the motion has begun, allowing enough time for any unwanted motion and vibration to be stabilized that may have been caused by the rapid acceleration of the tube and film. The exposure is then terminated just before the end of the movement to avoid any motion that may occur during the rapid deceleration of the tube and film.

Since the thicknesses of cassettes vary with each manufacturer, one type of cassette should be used throughout the entire examination. Otherwise, the focal plane images will not be successively consistent from level to level, because the height of the film and therefore the focal plane image will vary with each different cassette used.

The film-screen combination will greatly affect the tomographic image. Very low speed film-screen combinations will produce images with very good detail, but they require a prohibitive amount of radiation. A faster combination produces images with good detail and contrast with much less radiation. Other combinations using rare earth screens are available that produce films with excellent detail but slightly lower contrast.

EQUIPMENT

Tomography machines may be varied in appearance and function, but all have three basic requirements in common. Aside from the usual features of any radiographic machine, such as an x-ray source, timer, and mA and kVp selector, any x-ray machine capable of producing a tomographic image must have the following additional features: (1) the machine must have some type of linkage connecting the x-ray source and film carriage that will provide synchronous, vibration-free movement of the tube and film in opposite directions during the tomographic exposure; (2) there must be a means of imparting motion to the tube and film carriage for each tomographic movement; and (3) there must be a means of adjusting the fulcrum height for tomograms at different levels.

The simplest type of linkage is a mechanical connection formed by a long metal rod connected to the x-ray source at one end and the film carriage at the other. As the x-ray tube moves in one direction, the film carriage will always move in the opposite direction. The film will move synchronously with the movement of the tube, maintaining a constant relationship with each other as they move. This mechanical type of linkage is the basic type of linkage that most tomographic machines utilize, from the simplest machines to the highly sophisticated pluridirectional units. The major difference between the two is that in the multidirectional machines the simple metal rod is replaced by a heavier metal beam or a parallelogram of thick rods that attach at either end to the x-ray tube and film carriage. The heavier material used for the linkage is required to withstand the great centrifugal force created by the tube and film carriage as it swings rapidly through the complete motions.

There is another type of linkage that has been made possible by the recent advances in computer technology. One manufacturer has developed a radiographic machine capable of linear tomography with no direct mechanical linkage between the tube and film carriage. The x-ray tube is mounted on the ceiling and is electronically linked to the film carriage by a microcomputer. The microcomputer controls separate drive motors that maintain the tube and film in alignment throughout the linear motion. This revolutionary design allows for greater mobility of the x-ray tube for radiographic examinations, since it is free floating when not in the tomographic mode.

The second requirement is that there must be a means of imparting motion to the tube and film carriage for each tomographic motion. Modern machines employ motors that drive the tube and film for the blurring movement. The motor drive and the linkage mechanism must provide stable, vibration-free movement of the tube and film. Any unwanted motion may cause additional blurring of the focal plane image.

All tomographic machines must also have some means of adjusting the height of the fulcrum. In machines utilizing the adjustable or planigraphic principle, the motor drive alters the actual pivot point of the tube-film carriage assembly. Tomographic machines utilizing the fixed fulcrum or Grossman principle have a tabletop that is raised or lowered by a motor to the desired height.

Tomographic equipment has changed considerably since the early days of Vallebona and des Plantes. Their first machines were crude, although ingeniously designed contrivances operated with ropes, pulleys, and hand cranks. Present-day equipment is motor driven and ranges from simple radiographic tables that can change over to linear tomography to highly sophisticated machines designed primarily for pluridirectional tomography. The more elaborate tomographic machines offer several automatic functions, such as automatic fulcrum height adjustment and motorized cassette shift for multiple exposures on one film. The pluridirectional machines are capable of several different complex motions as well as the simple linear movement.

Testing of tomographic equipment

Tomographic equipment is carefully checked and calibrated by the manufacturer's service representative when it is installed. The tube-film movement must be stable and exactly balanced, and there must be synchronization of the travel time and exposure time at each of the exposure angles and tomographic movements. These are checked with a pinhole test device. The pinhole test device is a lead plate with a very small beveled hole in the middle, which is positioned on the tabletop directly in line with the central ray. Pinholes must be placed above or below the focal plane. The tomographic exposure is made, tracing on film the actual pattern of the tomographic motion used. Any mechanical instability or aberration in the correct exposure time can be noted on the pinhole tracing. Examples of pinhole tracings can be found in the section on blurring motions.

Another test device called a tomographic test phantom is used to determine the accuracy of the fulcrum height indicator and the section thickness of the different exposure angles and blurring motions. The blurring characteristics of the different motions may be determined with the phantom also (see the section on blurring motions). Different phantoms are available, but most manufacturers of tomographic equipment recommend the test phantom developed by Dr. J.T. Littleton.

CLINICAL APPLICATIONS

Tomography is a proven diagnostic tool that can be of significant value when an accurate interpretation cannot be made from conventional radiographs, since confusing shadows can be removed from the point of interest. Tomography may be used in any part of the body but is most effective in areas of high contrast, such as in bone and lung. Body-section radiography is used to demonstrate and evaluate a number of different pathologic processes, traumatic injuries, and congenital abnormalities. A basic familiarization of the clinical applications of tomography will help the tomographer to be more effective in the performance of his job. Some of the major areas of clinical applications are described below, although the versatility of tomography lends itself to other applications.

Pathologic processes in soft tissues

One of the most frequent uses of tomography is to demonstrate and evaluate benign processes and malignant neoplasms in the lungs. Differentiation between benign lesions and malignancies cannot always be made with conventional chest radiography. With tomography, it is possible to define the location, size, shape, and marginal contours of the lesion. Differentiation between benign and malignant tumors depends on the characteristics of the lesion itself. Benign lesions characteristically have smooth, well-marginated contours and frequently contain bits of calcium. The presence of calcium in a chest lesion usually confirms it as being benign. The benign lesions most commonly found in the lungs are granulomas, which form as a tissue reaction to a chronic infectious process that has healed.

Conversely, carcinogenic neoplasms characteristically have ill-defined margins that feather or streak into the surrounding tissue and rarely contain calcium. Lung cancers may originate in the lung, in which case the neoplasm would be termed a primary malignancy. Bronchogenic carcinoma is an example of a primary malignancy that may develop in the chest. Lung cancers may develop as the result of the spread of cancer from another area of the body to the lungs. These malignancies are termed secondary or metastatic tumors. Breast cancer and testicular cancer, as well as others, may metastisize to the lungs.

When a patient has a known primary malignant neoplasm, general tomographic surveys of both lungs are frequently performed to exclude the possibility of metastatic disease. Frequently these lesions cannot be visualized by conventional radiographic methods, and tomography is the only means to identify these occult nodules. The demonstration of the number of tumors, their location, and the size is crucial to the physician's plan of treatment and the prognosis for the patient. Reexamination by tomography may be performed at a later date to check on the progress of the disease and the effectiveness of the therapy.

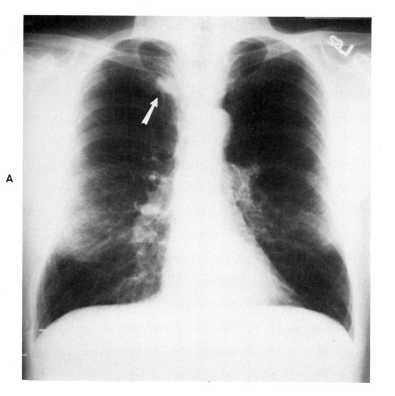

A

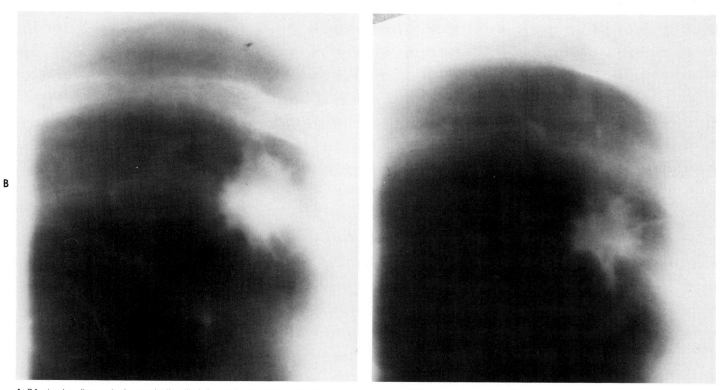

B

C

A, PA chest radiograph demonstrating ill-defined density (*arrow*) in right upper chest. **B** and **C,** Coned-down AP tomograms of patient in **A** demonstrating lesion in posterior chest plane with ill-defined margins that feather or streak into surrounding lung tissue, characteristic of malignant chest neoplasm.

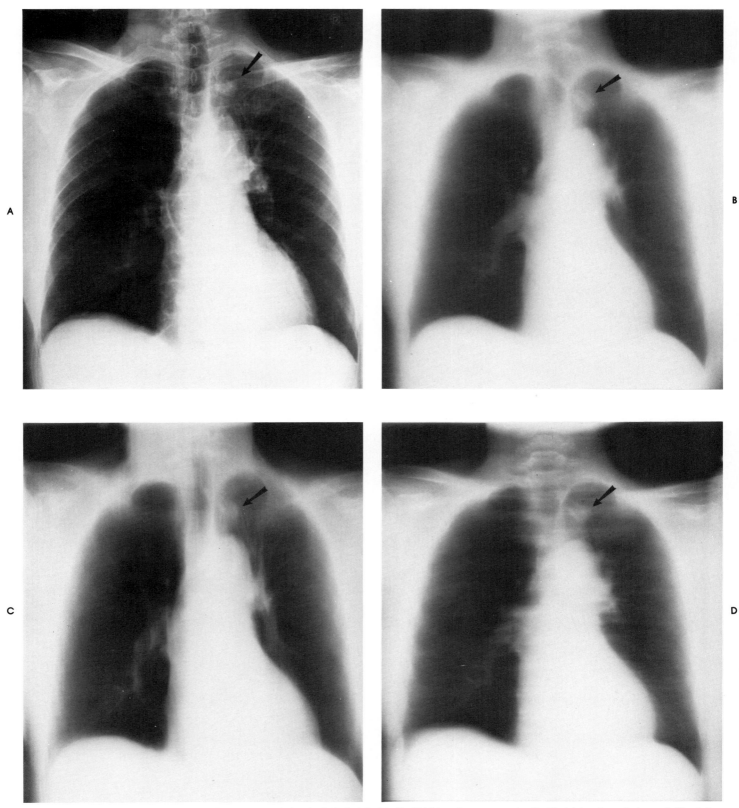

A, AP chest radiograph with vague density (*arrow*) over medial end of left clavicle. **B** to **D,** AP full lung tomograms of patient in **A** taken to exclude possibility of other occult lesions. **B,** Trispiral tomogram 1 cm anterior to hilar plane at level of tumor. Radiographic appearance of lesion (*arrow*) is consistent with malignant chest neoplasm. **C,** Longitudinal linear tomogram of 40 degrees at same fulcrum level as **B.** Visualization of lesion (*arrow*) is decreased because of linear streaking and incomplete blurring of other structures outside focal plane. **D,** 40-degree transverse linear tomogram at same level as **B** and **C,** again demonstrating poor visualization of lesion (*arrow*) because of linear blurring characteristics. Blurring of anterior ribs is incomplete.

Pulmonary hila

Neoplasms involving the pulmonary hila are most effectively evaluated by tomography. It is possible with tomography to determine if and to what degree the individual bronchi are patent or obstructed. This partial or complete obstruction may occur when a neoplasm develops within the bronchus and bulges into the bronchial airspace or if a tumor grows adjacent to the bronchus. As the lesion grows, it may press against the bronchus, causing a reduction in the size of the lumen and restricting or obstructing the airflow to that part of the lung. Pneumonia, atelectasis, and other inflammatory or reactive changes that may occur with the obstruction may further hinder conventional imaging of this area. Demonstration of bronchial patency through a density is strong evidence that the lesion is inflammatory and not malignant.

Soft tissue lesions affecting bony structures

Another major application of tomography is to demonstrate and evaluate soft tissue neoplasms in the presence of bony structures. Because of the high density of bone and the relatively low density of the soft tissue neoplasms, it is usually not possible to demonstrate the actual lesion, but it is possible to demonstrate with great clarity the bony destruction caused by the presence of the tumor.

For example, neoplasms involving the pituitary gland usually cause bony changes or destruction of the floor of the sella turcica, which would indicate the presence of a pituitary adenoma. In addition to demonstrating destruction caused by the tumor, it is possible with tomography to demonstrate the bony septations in the sphenoid sinus, which aids the surgeon in removing the neoplasm.

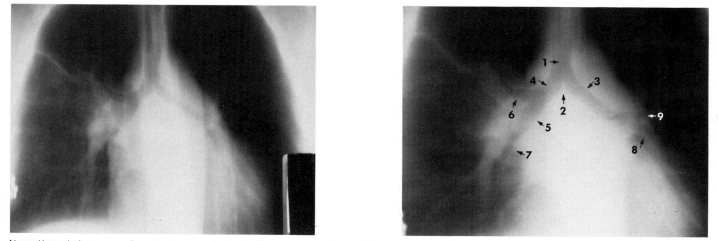

Normal bronchotomograms through midplane of hilum. **A,** Linear tomogram. **B,** Trispiral tomogram demonstrating more clearly the hilar structures: *1,* trachea; *2,* carina; *3,* left main stem bronchus; *4,* right main stem bronchus; *5,* intermediate bronchus; *6,* right upper lobe bronchus; *7,* right lower lobe bronchus; *8,* left lower lobe bronchus; *9,* left upper lobe bronchus.

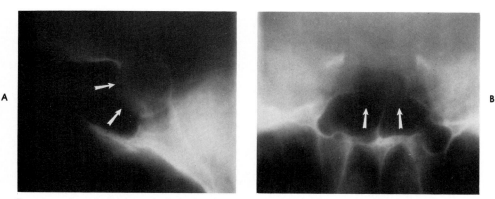

Tomograms through midplane of sella turcica demonstrating destruction of floor (*arrows*) caused by presence of pituitary adenoma. **A,** Lateral tomogram. **B,** AP tomogram.

Lesions in bone

Subtle changes that may occur as a result of a pathologic process in bone tissue may be noted on conventional radiographs, but in many instances only with the aid of tomography can the true nature and extent of the involvement be determined. Pathologic processes involving bony structures are normally characterized by bone destruction and/or changes in the bone tissue or the surface margins. More specifically, in tomography the attempt is made to identify the extent of bone destruction, the status of the cortex of the bone (i.e., whether destruction extends through the cortical bone), the presence of any periosteal reaction to the lesion, changes in the bone matrix, new bone formation, and the status of the zone of the bone between the diseased and normal bone.

Destruction of bone or other alterations in the bone may be the result of a multitude of different benign or malignant processes that manifest themselves in different ways. Some benign processes such as osteomyelitis are presented as areas of bone destruction, whereas others such as osteomas are presented as abnormal growths of bone from bone tissue. Some processes may exhibit a combination of bone destruction and new growth, as occurs in Paget's disease and rheumatoid arthritis.

Malignant neoplasms in bone tissue may occur in the form of primary lesions or secondary lesions resulting from the metastatic spread of cancer from another area of the body.

Some forms of cancer occurring in bone will exhibit areas of both destruction and new growth, whereas others exhibit only areas of extensive destruction.

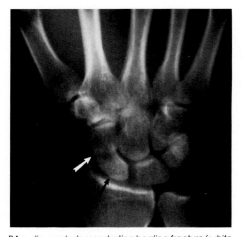

PA radiograph demonstrating healing fracture (*white arrow*) of navicular bone and increased density (*black arrow*) of proximal end.

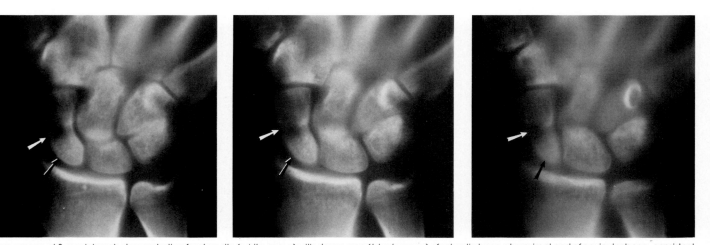

Tomograms at 3-mm intervals demonstrating fracture site (*white arrows*) with dense area (*black arrows*) of sclerotic bone at proximal end of navicular bone, consistent with aseptic necrosis.

Fractures

The three major clinical applications for tomography when dealing with known and suspected fractures are (1) identification and evaluation of occult fractures, (2) better evaluation of known fractures, and (3) evaluation of the healing process of fractures.

If a fracture is suspected clinically but cannot be ruled out or identified by conventional imaging methods, tomography may be indicated. Tomography is often used when fractures are suspected in areas of complex bone structures such as the cervical spine. The cervical spine projects a myriad of confusing shadows, often hiding fracture lines, making an accurate diagnosis impossible. With tomography it is possible to identify and evaluate these occult fractures. Knowledge of these fractures can be crucial to the patient's plan of treatment and prognosis. Another area that frequently requires tomographic evaluation for occult fractures is the skull. The skull has many complicated bone structures that often make identification and evaluation of fractures in some areas extremely difficult without the use of tomography. The facial nerve canal that courses through the temporal bone is just one of many areas in the skull that is difficult to evaluate for fractures without tomography. Blowout fractures of the orbital floor also frequently require tomographic evaluation because of the difficulty in identifying and evaluating fractures and fragments of the thin bone of which the floor and medial wall of the orbit are composed.

Tomography may also be used to evaluate known fractures with greater efficiency than is possible with conventional radiography. In some instances a fracture may be visualized on a conventional radiograph, but, because of the complex nature of the fracture or superimposition of shadows from adjacent structures, the fracture site cannot be adequately evaluated without the use of tomography. This often is the case in fractures of the hip involving the acetabulum. In acetabular fractures portions of the actabulum are often broken into many fragments. These fragments may be difficult to identify, but with tomography the fragments and any possible femoral fracture can be evaluated before any attempt to reduce the fracture.

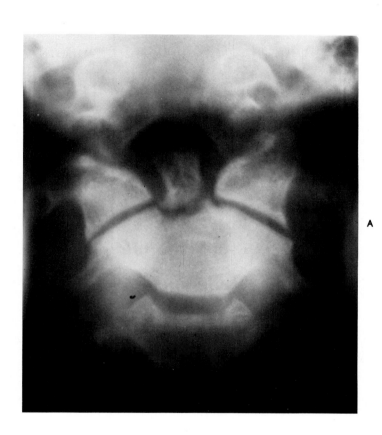

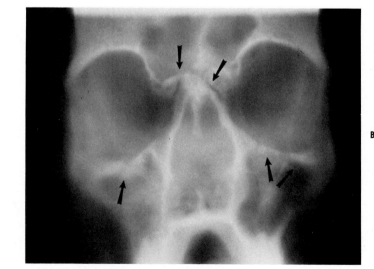

A, AP tomogram of C1-C3 demonstrating complete fracture at base of odontoid process. **B,** Frontal tomogram in reverse Caldwell projection demonstrating multiple facial fractures (*arrows*).

Healing fractures

Tomography may also be used to evaluate the healing process of fractures when, because of overlying shadows of fixation devices, adjacent structures, or the bone callus, conventional imaging methods may prove inadequate. In these cases it may be impossible to tell if the bone is healing properly throughout the fracture site without the use of tomography. With tomography it is possible to identify the areas of the fracture when incomplete healing exists.

Abdominal structures

Because of the relatively homogeneous densities of abdominal structures both radiographic and tomographic imaging of this area are most effectively performed in conjunction with the use of contrast materials. Narrow-angle tomography, or zonography, is usually preferred for tomographic evaluation of these organs. As previously stated, zonography produces focal plane images of greater contrast than is possible with thin-section tomography. This increased level of contrast aids in the visualization of the rela-

tively low-density organs of the abdomen. The extensive blurring of remote structures that occurs with wide-angle tomography is not necessary in the abdomen, since there are relatively few high-density structures in this area that would compromise the zonographic imaging of the abdominal structures. Thick sections of organs are depicted with each zonogram, and entire organs can be demonstrated in a small number of tomographic sections.

A circular motion with an exposure angle of 8 or 10 degrees is recommended for use in the abdomen. Occasionally, an angle of 15 degrees may be necessary to eliminate bowel gas shadows if the smaller angle does not provide adequate effacement (blurring) of the bowel.

Zonography using a linear movement is not recommended, because it does not provide adequate blurring of structures outside the focal plane. If a linear movement is used, an exposure angle of 15 degrees should be used to provide adequate blurring. It should be remembered that linear tomography does not produce accurate focal plane images because of the incomplete blurring effect of structures

oriented parallel to the tube movement. Although the possibility of false image formation does exist with circular tomography, the image of the focal plane is far more accurate than with linear tomography. Linear tomograms are higher in contrast than circular tomograms, but this is actually because of the linear streaking caused by the incomplete blurring characteristics of the linear motion. The circular motion, on the other hand, will produce an accurate focal plane image with slightly less but even contrast.

The most common tomographic examinations of the abdomen are of the kidneys and bile ducts. These examinations are normally performed with contrast material.

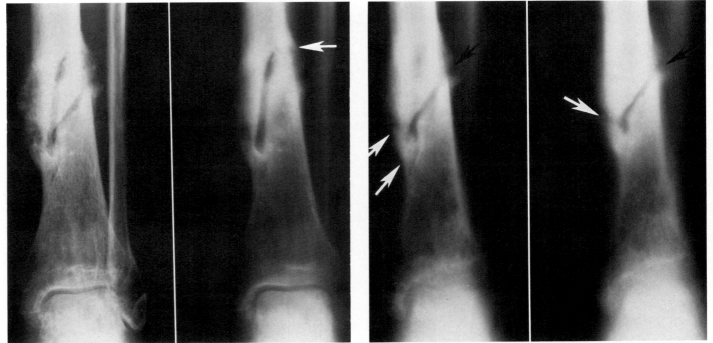

A, AP radiograph of distal tibia demonstrating questionable complete union of fractures. **B,** AP tomogram of same patient as in **A,** demonstrating incomplete union of longitudinal fracture (*arrow*). **C** and **D,** Tomograms demonstrating incomplete union of oblique fractures (*arrows*) through shaft of tibia of same patient as in **A** and **B**. **C,** 0.5 cm and, **D,** 1 cm posterior to **B**.

Renal tomography

Many institutions routinely include tomography of the kidneys as part of the procedure for intravenous pyelograms (IVP). The tomograms are usually taken immediately following the bolus injection of the contrast material. At this time the kidney is entering the nephrogram of the IVP in which the nephrons of the kidney begin to absorb the contrast material, causing the parenchyma of the kidney to become fairly radiopaque. It is then possible to demonstrate with zonography lesions in the kidney that may have been overlooked with conventional radiography.

Another typical renal tomographic examination is the nephrotomogram. The major difference between this and the IVP is the method of introduction of the contrast material. In nephrotomography the contrast material is drip-infused throughout the examination instead of introduced in a single bolus injection. This method allows for a considerably longer nephrographic effect, since the nephrons continuously absorb and excrete the contrast material as it is being infused and opacify the kidney.

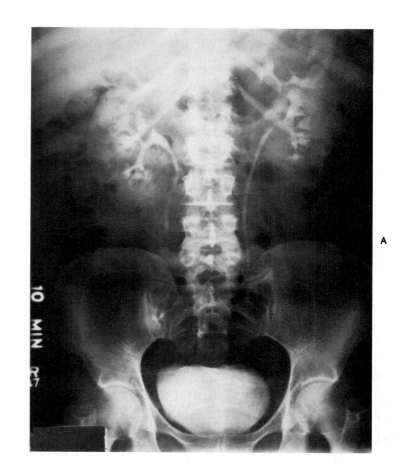

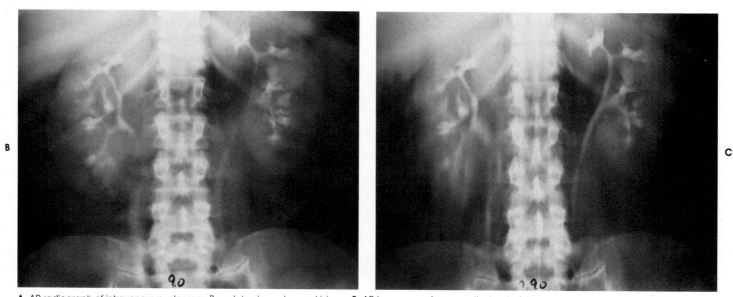

A, AP radiograph of intravenous pyelogram. Bowel shadows obscure kidneys. **B,** AP tomogram of same patient as in **A** through midplane of kidneys using 8-degree circular motion. Bowel shadows are absent, and visualization of kidneys is improved over **C. C,** AP tomogram of same patient as in **A** and **B** and at same levels as in **B,** but employing 20-degree linear motion. Note linear streaking and loss of detail of collecting systems and kidney borders.

Intravenous cholangiograms

The biliary tract is another organ system that may require tomography for adequate evaluation. If an oral cholecystogram does not yield sufficient information for a diagnosis or if biliary ductal disease is suspected in a cholecystectomized patient, then an intravenous cholangiogram (IVC) may be indicated. The IVC is performed by infusing a solution of the contrast material Cholegrafin into the bloodstream, where it is first absorbed into and then excreted by the liver into the biliary ducts. The drip infusion should be administered slowly over approximately 20 to 30 minutes to reduce the possibility of anaphylactic shock. Opacification of the ducts is generally not dense enough for adequate evaluation with conventional radiography alone. The ducts may also be partially or completely obscured by the superimposition of shadows or other structures in the abdomen. Even though the ducts may be well opacified on conventional radiographs, tomography should be performed to provide additional information not available with conventional radiography. Zonography is normally used for IVCs; however, there may be instances in which a more complex movement such as trispiral or hypocycloidal movement may be preferred. If a linear motion is to be employed, an exposure angle of 15 or 20 degrees should be used.

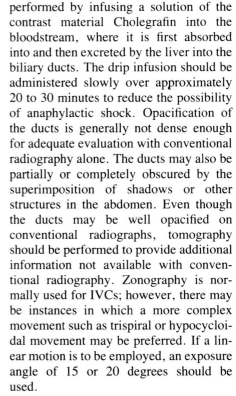

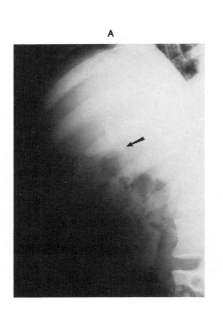

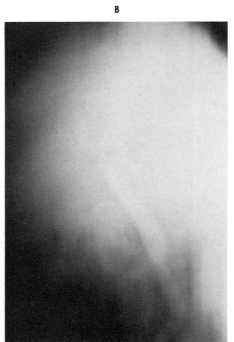

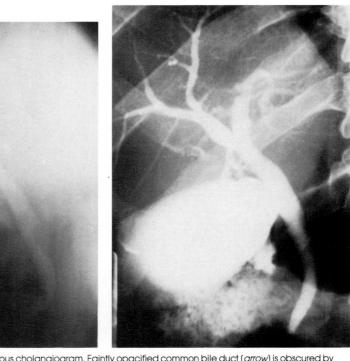

A, RPO radiograph of intravenous cholangiogram. Faintly opacified common bile duct (*arrow*) is obscured by bowel gas and liver. **B** and **C,** RPO tomograms of same patient as in **A** through level of common bile duct. Visualization of duct is improved over plain film study (**A**). **D,** Transhepatic cholangiogram of same patient as in **A** to **C.**

BASIC PRINCIPLES OF POSITIONING

In conventional radiography rarely does one single projection contain all the diagnostic information necessary to make an accurate diagnosis. This is also true in tomography; one series of tomograms in a single projection usually does not contain enough information to make an accurate diagnosis. As in radiography, two or more projections are usually required for most tomographic examinations. In the case of bilateral structures, such as the internal auditory canals, only one projection may be used. In such cases, tomograms of the contralateral side are made for comparison.

Many standard radiographic positions are used in tomography. The AP and lateral projections are basic to most tomographic examinations. Occasionally, a special oblique projection may be necessary to optimally visualize the part under investigation. Basically, in tomography the structures to be tomographed should be oriented parallel or perpendicular to the tomographic plane. For example, when evaluating structures in the base of the skull the patient's head should be positioned in a basal projection so that the base of the skull will be oriented parallel to the section plane. This parallel position not only will produce images that are more anatomically correct but also will reduce the total number of tomograms necessary to cover the area of interest. If the base of the skull is not parallel but is slightly obliqued, more tomograms are required to adequately evaluate the area of interest. This also pertains to other areas of the body in which large, relatively flat surfaces occur, such as in long bones. When tomographing long bones such as the femur the long axis of the bone should be adjusted to be parallel to the tomographic plane. Some structures, such as the sella turcica, are better suited to a perpendicular orientation for tomography. Since the presence of a pituitary adenoma usually affects the floor of the sella, it should be oriented to be perpendicular to the section plane. The AP and lateral projections are routinely used for this examination, and in both positions the floor will remain perpendicular to the tomographic plane.

There are very few areas in radiology in which the demand placed on the knowledge and ability of the technologist are as great as in the field of tomography. The tomographer must possess a better than average knowledge of anatomy and of the spatial relationships of the structures of the body. The tomographic technologists must know where certain structures of the general body parts are located, how to best position those structures for tomographic examination, at what depth the particular structures are located, and how the tomographic image should look. There are many occasions when even the experienced tomographer must rely heavily on the knowledge and instruction of the radiologist monitoring the examination. A close working relationship between the technologist and the radiologist should exist, since no two tomographic examinations are exactly alike, and each case must be considered individually.

It is necessary to provide the radiologist with an adequate clinical history of the patient. This information may be obtained from the patient's medical records if it is not provided on the examination requisition or by interviewing the patient. This clinical information and any pertinent radiographs should be reviewed and discussed with the radiologist before beginning the examination. After reviewing this information the radiologist and technologist can then decide on the area of interest, the optimum position, the size of the field of exposure, the type of blurring motion and exposure angle to be used, the separation intervals between tomographic sections, and the parameters for the fulcrum height.

All equipment preparation should be accomplished before positioning the patient. This will reduce the amount of time that the patient is required to maintain an often uncomfortable position. The technologist should briefly and simply explain the procedure to the patient and offer a rough estimate of the expected length of the examination. Many patients are under the mistaken impression that the procedure consists of just a few x-rays that can be taken in a matter of a few minutes and that they will then be permitted to leave. They are not aware that they will be required to maintain a certain position throughout the procedure. If the patient knows beforehand what to expect, he will be in a better frame of mind to cooperate throughout the lengthy examination.

The use of a suitable table pad is recommended for tomographic examinations. A table pad that is 4 cm thick will add an insignificant amount of distance to the overall patient thickness and will greatly increase the patient's comfort. Patient comfort is extremely important, and all attempts should be made to ensure this. If the patient is not comfortable, he simply will not hold still for the examination. Angle sponges and foam blocks should be used to assist the patient in maintaining the correct position wherever applicable. However, foam sponges are not recommended for use in tomographic examinations of the head. Section intervals of 1 or 2 mm are often employed in this area, and foam sponges do not give firm enough support of the head. With little change in pressure the head may move, drastically altering the desired focal plane levels. Folded towels may be used to support the head; they offer greater resistance to any downward pressure of the head.

IMMOBILIZATION TECHNIQUES

The most effective immobilization technique is the technologist's instructions to the patient. No amount of physical restraint will keep a patient from moving if he does not fully understand the importance of holding still from the first preliminary film to the end of the tomographic series.

Although suspension of respiration is not necessary in many tomographic examinations, it is mandatory in examinations of the chest and abdomen. Explicit breathing instructions must be given to the patient for examinations of these areas. In chest tomography the patient should be instructed to take the same fairly deep breath for each tomogram. This not only allows for optimum inflation of the lungs but also provides consistency between the focal plane levels throughout the tomographic series. This consistency in inspirations is vitally important if the area of interest is located near the diaphragm. Slight variations in the amount of air taken in may result in obscuring the area of interest by the elevated diaphragm. Suspension of respiration is also necessary to prevent blurring of structures by the breathing motion.

Respiration should be suspended in the expiratory phase in examinations of the abdomen to elevate the diaphragm and visualize more of the abdomen. As in chest tomography, the suspension of respiration will assist in maintaining consistency in tissue planes and reduce motion artifacts.

Occasionally, suspended respiration techniques may be necessary in tomographic examinations of the head. Unwanted motion of the head may occur when obese people or females with large breasts are positioned in the RAO position for lateral skull tomography. This problem may be resolved by having the patient suspend respiration during the exposure or by turning the patient over into an RPO position.

It is helpful to mark the entrance point of the central ray on the patient's skin. If the patient does happen to move, he can easily be repositioned using this mark as a reference mark. This will eliminate the need to take another scout film to recheck the position. If the mark is made with a grease pencil, it can easily be removed at the completion of the examination. When performing tomographic examination of the skull in the lateral position it is helpful to place a small midline mark on the patient's nasion to facilitate measuring for the midline tomogram and to recheck the position between the scout films and the actual tomographic series. By ensuring that this mark is still at the same level from the tabletop, that the interpupillary line is still perpendicular to the tabletop, and that the central ray is still entering at the reference mark, the correct position can be maintained throughout the entire examination.

SCOUT TOMOGRAMS

Three preliminary tomograms are usually taken to locate the correct levels for the tomographic series. One tomogram is taken at the level presumed to be at the middle of the structure or area to be examined. The other two scout tomograms are taken at levels higher and lower than this midline tomogram. The separation interval between these tomograms depends on the thickness of the structure. Small structures, such as those found in the skull, may be tomogrammed at 5 mm or 1 cm intervals for the preliminary films. Once the correct planes have been determined, the tomographic series will be taken at smaller intervals. When the total depth of the area of interest is several centimeters thick, the separation interval for these scout tomograms is increased to 2 cm or more. Table II includes separation intervals for the preliminary tomograms and the tomographic series.

GENERAL RULES FOR TOMOGRAPHY

1. Know the anatomy involved.
2. Position the patient as precisely as possible.
3. Utilize proper immobilization techniques.
4. Use a small focal spot for tomography of the head and neck and extremities.
5. Use a large focal spot for other areas of the body where fine detail is not critical.
6. Use low kVp when high contrast is desired.
7. Use high kVp when it is necessary to reduce contrast differences between structures; for example, whole lung tomography requires high kVp (80-90) in conjunction with a trough filter.
8. Use water or flour bags in other areas when necessary to absorb primary or secondary radiation; for example, in lateral cervical spine tomography place the filter bags on the upper cervical spine area to reduce the density difference between the spine and dense shoulders.
9. Collimate the beam as tightly as possible to reduce patient exposure and improve contrast.
10. Shield the patient, especially the eyes, in examinations of the skull and upper cervical spine.
11. Use the proper blurring motion. In general, use the most complex blurring motion available. Where zonography is required, a circular motion should be used. If linear motion is the only one available, care must be taken to orient the part correctly to the direction of the tube.
12. Mark each tomogram with the correct layer height. This may be done by directly exposing lead numbers on each tomogram or by marking each tomogram after it is processed. Another method is to vertically shift the right or left marker used on each successive film. By knowing the level of the first film the technologist can determine the correct level for each successive film. If multiple tomograms are taken on one film, the same shift sequence must be followed to avoid confusion in marking the layer heights.

Tomography of skull

Strict immobilization techniques must be utilized for any tomographic examination of the skull. Reference points should be marked on the patient for rechecking the position.

The basic skull positions are outlined below and are to be used in conjunction with Table 11.

AP position. The patient's head should be adjusted to align the orbitomeatal line and the midsagittal plane perpendicular to the tabletop. The distances from the tabletop to each tragus (the tonguelike projection of the ear just in front of the external auditory meatus) should be equal if the head is positioned perfectly straight.

Reverse Caldwell position. The infraorbitomeatal line should be perpendicular to the tabletop as well as to the midsagittal plane. The tragi should be equidistant from the tabletop.

Lateral position. The midsagittal plane should be parallel to the tabletop. The interpupillary line should be perpendicular to the tabletop. The orbitomeatal line should be approximately parallel to the lower border of the film.

Table 11. Positions for tomography

Examination part	Position	Central ray position	Preliminary tomographic levels	Separation intervals	Comments
Sella turcica	AP	Glabella	1.5, 2.5, and 3.5 cm anterior to tragus	2 mm	Shield eyes.
	Lateral	2.5 cm anterior and superior to tragus	−1, 0, and +1 cm to midline of skull	2 mm	Place water bag under patient's chin for support.
Middle ear (internal auditory canal, facial nerve canal, etc.)	AP	Midpoint between inner and outer canthi	−0.5, 0, and +0.5 mm to tip of tragus	1 or 2 mm	Shield eyes.
	Lateral	5 mm posterior and superior to external auditory canal	At level of outer canthus and 1 and 2 cm medial	1 or 2 mm	Place water bag under patient's chin for support.
Paranasal sinuses (general survey) and orbital floors	Reverse Caldwell	Intersection of mid-saggital plane and infraorbital rims	−2, 0, and +2 cm to level of outer canthus	3 or 5 mm	Infraorbitomeatal line should be perpendicular to the tabletop.
	Lateral	2 cm posterior to outer canthus	−3.0 and +3 cm to midline of skull	3 or 5 mm	Place water bag under patient's chin for support.
Base of skull	Submentovertex	Midpoint between angles of mandible	+1, 0, and −1 cm	2 or 3 mm	Orbitomeatal line should be parallel to tabletop.
Cervical spine	AP	To vertebral body(ies) of interest	0, −2, and −4 cm to external auditory meatus	3 or 5 mm	
	Lateral	To vertebral body(ies) of interest	−2, 0, and +2 cm	3 or 5 mm	Place water bag under patient's chin for support and two or more on neck to equalize density for entire cervical spine.
Thoracic spine	AP	To vertebral body(ies) of interest	3, 5, and 7 cm from tabletop	5 mm	Flex knees slightly to straighten spine.
	Lateral	To vertebral body(ies) of interest	−2.0 and +2 cm from midline of back	5 mm	Flex knees and place sponge against patient's back for support.
Lumbar spine	AP	To vertebral body(ies) of interest	4, 7, and 10 cm from tabletop	5 mm	Flex knees slightly to straighten spine.
	Lateral	To vertebral body(ies) of interest	−2, 0, and +2 cm from midline of back	5 mm	Flex knees and place sponge against patient's back for support.
Hip	AP	Head of femur	−2, 0, and +2 cm from greater trochanter	5 mm	Place water bag over area of greater trochanter to equalize density in hip.
	Lateral (frog leg)	Head of femur	5, 7, and 9 cm from tabletop	5 mm	Place water bag over area of femoral neck to equalize density.

Continued.

Table 11. Positions for tomography—cont'd

Examination part	Position	Central ray position	Preliminary tomographic levels	Separation intervals	Comments
Extremities	AP and lateral	At area of interest	5 mm to 1.5 cm depending on size of extremity	2-5 mm	Adjust extremity to be parallel to tabletop.
Chest (whole lung and hila)	AP	9-12 cm below sternal notch	10, 11, and 12 cm above tabletop	1 cm	Use trough filter (80-90 kVp).
	Lateral	Midchest at level of pulmonary hila	−5, 0, and +5 cm	1 cm	Place sponge against patient's back for support.
Chest (localized lesion)	AP and lateral	Measure distance to lesion from chest wall on plain radiographs and center at this point on patient.	Measure distance to lesion on lateral chest x-ray and add thickness of table pad; −2, 0, and +2 cm from measurement	2, 3, or 5 cm	Use low kVp (50-65) for high contrast.
Nephrotomogram	AP	Midpoint between xiphoid process and top of iliac crests	7 cm for small patient; 9 cm for average patient; 11 cm for large patient	1 cm	Use 8-10 degrees circular movement or 15-20 degrees linear movement.
Intravenous cholangiogram	20 degrees from RPO	10 cm lateral to lumbar spine	10, 12, and 14 cm for small patient; 12, 14, and 16 cm for average patient; 13, 16, and 19 cm for large patient	5 mm to 1 cm	Use 8-10 degrees circular movement or 15-20 degrees linear movement.

Tomography of other body parts

Standard radiographic positions (AP, lateral, and oblique) are utilized for most areas of the body. The same general rules of tomography apply to all areas. In general, the position that best shows the area of interest in a conventional radiograph is usually the best position for tomography.

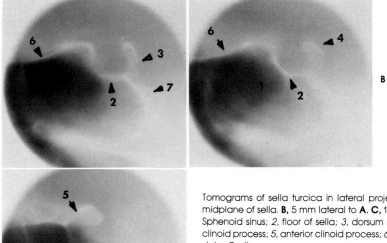

Tomograms of sella turcica in lateral projection. **A,** Through midplane of sella. **B,** 5 mm lateral to **A. C,** 1 cm lateral to **A.** *1,* Sphenoid sinus; *2,* floor of sella; *3,* dorsum sellae; *4,* posterior clinoid process; *5,* anterior clinoid process; *6,* planum sphenoidale; *7,* clivus.

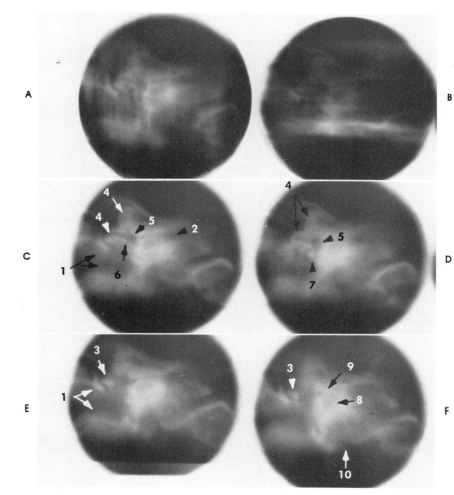

Tomograms of middle ear in AP projection. **A,** Longitudinal linear; **B,** transverse linear; and **C,** trispiral motion are at same posterior level of middle ear. Note improved visualization of structures with trispiral motion **(C). D** to **F,** Anterior to level of **C** by 2, 4, and 6 mm respectively. 1, External auditory canal; 2, internal auditory canal; 3, ossicular mass including malleus, incus, and lateral and superior semicircular canals; 5, vestibule; 6, oval window; 7, round window; 8, cochlea; 9, cochlear portion of facial nerve canal; 10, carotid canal.

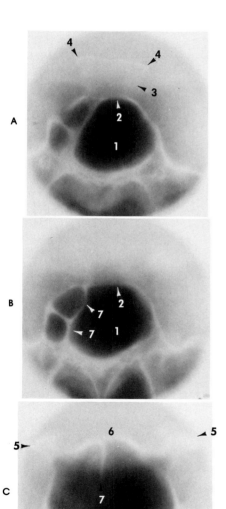

Tomograms of sella turcica in frontal projection. **A,** Posterior plane of sella turcica. **B,** 1 cm anterior to **A** demonstrating floor of sella. **C,** 2 cm anterior to **A** demonstrating anterior clinoid processes. 1, Sphenoid sinus; 2, floor of sella; 3, dorsum sellae; 4, posterior clinoid processes; 5, anterior clinoid processes; 6, planum sphenoidale; 7, septations of sphenoid sinus.

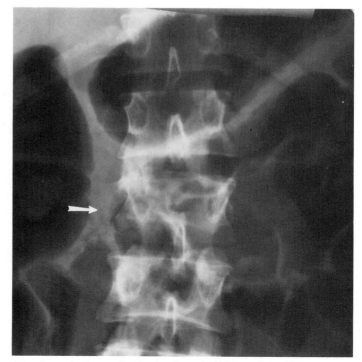

AP radiograph of suspected fracture (*arrow*) of L2 (see also p. 280)

279

A

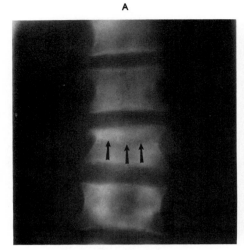

B

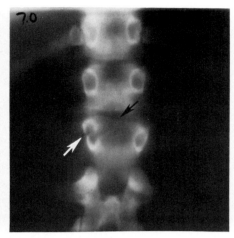

C

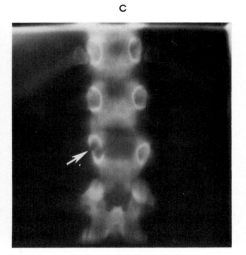

AP tomograms **A** to **D** further delineate fracture site shown in AP radiograph on p. 279. **A,** AP tomogram through anterior plane of vertebral body. *Arrows,* Wedging of vertebral body of L2.

B, AP tomogram 2 and 5 cm posterior to **A** through plane of pedicles. Fracture line extends through right pedicle (*white arrow*) and vertebral body (*black arrow*).

C, AP tomogram 3 cm posterior to **A** demonstrating displacement of fracture fragment (*arrow*).

D

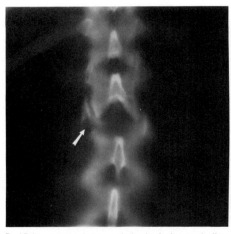

A

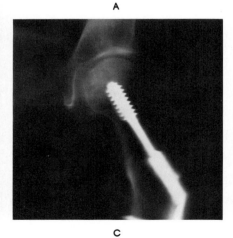

B

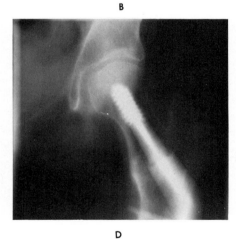

D, AP tomogram 4 cm posterior to **A** demonstrating displaced fracture (*arrow*) of superior articular process of L3.

C

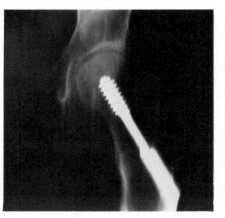

D

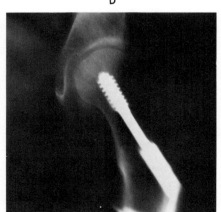

For information on *panoramic tomography,* which is used to radiographically demonstrate the entire mandible and temporomandibular joint on one film, see Volume Two, Chapter 18.

AP tomograms of hip with fixation device at same level comparing different blurring motions: **A,** trispiral; **B,** circular; **C,** longitudinal linear; **D,** oblique linear.

14

Pediatric radiography

JOHN P. DORST
ANN B. HRICA
MARY J. BLOME
THOMAS J. BECK
JANE WARD

Radiographic examinations are fundamentally the same whether the patient is an adult or a child. Consequently, when judiciously modified, most of the techniques described in these three volumes are applicable to children and infants. Pediatric radiography, however, does differ from adult radiography in one important way—many of the patients are either too young or too frightened to cooperate with the examination.

If physicians and nurses are to provide quality care for infants and children, they must perform unpleasant or painful procedures on these patients at many of their medical visits during their early, impressionable years. For example, they must give hypodermic injections for the routine immunizations and perform throat cultures, which make many children gag and some vomit. Therefore many young children begin to cry when they are approached by anyone in a white uniform or jacket. Indeed, in many pediatric centers the nurses and technologists no longer wear uniforms for just this reason.

Fortunately, most of the radiologic procedures necessary for children are not painful. Yet, small children often furiously fight even the painless radiograph because of fear of imagined hurt during *any* medical procedure. Their fear increases if they are taken from the security of their parents and increases again when they see the large size of the x-ray machine.

Does the taking of a radiograph have to be so unpleasant for a small child? Usually not. Most children are reasonably adaptable patients when approached on their terms. This takes time, but usually less time than is needed when the child is frightened and uncooperative.

APPROACH TO CHILD

The first prerequisite for a successful relationshp with children is to like them—not just happy, well children but also tired, cranky, and frightened sick children.

The next prerequisites are understanding, patience, and honesty. One must understand as well as possible the fears, needs, and desires of children. One must recognize that a child's immature concept of the world and of illness frequently leads to frightening misconceptions of what may happen in a hospital or a physician's office. Indeed, what is a small child to think of the "very large camera that takes pictures of what is inside him"? Also, certain words may frighten children. If one technologist calls "shoot" to another to indicate the moment to make the exposure, the child is likely to be startled and cry, because the word *shoot* often connotes a hypodermic injection or a gunshot. Other words that may upset children, depending on their ages, include needle (same connotation as shot), hurt, pain, remove, cut out, cut off, dye (misinterpreted as die) surgery, operation, cancer, and leukemia.

Patience is required to greet each child in the waiting room, to learn what name or nickname is preferred, to learn the child's interests, and then to explain in simple terms what the child will experience. It is most effective if one communicates at the child's eye level, which means that one might kneel for small children. Frequently the child will ask for a description of the procedure a number of times, and such repetitions may indeed test one's patience.

Understanding and patience will be of little value, however, if one is not honest when the procedure is likely to be disagreeable or painful, such as drinking a barium suspension, having an enema, or receiving an injection for an intravenous urogram. *Never tell a child that a painful procedure will not hurt.* Children old enough to understand should have advance explanation. To help parents, physicians, and nurses prepare children, some hospitals have illustrated pamphlets that describe in age-appropriate language intravenous urography and the common fluoroscopic procedures.[1] It is perhaps best left to the parents to decide when to tell a child about a forthcoming examination. If told too early, many children will fret and lose sleep worrying about an only moderately or briefly unpleasant examination. Yet, most children do better if they are told what is in store for them before they leave home or their hospital bed.

Technologists need to learn to observe and quickly evaluate each child's level of maturity and ability to communicate. The following vignettes of children of various ages may help to determine a child's maturity. To find a much more detailed discussion see Whaley and Wong.[2]

Young infants

Infants to about 6 months of age do not make a sharp distinction among persons who care for them. They often are playful or sleepy when warm and well fed. Reaction to pain stimulates total body movement and loud crying that may cease upon distraction—a pacifier is frequently most successful. When there is time, prolonged crying can be quieted by taking the child from the room so that others may be examined. Ask the mother or an aide to hold the child, speak softly and soothingly, and offer a bottle of water or formula if not contraindicated.

[1]Examples of pamphlets are available without charge from Dr. J. Dorst, Department of Radiology, The Johns Hopkins Hospital, 600 N. Wolfe Street, Baltimore, MD 21205.
[2]Whaley, L.F., and Wong, D.L.: Nursing care of infants and children, St. Louis, 1979, The C.V. Mosby Co.

Infants to 3 years of age

The principal stress factors for children 6 months to 3 years are (1) pain, (2) separation from parents, (3) limitation of by now impressive motor skills, and (4) loss of routines and rituals involving eating, sleeping, bathing, and play. A pacifier or baby bottle may often calm the infant. The technologist should approach the toddler with a smiling, friendly manner and talk with a gentle voice, possibly offering a simple toy. Immobilization is almost always necessary, and it is less disturbing to a child than the combined restraint of several people at one time. Once immobilized, most children become calm, and a diagnostic examination can be completed. *A major precaution—an immobilized child must never be left alone in a room except for the moment the exposure is made.*

Three to five years of age

Preschoolers can understand instructions and explanations if they are offered with an understanding of the child's likely perceptions; for example, ''Does your mommy or daddy take pictures of you with a camera? . . . She does? . . . Good! We are going to take pictures of you too. We have a big and special camera—bigger than your mommy's. There it is. Isn't it big? But it won't hurt. It takes a special kind of picture that will help your doctor make you well. They have to be really good pictures. So you have to lie very still on this table so that we can make a really good picture that will help your doctor. I will bring the camera over you while you lie on the table, but it will not touch or hurt you.''

Preschoolers are eager to please, and a gamelike atmosphere can facilitate your work. Often the child can be ''talked through'' a procedure. Praise must be given when the child tries to cooperate. It will serve to reduce the child's anxiety, and it is a highly valued reward. Even with the most cooperative preschoolers, immobilization often is required, because they do not understand the need to hold still in a fixed position.

Immature conceptions relating to illness, the feared ''invasion'' of their bodies, and the possible loss of any body part are paramount at this age. Thus Band-Aids are very important to preschoolers, since they fear that any intrusion of the body will result in their ''insides leaking out''; make liberal use of Band-Aids.

School-aged children

The suggestions in the preceding section also apply for schoolchildren. To gain their confidence, technologists should offer full explanations of the expected experience to these older, more sophisticated children. Naturally, the explanations should be modified as the children get older; for example, ''We are going to take your picture with an x-ray machine. It is like your mother and father's camera, but much bigger. It doesn't hurt when your father takes your picture, does it? Well, it won't hurt when we . . .''

Children in this age group are better able to cope with hospitalization, because as they socialize in school and form attachments to their peers they are loosening their bonds with home and parents. Indeed, attaining independence is important to them, and they should be allowed freedom of choice whenever possible— for example, a choice of which projection of the chest to do first or the injection site for an intravenous urogram. They will have less time to worry about their strange surroundings and feelings of helplessness if the technologist talks to them throughout the procedures. Keep up your chatter, but do not demean the children or forget their ''personhood.'' *Many grade-school children are surprisingly modest, and lack of respect in this regard can cause stress and intense embarrassment.*

Restraints are often necessary if good radiographic examinations of infants and young children are to be obtained. However, any child older than 7 or 8 years should not be forced to have an examination, except during an emergency. When older children are recalcitrant, they should be taken from the radiographic room, a now-threatening atmosphere, and the parents should be enlisted for calm reassurance. Speak to the parents to make certain that they understand the procedure so that they may explain it and allay fear. Sometimes the radiologist may offer support for the technologist and share the conversation with the parents and child. The presence of a nurse or physician trusted by the child eases the trial of the moment and enables many examinations to be performed without force.

Adolescents

Adolescent patients have often developed successful mechanisms of coping with the stress of hospitalization. Yet, because many of them have a great deal of misinformation about illness and medical care, their responses to a particular examination may seem quite inappropriate. Occasionally an adolescent child will refuse an examination. Parents, older siblings, nurses, or physicians may, in that event, be of some help and should be invited to join in the discussion. *Only in life-threatening emergencies and when all explanations and arguments have failed should an adolescent patient be forced to have an examination.*

The rapidly changing body image during pubertal development causes adolescents to be quite concerned about privacy and modesty, and technologists should respect these feelings.

Mentally retarded children

Some mentally retarded children can be examined without problem if they are treated in accordance with their mental age rather than their chronologic age. Others can be examined with the help of their parents, teachers, or hospital attendants. Although a few can be examined only when sedated, sedation may often compound the problem, as discussed in the next section, and should be the last resort. Meperidine hydrochloride and promethazine hydrochloride are the drugs usually employed, since chlorpromazine hydrochloride occasionally is epileptogenic in children who have seizures, and some mentally retarded children require unusually large doses of chloral hydrate for sedation.

Sedation

Most children, especially those who are not mentally retarded, are usually more difficult to examine after they have been sedated. They may arrive in the radiographic room sleeping peacefully, but they usually awaken when they are transferred to the table and are positioned for the examination. They may at this point be much more difficult to manage than without sedation, since it decreases the ability to cooperate, to understand explanations and instructions and to control fear.

Moreover, sedation is hazardous. The child may vomit and aspirate the vomitus. Occasionally, the standard dose may prove excessive for a particular child and may cause respiratory arrest. Sedated children must be watched carefully by a nurse or other qualified individual throughout the trip to the radiology department, the time there, and the trip back to the bed. *Therefore sedation should be used only in those rare instances when it has been proved impossible to examine a child without it.*

Parents in radiographic room

Many pediatric radiologists and technologists of the past would virtually forbid parents to accompany their children into radiographic rooms. Today quite a few believe that parents should be permitted to accompany the child when they wish to do so. Indeed, it has already been suggested that parents provide important support to the child who is unduly apprehensive—especially one who has had prolonged hospitalization. On the other hand, it is not uncommon for parents to be more concerned than the child. The technologist's explanation of the procedure may not satisfy them, and there may be a desire for assurance that the child will not be injured. Such parents probably should be permitted to watch the examination.

It is best then if parents watch from the control booth. Indeed, unless the mother is certain that she is not pregnant, she *must* be in the control booth or *out* of the radiographic room when the exposure is made. If the parent becomes upset by any feature of the examination and is not reassured by the technologist's explanation, the examination should be discontinued until the radiologist, a trusted nurse or attendant, or the referring physician has allayed the fears.

NURSING CARE
General principles

Technologists should know how to provide basic patient care for the infants and children entrusted to them. When a child arrives in the department, the competent technologist notes a number of things: Are there specific instructions for the child's care while in the department? Does the child have physical problems that will interfere with the examination, possibly requiring use of unusual positions? Is the intravenous solution flowing at the proper rate and on time? Does the child's condition suggest the possibility of emergency treatment or other special care?

Many sick infants and children have conditions that require *special diets* or *the collection of all urine or stool*. Before giving a child anything to eat or drink or discarding a specimen, check with the nursing unit or, if the child is an outpatient, with the parents.

When a child arrives in the radiology department with an *intravenous infusion* running, it is important to check that the infusion is on time and has not infiltrated the soft tissues and that there is enough fluid in the bottle to last until the child returns to the nursing unit. When restraining the child for a radiographic examination, care is required to ensure that the tubing does not become blocked or the needle dislodged. The radiologist or the child's nurse should be notified as soon as any such problem develops.

Technologists must know how to care for a child with a *colostomy* or *ileostomy*—how to remove and replace the bag and how to protect the stoma. Consult the attending physician or radiologist about removing a bag before the examination begins. Most should be removed before taking any radiograph of the abdomen, since the attachment to the skin requires a radiopaque ring that can hide calculi or other abnormalities. Some bags have radiolucent rings and therefore do not require removal.

Children are especially likely to have *contagious illnesses*. The radiology department should not be the place where children "catch" each other's infections. Most of the measures to avoid the spread of infection are simple and effective and should be scrupulously observed in the department and during bedside (portable) examinations: Wash hands before and after examining each child, clean the radiographic table and restraining devices with a mild disinfectant solution immediately after use, and keep the department clean and neat. *The most important precaution is hand washing, but unfortunately it is the most neglected.*

When children have been placed in *respiratory or enteric isolation* or on *wound or blood precautions* and they cannot be radiographed in bed, they should be brought to the department when few or no other patients are present. They must be kept separate from other patients, examined quickly, and returned to their nursing unit promptly. Depending on the type of illness, technologists and physicians may be required to wear protective gowns, gloves, or face masks, as specified by hospital protocol. After the examination the radiographic room, table, and equipment used must be disinfected as specified by protocol.

Severely burned children and children who have immunologic deficiencies, either innate, such as dysgammaglobulinemia, or associated with chemotherapy for cancer, are likely to get serious and sometimes fatal infections. They require *protective isolation,* which should be provided as specified by the hospital protocol. In general, this consists of precautions taken to protect the patient from contracting an infection. These children should be examined, whenever possible, when no other patients are in the department—particularly any with infectious diseases. The radiographic room and equipment must be carefully cleaned before the patient is admitted. Technologists and physicians must wear face masks when with the patient.

Smith et al.[1] have published a practical guide to handling children in the radiology department who are known to have specific infections.

Respiratory distress may develop rapidly in children. Children restrained for an examination must never be left alone. If distress develops while the child is restrained, release him immediately. Generally this remedies the situation. Sometimes it helps to raise the child into a semierect position and extend the head slightly. Periodic classes should be held to educate and reeducate all personnel who deal with pediatric patients in the recommended methods of cardiopulmonary resuscitation.

Care of premature infants

In the radiology department, *hypothermia* is the greatest hazard to premature infants and to some full-term infants. Hypothermia is likely to intensity their illnesses and may prove fatal.[2] Since small infants may rapidly become hypothermic even in rooms most people consider uncomfortably warm, they should be examined whenever possible in the nursery with the infant in an incubator or infant warmer. When the examination must be done in the radiology department, the infant should be transported in a warm incubator by a health professional. The infant may be prepared for the examination while still in the incubator; for example, an enema tube or a nasogastric tube may be inserted or simple restraints may be applied. Removal from the incubator should be for as short a period as possible, and the infant should be returned during pauses in the examination if there is any evidence of hypothermia. Immobilization is rarely needed for these infants; when it is, a gentle, simple method that can be applied quickly should be chosen.

[1]Smith, W.L., et al.: Minimizing the risk of infectious diseases in the radiology department, Appl. Radiol. **10**(4):70-73, 1981.

[2]Avery, M.E., Fletcher, B.D., and Williams, R.Y.: The lung and its disorders in the newborn infant, ed. 4, Philadelphia, 1981, W.B. Saunders Co., pp. 251, 306, 339.

No completely satisfactory method of keeping an infant warm during fluoroscopy appears to have been developed. One method is to place the infant on a relatively radiolucent warming pad and under a portable infrared heat lamp or similar warmer. The lamp must be kept a suitable distance from the infant, usually at least 3 feet. Most heat lamps become inefficient during fluoroscopy, because the fluoroscope shields them from the infant. The warmers designed by Newman and Poznanski,[1] however, remain effective since they are placed on each side of the infant.

The infant's temperature should be monitored while he is out of the incubator. A remote reading thermometer with a skin probe is the most accurate method. If a separate unit is not available, the one in an incubator can be used. The skin probe is placed over the liver, where the skin temperature should be about 36.5° C. If the skin temperature drops below 35° C, the examination should be interrupted and the infant returned to the incubator.[2]

Special nursing problems

Several pediatric conditions may present problems to radiologic technologists.

Myelomeningocele. *Myelomeningocele* is a birth defect characterized by a cystic protrusion of meninges and nerve roots or spinal cord from the back that causes varying degrees of permanent paralysis and is often associated with hydrocephalus. Most infants with myelomeningoceles should be examined prone until the defect has been surgically repaired and the wound healed.

[1]Newman, D.E., and Poznanski, A.K.: A simple device for infant warming during radiography, Radiology **97**:439, 1970.

[2]Poznanski, A.K.: Practical approaches to pediatric radiology, Chicago, 1976, Year Book Medical Publishers, Inc., pp. 14-16.

Omphalocele. An *omphalocele* is a birth defect that resembles an enormous umbilical hernia. It has a thin, translucent wall and contains bowel and liver. It must be carefully supported so that the sac is not broken, and it must be kept moist and warm. In *gastroschisis,* a similar congenital anomaly, a portion of bowel protrudes through a defect near the naval. It is even more important that this bowel be kept moist and warm, since it is not contained in a sac. Whenever possible, the referring physician or a specially trained nurse should remain with such infants in the radiology department, since they may rapidly become hypothermic.

Osteogenesis imperfecta. *Osteogenesis imperfecta* is an inherited condition characterized by bones that are likely to break. There is great variation in severity, from individuals who suffer only a few fractures during their lives and often do not realize that they are different from anyone else to infants who are born with multiple fractures. All infants and children with osteogenesis imperfecta must be handled with extreme care; otherwise, a fracture may be caused. The technologist should explain to the attendant (parent, nurse, or physician) the correct position for each radiograph, and the attendant should help the child assume the proper position. If the attendant believes that the child cannot safely assume this position, the technologist may be able to obtain a properly positioned radiograph by angling the x-ray tube, the film, or both. If the technologist does not believe that he will be able to make a satisfactory radiograph or has any questions about handling the child, he should consult the radiologist promptly.

Child abuse. The technologist may be the first person to suspect a case of child abuse when preparing a child for an examination or viewing the radiographs. Many states require all health professionals to report suspected cases of abuse. The technologist should speak with the radiologist, if available, or the attending physician. The decision to report the suspicion then rests with the physician.

Identification of an abused child will be aided by familiarity with the list of typical types and sites of abuse given in the outline below. The technologist should not be reassured if the child appears clean and well dressed, since the parents of an abused child may feel remorse and guilt following the incident and may therefore bathe and dress the child in clean clothes to make a good impression.[1] Helfer and Kempe[2] have published two helpful lists of features that should sensitize health professionals to the possibility of child abuse.

The victims of child abuse and their parents must be accorded kindness and understanding. An initial critical or derogatory approach to the parents may seriously jeopardize the child's opportunity to grow up to be a socially productive and reasonably normal adult.

Child abuse may occur at any age but is probably most common in infancy. Certainly, fractures occur most often in that period, and it is in infants that the fractures are most likely to have characteristics that permit a definite diagnosis of abuse. Radiologic examination, however, can never exclude abuse, since 80% to 90% of significantly abused children do not have fractures or dislocations.[3]

The usual radiographic examination of an infant or young child for possible fractures caused by abuse includes projections of the skull (frontal, Towne, and lateral projections), chest (frontal projection with good rib detail), spine (lateral projections of the cervical, thoracic, lumbar, and sacral spine), and upper and lower limbs (frontal projections that include the hands, pelvis, and feet).

Abused children may suffer from injuries other than fractures, which are best diagnosed by radiography or the newer imaging modalities (Table 12).

[1]Weston, J.T.: The pathology of child abuse. In Helfer, R.E., and Kempe, C.H., editors: The battered child, ed. 2, Chicago, 1974, University of Chicago Press, pp. 69-70.

[2]Helfer, R.E., and Kempe, C.H.: The child's need for early recognition, immediate care and protection. In Kempe, C.H., and Helfer, R.E., editors: Helping the battered child and his family, Philadelphia, 1972, J.B. Lippincott Co., p. 73.

[3]Rodriquez, A.: Handbook of child abuse and neglect, Flushing, N.Y., 1977, Medical Examination Publishing Co., Inc., p. 22.

Visual diagnosis of nonaccidental trauma[1]

I. Typical sites
   Buttocks and lower back (paddling)
   Genitals and inner thighs (sexual abuse)
   Cheeks (slap marks)
   Ear lobes (pinch marks)
   Upper lip and frenulum (forced feeding)
   Neck (choke marks)
II. Inflicted bruises
   A. Human hand marks (pressure bruises)
      Oval grab marks (fingertips)
      Trunk encirclement bruises
      Linear marks (fingers)
      Handprints
      Pinch marks
   B. Human bite marks
   C. Strap marks
      Linear bruises (belt or whip)
      Loop mark bruises (doubled-over cord)
   D. Bizarre marks
      Bruises from blunt instruments
      Tattoos and fork mark punctures
      Circumferential tie marks (ankle, wrist)
      Gag marks
   E. Bruises at different ages of healing:

Age	Color
0 to 2 days	Swollen, tender
0 to 5 days	Red, blue
5 to 7 days	Green
7 to 10 days	Yellow
10 to 14 days	Brown
2 to 4 weeks	Clear

[1]Prepared by Barton D. Schmitt, M.D., Department of Pediatrics, University of Colorado Medical Center, Denver, 1978.

III. Normal bruises
   Facial scratches on babies with long fingernails
   Knee and skin bruises
   Forehead bruises
   Bruises over bony prominences
IV. Other types of abuse
   A. Inflicted burns
      Cigarette burns
      Match tip or incense burns
      Dry contact burns (from forced contact with heating devices, e.g., electric hot plate)
      Branding burns (from heated metals)
      Scalds (from forced immersion)
   B. Head injuries
      1. From direct blows
         Skull fractures
         Scalp swelling and bruises
         Retinal hemorrhages
      2. From violent shaking
         No skull fractures
         No scalp swelling or bruises
         Retinal hemorrhages
   C. Abdominal injuries (from being kicked or hit)
      Ruptured liver or spleen
      Ruptured blood vessel
      Intestinal perforation
      Kidney injury
      Pancreatic injury
      Intramural hematoma of duodenum or proximal jejunum
   D. Bone injuries
      Usual fractures
      Fractures at different stages of healing
      Repeated fractures at same site
      Unusual fractures (ribs, scapula, sternum)

PROTECTION OF CHILD
Protection from injury

It is the responsibility of the radiology department to see that a child neither injures himself nor is injured while in the department. To avoid injury the department must provide supervision of all children while in the department and frequently during their passage to and from the department. Infants and young children must be watched with particular care. Even the best available methods of immobilizing infants and young children are slightly hazardous; thus immobilization should be done only by experienced technologists.

Protection from unnecessary radiation

Children are more sensitive than adults to both the latent somatic effects and the genetic effects of radiation.

The *latent somatic effects* of radiation are those that may occur months or years later in the person who is irradiated. They include nonspecific life shortening and the induction of malignancies. Immature growing tissues in many of the child's organs are considerably more sensitive to radiation damage than the mature tissues of an adult. Moreover, a child is more likely than an adult to live long enough to develop a malignancy or other change induced by radiation administered possibly 30 years earlier.

The malignancies most likely to be induced by irradiating a child are leukemia and thyroid cancer.[1] Consequently, the tissues at greatest risk are the thyroid gland and the hematopoietically active bone marrow, which in the child younger than 7 years is present throughout most of the skeleton.

Although *genetic effects* are caused by irradiation of a person's testicles or ovaries, they cause no recognizable damage in the irradiated person. The damage usually takes the form of mutations in that person's sperm or ova that increase the likelihood that his or her future children or their descendants will have a serious disease. Because their entire reproductive periods lie ahead, children are particularly susceptible to the genetic effects of radiation.

Provided that reasonable precautions are taken, the likelihood that a diagnostic x-ray examination will cause a harmful somatic or genetic abnormality is quite small. For example, if 1 million small children are each given 1 rad to their hematopoietic bone marrow, 32 to 68 more cases of leukemia are likely to result during the next 25 years than if they had received no radiation.[2] To put this into perspective, if 10 million 1-year-old children have one AP abdominal radiograph each, one of them is likely to develop radiation-induced leukemia within 25 years.[3]

Table 12. Examples of injuries caused by child abuse that may be diagnosed by radiography, ultrasound, and nuclear imaging

Lesions	Imaging methods
Fractures	SR, IS
Subdural hematoma or hygroma	CT, CA
Cerebral contusion	CT, CA, US (infants)
Intraventricular hematoma	CT, US (infants)
Pulmonary contusion	Chest films
Pleural effusion	Chest films
Pericardial effusion	US, chest films
Hematoma of bowel wall (usually duodenum)	UGI
Laceration of bowel	AR, UGI (WS)
Laceration of kidney	IVU, CT, US, IS
Laceration of liver or spleen	AR, CT, US, IS
Pancreatic pseudocyst	AR, CT, US, UGI
Pancreatitis	CT, US

AR, Abdominal radiography; CA, carotid arteriography; CT, computed tomography; IS, isotope scan; IVU, intravenous urogram; SR, skeletal radiography; UGI, upper gastrointestinal series; US, ultrasonography; WS, with a water soluble contrast material.

[1]The effects on populations of exposure to low levels of ionizing radiation. Report of the Advisory Committee on the Biological Effect of Ionizing Radiation. National Academy of Science, 1980.

[2]The effects on populations of exposure to low levels of ionizing radiation. Report of the Advisory Committee on the Biological Effect of Ionizing Radiation. National Academy of Science, 1980.

[3]Technique: 10 mAs, 65 kVp, single phase, 8:1 grid, Kodak Lanex regular screens with Ortho G film; estimated marrow dose 0.002 rads. Computed from Rosenstein, M., Beck, T.J., and Warren, G.G.: Handbook of selected organ doses for projections common in pediatric radiology, HEW Publication (FDA) 79-8079, May 1979.

When the gonads lie within the x-ray field, shielding must be considered. The testicles are more easily shielded than the ovaries. In radiographs of the abdomen or pelvis a lead rubber shield (0.5 mm lead equivalent or greater) can be positioned over the testicles so as not to obscure pertinent anatomy. An ovarian shield, however, almost always obscures important portions of the body. Fortunately the unshielded ovaries lie near the midplane of the body and receive significantly less radiation than the superficial testicles in similar examinations.

Intravenous urograms should be tailored so that the ovaries are outside the x-ray field on as many of the radiographs as possible. Similar tailoring occasionally is possible with other abdominal examinations.

Once girls begin to menstruate they can become pregnant, and the immature tissues of the embryo and fetus are even more sensitive to radiation damage than the tissues of the child. To avoid unnecessary irradiation of an unborn child, elective radiographic examination of the abdomen, pelvis, and thighs should only be done during the first 10 days of the menstrual period. All girls older than 11 years or their parents should be questioned about their menstrual history, and if indicated the girls should be spoken to privately to learn if they are sexually active and use effective birth control. Because of the adolescent's concern for modesty, gentle questioning by a sympathetic woman is most likely to elicit true responses.

Suggestions for minimizing radiation to parents are given in an earlier section about parents in the radiographic room.

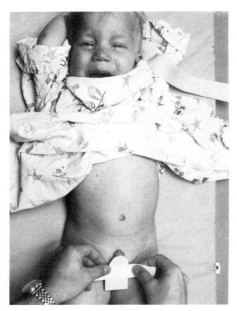

Positioning male gonad shield

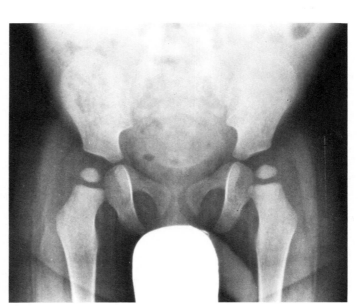

Radiograph showing correctly positioned male gonad shield that covers the testicles but does not obscure any of the bones

THE PRINCIPAL PROBLEM: PATIENT MOTION

Infants and young children are charming wigglers at best, screaming fighters at worst. The secrets of making good radiographs are (1) establishing a good rapport, which was previously discussed under "Approach to Child," (2) equipment that permits fast exposures with appropriate factors, and (3) proper positioning aids, with immobilization when necessary.

Appropriate x-ray equipment

Appropriate, fast exposures are largely dependent on suitable radiographic equipment and technical factors. Generators used for pediatric examinations should permit exposure times as brief as 1 or 2 milliseconds. Kilovoltages up to 140 are useful, but 125 kV is adequate for all but a few studies. Such generators offer optimum exposure flexibility when used with fast film-screen systems.

Field size and patient thickness are frequently smaller in pediatric than in adult radiology. When they are, less scattered radiation is produced. Consequently, grid ratios greater than 8:1 are rarely necessary. Depending on the kilovoltage, the replacement of a 12:1 grid with an 8:1 grid approximately halves the patient dose.[1] Abdominal radiographs of hypersthenic or obese adolescents may require a higher grid ratio. A 10:1 grid is a good compromise. Fine-line stationary grids or high-speed Potter-Bucky mechanisms are necessary for the short exposures that are used in many examinations.

Further dose reduction can be accomplished by replacing cassettes with metal fronts by cassettes with carbon fiber fronts. With infants and small children the dose reduction can be as much as 25%.[2]

[1] Nickoloff, E.L., Beck, T.J., and Leo, F.P.: Variations in patient entrance exposures for selected x-ray procedures, Proceedings of Medicine VIII Meeting of Society of Photo Optical Engineers, April 20-22, 1980, Las Vegas, Nevada.

[2] Jordan, D.A.: Graphite: wonder material for radiology, Appl. Radiol. **9**:61-64, 1980.

Radiographic machines now sold in the United States must have collimators that automatically adjust the x-ray beam to the same size as the film. Although selection of the proper film size and collimation to the margins of that film is usually adequate for adults, this practice almost always results in excessively large fields for infants and children, because small errors in collimation gives unnecessary radiation to a proportionately much greater amount of their small bodies. Therefore in pediatric radiography the collimator almost always needs to be adjusted further so that the radiograph includes only the pertinent anatomy.

The highest kilovoltages consistent with the desired level of contrast should be used to minimize dose and allow the shortest exposure times. New film-screen systems using rare earth phosphorus have allowed shorter exposure times and significant dose reductions without sacrificing image resolution or prohibitively increasing quantum mottle.

A rigorous quality control program is required to ensure optimum performance from radiographic machines, cassettes, film, and film processors over the years.

Immobilization

Even the best available methods of immobilizing infants and young children have a slight potential for harm. Therefore immobilization should only be performed by experienced technologists. Before starting, the procedure should be explained to the parents and to any child old enough to understand. The immobilized child must not be left unattended at any time, except for the instant when the exposure is made, and even then a technologist or another trained medical person must always watch the child.

Immobilization is used to ensure correct patient position and to minimize, but *not* completely stop, voluntary motion; other motion is minimized by fast exposures. *An infant or child must never be immobilized so tightly that small movements are impossible.*

The following items are useful for positioning and immobilizing children, and most of them should be available: bed sheets, diapers, adhesive tape, stretch gauze bandages, elastic bandages, orthopedic stockinettes, sponges, sandbags, compression bands, plastic compression panels, and head clamps. If many infants and young children are studied in a department, there are a number of commercial immobilizing devices that are well worth their cost.

Adhesive tape is used in many ways for immobilization. One way is to attach one end of the tape to the edge of the x-ray table, pass the tape over the child, and attach the other end of the tape to the other side of the table (see photograph on p. 291). It is best not to let the adhesive surface of cloth adhesive tape touch a child's skin or hair. Either the skin or hair is covered by a cloth or by a paper napkin or the tape is turned as it crosses the child so that the smooth side is next to the skin or hair. When it is necessary to *attach* cloth adhesive tape to a child's skin, first attach a piece of paper tape or a special plastic tape that causes minimal skin irritation, and then attach the cloth adhesive tape to the tape on the skin.

Sandbags should be available in many sizes: small, firm sandbags weighing 3 to 7 pounds; long, firm sandbags weighing 10 to 30 pounds; and long, floppy sandbags of the same weight. All should have covers that can be cleaned or changed after each use. The long, firm sandbags are placed on each side of an infant or young child to help ensure that he does not roll off the table. They can also be used to anchor the ends of a diaper or towel that is stretched over the child to hold him in the correct position. The long, floppy sandbags can be used for the same purpose; the sand is run into the ends of the bag, which are placed on each side of the child, and the empty portion of the bag is stretched over the child.

The technique known as *mummifying;* with a bed sheet held together by adhesive tape, is invaluable in certain situations.

Involuntary movement (for example, respiration) and small body movements are best minimized by *short exposures.* Even with equipment that permits exposures of 1 to 2 milliseconds (0.001 to 0.002 second), the technologist must make the exposure at the right instant, as explained in the following section.

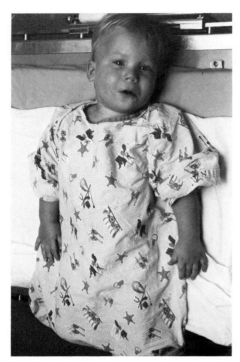

The child is placed in the center of a sheet folded lengthwise to extend from axillae to between the knees and ankles.

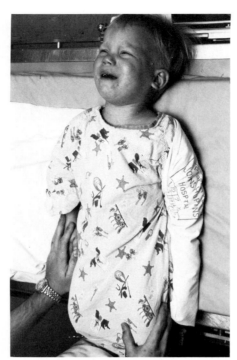

One end of the sheet is brought over the child's left arm and under his body.

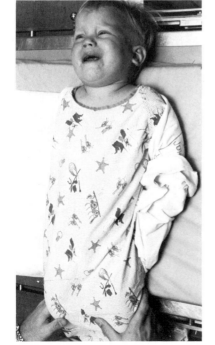

The same end of the sheet is next brought over the child's right arm and back under his body.

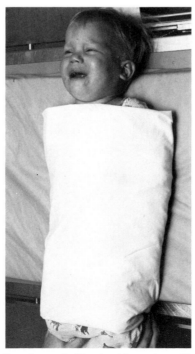

The other end of the sheet is now brought over the child, under him, over again, and secured with adhesive tape.

COMMON PEDIATRIC EXAMINATIONS
Chest radiography

Infants and children younger than 4 years old are best examined supine, unless a special device is used to hold them erect.[1] The arms are held next to the ears within a sleeve formed by a diaper, pillowcase, or orthopedic stockinette that passes behind the head. The legs and pelvis should be encased in a similar sleeve, this one conveniently made of stretch gauze bandage or elastic bandage *not* wrapped too tightly. The patient is placed supine on the x-ray film cassette, a compression band is placed over the pelvis, and a second band or adhesive tape is used to immobilize the legs. The head and arms are cradled between two sandbags. The head must not be turned even slightly to the side, because often this will oblique the chest. The head can be held straight by a head holder or by a length of cloth adhesive tape attached to paper adhesive tape on the child's forehead and to the sides of the x-ray table. For the lateral radiograph the child is turned on his side and immobilized in a similar manner.

[1]Poznanski, A.K.: Practical approaches to pediatric radiology, Chicago, 1976, Year Book Medical Publishers, Inc., pp. 30-34.

Children who are old enough to stand straight for the examination, without turning to the side or twisting their bodies, and to take a deep breath when requested, yet young enough to be apprehensive, are best examined in the AP position with their arms held over their heads, so that they may watch the technologist. Older children and adolescents may be examined in the PA or AP position; the AP position delivers less radiation to the bone marrow.[1] It seems to work best if children and adolescents hold their arms over their heads or drape their arms over the x-ray cassette holder, since they often have trouble holding the usual adult position (hands on hips with elbows and shoulders rotated forward) as they take a deep breath.

[1]Archer, B.R., et al.: Bone marrow dose in chest radiography: the postero-anterior vs. anteroposterior projection, Radiology **133:** 211-216, 1979.

Precise timing is especially important in chest radiography. *To obtain a film in deep inspiration* of an infant or child too young to follow directions the technologist should start the exposure at the beginning of expiration. This sounds paradoxical, yet it works because expiration is considerably longer than inspiration. The technologist watches the child breathe a number of times, moving his hand in time with the respirations. Then when he sees the child take a deep inspiration, he makes the exposure at the instant that expiration starts.

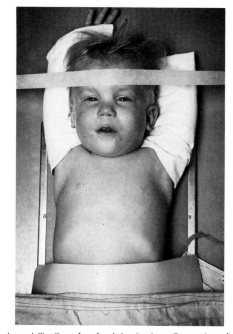

Immobilization for frontal chest radiography. A sleeve, made with a pillowcase in this instance, passes around each arm and behind the head and is fastened with three strips of adhesive tape. A lead shield covers the lower abdomen, pelvis, and upper thighs. A compression band holds the child in position. The center of a length of adhesive tape is attached to paper tape on the forehead, and the ends are attached to the edges of the x-ray table to keep the head straight. If the child struggles, a sandbag can be placed tightly against each arm, or a head clamp can be substituted for the adhesive tape.

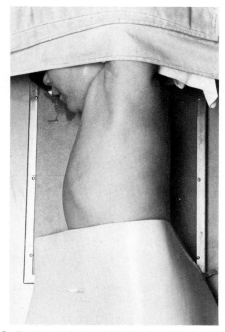

Positioning and immobilization for lateral chest radiographs

Abdominal radiography

Frontal radiographs of the abdomen should be made with the feet inverted about 20 degrees, which places the hips in a true AP position. Otherwise, positioning for a supine abdominal radiograph is much the same as for a supine chest radiograph. There are a number of advantages to taking the frontal radiograph with the child prone (PA) rather than supine: (1) the air is redistributed in the colon so that it is less likely to obscure the kidneys and adrenal glands and so that it often becomes possible to exclude a bowel obstruction; (2) A small pneumoperitoneum may be recognized; and (3) Duodenal obstruction may be disclosed.[1] The disadvantages are that young children may be frightened when placed prone and it is somewhat difficult to place the lead rubber testicular shield correctly.

[1]Berdon, W.E., Baker, D.H., and Leonidas, J.: Advantages of prone positioning in gastrointestinal and genitourinary radiographic studies in infants and children, Am. J. Roentgenol. Radium Ther. Nucl. Med. **103**:444, 1968,.

Abdominal radiographs of young children and infants standing or held erect are difficult to make. The lateral decubitus projection, made with the child's left side down and the x-ray beam horizontal, is easily made and gives as much information. Indeed, small amounts of free intraperitoneal air are more likely to be shown on the decubitus projection.

Except when examining premature infants, *all abdominal radiographs should be made with a stationary grid or a Potter-Bucky diaphragm.* Technologists inexperienced in pediatric radiology frequently think that an infant's or child's abdomen is so small that a grid is unnecessary, but radiation fog often obscures important detail on such radiographs.

When a newborn infant has an *anorectal malformation* (imperforate anus), it is important to determine whether the colon ends above or below the levator ani muscle. In the past this assessment was usually made on a lateral projection of the abdomen obtained with the infant held inverted and a lead marker placed on the anal dimple. This examination is seldom done today, since most pediatric surgeons believe that physical examination provides a more accurate assessment of where the colon ends.[1]

Skull radiography

Until a child is old enough to cooperate, skull radiography is best performed with the child supine on the radiographic table. If the infant or young child is "mummified" (see left) and secured between two long, firm sandbags with a compression band, it is relatively simple to position the head correctly and hold it with a head clamp or between two large, firm, clean sponges. When the skull is deformed and asymmetrical, best results usually are obtained if the skull is positioned with the line through the external auditory meatuses parallel to the tabletop for all frontal projections and perpendicular to the tabletop for all lateral projections.

[1] Berdon, W.E., et al.: A radiographic evaluation of imperforate anus: an approach correlated with current surgical concepts, Radiology **90**:466-471, 1968.

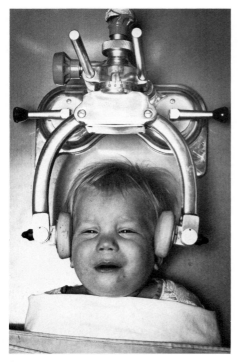

Frontal

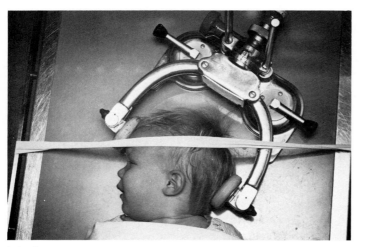

Lateral

Use of head clamps for frontal and lateral skull radiographs. The child has been "mummified" and is held by a restraining band. On the lateral projection, a length of adhesive tape secured to the edges of the x-ray table supplements the head clamp. The center of the tape has been twisted so that the adhesive does not touch the child and will not stick to his hair.

Limb radiography

When the child is too young to cooperate, the limbs can be held in position with a plastic panel held by sandbags. A true lateral radiograph of the elbow or forearm may be obtained with a child supine if the arm is abducted 90 degrees, the elbow is flexed 90 degrees, and the lateral aspects of the forearm and hand are placed against the radiographic table.

An *examination for a possible fracture* requires special care. Rough handling can increase the displacement of the bone fragments, causing further damage to blood vessels and other soft tissues and possibly causing a portion of the bone to break the skin. While positioning the limb, the technologist must be sensitive to the child's responses and never *force* the limb into the desired position. If there is any question, only one exposure should be made. By using a horizontal x-ray beam or by putting the film in the Bucky tray, it is often possible to make this exposure without moving the limb. Otherwise, the technologists will have to lift the limb gently and slip the cassette underneath. If the radiologist or attending physician does not find a gross fracture on this first radiograph, additional exposures can be made with the limb properly positioned under the physician's supervision. The limb should be moved extremely slowly and gently into the desired positions, stopping if the child has more than mild pain.

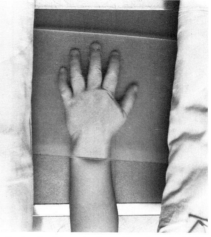

Positioning for PA projection of hand and wrist. The hand is held by a plastic panel weighted at the ends by sandbags.

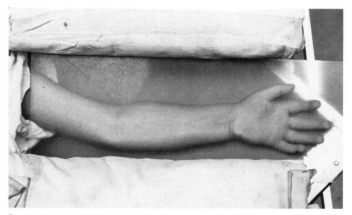

Positioning and immobilization for AP radiograph of forearm and elbow. The plastic panel is held in position by a sandbag along each edge and a third, smaller sandbag at the end (not shown on photograph).

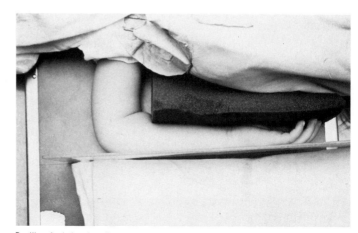

Position for lateral radiograph of elbow, forearm, and hand. The child is supine, the arm is abducted 90 degrees, and the elbow bent 90 degrees. The forearm and hand are held lateral by a sponge and a plastic panel, which in turn are held in place by two sandbags.

Intravenous urography

Although infants and children should have an empty stomach at the start of an intravenous urogram, *they must not be permitted to become dehydrated*. Infants should be scheduled so that the study is started at the time they would normally be fed. They may be fed after the contrast material has been injected and certainly should be fed if the examination lasts longer than 1 hour. Most young children tolerate going without fluids for 6 to 8 hours. The amount of contrast material injected is determined by the child's weight (Table 13).

To minimize radiation to the gonads many of the radiographs made during intravenous urography can often be limited to the kidneys. Unless the history or radiographic findings indicate a reason to obtain more radiographs of the pelvis and urinary bladder, they are included on only two radiographs—the preliminary radiograph and one late radiograph.

Table 13. Intravenous urography—dose of Conray 60, Hypaque 50, Renografin 60, and similar contrast agents

Weight of child (lbs)	Dose of contrast agent
0 to 4	Use ultrasound instead
5 to 15*	1 ml per pound*
16 to 50	1 ml per pound
51 to 100	50 ml
Over 100	0.5 ml per pound

Data from Berdon, W.E.: Pulmonary edema in infants who receive contrast media, Radiology **139**:507, 1981.
*When small infants have heart disease, serious congenital abnormalities, chromosomal anomalies, or other serious illnesses, use another method to evaluate their urinary tracts when possible.

Fluoroscopy

During fluoroscopic examinations of small children it is good practice to cover most of the radiographic tabletop with lead rubber (0.5 mm lead equivalent). Properly positioned, the lead will shield from radiation exposure the parts of the child one does not wish to examine and the people holding and feeding the child. For example, during a barium enema only the abdomen and pelvis are not protected by lead. Once the rectum and low sigmoid colon of a boy have been examined, he can be moved down slightly so that his testicles are shielded during the rest of fluoroscopy.

SPECIAL PEDIATRIC EXAMINATIONS
Bone age

Most children are evaluated using the Greulich and Pyle method[1] or the Tanner-Whitehouse 2 method.[2] Both methods require a single frontal radiograph of the left hand and wrist. The hand is placed palm down with the fingers slightly separated so that they do not touch and the thumb making an angle of about 30 degrees with the second metacarpal. The SID is 30 inches, and the x-ray tube is centered to the head of the third metacarpal.[2]

For children younger than 3 years of age, the Sontag, Snell, and Anderson method, modified to minimize gonadal radiation, can be used.[3] The following radiographs are needed: (1) an AP projection of the left humerus that includes the distal one half of the clavicle, the shoulder, and the elbow, (2) a PA projection of the left hand and wrist, (3) AP and lateral projections of the left knee, and (4) AP and lateral projections of the left foot and ankle. If the radiologist is available to check the radiographs before the child leaves the department, (3) and (4) are modified. A single lateral projection of the knee and a single oblique projection of the foot and ankle are made and checked by the radiologist to determine whether an AP projection of the knee or an additional projection of the foot and ankle is needed.

[1]Greulich, W.W., and Pyle, S.I.: Radiographic atlas of skeletal development of the hand and wrist, ed. 2, Stanford, Calif., 1959, Stanford University Press.
[2]Tanner, J.M., et al.: Assessment of skeletal maturation and prediction of adult height (TW2 method), New York, 1975, Academic Press, Inc.
[3]Schuberth, K.C., and Zitelli, J., editors: The Harriet Lane handbook, ed. 8, Chicago, 1978, Year Book Medical Publishers, Inc., pp. 261-262.

Clubfoot films

Reproducible positioning on serial radiographic examinations at intervals of months are required for evaluation and correction of many foot deformities.

The frontal, or dorsoplantar, radiograph should be made with the foot in its usual weight-bearing position and the *leg* (knee to ankle) *absolutely perpendicular to the x-ray cassette*. The x-ray beam is angled about 15 degrees posteriorly. Some surgeons like a second frontal study done with as much correction of the foot deformity as possible, but again with the leg perpendicular to the cassette.

The lateral radiograph is made with the leg parallel to the cassette and gentle force applied against the plantar surface of the foot with a plywood or plastic panel to simulate weight bearing. With older children this radiograph is made with the foot in its weight-bearing position. The child stands on a stable, raised platform with a handrail or other secure hand hold, the x-ray cassette is placed vertically beside the foot and leg, and the x-ray beam is directed horizontally.

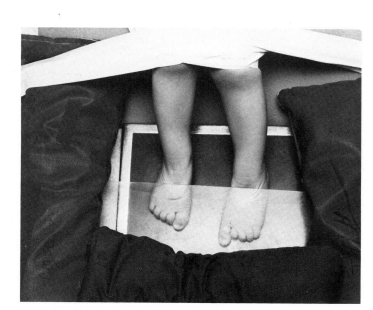

Clubfoot positioning (illustrated on a normal subject): frontal film made with patient sitting and the *legs perpendicular* to the x-ray cassette

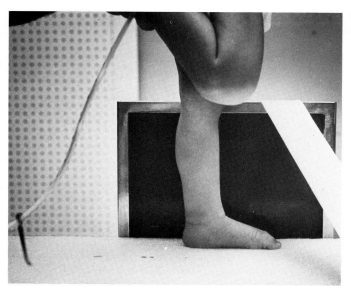

Lateral film with actual weight bearing (patient standing)

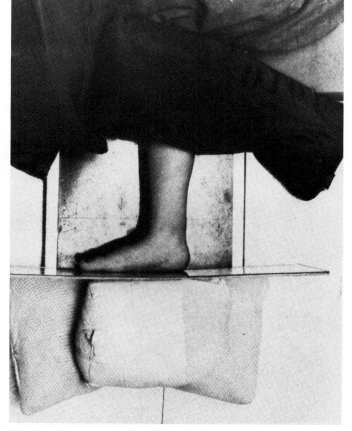

Lateral radiograph made with patient recumbent and weight bearing simulated

Trachea and larynx

Radiographic studies of the trachea and larynx are obtained to evaluate acute and chronic upper respiratory problems in infants and children. Examples of acute problems include croup and acute epiglottiditis; the most common chronic problems are complications of previous endotracheal intubation. Children with either type of problem can suddenly develop severe respiratory distress during the examination. They must be watched carefully at all times. Restraints should be used only if necessary and removed immediately if there is any evidence of increased respiratory difficulty. If a child is examined for possible *acute epiglottiditis,* a single soft tissue lateral projection is made of the neck centering on the larynx with the *child sitting erect and his physician in attendance.* Only if evaluation of this radiograph shows no evidence of epiglottiditis is it safe to proceed with the usual study (below), and this child must be watched particularly carefully for any evidence of increasing distress.

AP projections. *A special Thoraeus filter* of 0.40 mm tin, 0.50 mm copper, and 0.75 mm or 1.0 mm aluminum is placed in front of the x-ray collimator for the frontal, but not for the lateral, projections. The *tin side of the filter must face the x-ray tube,* and the aluminum side must face the patient. Exposures are made using as high kilovoltage as is available—140 kVp probably is optimum.[1]

Correct positioning is critical. The child is placed supine with the shoulders supported by a folded sheet or a sandbag to extend the neck so that a line joining the inferior aspect of the body of the mandible and the most inferior portion of the occipital bone (which can be identified fairly well by palpation) is perpendicular to the x-ray film. The central ray is centered just below the larynx if the examination is limited to the cervical airway; it is centered to the suprasternal notch if the examination includes the larynx, all of the trachea, and the central bronchi.

Two radiographs are taken, one with the patient phonating and the second during quiet inspiration.

[1] Joseph, P.M., et al.: Upper airway obstruction in infants and small children: improved radiographic diagnosis by combining filtration, high kilovoltage and magnification, Radiology 121:143, 1976.

Lateral projection. The patient is not moved. The Thoraeus filter is removed, and the x-ray tube is positioned for a horizontal beam lateral exposure of the neck. The cassette is positioned vertically beside the neck. A soft tissue technique is used for this projection, which is best made during phonation. It should *not* be made as the child swallows.

Defecography

Defecography is used principally to evaluate the rectum and anal canal of children who are incontinent of feces, especially children who previously had surgical repair of an anorectal malformation (imperforate anus) or Hirschsprung's disease. The child is examined while sitting on a radiolucent potty or toilet seat. Barium paste is smeared on the anal verge, and the enema tube is inserted. The tube is not secured to the patient but held in place by means of a long sponge forceps. Barium is run in, and, when the child indicates a desire to defecate, the enema tube is removed. The child is told to start defecating, stop, and start again as a recording is made on videotape. The examination sometimes is repeated, with one fluoroscopic spot radiograph made as the child defecates and another after he stops.[1]

A modified method is to put water-soluble contrast material into a long balloon on a catheter. A Foley catheter with a 30 cc balloon works fairly well. A pediatric or intermediate Blakemore esophageal tube works better, but it has one more balloon than is needed. A Nachlas esophageal tube may be the best. The balloon catheter is inserted into the upper rectum and the balloon *partly* filled with water-soluble contrast material. The catheter is slowly pulled out, positioning the balloon at various levels. A videotape recording is made at each level as the child pretends to defecate and to stop two or three times.[2]

[1] Kelly, J.H.: Cine radiography in anorectal malformations, J. Pediatr. Surg. 4:538-546, 1969.
[2] Shermeta, D.M., et al.: To be published.

Positive contrast peritoneography (herniography)

Herniography can be used to evaluate both abdominal wall and diaphragmatic hernias. The most common use is to search for an inguinal hernia on one side when a child is known to have an inguinal hernia on the opposite side.[1] After the child has voided, the lower abdominal wall is prepared by two applications of 1% tincture of iodine solution or povidone-iodine solution. The second application is permitted to dry and then removed with alcohol. A 1½ inch, short-bevel 18 or 20 French hypodermic needle is inserted into the midline a little below the umbilicus and aspirated to check for inadvertent puncture of bladder or bowel. If either has occurred, the needle is removed, and another needle is inserted in a slightly different site.

When the needle is in satisfactory position in the peritoneal cavity, the *same* volume of a 25% or 30% water-soluble iodinated contrast agent is injected as is used for intravenous urography (Table 13). (The amount of iodine injected is thus one half as much as for an intravenous urogram, where a 50% or 60% contrast agent is used.) The injection is started under fluoroscopic control, to make sure that the contrast material does not enter the bowel or infiltrate the abdominal wall. As soon as the injection is completed, the needle is removed, and a small sterile dressing is applied.

[1] Oh, K.S., et al.: Positive-contrast peritoneography and herniography, Radiology 108:647-654, 1973.

When an *inguinal hernia* is suspected, the patient is next turned prone and rocked from side to side for 2 to 3 minutes. The head of the fluoroscopic table is then raised 45 degrees for 2 or 3 minutes, which permits the contrast material to flow over the internal inguinal rings. A PA radiograph of the pelvis and scrotum is obtained and viewed promptly, in case additional projections with the child turned oblique are necessary. Gonad shielding cannot be used for this examination. If the child has not had a recent excretory urogram, the urinary tract is evaluated with a radiograph of the abdomen made 1 hour after the intraperitoneal injection of the contrast material.

To evaluate a *diaphragmatic hernia*, the child is also turned prone and rocked from side to side for 2 or 3 minutes. This time, however, the head of the fluoroscopic table is lowered 45 degrees or more for 2 or 3 minutes, which permits the contrast material to flow under the inferior surface of the diaphragm.

FINAL THOUGHT

Our patients are our best teachers.

This chapter has a number of hints and suggestions about ways to make friends with children at the same time as one makes radiographs of them. The best teachers, however, are our young patients. If we pay careful attention to them, we will learn from their words and their actions what they like and dislike. They will teach us the best way to do our work.

Technologists who make the effort to learn from children will find working with them a richly rewarding experience.

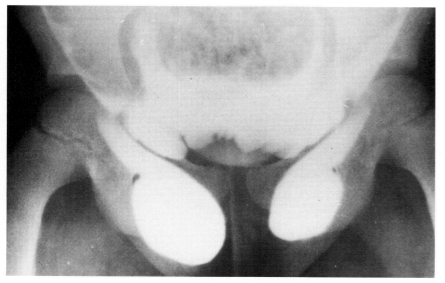

Herniogram showing bilateral inguinal hernias filled with contrast medium

15

Foreign body localization

Regions other than eye

Any alien object that has entered the body by any route is called a *foreign body*. A wide variety of foreign materials enter the body under many different circumstances—some by way of a puncture wound, others by way of a natural orifice. A majority of these objects must be removed by a surgical procedure. The referring physician depends on the radiology department to verify the presence of and to determine the nature and the exact site of any existent alien object or objects, so that he can determine the best procedure required for its removal.

The aim in this discussion is to present a description of the most commonly employed radiologic examinations used for the detection and localization of foreign bodies in regions other than the eye (for which see Volume Two, pp. 414 to 424). The bibliography contains a listing of papers detailing other methods of foreign body localization.

In civilian practice the most frequently encountered foreign bodies are those that have been aspirated or swallowed and tissue-penetrating materials such as needles, broken glass, and wood and metal splinters. Children sometimes insert a foreign object into the nose, the ear, or the genital orifice. An object lodged in one of these areas can usually be removed without referring the patient to the radiology department. When this is necessary, the examination consists of obtaining routine films made in at least two planes. Industrial areas and high crime areas frequently give rise to foreign body traumas comparable to those sustained on battlefields. These injuries often cause extensive bone and/or soft part damage by the impact of high-velocity objects.

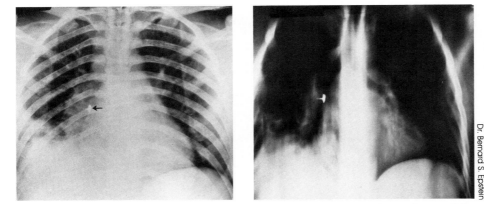

Patient treated for chronic pneumonia for 2 years, with symptoms of cough, foul-smelling sputum, and intermittent fever. The conventional film reveals pneumonia in the right lower lung and the presence of a foreign body. Tomography profiled a thumbtack lodged in the right lower lobe main bronchus adjacent to the hilum. The thumbtack was removed bronchoscopically.

Dr. Bernard S. Epstein

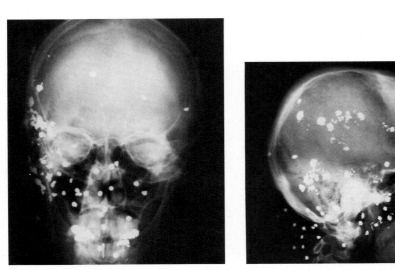

Battlefield injury resulting in multiple shell fragments lodged in the superficial tissues of the cranium, face, and neck

Dr. Peter Kuum

Aspirated and swallowed foreign bodies are discussed under this heading because the examinations employed for the detection and localization of objects entering by way of the mouth are limited to the two systems involved.

Penetrating foreign bodies are localized by both radiographic and fluoroscopic methods. The radiographic techniques are generally preferred because they afford a permanent record, and, after preliminary screening by the radiologist, they can be carried out by the technologist. During screening the radiologist places a mark on the skin surface, anteriorly or posteriorly, immediately over the center of the image of the foreign body. Then, by turning the patient or by the parallax method, he places a mark on the body at the exact site of the object to indicate its depth. These marks are used by the technologist as centering points in filming the patient and by the surgeon as reference points for operation.

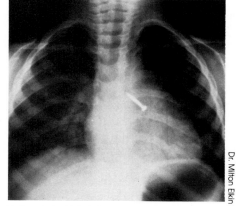

Nail aspirated into left main-stem bronchus

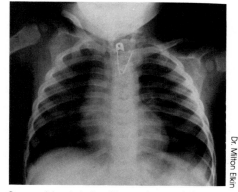

Open safety pin lodged in esophagus of 13-month-old boy

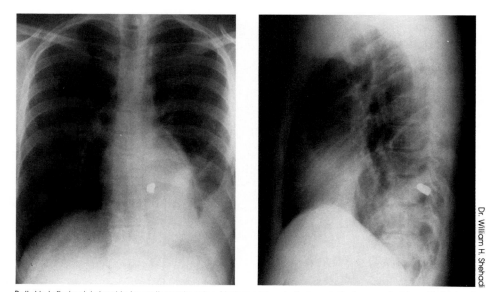

Bullet in left chest, lateral to lower thoracic spine. No bone injury. Left pleural effusion seen in PA and left lateral projections. Fluid mostly lateral and posterior.

301

PRELIMINARY CONSIDERATIONS

Careful attention to each of the factors affecting maximum radiographic detail is important in every examination, but it is nowhere more crucial than for the detection of low-density foreign bodies. The factors discussed here are of particular importance.

Focal spot

A perfect focal spot is a prerequisite for maximum radiographic detail. Pitting, cracking, and rippling of a focal spot result from overloading and overheating. These irregularities on the face of the target produce radiation emitted in all directions, causing serious blurring of detail. Using the tube within the limits shown on its rating chart, which should be prominently displayed in every control booth, will prevent target damage.

Screens

Dust and other extraneous particles, nicks, scratches, and stains produce shadows that can simulate small foreign bodies. Imperfect screen contact produces blurring similar to that produced by motion. These imperfections are the result of careless handling of cassettes and improper care of the contained screens.

Exposure factors

The exposure factors must be adjusted according to the tissue density of the part examined, and involuntary motion must be compensated for by the appropriate technique. For the demonstration of both bony and soft tissue structures in thick parts, a long scale of gray tones is generally desirable.

Fragments of low-density materials such as plastic, wood, and glass are most frequently found in the superficial tissues. The detection of these materials may require a short-scale contrast. It is important that thick surgical dressings be removed for the x-ray exposures, leaving only a thin layer of sterile gauze. However, only remove the dressings if so permitted.

The detection of glass fragments presents the greatest problem. There are at this time approximately 70,000 types of glass, each of which has a particular chemical composition. Many of the glasses contain a high enough percentage of lime and/or metallic oxide (iron, gold, lead, copper, etc., added to obtain specific colors) to render them sufficiently opaque to cast a shadow through the surrounding tissues. Others are composed of a high percentage of silicon (silica glass) with a low lime and metallic content. Failure to detect this type of glass does not preclude its presence.

Positioning of patient

Positioning of the patient is of prime importance in foreign body localization where even slight rotation of the patient or part can result in erroneous depth measurements. The frontal (AP or PA) and lateral positions must be exact. Optimum oblique and tangential positions are usually determined under fluoroscopic control to enable the radiologist to place the skin mark tangent to the film.

Motion

Motion of the part, voluntary or involuntary, causes blurring and loss of detail. This can obscure the presence of objects of low density and/or small size. For maximum radiographic detail, every effort must be made to control motion of body parts before an exposure is made. This must be done by means other than compression. Compression reduces tissue thickness, which results in erroneous depth measurements. Speed of exposure is the only means of overcoming the problem of involuntary motion.

Equipment

Precision depth-measurement techniques require exact centering of the tube within its housing and the exact measurement of target-film and target-shift distances.

The distance markings on the tube stand must be checked for accuracy so that exact compensation can be made for any discrepancy. The source-to-image receptor distance used for precision depth localization must be exact.

Suitable metal rulers can be attached to the tube carriage for the measurement of exact transverse tube shifts and on the side of the table or other convenient location for accurate longitudinal shifts. Provision must be made for both transverse and longitudinal tube shifts, because the tube is shifted at right angles to the long axis of elongated foreign bodies.

PENETRATING FOREIGN BODIES
Initial examination

The purpose of the initial examination is to verify the presence of suspected single or multiple foreign bodies and to determine their nature, size, shape, and location and the extent of bony and/or soft part trauma. In the presence of severe injury one or more scout films may be all that can be obtained on the initial examination.

The smaller parts of the extremities do not usually require scout filming. The foreign body is most often near the site of entry, and the central ray may be directed exactly through the foreign body. Right-angle projections (AP or PA and lateral) are obtained. The site of the puncture wound may be indicated on these studies by placing a lead marker on the film exactly opposite the wound. Additional projections are taken as indicated.

The initial examination of thick parts may be carried out by scout filming or, preferably, by fluoroscopy when the chest or the abdominopelvic regions are involved. Scout films must be large enough to include the entire region under investigation. The angle of entrance of high-velocity objects such as bullets and fragments of metal must also be taken into account. High-velocity objects entering at an angle usually lodge some distance from the puncture wound.

Preliminary screening expedites the examination because it enables the radiologist (1) to quickly locate radiopaque foreign bodies, whether near or far from the site of entry, (2) to ascertain whether the object is located within deep structures or in the periphery of a rounded area where it is best shown by tangential projections, (3) to determine the localization technique best suited to the circumstances, and (4) to mark the skin overlying the shadow of the foreign body in two or more planes. When the foreign body is distant from natural reference points (joints or other bony parts), the radiologist attaches metal markers to the skin for the surgeon's use as reference points. Emergency radiology departments keep a supply of sterile wire rings and crosses for this purpose.

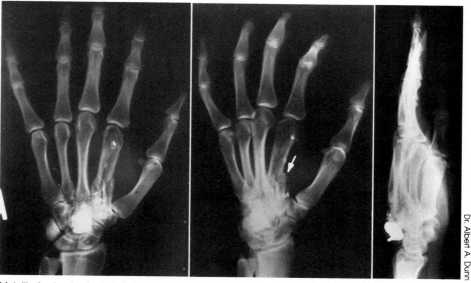

Dr. Albert A. Dunn

Metallic foreign body (bullet) in dorsal aspect of wrist, with comminuted fracture of second metacarpal

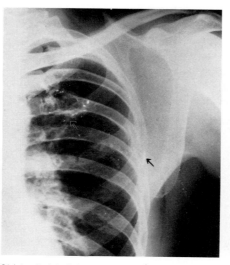

Old, healed, bullet wound fractures involving fifth rib laterally and posteriorly. Note track of lead deposits extending through soft tissues along path traveled by bullet.

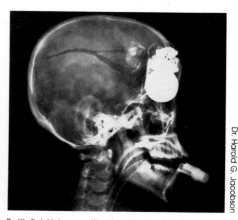

Dr. Harold G. Jacobson

Battlefield injury resulting in extensive bone and brain damage caused by hand grenade embedded in forehead

Radiographic localization techniques

The radiographic localization techniques are described as follows:
1. Stereoscopic projections
2. Oblique projections
3. Tangential projections
4. Right-angle projections
5. Single-film triangulation projection

Radiographic foreign body localization is performed after the surgeon has determined the route and the body placement to be used for the removal of the foreign body. The localization films are then made with the patient adjusted in the body position to be used for surgery. The films must always be large enough to include natural reference points, unless wire or other suitable markers have been attached to the skin or over a wound to serve this purpose.

Stereoscopic projections

The stereoscopic projection method simply consists in taking stereoscopic projections of the region under investigation.

This method is particularly applicable to regions that are not adaptable to exact right-angle projections. In addition to the stereoscopic studies, oblique and/or tangential projections and tomography are used as indicated.

Oblique projections

Oblique projections are used to separate overlapping shadows in any region. They are particularly useful in determining the relationship of superimposed bone and foreign body images to demonstrate whether the object is embedded in the bone or is lodged in the adjacent soft tissues.

Tangential projections

Tangential projections are useful in foreign body detection when the physical configuration of the body part allows the central ray to "skim" between the foreign body and the primary body part. It is most useful for the evaluation of superficial foreign bodies in extremities.

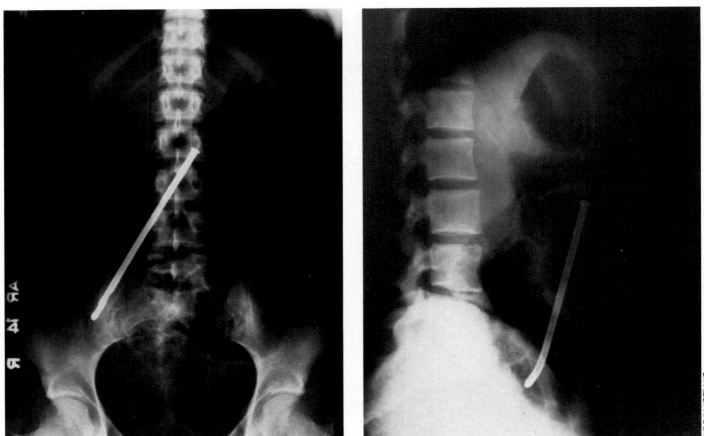

Intraperitoneal foreign body secondary to perforated uterus as a result of attempted criminal abortion

Dr. Albert A. Dunn

Right-angle technique

The right-angle technique of localization consists of taking exact right-angle projections (AP or PA and lateral), with the central ray directed through the foreign body.

Thick parts, particularly the chest and abdominopelvic regions, require (1) that the patient be adjusted in the body position to be used in the operating room for the surgical removal of the foreign body and (2) that the skin overlying the site of the foreign body be marked in both frontal and lateral planes. The central ray must be directed through the center of the foreign body for accurate localization of the object. If the centering is not accurate, the shadow of the foreign body will be cast by divergent radiation emitted from the periphery of the tube target. The distance of the image displacement and the resultant error in localization will depend on the distance between the foreign body and the film and on the source-to-image receptor distance as well as the distance of off-centering.

Except for the hands and feet, filming should, whenever possible, be obtained by biplane projections. This is particularly important in the presence of pointed and sharp-edged objects, where movement of the patient could result in deeper penetration of the object with further soft tissue trauma. It is also important when a foreign body is located where there is a possibility of a shift in its position, as in the mediastinum and the abdominopelvic areas. When there is a possibility of movement of a foreign body, resulting from its unstable location or from movement of the patient during his transfer from radiology to surgery, the location of the object should be verified with right-angle projections in the operating room immediately before the operation.

• • •

The foregoing methods are not only the simplest and most universally used procedures for the localization of penetrating foreign bodies; they are usually the only ones required.

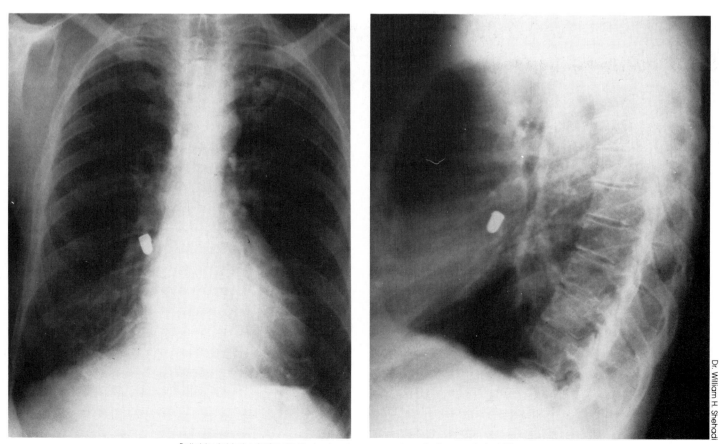

Bullet in right chest of patient who has been asymptomatic for a period of 15 years

Dr. William H. Shehadi

Single-film triangulation technique

The single-film triangulation technique is a precise method of depth localization. The only requirements are (1) that the *exact* source-to-image receptor distance (SID) and tube-shift distance (TSD) used be accurately measured and recorded, (2) that the patient and the film remain stationary for two exposures on one film, and (3) that the uppermost skin surface–to–film distance be accurately measured and recorded. The latter measurement is used in the final step of the depth calculation.

Any practical SID may be used—30, 36, or 40 inches. The TSD may be 4, 6, 8, or 10 inches. The greater the object-film distance, the greater will be the image shift distance (ISD). For this reason a shorter TSD can be used for near surface objects, but a longer TSD is more satisfactory for deep-seated objects, because it ensures adequate separation of the images. The tube is shifted at right angles to the long axis of elongated objects. This prevents possible difficulty in measuring the exact image-shift on partially superimposed shadows of slender or tapered objects.

Application of procedure

1. Adjust the patient in an exact AP or PA position as required to place him in the position to be used for the surgical removal of the foreign body.

2. Center the central ray to the skin mark overlying the site of the foreign body.

3. With the film in a Bucky tray, center it to the skin mark.

4. Carefully measure the uppermost skin-to-film distance in the plane of the foreign body, and record this measurement with the SID and TSD.

5. Make the first exposure using one half of the exposure time required for a conventional study of the part.

6. Shift the tube an exact distance, transversely or longitudinally as required, and, without disturbing the patient or the film, make the second exposure using the same factors as for the first exposure. These two "half exposures" produce a film density comparable to that obtained with a single full exposure of the region. When a wide tube shift is used the collimator must be adjusted for the second (off-center) exposure to avoid a cutoff, as shown by the transverse line on the right-hand illustration below. The upper right-hand corner cutoff was made by the gonad shield.

7. Process the film in the usual manner.

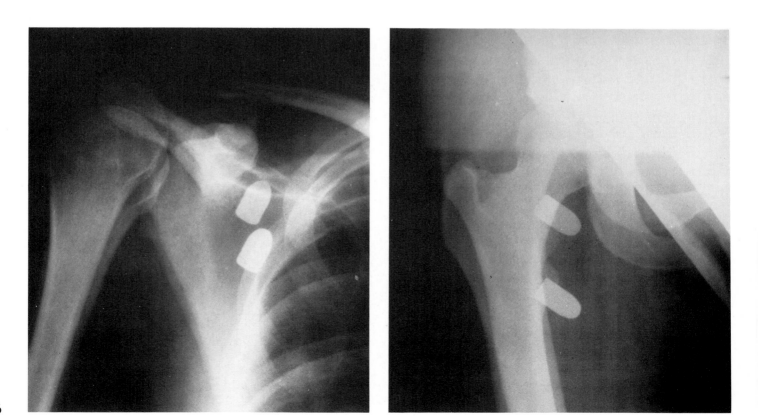

Depth calculation. From the same point on each image, the exact distance between the two images cast on the film by the foreign body are measured. With the three known factors, SID, TSD, and ISD, the foreign body–film distance is calculated by the following formula:

$$\frac{\text{SID} \times \text{ISD}}{\text{TSD} + \text{ISD}} = \text{Foreign body–film distance}$$

EXAMPLE: Assuming an SID of 40 inches, a TSD of 6 inches, and an ISD of 1½ inches, the foreign body–film distance =

$$\frac{40 \times 1\frac{1}{2}}{6 + 1\frac{1}{2}} = \frac{60}{7\frac{1}{2}} = 8 \text{ inches}$$

The depth of the foreign body below the skin surface is then calculated by subtracting the foreign body–film distance from the skin-film distance. Assume the latter measurement to be 10 inches. Using the result of the above example, 10 minus 8 equals 2, which places the foreign body 2 inches below the skin surface.

The measurements can be graphically reproduced on a sheet of paper by drawing a set of triangles, using a scale of ¼ inch to 1 inch as follows:

1. Draw a line representing the SID, line AB.
2. Draw a line representing the TSD, line AC.
3. Draw a line representing the ISD, line BD.
4. Draw a line from C to D.
5. Draw a line representing the skin surface, line SS.

The location of the foreign body is where line CD intersects line AB.

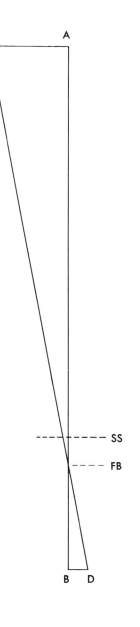

Fluoroscopic localization techniques

The fluoroscopic localization techniques are described as follows:
1. Parallax method
2. Right-angle method
3. Profunda method

The fluoroscopic methods of foreign body localization can be performed quickly and therefore are used when circumstances indicate that speed is of greater importance than the permanent record afforded by the somewhat more time-consuming radiographic methods.

Parallax method

The parallax method is based on the principle that the images cast by two objects equidistant from the fluoroscopic screen will move together at the same amplitude when the fluoroscope and tube are simultaneously moved back and forth across them. A metal indicator (a round-headed screw in the end of a wooden rod or stick serves the purpose well) is used for parallax localization of the depth of foreign bodies.

After locating the foreign body, the fluoroscopist closes the diaphragm shutters down to the size of the object to direct the central ray through its center. He marks the skin or tapes a suitable metallic marker in position to indicate the exact site of the foreign body in the frontal plane. He then places the metal indicator against the side of the body, and, holding it in an exactly horizontal position, he moves the screen back and forth as he raises or lowers the indicator until the images of the foreign body and the indicator move at the same amplitude. He then makes a mark on the side of the body to indicate the depth of the foreign body.

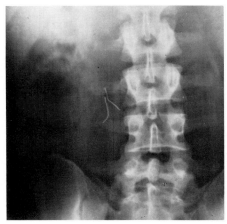

Initial frontal and lateral films

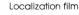

Localization film

The parallax method is the method of choice when the patient cannot be turned for right-angle projections. It is also used for depth localization in such regions as the shoulder, buttocks, and upper thigh.

Right-angle method

The right-angle method is applicable when turning the patient is not contraindicated by his condition or by the nature or location of the foreign body. It simply consists of locating and suitably marking the exact site of the foreign body in the frontal plane and then of repeating the procedure with the patient in the lateral position.

Profunda method

The profunda method consists of removing a foreign body under fluoroscopic guidance. The procedure can be time consuming, and because of the radiation dose to both patient and surgeon the use of this method is generally discouraged.

ASPIRATED AND SWALLOWED OBJECTS

Infants and young children instinctively investigate things by taste as well as by sight and touch. The result of this is that anything they can grasp they put into their mouth; therefore foreign bodies are frequently aspirated or swallowed. In adults the most frequent foreign body traumas under this heading may be fragments of bone (commonly fish or chicken bones), a bolus of solid food, and dental appliances. Adults are also prone to hold between their teeth such items as open safety pins (a habit of parents when changing diapers) and hair pins. Some craftsmen, most notably cobblers, carpenters, and those in the sewing trades, find it expedient to fill their mouth with such items as tacks, small nails, and pins, to be fed out for rapid use in their work. Many mentally disturbed patients have a compulsion to swallow objects and manage to swallow some of a surprisingly large size.

A foreign body that enters the mouth may start a gag reflex and be expelled immediately. When this occurs, a search should be made to recover and identify the object, thus obviating the necessity of futile and unnecessary radiologic examination of the patient.

More frequently the foreign body is retained and will be aspirated or swallowed. Rarely, it will be dislodged superiorly from the oral pharynx into the nasopharynx. If aspirated into air passages, the foreign body will be above the diaphragm in the neck or chest. If swallowed, the foreign body will pass beyond the oral pharynx and may lodge or become impacted in the cervical or thoracic portion of the esophagus, and/or it may travel on into the stomach and intestines.

The patient's symptoms will usually, but not always, indicate whether a foreign body has been aspirated or swallowed. When there is any doubt, particularly in the case of infants and young children, the preliminary radiographic survey should include the body of the patient from the level of the external auditory meatuses to the level of the anal canal—the neck, chest, abdomen, and pelvis—from the level of the highest external orifice to the level of the lowermost orifice. Once the location of the foreign body has been ascertained, accurate localization and follow-up films to determine its progress will depend on its size and shape and on the degree of impaction, if any.

About the only problem encountered in the detection of radiopaque foreign materials in the respiratory and alimentary tracts is the control of involuntary motion. This must be achieved by patient cooperation and/or rapid exposures.

Radiolucent foreign bodies require the use of a contrast medium to coat the object or localize the site of foreign body obstruction and to demonstrate the condition of the soft tissues at the site where the foreign body is lodged.

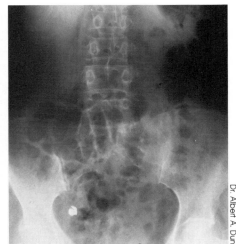

Coin in lower cervical esophagus

Tooth with splint in lower bowel

Dr. William H. Shehadi

Dr. Albert A. Dunn

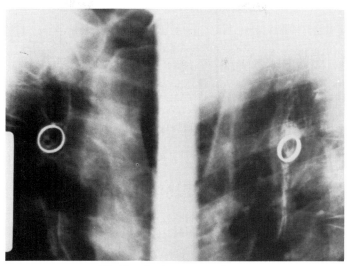
Wedding ring in upper esophagus

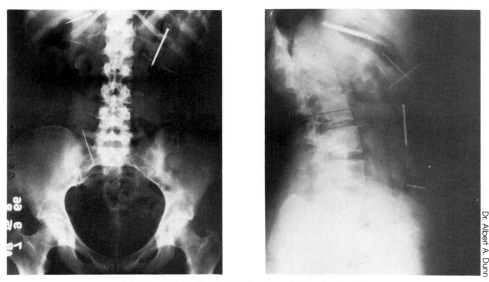
Multiple metallic foreign bodies in gastrointestinal tract

Dr. Albert A. Dunn

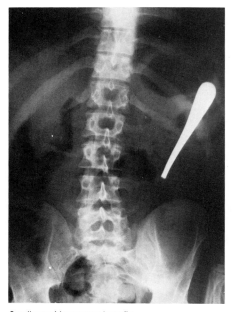
Swallowed teaspoon handle

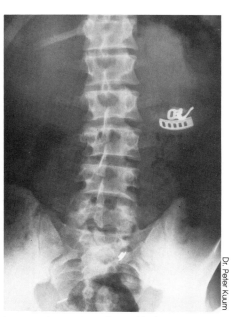
Swallowed storm-shoe clip and fastener

Dr. Peter Kuun

ASPIRATED FOREIGN BODIES
Infants and young children

Because an aspirated object can be quickly drawn into a distal branch of the airways, the initial films of infants and young children should be large enough to include the entire respiratory system. The upper edge of the films, a lateral projection of the neck and an AP projection of the neck and chest, should extend a little above the level of the external auditory meatuses for the inclusion of the nasopharynx. This is necessary for the detection of an object that rarely is, but may possibly have been, explosively dislodged from a lower level only to become lodged in the nasopharynx. The lower edge of the film used for the frontal projection of the neck and chest should extend well below the level of the diaphragm.

Unless old enough to sit or stand and to cooperate, the infant is placed in the supine position for greater ease in positioning and immobilization. The lateral projection of the neck is then obtained by cross-table projection. The routine infant technique, which is always based on the shortest possible exposure time, is employed for these studies. On viewing the scout films, the radiologist will determine if further studies are indicated.

Older children and adults

Aspirated foreign bodies may lodge in the larynx or trachea or in a main bronchus, most frequently in the right bronchus because of its larger diameter and more vertical direction. Small objects sometimes pass on to occlude one of the smaller bronchial branches where exact localization of the site of obstruction may require bronchoscopy.

Larynx and upper trachea. Radiopaque foreign bodies lodged in the larynx and upper trachea are clearly shown on AP and lateral films. The lateral retrosternal projection (Volume Three, p. 582) is sometimes useful, particularly with short-necked, high-shouldered subjects.

The films and the central ray are centered to the laryngeal prominence. The exposure technique should be decreased to better visualize the soft tissue structures.

Radiolucent foreign bodies require the use of a contrast medium. This procedure, laryngography, is carried out under fluoroscopic visualization, with spot films, conventional films, and tomography being used as indicated.

Trachea and bronchial tree. Filming of the intrathoracic respiratory system usually consists of two PA projections. A marker indicating the correct phase of respiration is placed on each film. The first film is taken on deep inspiration, and the second film on maximum expiration. Interference with air flow caused by bronchial obstruction will result in interference of airflow in the affected segment of the lung. Comparison of the two films will demonstrate this by showing no change in the radiolucency of the lung in the affected area. When the affected side is determined, a corresponding lateral projection is made. Depending on the nature of the foreign body and its site, further studies and/or bronchoscopy may be indicated.

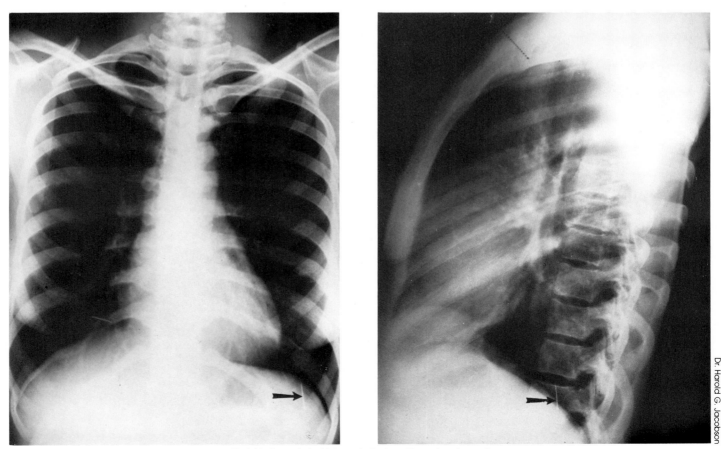

Straight pin aspirated into posterior basal bronchus *(arrows)*

Dr. Harold G. Jacobson

SWALLOWED FOREIGN BODIES
Infants and young children

Preliminary filming of infants and young children should include the entire alimentary canal, irrespective of the time lapse between the accident and the filming. As in aspirated foreign bodies, a lateral projection of the neck and nasopharynx is mandatory. This projection is best obtained by cross-table projection for ease of positioning and immobilization of small and/or uncooperative infants. A 14″ × 17″ film is large enough for the AP projection of the neck and body of small infants. Two films, one for the neck and chest areas and one for the abdominopelvic areas, are required for larger infants and young children. The routine rapid-exposure infant technique is employed for these studies.

The physician determines the nature and site of nonopaque objects under fluoroscopic visualization with the use of a contrast medium to coat the object or to localize the site of obstruction.

Smooth-surfaced foreign bodies such as coins and marbles are usually followed with 24-hour interval films to verify their clearance of the pylorus and the ileocecal valve, until a final film confirms that the foreign object is no longer in the body. An object presenting the possibility of perforation, such as an open safety pin, is followed at more frequent intervals.

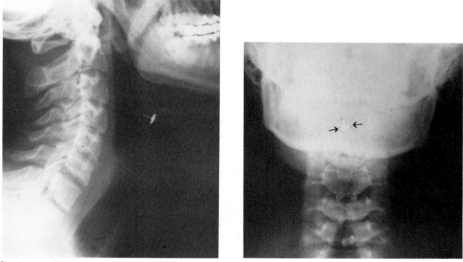

Thumbtack (aspirated) lodged on epiglottis. The tack was spontaneously expelled when the patient coughed.

Dr. William H. Shehadi

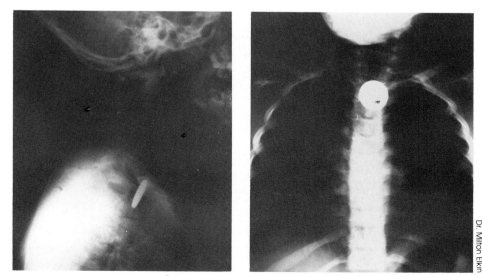

Coin in esophagus of 5-year-old boy

Dr. Milton Elkin

Older children and adults

Pharynx and upper esophagus. Radiopague foreign bodies lodged in the pharynx and upper esophagus can usually be clearly shown with one or two lateral soft tissue films of the neck. In the usual routine one film is taken on deep expiration to depress the shoulders and one at the height of deglutition to elevate the upper end of the esophagus (Volume Two, p. 545). Delineation of the upper end of the esophagus on short-necked, high-shouldered subjects usually requires a lateral retrosternal projection (Volume Three, p. 582).

As in infants and young children, nonopaque foreign bodies in this region are identified and localized with the use of a contrast medium administered under fluoroscopic control, followed by films made as directed by the radiologist.

Esophagus, stomach, and intestines. When a foreign body is not found in the pharynx, it is customary to take a right PA oblique projection (RAO) of the esophagus and an AP projection of the abdomen before fluoroscopy with the administration of a contrast medium. This precludes the possibility of obscuring a foreign object with the opaque medium.

Shehadi[1] recommends the use of one of the water-soluble iodinated media (Gastrografin or Oral Hypaque) for the investigation of esophageal foreign bodies. He states that the water-soluble medium localizes a nonopaque foreign body by giving an opaque coating, localizes the site of obstruction, and permits better evaluation of soft tissue trauma that may have occurred. The water-soluble medium does not adhere to the foreign body and therefore will not interfere with its endoscopic removal; barium mixtures adhere to a foreign body, rendering it slippery and difficult for the physician to grasp and remove with an esophagoscope.

Foreign bodies that have reached the stomach but present no danger of perforation are followed with interval films to verify their passage through the pylorus and the ileocecal valve and then until a final film confirms that the object has been discharged from the body.

[1]Shehadi, W.H.: Personal communication.

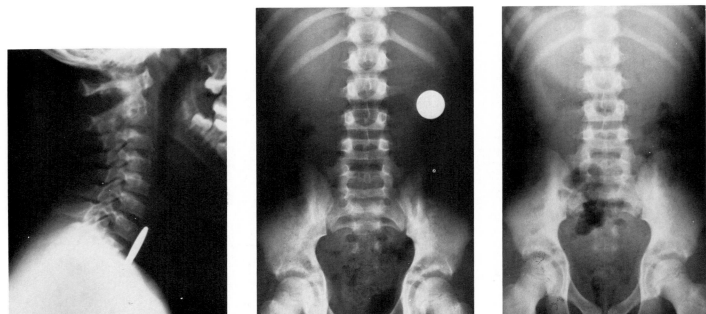

Twenty-five-cent piece in the lower cervical esophagus. Interval films show the coin (1) in the stomach and (2) to have been expelled.

Dr. William H. Shehadi

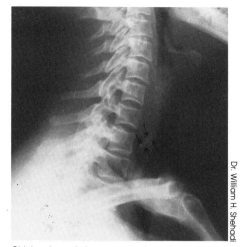

Dr. William H. Shehadi

Chicken bone in lower cervical esophagus

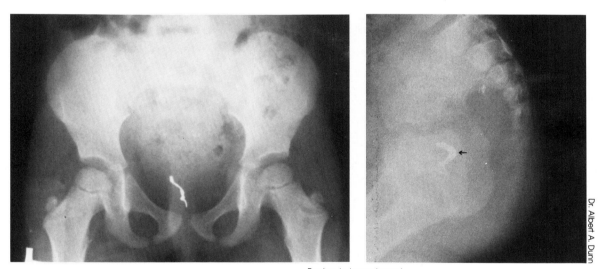

Dr. Albert A. Dunn

Earring in lower bowel

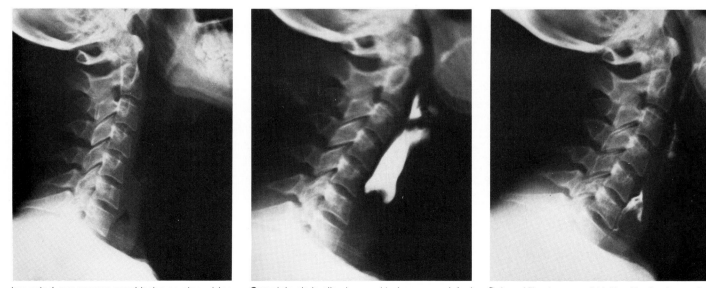

Impacted, nonopaque meat bolus causing widening of esophagus

Complete obstruction by meat bolus causes defect in barium column

Delayed film shows small trickle of barium bypassing the foreign body posteriorly.

Glossary

Anatomic and medical terms

Plurals of some of the more common Greek and Latin nouns are formed as follows:

Singular	Plural	Example
— a	— ae	maxilla — maxillae
— ex	— ces	apex — apices
— is	— es	diagnosis — diagnoses
— ix	— ces	appendix — appendices
— ma	— mata	carcinoma — carcinomata
— on	— a	ganglion — ganglia
— um	— a	antrum — antra
— us	— i	ramus — rami

A

a-, an- (before a vowel). Prefixes signifying without, lack of; as *atypical,* not characteristic of type, and *anemia,* lack of blood or of blood quality.

ab- Prefix signifying away from, departure; as *abduct,* to draw away from median plane or axis, and *abnormal,* deviation from usual structure or condition.

abdomen (ab-dō'men). Part of body lying between thorax and pelvis; cavity extending from diaphragm to pelvic floor.

abduct (ab-dukt'). To draw away from midsagittal plane, as in moving an arm or leg laterally.

abnormal (ab-nor'-mal). Irregular; deviation from usual form or condition.

abrade (ab-rād'). To rub or scrape off outer layer of a surface.

abrasion (ab-ra'zhun). Act of abrading; an area where skin or mucous membrane has been abraded.

abscess (ab'ses). Localized pus collection in a cavity, resulting from tissue disintegration.

absorb (ab-sorb'). To suck in, as a sponge, to assimilate fluids or other substances from skin, mucous surfaces, or absorbing vessels.

absorption (ab-sorp'shun). Sucking up or assimilation of fluids, gases, or other substances by absorbing tissues and vessels of body.

acanthiomeatal line (a-kan"the-o-me-ā'tal). Imaginary line extending from external auditory meatus to acanthion.

acanthion (a-kan'the-on). Point at center of base of anterior nasal spine.

accessory (ak-ses'or-e). Additional, supplementary; as an *accessory* organ that contributes subordinately to function of a similar but more important organ.

acinus (as'i-nus). Any one of smallest lobules of a racemose gland; one of saclike terminations of a passage, as air sacs, or alveoli, of lungs.

acoustic (a-koos'tik). Pertaining to sound or to organs of hearing.

acromegaly (ak"ro-meg'al-e). Chronic disease characterized by permanent enlargement of bones and soft tissues of face as well as of hands and feet.

acute (a-kūt'). Having a sudden onset and running a short but relatively severe course, as an *acute* disease; opposed to chronic.

ad- Prefix signifying toward; as *adduct,* movement toward central axis of body.

Addison's planes (ad'i-sonz). Imaginary planes used to divide abdomen into nine regions for descriptive purposes.

adduct (a-dukt'). To draw toward median plane or axis, as drawing an extremity medially.

adeno- (ad'en-o-), **aden-** A gland; of or pertaining to a gland; as *adenitis,* inflammation of a gland.

adenoma (ad"e-no'mah). Benign tumor of glandular origin.

adenopathy (ad"e-nop'ath-e). Any disease of glands.

adherent (ad-hēr'ent). Clinging or sticking to or together; that which adheres, as a covering membrane.

adhesion (ad-he'zhun). Union or sticking together of two surfaces as result of inflammatory process, as pleural *adhesions.*

adipose (ad'i-pōs). Fat; of a fatty nature; fat in cells of adipose tissue.

adnexa (ad-nek'sah). Appendages or conjoined parts; as *adnexa* uteri, the ovaries and oviducts.

adrenal (ad-re'nal). Situated adjacent to kidneys; pertaining to adrenal glands or bodies, also called suprarenal glands.

aer- (ā'er-), **aer-i, aer-o** Air; combining forms denoting relation to air or gas.

aerated (ā'er-at-ed). Filled with air, as lungs; charged with air or gas.

afferent (af'er-ent). Conveying inward from periphery to center; applied to nerves and to blood and lymphatic vessels; opposed to efferent.

aggregate (ag're-gāt). Grouped or clustered together; as an *aggregate* gland.

ala (ā'lah). Wing; winglike process or part.

alar (ā'lar). Pertaining to an ala or alae; as *alar* processes of sacrum.

-algia (-al'ji-ah). Suffix denoting pain; as *arthralgia,* pain in a joint.

aliment (al'i-ment). That which nourishes; food or alima (a-li'mah); any nutritive substance.

alimentary (al"i-men'ta-re). Of or pertaining to nutrition or aliment; as *alimentary* canal, the gastrointestinal tract.

alveolar (al-ve'o-lar). Pertaining to an alveolus or alveoli of mandible or lungs.

alveolus (al-ve'o-lus). Small cavity or pit; socket for tooth, acinus, or compound gland; terminal air sac of a bronchiole.

ambi- (am'be-). Prefix meaning both; as *ambilateral,* pertaining to or affecting both sides; bilateral.

amnion (am'ne-on). Thin, inner membrane of closed sac; bag of waters surrounding fetus in utero.

amphiarthrosis (am-fe-ar-thro'sis). Articulation admitting but little motion, as between vertebral bodies.

amplitude Length of travel described by tube during a tomographic motion; 45-degree circular tomographic motion will have greater amplitude than linear motion of same degree.

ampulla (am-pul'ah). Any flasklike or saccular dilatation of a canal; as rectal *ampulla.*

anal (ā'nal). Pertaining to anus.

analgesia (an"al-je'ze-ah). Diminished sensibility to pain.

analogous (a-nal'o-gus). Having analogy; corresponding in function in certain particulars to an organ or part of different structures; cf. homologous.

anatomic (an"a-tom'ik). Of, pertaining to, or dealing with body structure.

anatomy (a-nat'o-me). Science dealing with structure of body and relation of different parts.

anesthesia (an"es-the'ze-ah). Local or general loss of feeling or sensation; anesthesia may be produced by administration of anesthetic agent or by disease.

anesthetic (an"es-thet'ik). Agent capable of producing anesthesia.

aneurysm (an'ū-rizm). Abnormal, saccular dilatation of wall of blood vessel, containing blood and usually forming pulsating tumor.

angiography (an"je-og'ra-fe). Study of blood and lymphatic vessels; radiographic depiction of blood vessels after injection of radiopaque contrast substance.

angioma (an"je-o'mah). Tumor composed largely of blood or lymph vessels.

ankylosis (ang"ki-lo'sis). Abnormal union of two or more normally separate bones; immobility of a joint.

anomaly (a-nom'al-e). Marked irregularity or deviation from normal standard of structural formation.

ante- (an'te-). Prefix denoting before; as *anteversion,* forward displacement of an organ, and *antenatal,* occurring before birth.

anterior (an-ter'i-er). Pertaining to, designating, or situated in forward part of body or of an organ.

anteroposterior (AP) (an"ter-o-pos-ter'i-er). Directed or extending from front to back.

anthropologic base line As established at Munich Congress in 1877, anthropologic base line of skull passes from lowest point of inferior margin of orbit to center of superior margin of external auditory meatus; line is also known as Frankfurt horizontal plane, German horizontal plane, Reid's base line, and eye-ear plane; infraorbitomeatal line, or Virchow's plane *(which see),* is more widely used in radiographic positioning, because it is more easily localized and it parallels anthropologic base line closely enough for radiographic purposes.

anti- (an'ti-). Prefix signifying against, counter, opposite; as *antitoxin,* against poison.

antiseptic (an"ti-sep'tik). Opposing decay or putrefaction; any substance that will prevent or arrest growth of microorganisms without necessarily destroying them; cf. disinfectant.

antrum (an'trum). Cavern or cavity within a bone, especially maxillary air sinus.

anus (ā'nus). Terminal opening of alimentary canal; orifice through which fecal material is expelled.

aperture (ap'er-chūr). Opening, orifice, or mouth.

apex (a'peks). Tip or pointed extremity of any conical structure.

apnea (ap-ne'ah). Suspended respiration; transient cessation of breathing following forced respiration; as deglutition *apnea,* temporary cessation of respiration activity during swallowing.

apophysial (ap-of-iz'e-al). Of or pertaining to an apophysis; apophyseal.

apophysis (a-pof'i-sis). Any outgrowth or offshoot; process of bone, especially articular processes of vertebral arches.

appose (a-pōz'). To bring two surfaces in juxtaposition or proximity, as in reduction of a fracture.

apposition (ap"o-zish'un). Contact of adjacent parts; act of apposing or state of being apposed.

aqua (ak'wah). Latin for water; used in pharmacy in sense of liquid or solution.

aqueduct (ak'wē-dukt). Canal for transmission of a liquid; as *aqueduct* of Sylvius, passage connecting third and fourth ventricles of brain.

aqueous (a'kwe-us). Of or of the nature of water; watery.

areola (a-re'-lah). Minute space or interstice in a tissue; colored ring around mammary nipple.

areolar (a-re'o-lar). Of or pertaining to areola; containing interstitial areolae.

arteriography (ar-ter"e-og'ra-fe). Radiographic examination of arteries during injection of contrast medium.

artery (ar'ter-e). Any one of vessels conveying blood from heart to various parts of body.

arthritis (ar-thri'tis). Inflammation of joints.

arthrosis (ar-thro′sis). Any joint or juncture uniting two bones.

articulation (ar-tik″u-la′shun). Joint between bones.

ascites (a-sītēz). Collection of serous fluid in peritoneal cavity; abdominal dropsy.

asepsis (a-sep′sis). Methods of preventing and of maintaining freedom from infection; state of being free from septic or putrefactive matter.

aseptic (a-sep′tik). Free from septic material; substances capable of destroying pathogenic germs; cf. antiseptic.

-asis (-ă-sis). Combining form from -sis, used after nouns ending in *a* to denote action; as *metastasis*, transfer of a disease from a primary site of infection to another part or parts of body.

aspirate (as′pi-rāt). To remove or draw off by suction; to tap; to treat by aspiration.

aspiration (as″pi-rā′shun). A drawing out by suction; removal of fluids from a cavity by means of an aspirator; commonly called tapping.

assimilation (a-sim″i-lā′shun). Conversion or absorption of nutritive material into living tissue; anabolism or constructive metabolism.

asthenia (as-thē′ne-ah). Loss of strength; general debility.

asthenic (as-then′ik). Pertaining to asthenia or weakness; a bodily habitus characterized by slender build and poor muscular development.

asthma (az′mah). Disease characterized by recurrent attacks of paroxysmal breathing, with sense of suffocation.

ataxia (a-tak′si-ah). Condition characterized by inability to coordinate voluntary muscular movements.

atelectasis (at″e-lek′ta-sis). Defective aeration of pulmonary alveoli at birth; collapse or partial collapse of one or more of pulmonary lobes after birth.

atony (at′o-ne). Lack of normal tone or vitality; weakness; especially, deficient tonicity of contractile muscles.

atresia (ah-trē′zhe-ah). Absence or closure of a natural passage.

atrophic (a-trof′ik). Wasted; pertaining to or characterized by atrophy.

atrophy (at′ro-fe). Wasting away, or emaciation, of body or of any part; diminution in size of an organ or part.

atypical (a-tip′i-kal). Unusual; not characteristic of the type.

auditory (aw′di-tō″re). Of or pertaining to sense or organs of hearing.

auricle (aw′rik′l). Protruding portion of external ear; pinna or flap of ear; small, pouched portion of each of two atria of heart.

auricular line (aw-rik′u-lar). Line passing through external auditory meatuses and perpendicular to Frankfurt horizontal plane.

auricular point Center of external auditory meatus.

auto- (aw′tō). Prefix signifying self; as *autointoxicant*, a virus generated within body.

axial (ak′se-al). Pertaining to axis of a body, part, or thing; directed along axis, or center line.

axilla (ak-sil′ah). Armpit or fossa beneath junction of arm and shoulder.

axillary (ak′si-ler″e). Of or pertaining to armpit, or axilla.

axis (ak′sis). Straight line, real or imaginary, passing through center of a body or thing and around which body or part revolves or is supposed to revolve; second cervical vertebra.

azygos (az′i-gos). An unpaired part, especially an azygous vein or an azygous lobe of lung.

B

barium (bâr′e-um). Chemical element belonging to alkaline earth metals; symbol, Ba; atomic weight 137.36. The soluble compounds or salts of barium are poisonous. Chemically pure (USP) barium sulfate ($BaSO_4$) is a heavy, white, insoluble compound of barium and sulfuric acid and is used as a contrast medium in roentgenography because of its high radiopacity.

basion (bā′se-on). Center of anterior margin of foramen magnum.

benign (be-nīn′). Of mild character; as *benign* tumor, not malignant.

bi- (bī) [bis-, twice; di-, twice]. Prefix signifying two or twice; as *bilateral*, having or pertaining to two symmetric sides, and *biarcuate*, twice curved.

bifurcate (bī′fur-kāt). To fork, or divide into two branches.

bifurcation (bī″fur-kā′shun). Division into two branches; point of division.

bilateral (bīlat′er-al). Two-sided; pertaining to two sides.

bio- (bī′o-) [Gr. *bios*, life]. prefix signifying relation to life; as *biology*, science dealing with living organisms.

bismuth (biz′muth). Metallic element, the salts of which are used chiefly in medicine, by mouth in treatment of certain gastrointestinal conditions and by intramuscular injection in treatment of syphilis. Bismuth salts are radiopaque.

BNA Abbreviation for Basle Nomina Anatomica or for anatomic terminology adopted by Anatomical Society at Basel, Switzerland, in 1895.

body-section radiography Technical procedure in which any selected plane of body is depicted distinctly by moving film and x-ray tube in opposite directions to blur superjacent and subjacent structures; also called planigraphy, laminagraphy, stratigraphy, and tomography.

bolus (bō′lus). Round mass of anything, especially a soft mass of masticated food ready for swallowing.

bougi (bōō-zhē′). Tapering instrument used to dilate tubular passages.

brachial (brāke-al). Pertaining to arm; as *brachialgia*, pain in arm.

brachiocubital (brā″ke-o-kū′bit-al). Pertaining to arm and forearm.

brachy- (brak′e-). Prefix meaning short; as *brachyfacial*, a short, broad face.

brachycephalic (brak″e-se-fal′ik). A head of short, broad type.

brady- (brad′e-). Prefix meaning slow; as *bradycardia* (also called brachycardia), abnormal slowness of heart action.

bregma (breg′mah). Point on surface of cranium at junction of coronal and sagittal sutures.

bronchiectasis (brong″ke-ek′ta-sis). Dilatation of a bronchus or bronchi, which may be saccular or cylindrical.

bronchiogenic (brong″ke-o-jen′ik). Of bronchial origin.

bronchitis (brong-kī′tis). Inflammation, acute or chronic, of bronchial passages.

bronchography (brong-kog′ra-fe). Radiographic examination of lungs and bronchial trees after bronchi have been filled with radiopaque contrast substance.

buccal (buk′al). Of or pertaining to a bucca, or cheek; as *buccal* cavity, space between teeth and cheeks.

bursa (bur′sah). Small, fluid-containing sac interposed between surfaces that glide on each other and that would otherwise cause friction.

bursitis (bur-sī′tis). Inflammation of a bursa, sometimes attended with formation of concretions or calculi.

C

c Symbol for Latin *cum*, with.

calcareous (kal-kar′e-us). Consisting of or containing lime or calcium.

calcific (kal-sif′ik). Having or forming lime or calcium salts.

calcification (kal″si-fi-kā′shun). Deposition of lime salts in a tissue; preliminary process in formation of bone; a calcified part or calcific deposit.

calculus (kal′ku-lus). Abnormal concretion formed in any part of body, usually in various reservoirs of body and in their passages; as biliary *calculi*, or gallstones, located mainly in gallbladder and biliary ducts, urinary *calculi*, located in any part of urinary tracts, and renal *calculi*, occurring in kidneys.

callous (kal′us). Hard, horny; as thickened area of skin; a callosity.

callus (kal′us). Plastic substance exuded around fragments of fractured bone and ultimately converted into bone as it repairs break.

Camper line (Pieter Camper, Dutch physician, 1722-1789). Line extends from lower posterior border of wing of nose to center of tragus.

cancer (kan′ser). Malignant growth or tumor; cf. carcinoma.

cannula (kan′u-lah). Small, tubular instrument used for insertion, usually with a trocar, into a body cavity, as in a paracentesis.

canthus (kan′thus). Angle on each side of eye where upper and lower eyelids meet.

capillary (kap′i-ler-e). Any one of minute, thin-walled vessels that connect arterioles with venules to form networks in practically all parts of body.

carcinoma (kar″si-nō′mah). Malignant tumor originating in epithelial tissue and tending to spread, or metastasize, to other parts of body; a cancer.

cardia (kar′de-ah). Upper, or esophageal, orifice of stomach; pertaining to or in relation to heart.

cardio- (kar′de-ō-), **cardi-** (kar′de-). Prefix indicating relation to heart.

cardioangiography (kar″de-o-an″je-og′ra-fe). Radiographic demonstration of heart and great vessels during injection of opaque contrast medium; angiocardiography.

cardiospasm (kar′de-o-spazm). Spasmodic contraction of cardiac sphincter of stomach.

caries (kā′ri-ēz). Molecular decay and subsequent suppuration of bone; gradual disintegration, as distinguished from mass destruction from necrosis; tooth decay.

cata- (kat´ah-). Prefix signifying down, lower, against, in accordance with; as *catabasis*, stage of decline of a disease, and *catastaltic*, restraining, as an agent that tends to check a process.

cathartic (ka-thar´tik). Medicine producing evacuations by stool or catharsis; mild purgative.

catheter (kath´e-ter). Tubular instrument for passage through a canal to withdraw fluid from a cavity or to distend canal.

cauda (kaw´dah). Tail or tail-shaped appendage; as *cauda equina*, taillike termination of spinal cord, which consists of sacral nerves.

caudad (kaw´dad). In a caudal direction; toward tail; opposed to cephalad.

-cele (-sēl). Suffix signifying tumor or hernia; as *cystocele*, hernial protrusion of urinary bladder.

celiac, coeliac (sē´le-ak). Pertaining to abdomen; as *celiotomy*, surgical incision into abdominal cavity.

celiocentesis (sē″le-o-sen-tē´sis). Surgical puncture of abdomen; tapping.

cellulitis (sel″u-lī´tis). Inflammation of cellular tissue, especially of subcutaneous areas.

centesis (sen-tē´sis). Surgical puncture of a cavity; tapping.

centi- (sen´ti-). Prefix denoting a hundred or a hundredth part; used chiefly in metric system, as in *centimeter*.

centigrade (sen´ti-grād). Graduated into 100 equal divisions called degrees; centigrade thermometer (also called Celsius thermometer), a thermometer having 0° as freezing point of water and 100° as boiling point of water. For conversion to degrees Fahrenheit, multiply degrees centigrade by ⅘ and add 32.

cephalad (sef´al-ad). In a cranial direction, toward head; opposed to caudad.

cephalic (se-fal´ik). Of or pertaining to cranium; directed toward head end of body.

cephalo- (sef´al-o-), **cephal-** Prefix indicating relation to cranium; as *cephalotrypesis* (sef″al-o-tri-pē´sis), trephination of cranium.

cerebellum (ser-e-bel´um). The little brain; part of brain lying in inferior occipital fossae below cerebrum and behind fourth ventricle, pons, and upper part of medulla.

cerebral (ser´e-bral). Of or pertaining to brain, specifically to cerebrum.

cerebro- (ser´e-bro-). Prefix indicating relation to brain; as *cerebrospinal*, pertaining to or affecting brain and spinal cord.

cerebrum (ser´e-brum). Largest and main part of brain, its two hemispheres filling upper and greatest portion of cranial cavity.

cervical (ser´vik-al). Of or pertaining to neck or any necklike part.

cervico- (ser´vi-ko-), **cervic-** Prefix indicating relation to neck or to cervix of any organ; as *cervicooccipital*, pertaining to neck and occiput, and *cervicitis*, inflammation of neck of uterus.

cervix (ser´viks). Neck or necklike portion of any organ; as *cervix uteri*, narrow lower portion of uterus.

cholangeitis, cholangitis (kol″an-jī´tis). Inflammation of bile ducts.

cholangiography (ko-lan″je-og´ra-fe). Radiograhic demonstration of bile ducts after they have been filled with radiopaque medium; cholangiography may be performed in operation room while biliary tract is exposed or later in radiology department.

chole- (kol´e-), **cholo-** Prefix signifying relation to bile or to biliary tract; as *cholecyst*, gallbladder, and *cholecystectomy*, surgical removal of gallbladder.

cholecystitis (kil″e-sis-tī´tis). Inflammation of gallbladder.

cholecystography (kol″e-sis-tog´ra-fe). Radiographic demonstration of gallbladder following administration of substance that will render organ radiopaque.

choledochogram (ko-led-o´ko-gram). Radiograph of common bile duct while it is filled with contrast medium.

choledochography (ko-led-o-kog´ra-fe). Radiographic demonstration of common bile duct while it is filled with opaque medium administered by ingestion or injection.

choledochus (ko-led´o-kus). Common bile duct.

cholegraphy (ko-leg´ra-fi). Radiologic examination of biliary tract by means of contrast medium.

cholelithiasis (kol″e-li-thī´a-sis). Condition favoring formation of or of being affected with biliary concretions or calculi.

cholesteatoma (ko″les-te-a-tō´mah). Tumor containing cholesterol and fatty tissue, occurring in connection with middle ear.

chondro- (kon´dro-), **chondr-** Prefix signifying relation to cartilage; as, *chondroma*, benign tumor composed of cartilage, and *chondrocostal*, pertaining to ribs and rib cartilages.

chorea (ko-rē´ah). St. Vitus' dance, a nervous disease characterized by spasmotic twitching of muscles; most common in children.

chorion (ko´re-on). Outer membrane of protective covering that envelops fetus.

chronic (kron´ik). Continuing for a long time; as a *chronic* disease, one which is characterized by a protracted course; opposed to acute.

cicatricial (sik″a-trish´al). Pertaining to or having character of a scar or cicatrix.

cicatrix (sik´a-triks). Scar or scarlike mark; contracted fibrous tissue that forms at site of a wound during process of healing.

cirrhosis (sir-ō´sis). Disease associated with increase in fibrous tissue followed by contraction; specifically, chronic disease of liver in which organ may diminish in size (atrophic cirrhosis) or may increase in size (hypertrophic cirrhosis).

cleido- (kli´do-), **cleid-** Prefix indicating relation to clavicle; as *cleidocostal*, pertaining to clavicle and ribs, and *cleidarthritis*, gouty pain in clavicular region.

clysis (klī´sis). Washing out of a body cavity, as by lavage; an irrigation.

coagulation (ko-ag″u-lā´shun). Act or state of changing from liquid to gelatinous or solid mass; as clotting or coagulation of freshly drawn blood.

coalescence (ko″a-les´ens). Growing together or fusion of parts, as in a wound.

cohesion (ko-he´zhun). Molecular attraction or force that causes particles of a substance to cohere or cling together as in a mass.

colitis (ko-lī´tis). Inflammation of colon.

collateral (ko-lat´er-al). Having indirect relation to; secondary or accessory in function.

colo- (ko´lo-; kol´o-). Prefix denoting relation to colon; as *colocentesis*, surgical puncture of colon.

columella (kol″u-mel´ah). A little column; any part likened to a column; as *columella nasi*, nasal septum.

coma (ko´mah). State of profound unconsciousness caused by disease or injury and from which patient cannot be aroused.

comatose (kōm´a-tōs). Resembling or affected with coma; lethargic.

comminuted (kom″i-nūt´ed). Broken into small pieces; splintered, as in a *comminuted* fracture.

compound (kom´pound). Distinct, homogeneous substance composed of two or more chemically combined elements that have lost their original identity and cannot be separated by other than chemical means; cf. mixture, solution.

compound fracture Fracture having an open wound extending into site of fracture.

concentric (kon-sen´trik). Having a common center, as graduated circles, one within the other; directed toward or converging at a common center; opposed to eccentric.

condyle (kon´dīl). Rounded, knucklelike articular process on a bone; applied mainly to rounded articular eminences that occur in pairs, as those of occipital bone, mandible, and femur.

confluent (kon´flu-ent). Coming together; meeting or merging.

congenital (kon-jen´i-tal). Existing at birth; acquired or developed in uterus.

congestion (kon-jes´chun). Abnormal accumulation of blood in any part or organ; hyperemia.

coniosis (ko″ne-ō´sis). Pulmonary disease caused by inhalation of dust.

consolidation (kon-sol″i-dā´shun). Process of solidification in porous tissue as result of disease, as of lung in pneumonia and tuberculosis.

constriction (kon-strik´shun). Narrowing of lumen or orifice of a passage; a stricture.

contagion (kon-tā´jun). Communication of disease by direct or indirect contact; contagious disease, one that is readily transmissible from one to another without immediate contact.

contagious (kon-tā´jus). Transmissible by mediate or immediate contact; generating disease; conveying contagion.

contra- (kon´trah-). Prefix signifying against, in opposition; as *contraindication*, a symptom that opposes a treatment otherwise advisable.

contralateral (kon″tra-lat´er-al). Occurring on or associated in function with a similar part on opposite side.

contusion (kon-tū´zhun). Bruise; injury to subcutaneous tissue, with effusion of blood throughout area, but without breaking the skin.

coracoid (kor´a-koid). Process of bone projecting upward and forward from upper part of neck of scapula, called coracoid process because of its resemblance to a crow's beak.

coronal plane (ko-rō´nal). Plane or section passing from side to side parallel with coronal suture, at right angles to midsagittal plane of body.

coronoid (kor´o-noid). Shaped like beak of a crow; process on anterior surface of upper extremity of ulna.

corpus (kor´pus). Latin for body; main part of any organ; mass of specialized tissue.

costal (kos´tal). Of or pertaining to a rib or ribs.

costo- (kos´to-). Prefix signifying relation to ribs; as *costogenic*, originating in a rib.

319

costophrenic (kos″to-fren′ik). Pertaining to ribs and diaphragm; as *costophrenic* angle, angle formed by ribs and diaphragm and occupied by phrenicostal sinus of pleural cavity.

cox- (koks), **coxo-** Prefixes denoting relation to hip or hip joint; as *coxalgia*, pain in hip, and *coxofemoral*, pertaining to hip and thigh.

coxa (kok′sah). Hip or hip joint.

cranial (kra′ne-al). Of or pertaining to cranium.

cranio- (kra′ne-o-). Prefix denoting relation to cranium; as *craniofacial*, pertaining to cranium and face.

craniotrypesis (cra″ne-o-tri-pē′sis). Trephination of cranium, as in preparation for pneumoventriculography.

crater (kra′ter). A pit; a bowl-shaped depression.

crepitation (krep″i-ta′shun). Crackling or grating sound, such as that produced by rubbing together two ends of a fractured bone; crepitant râles, crackling sound heard on auscultation in certain lung diseases.

crepitus (krep′i-tus). Crackling noise; crepitation; noise produced by rubbing fragments of fractured bones.

crisis (kri′sis). Turning point in a disease; change that indicates whether symptoms will begin to subside or to increase in severity.

cum (kum). Latin for with; symbol is c̄.

cumulative (kū′mu-lā″tiv). Composed of added parts; increasing in intensity of action after successive additions; cumulative force or action.

cutaneous (kū-tā′ne-us). Of or pertaining to skin or cutis.

cutis (kū′tis). Corium or dermis; true skin as distinguished from epidermis.

cyanosis (sī″a-nō′sis). Bluish or purplish coloration of skin and mucous membrane resulting from deficient oxygenation of blood.

cyst (sist). Any normal fluid-containing sac or pouch, such as gallbladder and urinary bladder; any encapsulated or encysted collection of fluid or semifluid material formed as a result of disease.

cystitis (sis-tī′tis). Inflammation of urinary bladder.

cystography (sis-tog′ra-fe). Radiographic examination of urinary bladder after it has been filled with contrast medium.

cystoscopy (sis-tos′ko-pe). Visual inspection of interior of urinary bladder by means of cystoscope.

D

dacryo- (dak′ri-o-), **dacry-** (dak′ri-). Combining form denoting relation to tears or to lacrimal apparatus; as *dacryocyst*, lacrimal sac, and *dacryocystography*, radiography of lacrimal drainage system.

debility (de-bil′i-te). Weakness; lack or loss of strength.

deciduous (de-sid′u-us). Temporary; that which falls off or is shed, as *deciduous* teeth.

decubitus (de-kū′bi-tus). Lying down; as dorsal *decubitus*, lying on back.

defecation (def″e-kā′shun). Act or process of expelling fecal material from bowel.

deglutition (de″glū-tish′un; deg″lu-tish′un). Swallowing; act or process of swallowing.

demarcation (dē″mar-kāshun). Act or process of marking off boundaries; line of separation, as between healthy and diseased tissue.

dens (denz). Odontoid process of second cervical vertebra; a tooth.

dentition (den-tish′un). Eruption, or cutting, of teeth; form and general arrangement of teeth.

denture (den′tūr). Full set of teeth; artificial teeth.

depression (de-presh′un). Hollow area; concavity; decrease of functional activity or mental vitality.

dermato- (der′ma-to-). Prefix denoting relation to skin; as *dermatoma*, a skin tumor.

dermis (der′mis). Skin; specifically, corium, or true skin.

detergent (de-ter′jent). Any cleansing agent; a medicine used to cleanse wounds.

dextral (deks′tral). Of or pertaining to right side; opposed to sinistral.

dextro- (deks′tro-). Prefix denoting relation to right side; as *dextrocardia*, transposition of heart to right side of chest.

dextrosinistral (deks″tro-sin′is-tral). Extending from right to left; as *dextrosinistral* plane.

diagnosis (dī″ag-nō′sis). Art or act of determining character of a disease from existing symptoms; also, conclusion reached.

diaphysis (dī-af′i-sis). Shaft, or main part, of a long bone.

diarrhea (dī″a-rē′ah). Frequent discharge of loose or fluid fecal material from bowels.

diarthrosis (dī″ar-thrō′sis). Joint that permits free movement, such as hip or shoulder joint.

diastole (dī-as′to-lē). Phase of rhythmic dilatation or relaxation of heart and arteries; correlative to systole.

digestion (di-jes′chun). Process of converting food into chyme and chyle so that it can be absorbed and assimilated.

diploë (dip′lo-ē). Cancellous osseous tissue occupying space between two tables of cranial bones.

dis- (dis-). Prefix denoting absence, reversal, or separation.

disarticulation (dis″ar-tik″u-la′shun). Amputation at a joint with separation of joint.

disinfectant (dis″in-fek′tant). Any agent (heat or chemical) that destroys disease microbes but does not ordinarily injure spores; cf. germicide.

dispersion (dis-per′shun). Act of separating or state of being separated, as finely divided particles of a substance dispersed through a suspension medium.

distal (dis′tal). Remote from origin or head of a part; as *distal* end of a long bone; opposed to proximal.

diverticulitis (dī″ver-tik″u-lī′tis). Inflammation of a diverticulum or diverticula.

diverticulosis (dī″ver-tik″u-lō′sis). Multiple diverticula of any cavity or passage, most commonly of colon.

diverticulum (dī″ver-tik′u-lum). A blind sac or pocket branching off from a main cavity or canal.

dolicho- (dol′i-ko-). Prefix meaning long and narrow; as *dolichofacial*, a long, narrow face.

dolichocephalic (dol″i-ko-se-fal′ik). Having a long, narrow head.

dorsal (dor′sal). Pertaining to or situated near back of body or an organ; opposed to ventral.

dose (dōs). Proper quantity of a medicine to be taken at one time or within a specified time; quantity of x-radiation administered therapeutically at one time or over a period of time.

dropsy (drop′se). Abnormal accumulation of fluid in cellular tissue or in a cavity of body.

drug (drug). Any chemical substance used, internally or externally, in treatment of disease.

dys- (dis-). Prefix denoting (1) difficulty or pain, as *dyspnea*, labored or painful breathing, or (2) abnormality or impairment, as *dysarthrosis*, malformation of a joint, and *dystrophia*, defective nutrition.

dyspnea (disp-nē′ah). Labored or painful breathing.

dysuria (dis-u′ri-ah). Difficult or painful urination.

E

ec- (ek-). Prefix meaning out or out of; as *eccyesis*, extra-uterine pregnancy, and *ecchymosis*, extravasation of blood; also, resulting discoloration of skin.

eccentric (ek-sen′trik). Situated off center; not having same center; opposed to concentric.

ecto- (ek′to-), **ect-** Prefix denoting without, on the outer side, external; as *ectopic*, out of normal position, and *ectocondyle*, external condyle of a bone.

-ectomy (ek′to-me). Suffix denoting surgical removal of; as *cholecystectomy*, removal of gallbladder.

edema (e-dē′mah). Abnormal accumulation of fluid in tissues or cavities of body, resulting in puffy swelling when present in subcutaneous tissues or in distention when in abdominal cavity; dropsy.

edentulous (e-den′tu-lus). Without teeth; edentate.

efferent (ef′er-ent). Conveying outward from center toward periphery; applied to nerves and to blood and lymphatic vessels; opposed to afferent.

effusion (ef-ū′zhun). Escape of fluid from vessels into tissues or cavities of body.

egest (e-jest′). To expel or excrete waste material from body; opposed to ingest.

elephantiasis (el″e-fan-tī′a-sis). Chronic disease in which affected part undergoes extensive enlargement and skin becomes thick, rough, and fissured, so that it resembles an elephant's hide.

em-, en- Prefixes meaning in; as *empyema*, pus in a cavity, and *encysted*, enclosed in a sac.

emaciation (e-mā″si-ā′shun). Wasted; condition of becoming lean or emaciated.

embolism (em′bo-lizm). Obstruction of a blood vessel by an embolus or plug carried in from a larger vessel, usually a blood clot.

embolus (em′bo-lus). Clot of blood, air bubble, or other obstructive plug conveyed by bloodstream and lodging in smaller vessel; cf. thrombus.

emesis (em′e-sis). Act of vomiting.

emetic (e-met′ik). Any means employed to produce vomiting; a medicine that causes vomiting.

emphysema (em″fi-sē′mah). Swelling produced by an accumulation of gas or air in interstices of connective tissues; dilatation of pulmonary alveoli.

empyema (em″pi-ē′mah). Accumulation of pus in a body cavity; most frequently in pleural cavity.

emulsion (e-mul′shun). Oily or resinous substance suspended in an aqueous liquid by mucilaginous or other emulsifying agent.

en-, em- Prefixes meaning in; as *empyema*, pus in a cavity, and *encysted*, enclosed in a sac.

encephalo- (en-sef′a-lo-). Prefix signifying relation to brain.

encephalography (en-sef″a-log′ra-fe). Radiographic examination of brain after ventricles have been filled with contrast medium; pneumoencephalography.

encysted (en-sist′ed). Enclosed in a sac or cyst.

endo- (en′do-). Prefix meaning within; occupying an inward position; as *endocarditis*, inflammation of lining membrane of heart, and *endoscope*, instrument that permits visual examination of interior of a hollow viscus, such as urinary bladder.

endocrine (en′do-krin). Secreting internally, as ductless glands; pertaining to endocrine glands such as pituitary, thyroid, thymus, pineal body, and spleen.

endoscopic retrograde cholangiopancreatography Radiographic examination of pancreatic and biliary duct performed by injection of contrast media into these ducts; contrast media is injected through a catheter positioned with use of fiberoptic scope.

endoscopy (en-dos′ko-pe). Visual inspection of gastrointestinal tract with fiberoptic scope.

endosteal (en-dos′te-al). Of or pertaining to endosteum, vascular tissue lining medullary cavity of bones.

enema (en′e-mah). Fluid injected into rectum for purpose of cleansing bowel or of administering food or a drug.

enteric (en-ter′ik). Of or pertaining to intestines.

enteritis (en-ter-i′tis). Inflammation of intestine, specifically of small intestine.

entero- (en′ter-o-), **enter-** Prefix denoting relation to intestine; as *enteroptosis,* a dropping or downward displacement of intestines.

enterostomy (en″ter-os′to-me). Surgical formation of an opening into intestine through abdominal wall; as gun-barrel *enterostomy,* operation in which each segment of divided intestine is brought to a separate opening on surface of abdominal wall.

enuresis (en″u-re′sis). Involuntary discharge of urine; incontinence of urine.

epi- (ep′i), **ep-** Prefix meaning on, above, on the outside, over; as *epicostal*, situated on a rib, *epigastric*, situated above stomach, and *epidermis*, outermost layer of skin.

epiphysis (e-pif′i-sis). Center of ossification separated during growth from main body of a bone by cartilage that subsequently ossifies to unite two parts of bone, epiphysis and diaphysis.

epiphysitis (e-pif″i-si′tis). Inflammation of an epiphysis or of cartilage separating it from diaphysis.

ERCP See endoscopic retrograde cholangiopancreatography.

erosion (e-ro′zhun). Irregular or uneven wearing or eating away, beginning at surface of a part, as an ulcerative or necrotic process.

eructation (e″ruk-ta′shun). Act of discharging or belching gas from stomach; a belch.

erythema (er′i-the′mah). Morbid redness of skin caused by capillary congestion resulting from irritation or any form of inflammatory process.

etiology (e″ti-ol′o-je). Science or doctrine of causation; investigation or assignment of cause of a disease.

eu- (u-). Prefix signifying well; as *eupnea*, normal breathing; opposed to dys-.

evagination (e-vaj″i-na′shun). Turned inside out; protrusion of a part or organ.

eventration (e″ven-tra′shun). Protrusion of intestines from abdomen.

eversion (e-ver′shun). Act of turning or state of being turned outward or inside out.

evert (e-vert′). To turn outward or inside out.

ex- (eks-). Prefix denoting out, out of, or away from; as *excavation*, a hollowing out, and *excrete*, throwing off of waste material.

excreta (eks-kre′tah). Waste materials excreted or separated out by an organ; waste products cast out from body.

excretion (eks-kre′shun). Throwing off of waste matter.

excretory (eks′kre-to″re). Of or pertaining to excretion.

exo- (ek′so-), **ex-** Prefix meaning outward or outside; as *exogenous*, growing from or on the outside of a part of body; originating outside body.

exostosis (eks″os-to′sis). Spur, or osseous outgrowth, from a bone or tooth.

extension (eks-ten′shun). Movement of a joint or joints that brings parts of an extremity or of body into or toward a straight line.

extra- (eks′tra-). Prefix meaning on outside, beyond, in addition; as *extragastric*, situated or occurring outside stomach.

extravasation (eks-trav″a-sa′shun). Escape of fluid from a vessel into surrounding tissues; said of blood, lymph, and serum.

extrinsic (eks-trin′sik). Originating outside of part involved.

exudate (eks′u-dat). Adventitious material exuded or thrown out on injured or diseased tissues.

F

facet (fas′et). Any plane, circumscribed surface; as an articular facet on a bone.

Fahrenheit (fah′ren-hit). Pertaining to thermometric scale invented by Gabriel Daniel Fahrenheit. On Fahrenheit thermometer, freezing point of water is 32° above zero point, and boiling point of water at 212°. Cf. centigrade.

febrile (fe′bril). Pertaining to fever; feverish.

fecal (fe′kal). Relating to or of nature of feces.

feces (fe′sez). Excrement, or waste products, of food digestion discharged from bowels.

fenestra (fe-nes′trah). Small aperture, or opening, as in certain bones.

fetid (fet′id). Having offensive smell.

fetography (fe-tog′ra-fe). Radiographic examination of fetus in utero.

fibroma (fi-bro′mah). Benign tumor composed mainly of fibrous tissue.

fibrosis (fi-bro′sis). Formation of fibrous tissue in any organ or region; replacement of normal tissue with fibrous tissue.

fissure (fish′ur). Any narrow furrow, cleft, or slit, normal or otherwise.

fistula (fis′tu-lah). Abnormal passage leading from an abscess cavity or from a hollow organ to surface of body or from one hollow organ to another.

flaccid (flak′sid). Without firmness or tone; flabby, as a *flaccid muscle.*

flatulence (flat′u-lens). Gaseous distention of stomach or intestines.

flatus (fla′tus). Gas generated in stomach or intestines.

flexion (flek′shun). Bending of a joint in which angle between parts is decreased; forward bending; opposite of extension.

flocculent (flok′u-lent). Containing soft flakes or shreds, as in a *flocculent* precipitate.

flux (fluks). Flow of a liquid; an excessive discharge, as from the bowels.

focal plane Plane of tissue that is maximumly in focus on a tomogram.

focal plane level Height from level of focal plane to tabletop.

fontanel (fon′ta-nel). Any one of intervals or soft spots between angles of parietal bones and adjacent bones of cranium in an infant.

formula (for′mu-lah). Prescribed ingredients, with proportions, for preparation of a medicine; prescription; combination of symbols to express chemical constituents of a body.

fossa (fos′ah). A pit, cavity, or depression; as acetabular *fossa*, supraclavicular *fossa*, and nasal *fossae.*

fovea (fo′ve-ah). Pit or cup-shaped depression.

Fowler's position (fow′lerz). Position in which head end of body is elevated, usually about 30 degrees.

Frankfurt plane or line See anthropologic base line.

fremitus (frem′i-tus). Palpable vibration or thrill; as tussive *fremitus*, vibration felt through head on humming with mouth closed.

frenulum (fren′u-lum). Small fold of mucous membrane serving to support or restrain movements of a part.

fulcrum Pivot point or axis about which tube and film rotate during a tomographic motion.

fundus (fun′dus). Base of a hollow organ; part farthest from opening, as cardiac end of stomach.

furuncle (fu′rung-k′l). A boil.

G

gall (gawl). Bitter, brownish or greenish yellow fluid secreted by liver; bile.

ganglion (gang′gle-un). Any aggregation of nerve cells forming a nerve center; small cystic tumor occurring on a tendon, usually about wrist or ankle.

gangrene (gang′gren). Necrosis of tissue caused by interference with blood supply to part, usually accompanied with putrefaction.

gas gangrene Gangrene occurring chiefly in lacerated wounds and in which tissues become impregnated with gas produced by a mixed infection of bacteria, including gas bacillus.

gastr- (gas′tr-), **gastro-** Prefix signifying relation to stomach; as *gastritis, gastroenterostomy.*

gastric (gas′trik). Of or pertaining to stomach.

gastroentero- (gas″tro-en′ter-o-), **gastroenter-** Prefix denoting relation to stomach and intestine; as *gastroenteroptosis*, prolapse or downward displacement of stomach and intestines.

gavage (gah″vahzh′). Feeding by stomach tube.

-genic (-jen′ik). Combining form meaning causing, giving origin to, or arising from; as *osteogenic*, originating in bone.

German horizontal plane Base line of cranium; anthropologic base line.

germicide (jer′mi-sid). Any agent that destroys germs; cf. antiseptic and disinfectant.

gingivae (jin-ji′ve); sing. **gingiva** (jin-ji′vah). Gums.

gingival (jin′ji-val). Of or pertaining to gums.

glabella (glah-bel′ah). Smooth space on forehead between superciliary arches, which correspond in position with eyebrows.

glabelloalveolar line (glah-bel″o-al-ve′o-lar). Imaginary line extending from glabella to upper alveolus; localization plane of face.

glabellomeatal line (glah-bel″o-me-a′tal). Imaginary line extending from glabella to external auditory meatus; localization line used in Caldwell sinus method.

glenoid (gle′noid). Smooth, shallow depression; specifically, glenoid fossa of scapula.

glioma (gli-o′mah). Malignant tumor originating in nerve tissue.

glossa (glos′ah). Greek for tongue.

glossal (glos′al). Of or pertaining to tongue; lingual.

gonion (go′ne-on). Tip of angle of mandible.

granulation (gran-u-la′shun). Formation of small grains or particles; any small, granulelike mass of abnormal tissue projecting from surface of an organ; formation in a wound of small, rounded granules of new tissue during healing process.

gravel (grav′el). Deposit of small, stonelike concretions in kidneys and urinary bladder; calculi.

groin (groin). Depression between lower part of abdomen and thigh, or region around depression; inguen, or inguinal region.

groove (groov). Shallow, linear depression, or furrow in a part, especially in bone.

Grossman principle Tomographic principle in which fulcrum or axis of rotation remains at a fixed height. The focal plane level is changed by raising or lowering the tabletop through this fixed point to the desired height.

gumma (gum′ah). Soft, gummy, granulomatous tumor of syphilitic origin, occurring in third stage of disease.

gynecology (gin″e-kol′o-je). Branch of medicine that treats women's diseases occurring in genital, urinary, and rectal regions.

H

habitus (hab′it-us) [Latin for habit]. Fixed practice established by frequent usage; bodily appearance; general form or architecture of body.

haustrum (haws′trum); pl. **haustra** (-trah). Any one of recesses formed by sacculations of colon.

hem-, haem-, hemo- Prefix denoting blood or relation to blood; as *hematuria,* presence of blood in urine.

hemangioma (he-man″je-o′mah). Tumor consisting of newly formed blood vessels.

hematoma (he″mah-to′mah). Tumor or swelling containing effused blood.

hemi- (hem′i-). Prefix signifying one half; pertaining to or affecting one side of body; as *hemiplegia,* paralysis of one side of body.

hemoptysis (he-mop′ti-sis). Presence of blood in sputum; expectoration of blood.

hemorrhage (hem′o-rij). Discharge of blood from vessels in any region; bleeding.

hemorrhoid (hem′o-roid). Vascular tumor situated at orifice of or within anal canal.

hepatic (he-pat′ik). Of or pertaining to liver.

hepato- (hep′a-to-), **hepat-** Prefix signifying relation to liver; as *hepatomegalia,* enlargement of liver.

hernia (her′ne-ah). Protrusion of a part of an organ through normal or abnormal opening in wall of its natural cavity; a rupture.

herniation (her-ne-a′shun). Hernial protrusion; formation of a hernia.

herpes (her′pez). Acute inflammation of skin or mucous membrane, in which clusters of small vesicles form and tend to spread.

hetero- (het′er-o-). Prefix signifying other, or other than usual; difference or dissimilarity between constituents; to or from a different source; opposite of homo-.

heterogeneous (het″er-o-je′ne-us). Differing in kind or nature; composed of unlike elements or ingredients or having dissimilar characteristics; opposed to homogeneous.

heterogenous (het″er-oj′e-nus). Arising or originating outside body; opposed to autogenous.

hiatus (hi-a′tus). An opening; a space, gap, or fissure for transmission of a nerve, vessel, or tubular passage.

hilum (hi′lum). Depression on a gland or organ that marks site of entrance and exit of nerves, vessels, and ducts; as *hilum* of kidney or of lung.

hilus (hi′lus). Same as hilum.

homeo-, homoeo- (ho′me-o-). Prefix meaning like, similar; as *homeomorphous,* of similar structure and form.

homo- (ho′mo-). Prefix meaning one and same, common, similar; as *homodox, homocentric, homologue;* opposed to hetero-.

homogeneous (ho″mo-je′ne-us). Of same kind or nature; composed of similar elements or ingredients or having similar uniform characteristics; opposed to heterogeneous.

homologous (ho-mol′o-gus). Corresponding in position or structure but not necessarily resembling in function; cf. analogous.

hydro- (hi′dro-). Prefix meaning water or denoting some relation to water or to hydrogen.

hydrocele (hi′dro-sel). An accumulation of fluid, usually in a sacculated cavity such as scrotum.

hydrocephalus (hi″dro-sef′a-lus). Condition characterized by excessive amount of cerebrospinal fluid in cerebral ventricles, accompanied by dilatation of ventricles, and causing atrophy of brain substance and enlargement of head.

hydronephrosis (hi″dro-nef-ro′sis). Accumulation of urine in pelvis of kidney, caused by obstruction of ureter, with resultant dilatation of pelvis and atrophy of organ itself.

hydrops (hi′drops). Excessive accumulation of fluid in a cavity of body; dropsy.

hyper- (hi′per). Prefix meaning over; above in position; beyond usual or normal extent or degree; excessive; opposite of hypo-.

hypermotility (hi″per-mo-til′i-te). Excessive movement or motility of involuntary muscles, especially those of gastrointestinal tract.

hyperpnea (hi″perp-ne′ah). Abnormally rapid respiratory movements.

hypersthenic (hi″per-sthen′ik). Excessive strength or tonicity of body or of any part; type of bodily habitus characterized by massive proportions.

hyperthyroid (hi″per-thi′roid). Pertaining to hyperthyroidism; excessive functional activity of thyroid gland.

hypertrophic (hi″per-trof′ik). Pertaining to or affected with hypertrophy.

hypertrophy (hi-per′tro-fe). Morbid increase in size of an organ or part.

hypo- (hi′po-). Prefix meaning under; below or beneath in position; less than usual or normal extent or degree; deficient; opposite of hyper-.

hyposthenic (hi″pos-then′ik). Lack of strength or tonicity; type of bodily habitus characterized by slender build, a modification of more extreme asthenic type.

hypothyroid (hi″po-thi′roid). Pertaining to hypothyroidism; deficient functional activity of thyroid gland.

hysteresis (his″ter-e′sis). Lagging or retardation of one of two associated phenomena; failure to act in unison.

hystero- (his′ter-o-), **hyster-** Prefix denoting relation to uterus; as *hysterectomy,* surgical removal of uterus.

hysterography (his″ter-og′ra-fe). Radiographic examination of uterus after injection of contrast medium; uterography.

hysterosalpingography (his″ter-o-sal-ping-gog′ra-fe). Radiographic examination of uterus and oviducts after injection of contrast medium; uterosalpingography.

I

-iasis (-i′a-sis). Suffix denoting morbid or diseased condition; as *elephantiasis, nephrolithiasis, dracontiasis.*

idio- (id′i-o-). Combining form denoting self-produced; as *idiopathic,* self-originated, of unknown cause.

ileac (il-e-ak). Pertaining to ileum or to ileus; cf. iliac.

ileo- (il′e-o-). Prefix denoting some relation to ileum; as *ileocolic, ileocecal, ileotomy.*

ileum (il′e-um). Terminal three fifths of small intestine, part extending from jejunum to cecum; cf. ilium.

ileus (il′e-us). Condition caused by intestinal obstruction, marked by severe pain in and distention of abdomen; volvulus.

iliac (il′e-ak). Of or pertaining to ilium; cf. ileac.

ilium (il′e-um). Wide upper one of three bones composing each half of pelvic girdle; cf. ileum.

im-, in- Prefixes meaning in, within, or into, as *immersion, injection;* also, not, non-, un-, as in *imbalance, inactive, incurable.*

impacted (im-pak′ted). Firmly wedged or lodged in position; forcibly driven together, as two ends of a bone in an *impacted* fracture.

incipient (in-sip′e-ent). Beginning to exist; commencing; as the *incipient* or initial stage of a disease.

incisura (in″si-su′rah). Notch or cleft; deep indentation.

incisure (in-sizh′ur). Notch; cut or gash.

incontinence (in-kon′ti-nens). Inability of any of organs to restrain a natural evacuation; involuntary discharges; as *incontinence* of urine or feces.

induration (in″du-ra′shun). Hardening or hardened tissue resulting from inflammation or congestion.

infarct (in′farkt). Circumscribed area of necrosis of tissue, resulting from obstruction of local blood supply by an embolus or a thrombus.

infection (in-fek´shun). Communication of disease germs to body tissues by any means.

infectious (in-fek´shus). Contaminated or charged with disease germs; readily communicable by infection but not necessarily contagious; cf. contagious.

inferior (in-fer´i-er). Situated lower or nearer to bottom or base; below.

inferosuperior (in″fer-o-su-per´i-er). Directed or extending from below upward; caudocranial.

infiltration (in″fil-tra´shun). Filtering into or penetration of tissues by a substance not normal to them.

inflammation (in″fla-ma´shun). Morbid condition produced in tissues by an irritant; natural reaction to irritation wherein plasma and blood cells are exuded at site of infection or injury in attempt to heal damage; it is manifested by redness, swelling, and pain.

infra- (in´frah-). Prefix meaning below; as *infraorbital*, situated below orbit.

infraorbitomeatal line (in″frah-or″bit-o-me-a´tal). Also known as Virchow's plane (ver´koz). A line that extends from center of inferior orbital margin to center of tragus and that is used in radiography for adjustment of base of cranium. Because this line closely parallels anthropologic base line, it is frequently denoted by this and other terms applied to anthropologic base line.

infundibulum (in″fun-dib´u-lum). Any conical or funnel-shaped structure or passage.

infusion (in-fu´zhun). Process of introducing a solution into a vessel or a hollow viscus by gravity pressure; cf. injection, instillation, insufflation.

ingest (in-jest´). To take in for digestion; to eat; to take anything by mouth.

inguinal (ing´gui-nal). Of or pertaining to region of inguen or groin, region between abdomen and thigh.

inion (in´i-on). External occipital protuberance.

injection (in-jek´shun). Forcible introduction, usually by syringe, of a liquid, gas, or other material into a part of body, a vessel, a cavity, an organ, or subcutaneous tissue; cf. infusion, instillation, insufflation.

inorganic (in″or-gan´ik). Not organic in origin; pertaining to or composed of substances other than animal or vegetable; inanimate matter; as *inorganic* elements.

inspissated (in-spis´a-ted). Thickened by evaporation or by absorption of fluid content; as *inspissated* plus.

instillation (in″stil-la´shun). To drop in; process of introducing a liquid into a cavity drop by drop; cf. infusion, injection, insufflation.

insufflation (in″su-fla´shun). Act of blowing air or gas (or a powder or vapor) into a cavity of body, as into colon for double-contrast enema; cf. infusion, injection, instillation.

inter- (in´ter-). Prefix signifying between; as *interlobar*, situated between two lobes; cf. intra-.

intercostal (in″ter-kos´tal). Pertaining to or situated in spaces between ribs.

interpediculate (in″ter-pe-dik´u-lāt). Of or pertaining to space between pedicles of neural arch.

interpupillary line (in″ter-pu´pi-ler″e). Imaginary line passing through pupils of eyes; used in radiography in adjustment of head in an exact lateral position.

interstice (in-ter´stis). Small gap or space in a tissue; an interval.

interstitial (in″ter-stish´al). Of or pertaining to spaces, or interstices, of a tissue.

intra- (in´trah-). Prefix meaning within or into; as *intralobar*, within a lobe, and *intravenous*, injected into a vein; cf. inter-.

intrinsic (in-trin´sik). Situated or originating entirely within an organ or part; opposite of extrinsic.

invaginated (in-vaj´i-nāt″ed). Condition of being drawn inward to become ensheathed, as a covering membrane turning backward to form a double-walled cavity.

invert (in´vert). To turn inward; as to *invert* foot.

involuntary (in-vol´un-ter″e). Movement not under control of the will, as that of cardiac, gastrointestinal, and other involuntary muscles.

ipsilateral (ip″si-lat´er-al) [L. *ipse*, self]. Located on or pertaining to same side.

-itis (-i´tis). Suffix signifying inflammation of specified part; as *arthritis, appendicitis, bronchitis*.

J

jaundice (jawn´dis). Morbid condition caused by obstruction of biliary passages; it is characterized by a yellowish discoloration of skin, eyes, and secretions of body resulting from absorption of accumulation of bile pigments from blood.

jejuno- (je-ju´no), **jejun-** Prefix signifying some relation to jejunum; as *jejunoduodenal, jejunitis, jejunectomy, jejunostomy*.

jejunum (je-ju´num). Middle division of small intestine, extending from duodenum to ileum.

joint mouse (joint mous). Small, movable calcific body in or near a joint, most commonly knee joint.

jugular (jug´u-lar). Of or pertaining to region of throat or neck, specifically to jugular vein.

juxta- (juks´tah-). Prefix meaning by side of, near; as *juxtaspinal, juxtapyloric, justa-articular*, situated or occurring near part specified.

juxtaposition (juks″tah-po-zish´un). A placing or being placed end to end or side by side; apposition.

K

keloid (ke´loid). New growth or tumor of skin consisting of dense, fibrous tissue, usually resulting from hypertrophy of cicatrix, or scar.

KUB Abbreviation for kidney, ureter, and bladder.

kymography (ki-mo´-gra-fe). Radiographic recording of involuntary movements of such viscera as heart, stomach, and diaphragm.

kyphoscoliosis (ki″fo-sko″li-o´sis). Backward and lateral curvature of spine.

kyphosis (ki-fo´sis). Acute curvature of spine, usually of thoracic region, with convexity backward; humpback.

kyphotic (ki-fot´ik). Relating to or affected with kyphosis.

L

labial (la´be-al). Of or pertaining to lips, or labia.

labium (la´bi-um). A lip; any lip-shaped part.

lacerated (las´er-āt″ed). Torn or mangled; not clean-cut; a wound inflicted by tearing.

lacrimal (lak´ri-mal). Pertaining to or situated near lacrimal, or tear, gland; as *lacrimal* duct, *lacrimal* bone.

lacuna (la-ku´nah). A small pit or depression; a minute cavity.

lambda (lam´dah). Eleventh Greek letter (Λ, λ); point of junction of lambdoidal and sagittal sutures of cranium, site of posterior fontanel.

lamina (lam´i-nah). Thin, flat plate or layer; flattened posterior portion of neural arch, which extends from pedicle to midsagittal plane, where it unites with contralateral lamina or neurapophysis.

laminagraphy (lam″i-nag´ra-fe). See tomography.

laminated (lam´i-nāt″ed). Separated into or made up of thin, flat plates or layers; arranged in layers.

laminectomy (lam″i-nek´to-me). Excision of posterior part of neural arch.

laminography See tomography.

laparo- (lap´a-ro-), **lapar-** Prefix signifying relation to flank, side of body extending between ribs and ilium or, more loosely, to abdominal wall; as *laparotomy*, surgical incision into abdominal wall.

laryngo- (lăr-in´go-), **laryng-** Prefix denoting relation to larynx; as *laryngotracheal, laryngitis*.

laryngogram (la-rin´go-gram). Radiograph of larynx.

larynogography (lăr″in-gog´ra-fe). Radiographic examination of larynx with aid of contrast medium.

larynx (lăr´ingks). Modified upper extremity of trachea; organ of voice.

latent (la´tent). Not apparent or manifest; dormant.

laterad (lat´er-ad). Directed toward side.

lateral (lat´er-al). Pertaining to side.

lavage (lah″vahzh´). Washing out of an organ, especially irrigation of stomach.

laxative (laks´a-tiv). Mild cathartic.

lesion (le´zhun). Injury or local pathologic change in structure of an organ or part.

lien (li´en). Latin for spleen.

lienal (li-e´nal). Of or pertaining to spleen.

lienitis (li″e-ni´tis). Inflammation of spleen.

lieno- (li-e´no-), **lien-** Prefix signifying relation to spleen; as *lienorenal*, pertaining to spleen and kidney.

lienography (li″en-og´ra-fe). Radiographic examination of spleen after injection of contrast medium.

linea (lin´e-ah). Latin for line; any normal strip, mark, or narrow ridge.

lingua (ling´gwah). Latin for tongue.

lingual (ling´gwal). Of or pertaining to tongue; glossal.

lipo- (lip´o-), **lip-** Prefix meaning fat, fatty; as *lipomyoma*, a tumor composed of muscular and fatty elements.

lipoma (li-po´mah). Tumor composed of fatty tissue.

-lith (-lith). Suffix meaning a concretion or calculus; as *phlebolith*, a concretion or calculus in a vein.

lithiasis (li-thi´a-sis). Formation of concretions or calculi in body, especially in urinary passages and gallbladder.

litho- (lith´o-), **lith-** Prefix meaning calculus or concretion; as *lithonephritis*, inflammation of kidney caused by presence of calculi.

lithotomy position (lith-ot´o-me). Position in which body is supine, legs flexed on thighs, and thighs flexed on abdomen and abducted; also called dorsosacral position.

323

localize (lō′kal-īz). To restrict or limit to one area or part.

localized (lō′kal-īzd). Restricted to a limited area; not general.

locular (lok′u-lar). Divided into small compartments or loculi; pertaining to a loculus or loculi.

loculus (lok′u-lus). Small cavity, compartment, or chamber; a recess or cell, as cells of ethmoidal sinuses.

longitudinal (lon″ji-tū′di-nal). Extending lengthwise, as distinguished from transverse; axial, as *longitudinal* plane of posterior teeth extends anteroposteriorly with long axis of mandible.

lordosis (lor-dō′sis). Curvature of spine with forward convexity.

lumbar (lum′ber). Of or pertaining to loin; vertebrae situated in region of loin.

lumen (lū′men). Cavity or clear space of a tubular passage such as an artery, a bronchus, or intestine.

luxation (luks-ā′shun). Act or condition of being dislocated or luxated; dislocation.

lymph (limf). Transparent, nearly colorless fluid contained in lymphatics.

lymphatics (lim-fat′iks). Lymphatic system; lymphatic glands and lymphatic vessels, which pervade body and which collect and convey lymph.

M

macerate (mas′er-āt). To soften and separate parts of by soaking or steeping, with or without heat.

maceration (mas″er-ā′shun). Process of becoming macerated.

macro- (mak′ro-), **macr-** Prefix signifying excessive development, especially elongation; as *macrocephalic*, an unusually large head; also, morbid enlargement; as *macrencephaly*, hypertrophy or enlargement of the brain; opposed to micro-.

magenblase (mah″gen-blah′zä). German term applied to radiographic shadow of gas-filled fundic portion of stomach.

mal- (mahl-). Prefix meaning ill, bad, badly; as *malalignment, malfunction, maldevelopment*.

mal (mahl). Disease; usually qualified, as *mal de mer, petit mal*.

malacia (mă-lā′shi-ah). Morbid softening of any tissue; as *osteomalacia*, softening of bone.

malignant (ma-lig′nant). Virulent; having a tendency to cause death; as a *malignant* tumor.

mammary (măm′ah-re) [L. *mamma*, breast]. Of or pertaining to breast, or mamma (măm′ah).

mammilla (mă-mil′ah). Mammary nipple; any nipple-shaped part.

mammillary line (măm′i-ler″e). Imaginary line passing vertically through mammilla or one passing transversely through mammillae.

mammography (măm-og′ra-fe). Radiologic examination of breasts; also called mastography.

masto- (mas′to-), **mast-** [Gr. *mastos*, breast]. Prefix denoting relation to breast, as in *mastocarcinoma, mastitis*.

mastography (mas-tog′ra-fe). Same as mammography.

maximum (mak′si-mal). Greatest appreciable or allowable; opposite of minimum.

meatus (me-ā′tus); pl. **meatuses** (-iz). Natural passage or canal, especially external orifice of such a passage.

mediad (mē′di-ad). Directed toward midsagittal plane.

medial (mē′di-al). Situated in or occurring near middle in relation to another part; nearer center, or midsagittal plane.

median (mē′di-an). Having a central position; in middle; mesial.

mediastinum (mē″di-as-tē′num). Space between pleural sacs of lungs, sternum, and thoracic spine; it contains heart and all thoracic viscera except lungs.

mediate (mē′di-it). Indirect; effected by a secondary or intervening cause or medium; not immediate.

mediate (mē′di-āt). To effect by mediation; to intervene.

medulla (me-dul′ah). Marrow of bones; inner substance of an organ, such as that of kidney; tapering terminal portion of brain, medulla oblongata.

medullary (med′ŭ-ler″e). Pertaining to any medulla; consisting of or resembling marrow.

mega- (meg′ah-), **meg-** Prefix meaning large, as in *megacephalic;* also, a million times, as in *megohm*.

megacolon (meg″ah-kō′lon). Abnormally large colon.

megalo- (meg′a-lo-), **megal-** Prefix meaning large, great, abnormal enlargement; as *megalo-esophagus, megalakria, acromegaly*.

meninges (me-nin′jēz). Three membranes (dura mater, arachnoid, and pia mater) that form protective covering of brain and spinal cord.

meniscus (me-nis′kus). Interarticular, crescent-shaped fibrocartilage, especially of knee.

mental (men′tal) [L. *mentum*, chin; *mens*, mind]. Of or pertaining to chin or mind.

mesati- (mes′ah-ti-). Prefix meaning medium, or mid-most; as *mesatipelvic*, having a medium-sized pelvis.

mesaticephalic (mes″ah-ti-se-fal′ik). Having a head of medium or average proportions; midway between brachycephalic and dolichocephalic; same as mesocephalic.

mesentery (mes′en-ter″e). Fold of peritoneum that invests intestines and attaches them to posterior wall of abdominal cavity.

mesial (mē′zi-al). Situated near or toward midsagittal plane; medial.

mesiodistal (mē″zi-o-dis′tal). Directed laterally or posteriorly from center or median line of dental arch.

mesion (mē′zi-on). Plane that divides body into right and left halves; midsagittal plane.

meso- (mes′o-). Prefix meaning medium, moderate, or middle; as *mesosoma*, having medium stature, *mesosyphilis*, secondary stage of syphilis, and *mesotropic*, located in center of a cavity.

mesocephalic (mes″o-se-fal′ik). Head of medium or average size; same as mesaticephalic.

meta- (met′ah), **met-** Prefix signifying change or transfer, as in *metabolism, metabasis;* along with, after, or next, as in metatarsus.

metaphysis (me-taf′ĭ-sis). Zone of spongy bone between cartilaginous epiphyseal plate and diaphysis of a long bone.

metastasis (me-tas′tah-sis). Transfer of a disease from one organ or region to another, as a malignant tumor spreading from initial location to secondary locations in body; secondary growth so produced.

metastasize (me-tas′tah-sīz). To form new or secondary sites of infection in other parts of body by metastasis, as a tumor.

metra (mē′trah). Uterus.

metro- (mē′tro-), **metr-** Prefix denoting relation to uterus, as in *metrocarcinoma, metritis*.

micro- (mī′kro-), **micr-** Prefix meaning small, minute, as in *microbe, microcephaly;* one millionth part of, as in *microfarad*.

microcephalic (mī″kro-se-fal′ik). Having an unusually small head.

micturition (mik″tū-rish′un). Act of urinating.

miscible (mis′i-b′l). Susceptible to being readily mixed; mixable.

mixture (miks′chur). Heterogeneous substance made up of two or more ingredients that retain their own properties and can be separated by mechanical means; cf. compound, solution.

mobility (mo-bil′i-te). Capacity or facility of movement of an organ, such as stomach, gallbladder, or kidney; cf. motility.

mono- (mon′o), **mon-** Prefix meaning one, single, alone; as *monoplegia*, paralysis affecting but one part of body.

morbid (mor′bid). Disease; of or pertaining to an abnormal or diseased condition.

moribund (mor′i-bund). Near death; a dying state.

mortification (mor″ti-fi-kā′shun). Death of a part or localized area of tissue; gangrene.

motility (mo-til′i-te). Capacity to move or contract spontaneously; contractility; cf. mobility.

mucoid (mū′koid). Resembling mucus.

mucosa (mū-kō′sah). Mucous membrane.

mucosal (mū-kō′sal). Of or pertaining to mucous membrane.

mucous (mū′kus). Of or pertaining to mucus.

mucus (mū′kus). Viscid, watery fluid secreted by mucous glands.

Müller maneuver (Johannes Peter Müller, German physiologist, 1801-1858). Forced inspiration against a closed glottis; maneuver is performed by closing mouth, holding nose, and attempting to breathe in.

multi- (mul′ti-). Prefix meaning many, much; as *multilobular*, composed of many lobes.

multipara (mul-tip′a-rah). Woman who has borne two or more children.

mummify (mum′mi-f ī). Term that, as used in nursing and radiographic procedures, means to wrap body in a mummy fashion with a sheet, binding arms to sides, to restrain movement during examination or treatment.

myel (mī′el). Spinal cord; myelon.

myelitis (mī″e-lī′tis). Inflammation of spinal cord or of bone marrow.

myelo- (mī′e-lo-), **myel-** Prefix denoting relation to bone marrow or to spinal cord; as *myeloma, myelomeningitis*.

myelography (mī″e-log′ra-fe). Radiographic examination of spinal cord following injection of contrast medium into spinal canal.

myo- (mī′o-), **my-** Prefix signifying relation to a muscle or muscles; as *myocarditis, myositis*.

myoma (mī-ō′mah). Tumor consisting of muscular elements.

N

nares (na′rēz); sing. **naris** (na′ris). Openings of nasal passages; anterior nares are commonly called nostrils.

nasion (na′zi-on). Midpoint of frontonasal suture.

naso- (na′zo-). Prefix denoting relation to nose; as *nasofrontal, nasopharyngeal.*

nates (na′tēz). Buttocks.

nausea (naw′she-ah). Feeling of sickness at stomach, associated with desire to vomit.

navel (na′vel). Cicatrix, or scar, in center of abdomen, marking point of attachment of umbilical cord; umbilicus.

necrosis (ne-kro′sis). Death or mortification of a part or of a circumscribed area of tissue.

necrotic (ne-krot′ik). Affected with or pertaining to necrosis, or death of tissue.

neo- (ne′o-). Prefix meaning new or recent; as *neonatus,* a newborn infant.

neoplasm (ne′o-plasm). Any new or morbid growth, such as a tumor.

nephro- (nef′ro-), **nephr-** Prefix denoting relation to kidney; as *nephrolith, nephritis, nephrectomy.*

nephrolithiasis (nef″ro-li-thi′a-sis). Condition caused by accumulation of calculi in kidney.

nephroptosis (nef″rop-to′sis). Abnormal dropping or downward movement of kidney.

neural (nū′ral). Pertaining to a nerve or nervous system.

neuro- (nū′ro-), **neur-** Prefix denoting relation to nerves, as in *neurofibroma, neuralgia, neuritis.*

niche (nich). Small recess or hollow space in a wall; abnormal saccular prominence on wall of stomach resulting from an ulcer crater.

nodular (nod′u-lar). Pertaining to or having form of a node or nodule.

nodule (nod′ūl). Small, rounded prominence; a little bump.

norm (norm). Fixed or authoritative standard; a rule; a pattern or model; a type.

normal (nor′mal). Conforming to an established norm or principle; regular; natural; functioning properly.

normal salt solution A normal or, more correctly, a physiologic salt solution is approximately isotonic with body fluids. It is a 0.9% solution of sodium chloride.

nullipara (nu-lip′ar-ah). Woman who has never borne a child.

O

obstetrics (ob-stet′riks). Science dealing with pregnancy and parturition; manangement of childbirth.

occiput (ok′si-put). Back part of cranium.

occlusal (o-klu′sal). Of or pertaining to biting surface of a tooth or teeth.

occlusal line Imaginary line passing through head at and parallel with biting surface of teeth.

occlusion (o-klu′zhun). Act of closing or occluding, or state of being closed or occluded, as in a stricture of a normal passage; bringing into contact of opposing surfaces of upper and lower teeth.

oedema (e-dē′mah). *See* edema.

-ology (-ol′o-je). Suffix meaning a science or branch of knowledge; as *radiology,* science dealing with diagnostic and therapeutic application of x-radiation.

-oma (-o′mah); pl. **-omata** (o′mah-tah) or **-omas** (-o′maz). Suffix denoting morbid condition of some type, usually a tumor, such as *carcinoma, fibroma, myoma, sarcoma.*

omentum (o-men′tum). Free folds of peritoneum that connect stomach with adjacent organs; apronlike great omentum hanging downward in front of small intestines.

optimum (op′ti-mum). Best; most conducive to success; condition that is best or most favorable; most suitable degree, quantity, or factor for attainment of a given end.

oral (o′ral). Of or pertaining to mouth or to speech sound.

orbitomeatal line (or″bi-to-me-ā′tal). Imaginary line extending from outer canthus to center of tragus; it is used in radiography for localization purposes.

organic (or-gan′ik). Of or pertaining to an organ or organs; consisting of or affecting organic structure; also (in chemistry) pertaining to carbon compounds, those of artificial origin as well as those derived from living organisms.

orifice (or′i-fis). Opening, or aperture, of any body cavity.

ortho- (or′tho-), **orth-** Prefix meaning straight or normal; correct or true; as *orthodontic, orthographic, orthuria,* and *orthostatic,* standing upright, caused by or pertaining to standing erect.

orthopedics (or″tho-pe′diks). Branch of surgery dealing with correction or prevention of deformities and with treatment of diseases of bones.

os (os); pl. **ora** (o′rah) [L. *oris,* mouth]. A mouth; any mouthlike orifice; as *os uteri.*

os (os); pl. **ossa** (os′ah) [L. *ossis,* bone]. A bone; as *os calcis, os coxae, os magnum.*

os innominatum (os in-nom″i-nā′tum). Innominate bone; os coxa.

-osis (-o′sis); pl. **-oses** (-o′sēz). Suffix denoting state or condition; as *psychosis, stenosis, sclerosis.*

ossification (os″i-fi-kā′shun). Formation of bone; process of changing into bone.

osteo- (os′te-o-), **oste-** Prefix denoting relation to bone; as *osteoma,* a benign bony tumor.

osteomalacia (os″te-o-mal-a′shi-ah). Chronic disease characterized by gradual softening of bones, with resultant deformities.

osteomyelitis (os″te-o-mi-el-i′tis). Inflammation of marrow and medullary portion of a bone.

oteoporosis (os″te-o-po-ro′sis). Condition characterized by absorption or rarefaction of bone so that tissue becomes thin and porous.

ostium (os′ti-um). Small mouthlike orifice, especially opening into a tubular passage such as an oviduct.

(o)-stomy [Gr. *stomos,* mouth]. Suffix signifying surgical formation of an artificial mouth or opening into some part or between two parts; as *enterostomy,* formation of an opening into intestines through abdominal wall, and *gastroenterostomy,* formation of an artificial opening between stomach and small intestine.

otic (o′tik). Of or pertaining to ear; auditory.

otitis (o-ti′tis). Inflammation of ear; as *otitis media,* inflammation of middle ear.

(o)-tomy [Gr. *-tomia,* cutting]. Suffix signifying surgical incision of, usually for the purpose of draining; as *cholecystotomy, nephrotomy, osteotomy.*

oviduct (o′vi-dukt). Duct, or passage, extending, one on each side, from uterus to ovary; fallopian tubes.

oxycephalic (ok″si-se-fal′ik). Having an unusually high vertex; a steeple-shaped head.

P

pachy- (pak′e-). Prefix meaning thick, dense; as *pachypleuritis,* inflammation of pleura attended with thickening of membranes.

pachycephalic (pak″e-se-fal′ik). Having unusually thick, dense cranial walls.

Paget's disease (paj′ets). Osteitis deformans; chronic disease of bones, characterized by irregular rarefaction and thickening, enlargement, and deformity.

palsy (pawl′ze). Loss of power of voluntary movement or sensation, partial or complete, of any part of body; paralysis.

para- (par′ah), **par-** Prefix denoting the following irregular or abnormal, as in *paranoia, parachroia, parachroma;* resembling in form (said of diseases), as in *paraparesis, parapneumonia, paratyphoid;* near, beside, alongside of, as in *paracystic, parathyroid;* accessory to, as in *paranasal sinuses.* Cf. peri-.

paracentesis (par″ah-sen-te′sis). Surgical puncture of a cavity of body for withdrawal of fluid; tapping.

paralysis (pah-ral′i-sis). Loss of function or sensation, partial or complete, in any part of body through injury or disease of nerve supply; palsy.

paralysis agitans (aj′i-tanz). Chronic, progressive disease of old age, characterized by muscular tremor, weakness, and peculiar gait; shaking palsy or Parkinson's disease.

parenchyma (pah-reng′ki-mah). Essential, functional tissue of an organ as distinguished from its stoma or framework.

paries (pā′ri-ēz); pl. **parietes** (pah-rī′e-tēz). A wall, especially wall of a hollow organ or cavity.

parietal (pah-rī′e-tal). Of or pertaining to parietes, or walls of a cavity.

parotid (pah-rot′id). Situated near ear; specifically, parotid gland, largest of salivary group, which is located on side of face in front of and below ear.

parotitis (par″ot-i′tis). Inflammation of parotid glands; mumps.

parturition (par″tū-rish′un). Process of bringing forth young; labor; childbirth.

patent (pā′tent). Open, patulous, unoccluded, as lumen of a vessel.

patho- (path′o-), **path-** Prefix denoting disease; as *pathogenic,* causing or giving origin to disease.

pathology (pah-thol′o-je). Science treating of essential nature of diseases, structural and functional alterations caused by them; condition or changes produced by disease.

p.c. Abbreviation for Latin *post cibum,* after food.

pediatrics (pe′de-at′riks). Science that treats diseases of children.

pedicle (ped′i-k'l) [L. *pediculus,* little foot]. Short stem or stalklike part; a pedicle or peduncle; specifically, anterolateral part of each side of neural arch, connecting laminae with body of vertebra.

pedicular (pe-dik′u-lar) [L. *pedicularis,* louse]. Pertaining to lice; lousy.

pediculate (pe-dik′u-lāt) [L. *pediculatus*]. Of or pertaining to a pedicle or pedicles.

325

peduncular (pe-dung'ku-lar). Of or pertaining to a peduncle or pedicle.

pelvimetry (pel-vim'e-tre). Measurement of size and capacity of pelvis.

peri- (per'i-). Prefix meaning around, about, all around, near; as *periapical*, around the apex of a tooth.

periosteum (per"i-os'te-um). Fibrous membrane that closely invests all parts of surface of a bone, except articular surfaces.

periphery (pe-rif'er-e). External part of an organ; circumference.

peristalsis (per"i-stal'sis). Rhythmic contractions by which tubular passages such as alimentary canal force their contents onward.

petrous (pet'rus; pē'trus). Resembling a stone or rock; specifically, pertaining to petrosa or petrous portion of temporal bone.

pH Symbol used to denote negative logarithm of hydrogen ion concentration in gram atoms per liter.

phleb- (fleb-), **phlebo-** Suffix denoting relation to a vein; as *phlebitis, phlebolith*.

phlebogram (fleb'o-gram). Radiograph of veins following injection of radiopaque substance; also called a venogram.

phonate (fō'nāt). To utter throaty or laryngeal, usually prolonged, vowel sounds with minimum aid from lips.

phrenic (fren'ik) [Gr. *phren, phrenos,* diaphragm, mind]. Of or pertaining to diaphragm or to mind; phrenic nerve.

phrenico- (fren'i-ko). Prefix signifying some relation to phrenic nerve; as *phrenicotomy.*

phreno- (fren'o-), **phren-** Prefix denoting relation to diaphragm, as in *phrenogastric, phrenohepatic,* or to mind, as in *phrenopathy, phrenoplegia.*

physiology (fiz"i-ol'o-je). Science that treats functions of tissues and organs, as distinguished from anatomy, which deals with their structure.

placenta (plah-sen'tah). Flat, cakelike mass; specifically, vascular organ through which fetus communicates with mother by means of umbilical cord.

placentography (plas"en-tog'ra-fe). Radiographic examination of gravid uterus for localization of placenta.

plane (plān). Any flat surface, real or imaginary.

planigraphic principle Tomographic principle in which fulcrum or axis of rotation is raised or lowered to alter level of focal plane; the tabletop height remains constant.

planigraphy (plah-nig'ra-fe). See tomography.

platy- (plat'i-), **plat-** Prefix meaning broad, flat; as *platycephalic,* having a broad, flat head.

pleural (ploor'al). Of or pertaining to pleura or pleurae.

pleurisy (ploor'i-se). Inflammation of pleura, usually attended with exudation into pleural cavity.

plica (pli'kah). A fold; as *plica sublingualis,* fold of mucous membrane on each side of floor of mouth overlying sublingual gland.

-pnea (-p'ne'ah). Suffix meaning breath; as in eupnea, dyspnea.

pneumo- (nū'mo-) [Gr. *pneumon,* lung; *pneuma,* air]. Prefix denoting relation to lungs or to air or other gas; as *pneumonia, pneumonic, pneumothorax, pneumocystography, pneumoperitoneum.*

pneumothorax (nū"mo-tho'raks). Accumulation of air or other gas in pleural cavity, usually induced for therapeutic purposes but, occasionally spontaneously as a result of injury or disease.

poly- (pŏl'e-). Prefix meaning many, much, often; as *polycystic, polygraph, polymorphous.*

polyp (pol'ip). Projection of hypertrophied mucous membrane in a body cavity such as nose, paranasal sinuses, and urinary bladder; a polypus.

popliteal (pop-lit'e-al). Of or pertaining to part of knee behind joint.

porus (pō'rus). Latin for pore or opening; meatus; as *porus acusticus internus,* internal auditory meatus.

post- Prefix meaning behind, after, later; as *postnasal, postpartum, postdiastolic.*

post cibum (post sī'bum). Latin for after food; abbreviation, p.c.

posterior (pos-ter'i-er). Pertaining to, designating, or situated in back part of body or of an organ.

posteroanterior (pos"ter-o-an-ter'i-er). Directed or extending from back to front.

pre- (prē-). Prefix signifying before in time or place; as *prenatal, prevertebral.*

primigravida (pri"mi-grav'i-dah). Woman pregnant for first time.

primipara (pri-mip'ah-rah). Woman who is bearing or has borne her first child.

pro- (prō-). Prefix signifying forward, to front, according to; as *project, progress, prolapse, proportion.*

procto- (prok'to-), **proct-** Prefix denoting relation to anus and rectum; as *proctopolypus, proctoscope, proctitis.*

prognosis (prog-no'sis). Forecast of course and probable outcome of a disease.

pronation (pro-nā'shun). Medial rotation of hand so that it faces downward or backward; act of lying face down; opposite of supination.

prone (prōn). Lying face down; having palm of hand facing downward or backward.

prophylaxis (pro"fi-lak'sis). Protection from or prevention of disease; protective or preventive treatment.

prostato- (pros'tah-to-) **prostat-** Prefix denoting relation to prostate gland; as *prostatocystitis, prostatitis.*

prostatography (pros"tah-tog'ra-fe). Radiographic examination of prostate gland.

protuberance (pro-tū'ber-ans). Any projecting part; a swelling; general term for a process or projection.

proximal (prok'si-mal). Toward beginning or source of a part; toward head end of body; opposed to distal.

pseudo- (sū'do-), **pseud-** Prefix meaning false; illusory; having a deceptive resemblance to; as *pseudoankylosis, pseudoparalysis, pseudoarthrosis.*

P.S.P. Abbreviation commonly used for a kidney function test with use of either phenolsulfonphthalein or indigo carmine.

psychiatry (sī'kī'ah-tre). Science that treats mental disorders, psychoses, and neuroses.

psycho- (sī'ko-), **psych-** Prefix denoting relation to mind or mental processes, as in *psychogenic, psychoneurosis, psychosis.*

psychology (sī-kol'o-je). Science that deals with mind in all its aspects; study of mental activity and behavior.

ptosis (tō'sis). Prolapse, or dropping, of an organ from its normal position; usually used as a suffix, as in *enteroptosis, gastroptosis, viseroptosis.*

puerile (pū'er-il). Of or pertaining to a child or children or to childhood; immature; juvenile.

puerperal (pū-er'per-al). Of or pertaining to childbirth; as *puerperal* sepsis, *puerperal* fever.

pulmonary, pulmonic (pul'mo-ner-e; pul-mon'ik) [L. *pulmo,* lung]. Of or pertaining to lungs.

purgative (pur'gah-tiv). Purging or cathartic medicine, causing extensive evacuations. These agents are more drastic in action than laxative or cathartic groups, which stimulate peristaltic activity and increase tendency to evacuate bowels with a minimum of irritation.

purulent (pū'rōō-lent). Consisting of or of nature of pus or matter; associated with suppuration; as a *purulent* lesion or wound.

pus (pŭs). Yellowish, greenish, or brownish matter generated by suppuration as a result of bacterial infection.

putrefaction (pū"tre-fak'shun). Decomposition of organic (animal or vegetable) matter, with formation of various foul-smelling products; decay.

putrescent (pū-tres'ent). Undergoing decomposition or decay; pertaining to putrefaction; as an offensive or *putrescent* odor.

pyelo- (pī'e-lo), **pyel-** Prefix denoting relation to pelvis of kidney, as in *pyelogram, pyelitis.*

pyo- (pī'o), **py-** Prefix signifying presence of pus; as *pyogenesis, pyonephrosis, pyuria.*

Q

quadrant (qwod'rant). A fourth; a quarter; any one of four equal parts or divisions, as of orbit or of abdomen.

quadrate (kwod'rāt). Square or almost square in form; cubical; quadrate lobe of liver.

quickening (kwik'en-ing). First movement of fetus in utero felt by mother, usually occurring about midterm.

R

racemose (ras'e-mōs) [L. *racemosus,* having clusters like a bunch of grapes]. Compound saccular gland (such as pancreas) having numerous branching ducts ending in acini arranged like grapes on a stalk.

rachio- (rā'ki-o), **rachi-** [Gr. *rachis,* spine]. Prefix denoting relation to spine, as in *rachiocentesis, rachioplegia, rachitis.*

radio- (ra'di-o) [L. *radius,* ray]. Prefix denoting (1) radial or radially, as lines radiating from a center, (2) radial, as in *radiomuscular,* (3) relation to lateral and larger of bones of forearm, as in *radioulnar, radiohumeral,* and (4) relation to radiant energy, especially to roentgen and radium radiation, as in *radioactive, radiosensitive, radionecrosis.*

radiodontia (ra"di-o-don'shi-ah). Roentgenographic examination of teeth and their supporting structures.

radiolucent (ra"di-o-lū'sent). Materials offering little resistance to passage of x-radiation; those that have insufficient physical density to cast an appreciable image on film when exposed to kilovoltages used in radiography of body; cf. radioparent.

326

radiopaque (ra″di-o-pāk′). Materials that are impenetrable to x-radiation generated by kilovoltages usually employed in medical radiography.

radioparent (ra″di-o-păr′ent). Materials wholly transparent to x-radiation; cf. radiolucent.

radius (ra′di-us). Line extending from center to periphery of a circle; semidiameter; lateral and larger bone of forearm.

ramus (ra′mus). Branch or branchlike process, as one of primary divisions of a nerve or blood vessel, or a projecting part of an irregularly shaped bone.

rarefaction (rar″e-fak′shun). State of being or process of becoming thin and porous or less dense without a diminution in size or volume; loss of substance; opposed to condensation and destruction.

recumbent (re-kum′bent). Reclining; lying down.

reflux (re′fluks). A flowing back, as return or reflux of a fluid.

regurgitation (re-gur″ji-ta′-shun). To flow or be cast backward, as blood from a heart chamber in insufficiency of a valve; egestion, or casting up, of incompletely digested food.

Reid's base line (rēdz) (Robert William Reid, Scottish anatomist, 1851-1938). See anthropologic base line.

renal (re′nal) [L. ren, kidney]. Of or pertaining to kidney or kidneys.

resorption (re-sorp′shun). Process of absorbing again; removal by absorption of an exudate or of bone.

respiratory (re-spīr′ah-tō″re; res′pi-rah-to″re). Of or pertaining to respiration or respiratory organs.

retro- (rē′tro-; ret′ro-). Prefix signifying backward, as in retroflexion; behind, as in retrosternal; reversed, or against natural course, as in retrostalsis.

retrograde (rē′tro-grad). Directed against natural course; specifically, retrograde pyelography, in which contrast solution is injected in a direction contrary to natural flow of urinary secretions.

rhinal (rī′nal). Of or pertaining to nose; nasal.

ruga (rōō′gah); pl. **rugae** (rōō′jē). Wrinkle or fold of mucous membrane; specifically, rugae or folds of gastric mucosa in empty or nearly empty stomach.

S

s̄ Symbol for Latin sine, without.

sac (săk). Soft-walled bag or pouch; any bladderlike organ.

sacculated (săk′u-lāt″ed). Having form of a sac or sacs; characterized by a series of pouched expansions or saccules.

sacralization (sa″kral-i-za′shun). Overdevelopment of one or both of transverse processes of last lumbar segment, with encroachment on or fusion with first sacral segment.

sagittal (saj′i-tal). Of or pertaining to sagittal suture of cranium, which lies in midsagittal plane of body; pertaining to any plane parallel with midsagittal plane.

sal (sal). Latin for salt.

saline (sā′līn). Consisting of or containing a salt or salts; salty; saline solution, especially a physiologic, or so-called normal, salt solution.

salpingo- (sal-ping′go-), **salping-** Prefix denoting some relation to an oviduct or, less commonly, to a eustachian tube.

salpinx (sal′pingks); pl **salpinges** (sal-pin′jēz) [Gr. salpinx, tube]. Oviduct; less commonly, a eustachian tube.

sarcoma (sar-ko′mah). Malignant tumor derived from tissue developed from mesoderm (connective and lymphoid tissue, bone, cartilage, muscle, and part of urogenital organs) and characterized by a fleshy consistency.

sclero- (skler′o-), **scler-** Prefix meaning hard, indurated, fibrous; also denotes relation to sclera.

sclerosis (skle-ro′sis). Hardening, or induration, of tissue, especially of interstitial connective tissue.

scoliosis (sko″li-o′sis) [Gr. skolios, crooked]. Abnormal lateral curvature of spinal column.

secreta (se-krē′tah). Any product of secretion; the secretions.

secrete (se-krēt′). To separate substances from blood and emit as a secretion.

secretion (se-krē′shun). Process of secreting; also, material secreted.

section thickness Width of plane of tissue that is maximumly in focus on a tomogram. The section thickness decreases as tomographic angle increases.

sedative (sed′ah-tiv). Soothing medicine.

semi- (sem′i-). Prefix meaning partly; half or approximately half; as semiflexion, semiprone, semicoma.

sepsis (sep′sis). Poisoning caused by absorption of pathogenic bacteria and their products from a putrefactive process.

septic (sep′tik). Putrefactive; produced by or caused by pathogenic bacteria.

septum (sep′tum). Any dividing wall or partition.

sequestrum (se-kwes′trum); pl. **sequestra** (se-kwes′trah). Piece of bone that has become detached as a result of trauma or necrosis.

shadowgram, shadowgraph (shad′o-gram, shad′o-graf). Radiograph; a roentgenogram.

sialaden (sī-al′ad-en) [Gr. sialon, saliva + aden, gland]. Salivary gland.

sialography (sī″al-og′ra-fe). Radiographic examination of a salivary gland or duct after injection of radiopaque contrast medium.

silicosis (sil″i-ko′sis). Condition of lungs caused by prolonged inhalation of dust particles of stone or silica; pneumonoconiosis.

Sim's position (simz). Position in which body is semiprone, lying on left side, with right knee drawn up.

sinciput (sin′si-put). Forehead; anterior part of cranium.

sine (sī′ne). Latin for without; symbol s̄.

sinistrad (sin′is-trad). Directed toward left; opposite of dextrad.

sinistro- (sin′is-tro-), **sinistr-** Prefix meaning left, as in sinistrocardia, sinistrocerebral.

sinus (sī′nus). Cavity or hollow space in bone or other tissue; a dilated channel for passage of venous blood; a suppurating tract.

skiagraph, skiagram (ski′ah-graf, ski′ah-gram). Old term for radiograph or roentgenogram.

solution (so-lū′shun). Homogeneous body (typically liquid but may be gaseous or solid) consisting of two parts: (1) solvent, or dissolving substance, and (2) solute, or dissolved substance. The molecules of the solute, or dissolved substance, are dispersed among those of the solvent and cannot be filtered out; nor will they settle out on standing.

The composition or concentration of a solution can be varied within certain limits. A solution is similar to a compound in that it is homogeneous and similar to a mixture in that its composition is variable.

spasm (spaz′m). Involuntary, convulsive contraction of a muscle or muscles.

specific gravity (spe-sif′ik grav′i-te). Abbreviation, sp. gr.; relative density or weight of any volume of a substance compared with that of an equal volume of water at same temperature and pressure.

sphincter (sfingk′ter). Circular muscle structure that serves to close one of orifices of body; as sphincter ani, sphincter of Oddi, pyloric sphincter.

spicule (spik′ūl). Minute, needlelike fragment, especially of bone.

spina bifida (spi′nah bif′i-dah). Congenital malformation of vertebral arch in which there is a cleft in a lamina, with hernial protrusion of spinal cord and meninges.

spina bifida occulta (o-kul′tah). Cleft in vertebral arch without herniation of spinal cord and meninges.

spondylitis (spon″di-li′tis). Inflammation of a vertebra or vertebrae.

spondylolisthesis (spon″di-lo-lis-thē′sis). Forward displacement of a lumbar vertebra, most frequently of last lumbar segment on sacrum.

stasis (sta′sis). Defective circulation of blood; a slackening or stoppage of normal flow of contents of vessels or of any organ of body.

stellate (stel′āt). Shaped or radiated like a star; as a stellate fracture of cranium.

stenosis (ste-no′sis). Stricture, or narrowing, of lumen or orifice of a passage.

sternal angle (ster′nal ang′l). Angle formed by junction of manubrium and gladiolus, or body, of sternum.

sthenic (sthen′ik). Strength; vigor; opposed to asthenia.

sthenic habitus Bodily type characterized by strong build; a modification of more massive hypersthenic type.

stoma (sto′mah). Minute, mouthlike aperture; surgically established opening into intestine through abdominal wall; opening established between two anastomosed portions of intestine.

strangulated (strang′gu-lat″ed). Compressed or constricted to arrest or congest circulation in a part; as a strangulated hernia, one in which protruding viscus is so constricted as to stop circulation.

stria (stri′ah); pl. **striae** (stri′ē). A strip or line; a streak, distinguished by color, elevation, or texture.

stricture (strik′tur). Circumscribed narrowing of a canal; a constriction.

stroma (stro′mah). Tissue that forms supporting framework of an organ, as distinguished from its parenchyma, or essential functional elements.

sub- (sub-). Prefix meaning below, under, beneath; as subnormal, sublingual, subdiaphragmatic.

subacute (sub′ah-kūt). Between acute and chronic; having some acute symptoms.

subcutaneous (sub″ku-ta′ne-us). Situated beneath skin.

submentovertex (sub″men-to-ver′teks). Directed from below chin to vertex; pertaining to region beneath chin and vertex; submentovertical.

subphrenic (sub-fren′ik). Situated or occurring below diaphragm.

sulcus (sul′kus). A furrow; a groove; a fissure; especially one of sulci on surface of brain.

super- (su′per-). Prefix meaning over, above, in excess; as *superimpose, supernumerary, supersaturate.*

supero- (su′per-o). Prefix meaning above; situated or directed from above.

superoinferior (su″per-o-in-fēr′i-er). Directed from above downward; craniocaudal.

supination (su″pi-na′shun). Rotation of hand and arm so that palm faces forward; act or state of lying face upward; opposed to pronation.

supine (su-pin′). Lying on back; opposite of prone.

suppuration (sup″u-ra′shun). Process of generating and discharging pus.

supra- (su′prah-). Prefix meaning above, higher in position; as *supraclavicular, suprarenal, supraorbital.*

symphysis (sim′fi-sis). Joint, or line of fusion, between paired bones; as *symphysis pubis, symphysis menti.*

synarthrosis (sin″ar-thro′sis). Immovable joint (such as a cranial suture) in which only fibrous connective tissue intervenes between bones.

syncope (sing′ko-pe). Temporary suspension of respiration and circulation with loss of consciousness; fainting.

systole (sis′to-le). Contraction phase of heartbeat; also contraction itself, by which blood is kept in circulation; correlative to diastole.

T

tachy- (tak′e-). Prefix meaning fast, swift; as *tachycardia,* rapidity of heart action.

tangent (tan′jent). Touching at a point; meeting a curve or surface at a point and then extending beyond without intersection; as a line or plane *tangent* to a curve, or a curve *tangent* to a line or a surface.

tangential (tan-jen′shal). Directed along or arranged in a tangent, as in adjustment of a structure or a mass so that one or more points of its surface will be tangent to central ray.

tele- (tel′e-; te′le-), **teleo-** Prefix meaning far, at a distance; as *telecardiography.*

teleoroentgenogram (tel″e-o-rent′gen-o-gram″). Radiograph made at a distance of 6 feet.

theca (thē′kah). Protective case or sheath; as *theca vertebralis,* dura mater of spinal cord.

thoracentesis (thō″rah-sen-tē′sis). Surgical puncturing of chest wall for removal of fluid in pleural effusion; tapping; also called pleuracentesis.

thoracic (tho-ras′ik). Pertaining to, or situated in region of chest.

thoracoplasty (tho′rah-ko-plas″te). Plastic surgery of thorax; especially, resection of a part of several ribs to collapse lung in advance unilateral tuberculosis.

thrombus (throm′bus). Plug or clot formed in heart or in a blood or lymphatic vessel and remaining at site of formation; cf. embolus.

tomographic angle/arc Angle described by tube and film during a tomographic motion.

tomography (to-mog′ra-fe). Special radiographic technique in which all planes of tissue above and

below a predetermined plane of tissue are blurred from view by means of synchronously moving the x-ray source and film in opposite directions during exposure.

tone (tōn). Healthy function; resiliency; normal vigor and elasticity; especially, tension of involuntary muscles; tonus.

tonic (ton′ik). Pertaining to or characterized by normal tone or tension, particularly muscular tension; an agent that tends to produce or restore a healthy condition.

topical (top′i-kal). Of or pertaining to a specific spot; local, or for local application; as a *topical* anesthetic.

torsion (tor′shun). Act of turning or twisting or state of being full of turns and twists.

torticollis (tor″ti-kol′is). Irregular contraction of cervical muscles, with twisting of neck and an unnatural position of head; commonly called wryneck.

tortuous (tor′tu-us). Winding; circuitous; full of curves or bends; twisted.

trabecula (trah-bek′u-lah); pl. **trabeculae** (trahbek′u-lē). Little beam or crossbar; one of septal membranes in framework of various organs; one of intersecting osseous plates, or cancelli, composing spongy, or cancellous, portion of a bone.

tragus (trā′gus). Cartilaginous projection in front of external auditory meatus.

trans- (trans-; also tranz-). Prefix meaning across, through, over; to pass across or through; as *transabdominal,* passing through or across the abdomen, and *transoral,* passing through or across mouth.

transverse (trans-verse′). Crosswise, from side to side; horizontal; opposed to lengthwise and longitudinal.

transverse plane Plane that divides body or any one of its parts horizontally at any level.

trauma (traw′mah). Injury; condition resulting from injury.

traumatic (traw-mat′ik). Of, pertaining to, or caused by a trauma.

tremor (trem′er; tre′mor). Involuntary trembling or shaking as result of undue strain, weakness, injury, or disease.

Trendelenburg position (tren-del′en-berg). Position in which body is recumbent on a plane inclined 45 degrees cranially.

trephine (tre-fīn′). Circular saw or trepan for removing a disk of bone, used chiefly in brain surgery for perforating cranium; also, to operate with a trephine or trepan.

trocar (tro′kar). Sharp-pointed, rodlike instrument that is fitted into and used for insertion of a cannula or catheter.

trochanteric (tro″kan-ter′ik). Pertaining to a trochanter or trochanters.

tubercle (tu′ber-k′l). Small nodule or prominence; small rounded process on a bone, serving for attachment of muscles or ligaments.

tuberculosis (tu-ber″ku-lo′sis). Infectious disease caused by tubercle bacillus and marked by production of tubercles, fever, night sweats, and progressive emaciation. The lungs are the most common site of infection, but such organs as the intestines, lymph nodes, larynx, kidneys, and bones are frequently involved.

tuberosity (tu″ber-os′i-te). Broad, roughened process on a bone, serving for attachment of muscles or ligaments.

tumor (tu′mor). Circumscribed swelling; any morbid growth, innocent or malignant; neoplasm.

U

ulcer (ul′ser). Open, suppurating sore occurring on surface of skin or a mucous membrane, as distinguished from an abscess, which is a sore of deepseated origin.

umbilical (um-bil′i-kal). Of or pertaining to navel, or umbilicus.

umbilicus (um-bil′i-kus; um″bi-lī′kus). Scar on center of abdomen marking site of attachment of umbilical cord; navel.

uni- (ū′ni-). Prefix meaning one, single, first; as in *unilocular, unidirectional, unigravida.*

unilateral (u″ni-lat′er-al). Affecting or situated on only one side.

uresis (u-re′sis). Discharge of urine; urination.

ureteral (u-re′ter-al). Pertaining to ureter.

ureterography (u-re″ter-og′ra-fe). Radiographic examination of ureter after injection of radiopaque solution.

urethral (u-re′thral). Pertaining to urethra.

urethrogram (u-re′thro-gram). Radiograph of contrast-filled urethra.

urethrography (u-re-throg′ra-fe). Radiographic examination of urethra during injection of contrast medium or during voiding.

-uria (u′ri-ah). Suffix denoting some relation to urine; as *hematuria, dysuria, pyuria.*

uro- (u′ro-), **ur-** Prefix denoting some relation to urine or to urinary tract, as in *urinalysis, urodynia, urolithiasis.*

urography (u-rog′ra-fe). Radiographic examination of urinary tract or of any of its parts with contrast medium.

urticaria (ur″ti-kā′ri-ah). Inflammatory skin disease characterized by transient, whitish wheals on a reddish base, causing intense stinging and itching; uredo; nettle rash; hives.

uterine (u′ter-in). Of or pertaining to uterus.

utero- (u′ter-o-), **uter-** Prefix denoting some relation to uterus; as *uterocele, uteroscope, uteritis.*

uterography (u″ter-og′ra-fe). Radiographic examination of uterus after injection of contrast medium.

uterosalpingography (u″ter-o-sal″pin-gog′ra-fe). Radiographic examination of uterus and oviducts after injection of contrast medium.

V

Valsalva maneuver (văl-săl′vă) (Antonio Mario Valsalva, Italian anatomist, 1666-1723). Act of forcing a deep breath against closed glottis. This is achieved by a straining action, as if trying to move the bowels, without blowing out the cheeks or filling the pharynx.

varices (văr′i-sēz); sing. **varix** (văr′iks). Permanently dilated and tortuous veins; varicosities.

varicose (văr′i-kōs). Irregularly dilated; enlarged and tortuous; pertaining to a venous varix or varices.

vas (văs); pl. **vasa** (vă′sah). Vessel or duct; specifically, a blood or lymph vessel.

vascular (vas′ku-lar). Pertaining to or composed of vessels; specifically, pertaining to blood or lymph vessels.

vena (vē′nah); pl. **venae** (vē′nē). Vein.

venogram (ven′o-gram). Radiograph of veins filled with contrast medium; a phlebogram.

venography (ve-nog′ra-fe). Radiologic examination of veins during injection of radiopaque solution.

ventrad (ven′trad) [L. *venter*, belly]. Situated or directed toward abdomen or anterior aspect of body; ventrally.

ventral (ven′tral). Pertaining to abdomen or to anterior aspect of body or a part; designating or situated near anterior aspect.

ventricle (ven′tri-k′l). Cavity of an organ, such as ventricles of brain or of heart.

ventriculography (ven-trik″u-log′ra-fe). Radiographic examination of brain following injection of radioparent medium into ventricles; pneumoventriculography.

vermiform (ver′mi-form). Resembling a worm; as *vermiform* appendix of cecum.

vertex (ver′teks). Top or highest part of head.

verticomental (ver″ti-ko-men′tal). Pertaining to vertex and chin; as a *verticomental* projection of facial bones.

verticosubmental (ver″ti-ko-sub-men′tal). Pertaining to vertex and region of throat below chin; as a *verticosubmental* projection of petrosae.

vesicle (ves′i-k′l). Fluid-containing cavity or sac; blister.

villi (vil′ī); sing. **villus** (vil′us). Minute, threadlike vascular processes that project from specialized mucous membrane, as from mucosa of small intestine.

Virchow's plane (vēr′koz) (Rudolf Virchow, German pathologist, 1821-1902). See infraorbitomeatal line.

virulent (vir′u-lent). Extremely poisonous or noxious; violent; malignant.

visceral (vis′er-al). Pertaining to a viscus or viscera.

visceroptosis (vis″er-op-to′sis). Falling or downward displacement of abdominal organs.

viscid (vis′id). Having a gelatinous or sticky consistency; adherent; viscous.

viscosity (vis-kos′i-te). State or quality of being thick and sticky; viscid; gluey; glutinous.

viscus (vis′kus). Internal organ, such as heart, kidney, or stomach.

vitiate (vish′i-āt). To render faulty or defective; to impair quality of; to contaminate; to make impure, as air by electrical corona or by products of respiration.

voluntary (vol′un-ter″e). Proceeding in obedience to will; acting according to choice.

vomit (vom′it). Spontaneous expulsion of contents of stomach by mouth; also, the vomited matter.

vomitus (vom′i-tus). Matter ejected from stomach through mouth; vomiting.

Z

zonography Tomographic technique that depicts thick sections or zones of tissue by utilzing tomographic angles of 10 degrees or less.

zoster (zos′ter). Acute inflammatory skin disease of nervous origin, causing tenderness, itching, and neuralgic pains; it is characterized by clusters of small vesicles on a reddish base following along course of a peripheral nerve; herpes zoster; zona; shingles.

zygapophysical (zīg″ap-of-iz′e-al). Of or pertaining to a zygapophysis or to zygapophyses.

zygapophysis (zīg″ah-pof′i-sis) [Gr. *zygon*, yoke + *apophysis*, process]. Yokelike articular process; specifically, one of articular processes of neural arch of a vertebra.

zygion (zig′i-on; zij′i-on). Point at either end of bregmatic diameter of skull.

zygoma (zi-go′mah). Arch formed by union of malar bone of face and zygomatic process of temporal bone of cranium; also, malar bone.

zygomatic (zi″go-mat′ik). Of or pertaining to zygomatic arch or to malar bone.

VOLUME ONE

Bibliography

Bibliography

HISTORY

1895 Röntgen, W.C.: Ueber eine neue Art von Strahlen. Part I, Sitzungsber. phys.-med. Gesellsch. Würzburg, pp. 132-141, 1895, English translation in Science 3:Feb. 14, 1896.

1896 Röntgen, W.C.: Ueber eine neue Art von Strahlen. Part II, Sitzungsber. phys.-med. Gesellsch. Würzburg, pp. 11-19, 1896, English translation in Science 3:May 15, 1896.

1897 Röntgen, W.C.: Weitere Beobachtungen über X-strahlen, Mitt. Sitzungsberichte Preuss. Akad. Wess., Physik. Math. K1., p. 392, 1897.

1905 Albers-Schönberg, H.E.: The development and present state of radiology, Arch. Roentgen Ray 10:105, 1905.

1909 Pfahler, G.E.: Notes from some of the roentgen laboratories in Europe, Am. Q. Roentgenol. 2:15-22, 1909-1910.

1923 Grashey, R.: Wilhelm Conrad Röntgen, Fortschr. Roentgenstr. 30:409, 1923.

1929 Memenov, M.I.: Das Staatsinstitut für Röntgenologie, Radiologie und Krebsforschung in Leningrad, Fortschr. Roentgenstr. 40:1069-1087, 1929.

1931 Brown, P.: Early American roentgenology: manners and men, Radiogr. Clin. Photogr. 7:2-6, 1931.

Glasser, O.: Dr. W.C. Roentgen and the discovery of the roentgen ray, A.J.R. 25:437-450, 1931.

Hickey, P.M.: The Caldwell lecture, 1928, A.J.R. 25:177-195, 1931.

1932 Glasser, O.: Reception of Roentgen's discovery in America, Radiogr. Clin. Photogr. 8:2-6, 1932.

O'Hara, F.S.: Looking backward, Radiogr. Clin. Photogr. 8:3-9, 1932.

1934 Crane, A.W.: The research trail of the x-ray, Radiology 23:131-148, 1934.

Curie, M.S.: An editorial by E.W. Hall, A.J.R. 32:395, 1934.

Donaghey, J.P.: Reminiscences of Röntgen, Radiogr. Clin. Photogr. 10:2-7, 1934.

Forssell, G.: Marie Curie—in memoriam, Acta Radiol. 15:685-688, 1934.

Glasser, O: Wilhelm Conrad Röntgen and the early history of roentgen rays, Springfield, Ill., 1934, Charles C Thomas, Publisher.

Schinz, H.R.: Röntgen und Zürich, Acta Radiol. 15:562-575, 1934.

1936 Brown, P.: American martyrs to science through the roentgen ray, Springfield, Ill., 1936, Charles C Thomas, Publisher.

1937 Glasser, O.: The life of Röntgen as revealed in his letters, Sci. Monthly 45:193-206, 1937.

1938 Pancoast, H.K.: Reminiscences of a radiologist, A.J.R. 39:169-186, 1938.

1939 Casey, F.S.: Early scientists in the field of radiology, Xray Techn. 11:88-92, 1939.

1944 Glasser, O., et al.: Physical foundations of radiology, New York, 1944, Paul B. Hoeber, Inc.

1945 Case, J.T.: Fifty years of roentgen rays in gastroenterology, A.J.R. 54:607-625, 1945.

Davidoff, L.M.: The development of modern neuroroentgenology, A.J.R. 54:640-642, 1945.

Glasser, O.: Chronology of Röntgen's life, A.J.R. 54:541-544, 1945.

Glasser, O.: Fifty years of roentgen rays, Radiogr. Clin. Photogr. 21:58-66, 1945.

Glasser, O.: Scientific forefathers of Röntgen, A.J.R. 54:545-546, 1945.

Glasser, O.: W.C. Röntgen, Springfield, Ill., 1945, Charles C Thomas, Publisher.

Hodges, P.C.: Development of diagnostic x-ray apparatus during the first fifty years, Radiology 45:438-448, 1945.

Kirklin, B.R.: Background and beginning of cholecystography, A.J.R. 54:637-639, 1945.

Lough, T.W.: Commemorating a great discovery and half a century of its development, Xray Techn. 17:325-330, 1945.

Reynolds, L.: The history of the use of the roentgen ray in warfare, A.J.R. 54:649-672, 1945.

Rigler, L.G.: The development of roentgen diagnosis, Radiology 45:467-502, 1945.

Roesler, H.: History of the roentgen ray in the study of the heart, A.J.R. 54:647-648, 1945.

Röntgen, W.C.: On a new kind of rays, Reprint from Röntgen's original papers, Radiology 45:428-435, 1945.

Shields, D.G.: Fashion parade of x-ray apparatus 1895-1945, Xray Techn. 17:348-360, 1945.

Spillman, R.: Early history of roentgenology of the sinuses, A.J.R. 54:643-646, 1945.

Wolcott, R.E.: X-ray horizons, Xray Techn. 17:337-347, 377, 1945.

1946 Chevalier, J.: Vie et travaux de Roentgen, J. Radiol. Electrol. 27:107-110, 1946.

Dariaux, A.: Hommage aux victimes des rayons X, J. Radiol. Electrol. 27:101-104, 1946.

Delherm, L.: Première communication en France, sur les applications médicales de la découverte de Roentgen, J. Radiol. Electrol. 27:105-106, 1946.

Lacharite, H.: The healing and lethal rays, Xray Techn. 18:111-115, 138, 1946.

Ledoux-Lebard, R.: Les rayons X dans le diagnostic médical, J. Radiol. Electrol. 27:116-125, 1946.

Pilon, H.: Cinquante ans de construction radiologique, J. Radiol. Electrol. 27:111-115, 1946.

Stolz, Sister M.F.: Contributions of some of Röntgen's predecessors, Xray Techn. 18:1-4, 1946.

1947 Fuchs, A.W.: Edison and roentgenology, A.J.R. 57:145-156, 1947.

1951 Scott, W.G.: The development of angiocardiography and aortography, Radiology 56:485-518, 1951.

1952 Leucutia, T.: Pneumoperitoneum and pneumoretroperitoneum (editorial), A.J.R. 68:655-658, 1952.

1954 Diehl, K.L.: Bronchography: study of its techniques and presentations of improved modification, Arch. Otolaryngol. 60:277-290, 1954.

Stevenson, C.A.: Development of colon examination, A.J.R. 71:385-397, 1954.

1955 Olson, L.G.: Roentgen's scientific forefathers, Xray Techn. 27:184-189, 1955.

1956 Caffey, J.: The first sixty years of pediatric roentgenology in the United States, A.J.R. 76:437-454, 1956.

Maluf, N.S.R.: Role of roentgenology in the development of urology, A.J.R. 75:847-854, 1956.

1958 Glasser, O.: W.C. Röntgen, ed. 2, Springfield, Ill., 1958, Charles C Thomas, Publisher.

Kincaid, O.W., and Davis, G.D.: Abdominal aortography, N. Engl. J. Med. 259:1017-1024, 1958.

1960 Scott, J.: Ancient and modern, Radiography 26:97-107, 1960.

1961 Bull, J.W.D.: History of neuroradiology, Br. J. Radiol. 34:69-84, 1961.

Cole, W.H.: Historical features of cholecystography, Radiology 76:354-375, 1961.

Gershon-Cohen, J.: Breast roentgenology: a historical review, A.J.R. 86:879-883, 1961.

Watson, W.: 1895 and all that, Radiography 27:305-315, 1961.

1964 Bruwer, A.J., editor: Classic descriptions in diagnostic roentgenology, Springfield, Ill., 1964, Charles C Thomas, Publisher.

Strain, W.H., et al.: Radiologic diagnostic agents: a compilation, Med. Radiogr. Photogr. 40(suppl.):1-110, 1964.

1965 Grigg, E.R.N.: The new history of radiology, Radiol. Technol. 36:229-257, 1965.

Grigg, E.R.N.: The trail of the invisible light, Springfield, Ill., 1965, Charles C Thomas, Publisher.

Schatzki, R.: Esophagus: progress and problems: the Caldwell lecture, A.J.R. 94:523-540, 1965.

1974 Kraft, E., and Finby, N.: Wilhelm Conrad Roentgen (1845-1923): discoverer of x-ray N.Y. State J. Med. 74:2066-2070, 1974.

1976 Morgan, K.Z.: Rolf M. Sievert: the pioneer in the field of radiation protection, Health Phys. 31:263-264, 1976.

Ramsey, L.J.: Luminescence and intensifying screens in the early days of radiography, Radiography 42:245-253, 1976.

1978 Eastman, T.R.: History of radiographic technique, Appl. Radiol. 7:97-100, 1978.

Lang, E.F.: From earlier pages . . . development of a name for radiology, A.J.R. 130:586-587, 1978.

1979 Fischmann, E.: Retracing Rontgen's discovery, Diagn. Imaging 48:294-303, 1979.

1980 Shampo, M.A., and Kyle, R.A.; Thomas A. Edison, J.A.M.A. 243:1719, 1980.

JOURNALS ON RADIOGRAPHY

Acta Radiologica, Stockholm, 1921-1962, and continued as both

Acta Radiologica: Diagnosis, Stockholm, 1962- and

Acta Radiologica: Therapy, Stockholm, 1962-1977, and continued as

Acta Radiologica: Oncology, Radiation, Physics, and Biology, 1978-

American Atlas of Stereo-roentgenology, Troy, 1916-1920.

American Journal of Anatomy, New York, 1901-

American Journal of Roentgenology, Pittsburgh, 1913-1923, and continued as

American Journal of Roentgenology and Radium Therapy, Pittsburgh, 1923-1952, and continued as

American Journal of Roentgenology, Radium Therapy, and Nuclear Medicine, Springfield, Ill., 1952-1975, and continued as

A.J.R. Baltimore, 1976-

American Journal of Surgery, New York, 1890-

American Quarterly of Roentgenology, Pittsburgh, 1906-1913.

American X-ray Journal, St. Louis, 1897-1904.

Anales del Instituto Municipal de Radiologia y Fisioterapia, Buenos Aires, 1934-1941, and continued as

Archivos del Instituto Municipal de Radiología y Fisioterapía, Buenos Aires, 1941-

Annales de Radiologie, Paris, 1958-

Annales de Roentgenologie et Radiologie: Journal de l'Institut d'état de Radiologie à Pétersbourg, Pétersbourg, 1922- , the international edition of Vestnik Rentgenologii i Radiologii

Annali di Radiologia e Fisica Medica, Bologna, 1934-

Annals of Otology, Rhinology and Laryngology, St. Louis, 1897-

Annals of Surgery, Philadelphia, 1885-

Applied Radiology, Los Angeles, 1976-

Archives of Radiology and Electrotherapy, London, 1915-1923.

Archivio di Radiologia, Naples, 1925-1956.

Archivos Uruguayos de Medicina, Cirugía y Especialidades, Montevideo, Uruguay, 1932-

Atti del Congresso Italiano di Radiologia Medica, Pavia, Italy, 1914-1959, and continued as

Atti del Congresso Nazionale di Radiologia Medicana Nucleare, 1959-

Australasian Radiology, Sydney, 1957-

British Journal of Radiology, London, 1928-

Bulletins et Mémoirs de la Société d'Electroradiologie Médicale de France, Paris, 1938-1939, and continued as

Journal de Radiologie, d'Electrologie et de Médicine Nucléaire, 1957-

CRC Critical Reviews in Diagnostic Imaging, Cleveland, 1970-

CT. The Journal of Computed Tomography, Baltimore, 1976-

Canadian Journal of Radiography, Radiotherapy, and Nuclear Medicine, Ottawa, 1943-

Canadian Association of Radiologists Journal, Montreal, 1973-

Computerized Tomography, Elmsford, N.Y., 1977-

Current Problems in Diagnostic Radiology, Chicago, 1971-

Diagnostic Imaging, Basel, 1974-

Fortschritte auf dem Gebiete der Röntgenstrahlen, Hamburg, 1897-1900, and continued as

Fortschritte auf dem Gebiete der Roentgenstrahlen und der Nuklearnmedizin, Stuttgart, 1956-

Gastrointenstinal Radiology, New York, 1976-

Health Physics, Elmsford, N.Y., 1958-

Investigative Radiology, Philadelphia, 1966-

Journal of the American Medical Association, Chicago, 1883-

Journal of Anatomy, Cambridge, England, 1866-

Journal Belge de Radiologie, Brussels, 1907-

Journal of Bone & Joint Surgery, Boston, 1922-

Journal of the Faculty of Radiologists, 1949-1959, and continued as

Clinical Radiology, Edinburgh, 1950-

Journal of Neuroradiology, Paris, 1978-

Journal de Radiologie, Paris, 1914-

Journal of the Röntgen Society, London, 1904-1923.

Journal of Thoracic Surgery, St. Louis, 1931-1959, and continued as

Journal of Thoracic and Cardiovascular Surgery, St. Louis, 1959-

Journal of Urology, Baltimore, 1917-

Klinische Wochenschrift, Berlin, 1922-

Laryngoscope, St. Louis, 1896-

Medical Imaging, Los Angeles, 1976-

Medical Journal of Australia, Sydney, 1914-

Medical Radiography and Photography, Rochester, N.Y., 1925-

Neuroradiology, New York, 1970-

Pediatric Radiology, New York, 1973-

Physics in Medicine and Biology, New York, 1956-

Presse Médicale, Paris, 1893-1971, and continued as

Nouvelle Presse Médicale, Paris, 1972-

Quaderni di Radiologia, Belluno, Italy, 1937-

Quarterly Bulletin of Sea View Hospital, New York, 1935-

Radiography . . . Society of Radiographers, London, 1935-

Radiography and Clinical Photography: Eastman Kodak Co., Rochester, N.Y., 1930-

Radiologe (Der), Berlin, 1961-

Radiología . . . órgano oficial de la Sociedad argentina de radiología, Beunos Aires, 1942-

Radiologia Diagnostica, Berlin, 1960-

Radiologia Medica . . . organo della Società italiana di radiologia medica, Pavia and Milano, 1914-

Radiologic Clinics of North America, Philadelphia, 1963-

Radiologica, Berlin and Leipzig, 1937-1939, and continued as

Fundamenta radiologica, Berlin, 1939-

Radiology: Radiological Society of North America, Easton, Pa., 1923-

Radiology, section 14 of Excerpta Medica, L. Paul, M.D., subeditor, Amsterdam, C., The Netherlands, International, 1948.

Röntgenpraxis, Leipzig, 1929-

Scritti Italiani di Radiobiologia Medica, Feltre, Italy, 1934-

Seminars in Roentgenology, New York, 1966-

Skeletal Radiology, New York, 1976-

Southern Medical Journal, Birmingham, Ala., 1908-

Surgery, St. Louis, 1935-

Surgery, Gynecology and Obstetrics, Chicago, 1905-

Urologic Radiology, Philadelphia, 1979-

Vestnik Rentgenologii i Radiologii, Moskva, 1921-

X-ray Technician: American Association of Radiological Technicians, St. Paul, Minn. 1929-1963, and continued as

Radiologic Technology, Baltimore, 1963-

X-ray Bulletin: Eastman Kodak Co., Rochester, N.Y., 1925-1930.

Year Book of Radiology: Year Book Medical Publishers, Inc., Chicago, 1932-1974, and continued as

Year Book of Diagnostic Radiology, Chicago, 1975-

TEXTBOOKS ON RADIOGRAPHY

1901 Williams, F.H.: The roentgen rays in medicine and surgery, New York, 1901, The Macmillan Co.

1903 Albers-Schönberg, H.E.: Die Röntgentechnik, Hamburg, 1903, Gräfe & Sillem.

1917 Christie, A.C.: A manual of x-ray technic, ed. 2, Philadelphia, 1917, J.B. Lippincott Co.

1919 Albers-Schönberg, H.E.: Die Röntgentechnik, ed. 5, Hamburg, 1919, Gräfe & Sillem.

1920 Hirsch, I.S.: The principles and practice of roentgenological technique, New York, 1920, American X-ray Publishing Co.

1924 Robertson, J.K.: X-rays and x-ray apparatus: an elementary course, New York, 1924, The Macmillan Co.

1926 Grashey, R.: Allgemeine Aufnahmetechnik und Deutung der Röntgenbilder, Berlin, 1926, Urban & Schwarzenberg.

1927 Fürstenau, R., Immelman, M., and Schutze, J.: Leitfaden des Röntgenverfahrens, ed. 5, Stuttgart, 1927, Ferdinand Enke.

Lilienfeld, L.: In Mayer, E.G., and Pardes, F., editors: Anordnung der normalisierten Röntgenaufnahmen des menschlichen Körpers, ed. 4, Berlin, 1927, Urban & Schwarzenberg.

1928 Jerman, E.C.: Modern x-ray technic, St. Paul, Minn., 1928, The Bruce Publishing Co.

1931 Jerman, E.C., et al.: X-ray studies in advanced radiographic technic, no. 1, Chicago, 1931, General Electric X-ray Corp.

1932 Pillsbury, H.C., editor: United States Army x-ray manual, ed. 2, New York, 1932, Paul B. Hoeber, Inc.

1934 Palazzi, S.: Roentgenografia, Milano, 1934, Ulrico Hoepli.

1936 Files, G.W., et al.: X-ray studies in advanced radiographic technic, no. 2, Chicago, 1936, General Electric X-ray Corp.

1938 Procher, P., and de Juguelier, A.: Précis de technique radiographique, Paris, 1938, Gauthier-Villars.

1939 Delherm, L., and Kahn, H.L.M.: Les principales positions utilisées en radiographie, ed. 2, Paris, 1939, Norbert Maloine.

1940 Bauer, K.: A B C der Röntgentechnik, Leipzig, 1940, Georg Thieme.

Davies, N., and Isenburg, U.: Standard radiographic positions, London, 1940, Bailliere, Tindall & Cox.

1941 McNeill, C.: Roentgen technique, ed. 2, Springfield, Ill., 1941, Charles C Thomas, Publisher.

Russell, J.J.: Outline of modern x-ray technic, ed. 3, New York, 1941, Picker X-ray Corp.

1942 Letterman General Hospital, San Francisco, Special Service School: Instructions in the use of roentgen rays and roentgen ray apparatus, San Francisco, 1942.

1943 Files, G.W., et al.: Medical radiographic technic, Springfield, Ill., 1943, Charles C Thomas, Publisher.

Rhinehardt, D.A.: Roentgenographic technique, ed. 3, Philadelphia, 1943, Lea & Febiger.

Sante, L.R.: Manual of roentgenological technique, ed. 10, Ann Arbor, Mich., 1943, Edwards Brothers, Inc.

1944 Castillo, E.: Técnica de la exploración roentgenoscópica roentgenográfica, vol. 1, Barcelona, Madrid, 1944, Editorial Labora, S.A., p. 745.

Military roentgenology: war department technical manual, TM 8-280, Washington, D.C., 1944.

Naval medical school: fundamentals of x-ray physics and technique. National Naval Medical Center, Bethesda, Md., 1944.

1945 Janker, R.: Röntgenaufnahmetechnik, II., vol. 1, Leipzig, 1945, Johann Ambrosius Barth.

1947 Hardman, G.L.: Guide to positioning, Radiography 13:42-43, 1947.

1948 Davies, N., and Isenburg, V.: Standard radiographic positions, ed. 2, Baltimore, 1948, The Williams & Wilkins Co.

1950 Porcher, P.: Précis de technique radiographique, ed. 3, Paris, 1950, Gauthier-Villars.

1955 Castillo, E.: Técnica de la exploración roentgenoscópica y roentgenográfica, ed. 2, Madrid, 1955, Instituto Radiologico Del Dr. Castillo.

1956 LeDoux-LeBard, R., and Garcia-Calderon, J.: Technique du radiodiagnostique, ed. 2, Paris, 1956, Masson & Cie.

Sante, L.R.: Manual of roentgenological technique, ed. 18, Ann Arbor, Mich., 1956, Edward Brothers, Inc.

Schlosshauer, B.: Röntgenaufnahmetechnik in der Hals-Nasen-Ohren-Heilkunde, Stuttgart, 1956, Georg Thieme.

Schoen, H.: Medizinische Röntgentechnik, ed. 2, Stuttgart, 1956, Georg Thieme.

1962 Schurtleff, F.E.: Children's radiographic technic, ed. 2, Philadelphia, 1962, Lea & Febiger.

1964 Bloom, W.L., Jr., et al.: Medical radiographic technic, ed. 3, Springfield, Ill., 1964, Charles C Thomas, Publisher.

Clark, K.C.: Positioning in radiography, ed. 8, New York and London, 1964, Grune & Stratton, Inc.

Jacobi, C.A., and Paris, D.Q.: X-ray technology, ed. 3, St. Louis, 1964, The C.V. Mosby Co.

Vennes, C.H., and Watson, J.C.: Patient care and special procedures in x-ray technology, ed. 2, St. Louis, 1964, The C.V. Mosby Co.

1965 Bauer, D.deF.: A textbook of elementary radiography for students and technicians, Springfield, Ill., 1965, Charles C Thomas, Publisher.

1968 Meschan, I., and Farrer-Meschan, R.M.F.: Radiographic positioning and related anatomy, Philadelphia, 1968, W.B. Saunders Co.

1969 Schmidt, J.E.: Paramedical dictionary: a practical dictionary for the semimedical and ancillary medical professions, Springfield, Ill., 1969, Charles C Thomas, Publisher.

1972 Cullinan, J.E.: Illustrated guide to x-ray technics, Philadelphia, 1972, J.B. Lippincott Co.

1973 Clark, K.C.: Positioning in radiography, ed. 9 (edited and revised by J. McInnes), Chicago, 1973, Year Book Medical Publishers, Inc.

1974 Watson, J.C.: Patient care and special procedures in radiologic technology, St. Louis, 1974, The C.V. Mosby Co.

1975 Snopek, A.M.: Fundamentals of special radiographic procedures, New York, 1975, McGraw-Hill Book Co.

1976 Schertel, L., et al.: Atlas of xeroradiography, Philadelphia, 1976, W.B. Saunders Co.

Snell, R.S., and Wyman, A.C.: An atlas of normal radiographic anatomy, Boston, 1976, Little, Brown & Co.

1977 Jacobi, C.A.: Textbook of radiologic technology, St. Louis, 1977, The C.V. Mosby Co.

Norman, D., Korobkin, M., and Newton, T.H., editors: Computed tomography, St. Louis, 1977, The C.V. Mosby Co.

1978 Abbott, M.K.: Invasive radiologic diagnostic procedures, Philadelphia, 1978, F.A. Davis Co.

Chesney, D.N., and Chesney, M.O.: Care of the patient in diagnostic radiography, Oxford, 1978, Blackwell Scientific Publications, Ltd.

Hiss, S.S.: Understanding radiography, Springfield, Ill., 1978, Charles C Thomas, Publisher.

1979 Bryan, G.J.: Diagnostic radiography, New York, 1979, Churchill Livingstone, Inc.

Thompson, T.T.: Cahoon's formulating x-ray techniques, Durham, N.C., 1979, Duke University Press.

Torres, L.S., and Moore, C.M.: Basic medical techniques and patient care for radiologic technologists, Philadelphia, 1979, J.B. Lippincott Co.

TEXTBOOKS ON POSITIONING

1905 Brühl, G.: Grundriss und Atlas der Ohrenheilkunde, ed. 2, Munich, 1905, J.F. Lehmann.

Grashey, R.: Atlas typischer Röntgenbilder vom normalen Menschen, Munich, 1905, J.F. Lehmann.

Schüller, A.: Die Schädelbasis im Röntgenbilde, Hamburg, 1905, Gräfe & Sillem.

1910 Köhler, A.: Grenzen des Normalen und Anfänge des Pathologischen im Röntgenbilde, Hamburg, 1910, Gräfe & Sillem.

1912 Denker and Brünings: Die Krankheiten des Ohres und der Luftwege, Jena, 1912, Gustav Fischer.

Grashey, R.: Atlas typischer Röntgenbilder vom normalen Menschen, ed. 2, Munich, 1912, J.F. Lehmann.

1914 Sonnenkalb, V.: Die Röntgendiagnostik des Hals-, Nasen-, Ohrenärztes, Jena, 1914, Gustav Fischer.

1918 Holzknecht, G.: Röntgenologie, ed. 2, Berlin, 1918, Urban & Schwarzenberg.

Rhese, H.: Die Kriegsverletzungen und Kriegserkrankungen von Ohr, Nase und Hals, Wiesbaden, 1918, J.F. Bergmann.

1920 Law, F.M.: Mastoids roentgenologically considered, Ann. Roentgenol. 1:1920.

Schaeffer, J.P.: The nose, paranasal sinuses, nasolacrimal passages, and olfactory organ in man, Philadelphia, 1920, P. Blakiston's Son & Co.

1923 Sonnenkalb, V., and Beyer, E.: Die Röntgendiagnostik von Ohr, Nase und Nebenhöhlen, Rachen, Kehlkopf, Mund und Zähne, Leipzig, 1923, Dr. Werner Klinkhardt, Handbuch Röntgendiagnostik, III, no. 3.

1924 Schüller, A.: Röntgen Diagnostik der Erkrankungen des Köpfes, Berlin, 1924, Urban & Schwarzenberg.

1928 Grashey, R.: Typische Röntgenbilder vom normalen Menschen. In Lehmann's medizinische Atlanten, ed. 5, vol. 5, 1928.

1929 Assmann, H.: Clinical roentgendiagnosis of internal diseases (Die klinische Röntgendiagnostik der inneren Erkrankungen), translated by New York Academy of Medicine Library, Bibliographic Department, March 1929.

Köhler, A.: Roentgenology, New York, 1929, William Wood & Co.

1930 Mayer, E.G., and Eisinger, K.: Otologische Röntgendiagnostik, Wien, 1930, Julius Springer, pp. 283-304.

1933 Busi, A.: Tecnica e diagnostica radiologica nelle malattie chirurgiche, Cl. T.E.T., 1933.

Davis, L.: Intracranial tumors, Ann. Roentgenol., 1933.

Engel, S., and Schall, L.: Handbuch der Röntgendiagnostik und Therapie im Kindesalter, Leipzig, 1933, Georg Thieme.

1934 Codman, A.E.: The shoulder, Boston, 1934, Little, Brown & Co.

1936 Harrison, B.J.M.: A textbook of roentgenology, Baltimore, 1936, William Wood & Co.

Hartman, E.: La radiographie en ophthalmologie, Paris, 1936, Masson & Cie.

1939 Ferguson, A.B.: Roentgen diagnosis of the extremities and spine, Ann. Roentgenol., 1939.

1940 Pancoast, H.K., Pendergrass, E.P., and Schaeffer, J.P.: The head and neck in roentgen diagnosis, Springfield, Ill., 1940, Charles C Thomas, Publisher.

1941 Golden, R., editor: Diagnostic roentgenology, ed. 2, New York, 1941, Thomas Nelson & Sons.

1945 Archer, V.W.: The osseous system, Chicago, 1945, Year Book Medical Publishers, Inc.

Ferguson, A.B.: Roentgen diagnosis of the extremities and spine, New York, 1945, Paul B. Hoeber, Inc.

1946 Pillmore, G.U., editor: Clinical radiology, Philadelphia, 1946, F.A. Davis Co.

1947 Ross, G., editor: Diagnostic roentgenology, ed. 3, New York, 1947, Thomas Nelson & Sons.

1948 Young, B.R.: The skull, sinuses, and mastoids: a handbook of roentgen diagnosis, Chicago, 1948, Year Book Medical Publishers, Inc.

1950 Chaumet, G.: Traité de radiodiagnostic, ed. 2, Paris, 1950, Vigot Frères.

Chaussé, C.: Premiers elements de radio-otologie, Paris, 1950, Masson & Cie.

1955 Bateman, J.E.: The shoulder and environs, St. Louis, 1955, The C.V. Mosby Co.

1956 Pendergrass, E.P., Schaeffer, J.P., and Hodes, P.J.: The head and neck in roentgen diagnosis, ed. 2, Springfield, Ill., 1956, Charles C Thomas, Publisher.

1957 Gamble, F.O.: Applied foot roentgenology, Baltimore, 1957, The Williams & Wilkins Co.

1961 Abrams, H., editor: Angiography, Boston, 1961, Little, Brown & Co.

1962 Bull, J.W., et al.: Atlas of myelography, New York, 1962, Grune & Stratton, Inc.

Darling, D.B.: Radiography of infants and children, Springfield, Ill., 1962, Charles C Thomas, Publisher.

1963 Stafne, E.C.: Oral roentgenographic diagnosis including an appendix on roentgenographic technic, ed. 2, Philadelphia, 1963, W.B. Saunders Co.

1964 Egan, R.L.: Mammography, Springfield, Ill., 1964, Charles C Thomas, Publisher.

Etter, L.E., et al.: Roentgenography and roentgenology of the middle ear and mastoid process, Springfield, Ill., 1964, Charles C Thomas, Publisher.

Taveras, J.M., and Wood, E.H.: Diagnostic neuroradiology, Baltimore, 1964, The Williams & Wilkins Co.

1972 Saxton, H.M., and Strickland, B.: Practical procedures in diagnostic radiology, New York, 1972, Grune & Stratton, Inc.

1979 Griffiths, H.J., and Sarno, R.C.: Contemporary radiology, Philadelphia, 1979, W.B. Saunders Co.

Kreel, L., and Steiner, R.E., editors: Medical imaging, Chicago, 1979, Year Book Medical Publishers, Inc.

Lodge, T., and Steiner, R.E., editors: Recent advances in radiology and medical imaging, New York, 1979, Churchill Livingstone, Inc.

NURSING PROCEDURES AND PATIENT CARE

1957 Furushiro, T.: Handling the handicapped patient, Xray Techn. 28:246-249, 1957.

1960 Chesney, M.O.: Emergency radiography, Radiography 26:277-286, 1960.

1961 Bentley, H.B.: Nursing points for students and radiographers, Radiology 27:75-84, 1961.

Reinhart, M.J.: Cross infection: the significance of efficient aseptic technique in the department of radiology, Xray Techn. 32:487-495, 1961.

1962 Chesney, D.N., and Chesney, M.O.: Care of the patient in diagnostic radiography, Philadelphia, 1962, F.A. Davis Co.

Howell, H.B.: Hospital practice and the care of the patient in x-ray departments, Radiology 28:2-10, 1962.

1964 Vennes, C.H., and Watson, J.C.: Patient care and special procedures in x-ray technology, ed. 2, St. Louis, 1964, The C.V. Mosby Co.

1965 Brinkbok, G.C.F.: Pathology for radiographers, London, 1965, Butterworth & Co., Ltd.

1966 Nelson, S.W.: Some important diagnostic and technical fundamentals in the radiology of trauma; with particular emphasis on skeletal trauma, Radiol. Clin. North Am. 4:241-259, 1966.

1973 Littleton, J.T.: Transportation of the traumatized patient, Radiol. Clin. North Am. 11:449-460, 1973.

1974 Watson, J.C.: Patient care and special procedures in radiologic technology, St. Louis, 1974, The C.V. Mosby Co.

1976 Laws, P.W.: How patients view the efficient use of diagnostic radiology, Radiol. Technol. 47:245-249, 1976.

Sweeney, R.J.: System designed to improve the communication process betwen patient and technologist, Radiol. Technol. 47:295-297, 1976.

1978 Bell, M.E.: Patient–radiologic technologist interpersonal relationship and how it can be improved, Radiol. Technol. 50:41-44, 1978.

Chesney, D.N., and Chesney, M.O.: Care of the patient in diagnostic radiography, Oxford, 1978, Blackwell Scientific Publications, Ltd.

Fengler, K.: The patient-care gap, Radiol. Technol. 49:599-600, 1978.

Neuhaus, B.: Our professional image: as we are seen, Radiol. Technol. 49:485-489, 1978.

Wedel, C.S.: Patient communication: the final step towards professionalism, Radiol. Technol. 50:27-31, 1978.

Wilson-Barnett, J.: Patients' responses to barium x-ray studies, Br. Med. J. 1:1324, 1978.

1979 Goldin, G.J.: Psychodynamic components in the role of the radiologic technologist, Radiol. Technol. 51:193-197, 1979.

Quinn, B.C.: Improving patient cooperation, Radiol. Technol. 51:68-71, 1979.

Torres, L.S., and Moore, C.M.: Basic medical techniques and patient care for radiologic technologists, Philadelphia, 1979, J.B. Lippincott Co.

1981 Warner, S.L.: Code of ethics: professional and legal implications, Radiol. Technol. 52:485-494, 1981.

RADIATION PROTECTION

1929 Goldstein, L., and Murphy, D.A.: Etiology of the ill health in children born after maternal pelvic irradiation and defective children born after postconception pelvic irradiation, A.J.R. 22:322-331, 1929.

1948 Frazer, M.D.: Protection in the radiological laboratory, Xray Techn. 19:170-173, 1948.

1949 Evans, D.R.: Quantitative inferences concerning the genetic effects of radiation on human beings, Science 109:299-304, 1949.

Tierney, R.B., and Deglow, R.E.: Radiation protection for the x-ray technician, Xray Techn. 21:140-149, 1949.

1952 Howard, A.: Radiation genetics. 1. Genetic aspects of radiation risks, Br. J. Radiol. 25:177-179, 1952.

Russell, L.B., and Russell, W.L.: Radiation hazards to the embryo and fetus, Radiology 58:369-377, 1952.

1954 Lachman, E.: Dangers of diagnostic radiation and protective measures, Xray Techn. 25:331-334, 1954.

1955 Stamford, R.W., and Vance, J.: The quantity of radiation received by the reproductive organs of patients during routine diagnostic x-ray examinations, Br. J. Radiol. 28:266-273, 1955.

1956 Ardran, G.M.: The dose to operator and patient in x-ray diagnostic procedures, Br. J. Radiol. 29:266-269, 1956.

1957 Ardran, G.M.: Dose reduction in diagnostic radiology, Br. J. Radiol. 30:436-438, 1957.

Ardran, G.M., and Crooks, H.E.: Gonad radiation dose from diagnostic procedures, Br. J. Radiol. 30:295-297, 1957.

Ardran, G.M., and Kemp, F.H.: Protection of the male gonads in diagnostic procedures, Br. J. Radiol. 30:280, 1957.

Billings, M.S.: Gonad dose during routine roentgenography, Radiology 69:37-41, 1957.

Laughlin, J.S., et al.: Bone, skin, and gonadal doses in routine diagnostic procedures, A.J.R. 78:961-982, 1957.

Merriam, G.R., Jr., and Focht, E.F.: A clinical study of radiation cataracts and the relationship to dose, A.J.R. 77:759-785, 1957.

Pyper, J.B.: An aid in the reduction of radiation hazard in the operating theatre, Lancet 2:1204-1205, 1957.

Sanford, R.W.: The use of cones and filters to reduce patient dosage in diagnostic radiology, Br. J. Radiol. 30:497-499, 1957.

Sowby, F.D.: Dose to the gonads during diagnostic procedures, J. Can. Radiol. Assoc. 8:57-59, 1957.

Stone, R.S.: Common sense in radiation protection applied to clinical practice, A.J.R. 78:993-999, 1957.

1958 Abram, E., Wilkinson, D.M., and Hodson, C.J.: Gonadal protection from x-radiation for the female, Br. J. Radiol. 31:335-336, 1958.

Braestrup, C.B., and Wyckoff, H.O.: Radiation protection, Springfield, Ill., 1958, Charles C Thomas, Publisher.

Jackson, W.: Ionizing radiations: their implications for radiographers, Radiography 24:53-62, 1958.

Lincoln, T.A., and Gupton, E.D.: Radiation dose to gonads from diagnostic x-ray exposures, J.A.M.A. 166:233-239, 1958.

Maitland, D.G.: Protection, Radiography 24:265-270, 1958.

Merriam, G.R., and Focht, E.F.: Radiation dose to the lens and adjacent structures: possibilities of cataract formation, Radiology 71:357-369, 1958.

Newell, R.R.: Common sense evaluation of radiation exposure in clinical radiology, A.J.R. 80:917-925, 1958.

Tievsky, G.: Ionizing radiation and a sense of proportion, J.A.M.A. 166:1667-1672, 1958.

1959 Madsen, E.T.: An adjustable mobile cassette holder for orthopaedic operations, J. Bone Joint Surg. 41-B:774-775, 1959.

Soule, A.B., Heilbronn, H., and Bannister, R.: The rational use of x-ray in medicine and dentistry with particular regard to protective measures, Xray Techn. 30:244-259, 1959.

1960 McRae, D.L.: Diagnostic x-ray exposures: the middle road, J. Can. Med. Assoc. 83:929-933, 1960.

Moos, W.S., and Harvey, R.A.: Development of radiation hazard control at the University of Illinois College of Medicine, Xray Techn. 32:33-38, 1960.

Tramm, E.: Minimum dosage radiography, Xray Techn. 31:619-622, 1960.

1961 Graham, D.: The limitation of the radiation dosage to patient in diagnostic radiography, Radiography 27:345-353, 1961.

Hammer-Jacobsen, E.: Radiation protection of personnel and patients in diagnostic departments, Radiography 27:210-217, 1961.

LaFond, J.V.: Restrictive cones in diagnostic roentgenology: an evaluation of their use, Xray Techn. 32:365-368, 1961.

1963 Sedlak, Sister M.P.: Some considerations of radiologic protection, Radiol. Technol. 35:176-180, 1963.

1966 Morgen, R.H., and Gehret, J.C.: The radiant energy received by patients in diagnostic x-ray practice, A.J.R. 97:793-810, 1966.

1970 Chin, F.K., Anderson, W.B., and Gilbertson, J.D.: Radiation dose to critical organs during petrous tomography, Radiology 94:623-627, 1970.

McGlone, W.E.: Radiation protection of the reproductive organs during radiography of the hip joints, Radiol. Technol. 41:277-279, 1970.

1972 Fischel, R.E.: Method of gonad protection, Acta Radiol. [Diagn.] 12:396-398, 1972.

1973 Grossman, H.: Radiation protection in diagnostic radiography of children, Pediatrics 51:141-144, 1973.

1974 Best, M.C., and Warrick, C.K.: The 10-day rule, Nurs. Times 70:1474, 1974.

Radiation protection: protection progress and exposure data, Radiol. Technol. 46:111-112, 1974.

Stephenson, S.K.: The diagnostic use of x-rays—physical aspects, Br. J. Radiol. 47:631, 1974.

1975 Purdy, J.A., et al.: Gonadal shield, Radiology 117:226, 1975.

Ryer, F.H.: The new health and safety act as it relates to occupational radiation exposure, Health Phys. 29:207-212, 1975.

1976 Douglas, S.J.: Protection of patients against the harmful effects of ionizing radiation, Ir. Med. J. 69:475-476, 1976.

Hinds, L.M.: Reducing radiation exposure to patient and operator, J. Natl. Med. Assoc. 68:115-116, 152, 1976.

Johnson, N.E.: Radiation protective shield for use during arthrography, Radiol. Technol. 48:35-38, 1976.

1977 Bergström, K., Jorulf, H., and Löfroth, P.O.: Eye lens protection for radiological personnel, Radiology 124:839-840, 1977.

Gross, G.P., et al.: Radiation protection requirements for a whole-body CT scanner, Radiology 122:825-826, 1977.

Seeram, E.: Protecting patients from radiation, Dimens. Health Serv. 54:40, 42, 1977.

Ziehm, D.J.: Guidelines for the diagnostic x-ray examination of fertile women, Ariz. Med. 34:762-763, 1977.

Bryant, T.H., and Julian, W.L.: Reduction of radiation dose to patients in xeroradiography, Br. J. Radiol. 51:974-980, 1978.

1978 Hemmingsson, A., and Löfroth, P.O.: Radiation protection in fluoroscopy with an image intensifier, Acta Radiol. 19:1007-1013, 1978.

ICRU submits new radiation unit system and reports, Radiol. Technol. 50:50-51, 1978.

Littleton, J.T., Durizch, M.L., and Perry, N.: Radiation protection of the lens for patients and users, Radiology 129:795-798, 1978.

1979 Manny, E.F., Brown, R.F., and Shaver, J.W.: Gonad shielding in diagnostic radiology: recommendation of the FDA and ACR, Postgrad. Med. 65:207-211, 1979.

Noz, M.E., and Maguire, G.Q.: Radiation protection in the radiologic and health sciences, Philadelphia, 1979, Lea & Febiger.

1980 Gloag, D.: Radiation exposure and the protection of the community, Br. Med. J. 281:1545-1548, 1980.

ANATOMY

1884 Kollman, J., Ranke, T., and Virchow, R.: Verständingung über ein gemeinsames craniometrisches Verfahren, Arch. Anthrop. 15:1-8, 1884.

Reid, R.W.: Relation of the principal fissures and convolutions of the cerebrum to the outer surface of the scalp, Lancet 2:539-540, 1884.

1901 Zuckerkandl, E.: Atlas der topographischen Anatomie, Munich, 1901, J.F. Lehmann.

1906 Addison, C. In Ellis: Demonstrations of anatomy, ed. 12, New York, 1906, William Wood & Co.

1914 Knox, R., and Salmond, R.W.: A system of topography for use in the radiography of the head, Arch. Roentgen Ray 19:393-398, 1914-1915.

1917 Mills, W.R.: The relation of bodily habitus to visceral form, position, tonus, and motility, A.J.R. 4:155-169, 1917.

1925 Goldhamer, K., and Schüller A.: Die Vertikalund die Horizontalebene des Kopfes, Fortschr. Roentgenstr. 33:183-190, 1925.

1926 Goldhamer, K., and Schüller, A.: Varietäten im Bereich der hinteren Schädelgrube, Fortschr. Roentgenstr. 35:1163-1189, 1926.

Hasselwander, A.: Anatomie des menschlichen Körpers in Röntgenbild, Munich, 1926, J.F. Bergmann.

1927 Mosher, H.P.: X-ray study of movements of tongue, epiglottis, and hyoid bone in swallowing, Laryngoscope 37:235, 1927.

1929 Ralph, S., Jr.: Radiographic appearance of anatomical landmarks, Xray Bull. 6:4-7, 11, 1929.

1930 Goldhamer, K.: Normal anatomy of the head, Radiologische Praktika 12-13:1930-1931.

1931 Camp, J.D., and Cilley, E.I.L.: Diagrammatic chart showing time of appearance of the various centers of ossification and period of union, A.J.R. 26:905, 1931.

1934 Reese, M.: The physiology of respiration—its relation to radiography, Xray Techn. 5:165-168, 1934.

Weski, O.: Röntgenanatomie des Schädels, der Kiefer und der Zähne, Berlin, 1934, Berlinische Verlag Anstalt.

1937 Benner, F.: Das Röntgenschnittaufnahmeverfahren und seine Beduetung für die Röntgendiagnostik des Kopfes, Berlin theses, 1937.

1939 McNeill, C.: Planos corrientes del craneo, Rev. Radiol. Fis. 6:297-302, 1939.

Sobotta, J.: Atlas of human anatomy, edited from 9th German ed. by McMurrich, J.P., New York, 1939, G.E. Stechert & Co.

1940 Cunningham, D.J.: In Brash, J.C., and Jameson, E.B., editors: Manual of practical anatomy, ed. 10, New York, 1940, Oxford University Press.

1942 Gray, H.: Anatomy of the human body, ed. 24, edited by Lewis, W.H., Philadelphia, 1942, Lea & Febiger.

Greisheimer, E.M.: Physiology and anatomy, ed. 4, Philadelphia, 1942, J.B. Lippincott Co.

1943 Williams, J.F.: A textbook of anatomy and physiology, ed. 7, Philadelphia, 1943, W.B. Saunders Co.

1945 Denley, K.C.: Importance of anatomical study in radiographic positioning, Radiography 11:82-84, 1945.

Vickers, A.A.: Radiographical investigation of diaphragmatic movements, Br. J. Radiol. 18:229-230, 1945.

1946 Appleton, A., Hamilton, W.J., and Tchaperoff, I.C.C.: Surface and radiological anatomy, ed. 2, Baltimore, 1946, The Williams & Wilkins Co.

Bishop, P.A., and Lindskog, G.E.: The diaphragm in relation to the thorax. In Pillmore, G.U., editor: Clinical radiology, vol. 1, Philadelphia, 1946, F.A. Davis Co.

Esposito, J.J.: The diaphragm in relation to the abdomen. In Pillmore, G.U., editor: Clinical radiology, vol. 1, Philadelphia, 1946, F.A. Davis Co.

Henderson, S.G., and Sherman, S.L.: Roentgen anatomy of the skull in the newborn infant, Radiology 46:107-118, 1946.

Mahoney, H.O., Anson, B.J., and Dent, R.F.: Roentgenographic preparations from gross anatomic sections, A.J.R. 56:49-54, 1946.

Sussman, M.L.: Cardiac roentgenography and anatomy. In Pillmore, G.U., editor: Clinical radiology, vol. 1, Philadelphia, 1946, F.A. Davis Co.

1947 Chalton, P., and Malcki, A.: Anatomie radiologique du poumon, J. Radiol. Electrol. 28:285-310, 1947.

1948 Brown, S., and Fine, A.: The diaphragm, Radiology 51:157-166, 1948.

1952 Girdany, B.R., and Golden, R.: Centers of ossification of the skeleton, A.J.R. 68:922-924, 1952.

1959 Meschan, I., and Farrer-Meschen, R.M.F.: An atlas of normal radiographic anatomy, ed. 2, Philadelphia, 1959, W.B. Saunders Co.

1960 Blewett, J.E., and Rackow, A.M.: Anatomy and physiology for radiographers, London and Washington, D.C., 1960, Butterworth & Co., Ltd.

1962 Mallet, M.: A handbook of anatomy and physiology for student x-ray technicians, Fond du Lac, Wis., 1962, American Society of Xray Technicians.

1975 McInnes, J.: Radiographic anatomy, New York, 1975, Appleton-Century-Crofts.

1976 Snell, R.S., and Wyman, A.C.: An atlas of normal radiographic anatomy, Boston, 1976, Little, Brown & Co.

1979 Wicke, L.: Atlas of radiologic anatomy, Baltimore, 1979, Urban & Schwarzenberg, Inc.

1980 Weir, J., et al.: X-ray anatomy, Nurs. Times 76:1-7, 1980.

Upper extremity

1916 Masmonteil, F.: Examen radiologique des fractures diaphysaires de l'avant-bras-position de choix, J. Radiol. Electrol. 2:704-709, 1916-1917.

1918 Laquerrière and Pierquin: De la nécessité d'employer une technique radiographique spéciale pour obtenir certains détails squelettiques, J. Radiol. Electrol. 3:145-148, 1918.

1921 Arcelin, F.: L'exploration radiologique du carpe, J. Radiol. Electrol. 5:349-361, 1921.

Staunig, K.: Die Darstellung der Hand in der Zitherspielerstellung, Fortschr. Roentgenstr. 28:464, 1921-1922.

1924 Buxton, D.: A radiographic survey of normal joints: the elbow joint, Br. J. Radiol. 29:395-410, 1924.

1925 Dress, L.C., and Payne, W.F.: Suggestions in making lateral roentgenograms of the hand, A.J.R. 13:292, 1925.

1926 McBride, E.: Wrist joint injuries: a plea for greater accuracy in treatment, J. Okla. Med. Assoc. 19:67-70, 1926.

1927 Buxton, D.: A radiographic survey of normal joints: the wrist joint and hand, Br. J. Radiol. 32:199-213, 1927.

1928 Belot, J., Lepennetier, F., and Pellizza, J.: Radiodiagnostic de quelques alterations osseuses de l'articulations du coude, J. Radiol. Electrol. 12:457-500, 1928.

1930 Schneider, C.C.: Mechanical devices for immobilizing the head and hand, Xray Techn. 1:70-71, 1930.

1931 Fiolle, J.: Le "carpe bossu," Bull. Soc. Chir. Paris 57:1687, 1931.

1932 Fiolle, J., and Ailland: Nouvelle observation de "carpe bossu," Bull. Soc. Chir. Paris 58:187-188, 1932.

Mills, R.E.: Some common errors in posturing, Radiogr. Clin. Photogr. 8:16-17, 1932.

1933 Archer, V.W., and Rawles, B.W.: Roentgenologic examination of injuries of the wrist joint, South. Med. J. 26:211-214, 1933.

1935 Hill, et al.: Radiography of the wrist and ankle, Radiogr. Clin. Photogr. 11:14-15, 1935.

1937 Stecher, W.R.: Roentgenography of the carpal navicular bone, A.J.R. 37:704-705, 1937.

1938 Alexander, O.M.: Radiography of the wrist, Radiology 4:181-183, 1938.

Perschl, A.: Zur röntgenologischen Diagnostik der frischen Kahnbeinbrüche der Hand, Röntgenpraxis 10:11-16, 1938.

1939 Schmitt, H.: Die röntgenologische Darstellung des Radiusköpfchens, Röntgenpraxis 11:33-36, 1939.

1940 Graziani, A.: L'esame radiologico del carpo, Radiol. Med. 27:382-392, 1940.

1941 Carter, R.M.: Carpal boss: a commonly overlooked deformity of the carpus, J. Bone Joint Surg. 23:935-940, 1941.

Hart, V.L., and Gaynor, V.: Roentgenographic study of the carpal canal, J. Bone Joint Surg. 23:382-383, 1941.

1942 Hart, V.L., and Gaynor, V.: Radiography of the carpal canal, Radiogr. Clin. Photogr. 18:23-24, 1942.

Whitehead, J.: Technique for obtaining a true posteroanterior and true lateral view of the carpal scaphoid bone, Radiology 8:105, 1942.

1943 Lewis, R.W.: Oblique views in roentgenography of the wrist, A.J.R. 50:119-121, 1943.

Shefferin, A.J.: An axial view of the head of the radius, Radiography 9:202-221, 1943.

1944 Burman, M.S., et al.: Fractures of the radial and ulnar axes, A.J.R. 51:455-480, 1944.

1945 Evans, M.E.: Rotational deformity in the treatment of fractures of both bones of the forearm, J. Bone Joint Surg. 27:373-382, 1945.

Holly, E.W.: Radiography of the pisiform bone, Radiogr. Clin. Photogr. 21:69-70, 1945.

1946 Roderick, J.F.: The roentgenographic examination of the carpus, Xray Techn. 18:8-11, 1946.

1947 Cleveland, M.: Fracture of the carpal scaphoid, Surg. Gynecol. Obstet. 84:769-771, 1947.

Perkins, B.: Radiography of the carpus, Radiography 13:8-10, 1947.

1948 Jacobs, L.G.: Isolated fracture of the pisiform bone, Radiology 50:529-531, 1948.

1949 Bridgman, C.F.: Radiography of the carpal navicular bone, Med. Radiogr. Photogr. 25:104-105, 1949.

1951 Alexander, O.M.: Radiography of the carpal scaphoid bone in inclined planes, Radiography 17:14-15, 1951.

1954 Wilson, J.N.: Profiles of the carpal canal, J. Bone Joint Surg. 36-A:127-132, 1954.

1956 Dorosin, N., and Davis, J.G.: Carpal boss, Radiology 66:234-236, 1956.

Holly, E.W.: Radiography of the radial head, Med. Radiogr. Photogr. 32:13-14, 1956.

1957 Lentino, W., et al.: The carpal-bridge view: a position for the roentgenographic diagnosis of abnormalities in the dorsum of the wrist, J. Bone Joint Surg. 39-A:88-90, 1957.

Viehweger, G.: Zum Problem der Deutung der knöchernen Gebilde distal des Epikondylus medialis humeri, Fortschr. Roentgenstr. 86:643-652, 1957.

1958 Burman, M.: Anteroposterior projection of the carpometacarpal joint of the thumb by radial shift of the carpal tunnel view, J. Bone Joint Surg. 40-A:1156-1157, 1958.

Stripp, W.J.: Radiography of the ulnar groove and of the carpal tunnel, Radiography 24:277-280, 1958.

1960 Bing, B.: Radiographic demonstration of the scaphoid fracture, Xray Techn. 31:380-381, 1960.

Russe, O.: Fracture of the carpal navicular, J. Bone Joint Surg. 42-A:759-768, 1960.

Vasilas, A., et al.: Roentgen aspects of injuries to the pisiform bone and pisotriquetral joint, J. Bone Joint Surg. 42-A:1317-1328, 1960.

1964 Templeton, A.W., and Zim, I.D.: The carpal tunnel view, Mo. Med. 61:443-444, 1964.

1965 Nørgaard, F.: Earliest roentgenological changes in polyarthritis of the rheumatoid type: rheumatoid arthritis, Radiology 85:325-329, 1965.

337

1966 Gramiak, R.: Oblique radiography of the hands, Med. Radiogr. Photogr. **42**:28-29, 1966.

1974 Gramiak, R.: Radiological case of the month: Monteggia fracture, Md. State Med. J. **23**:23-24, 1974.

Reichmann, S., et al.: Soft-tissue radiography of finger joints, Acta Radiol. **15**:439-448, 1974.

1975 Eto, R.T., Anderson, P.W., and Harley, J.D.: Elbow arthrography with the application of tomography, Radiology **115**:283-288, 1975.

Resnick, D.: Roentgenographic anatomy of the tendon sheaths of the hand and wrist: tenography, A.J.R. **124**:44-51, 1975.

1976 Rappoport, A.S., Sosman, J.L., and Weissman, B.N.: Spontaneous fractures of the olecranon process in rheumatoid arthritis, Radiology **119**:83-84, 1976.

1977 Horsman, A., et al.: Effect of rotation on radiographic dimensions of the humerus and femur, Br. J. Radiol. **50**:23-28, 1977.

Murphy, W.A., and Siegel, M.J.: Elbow fat pads with new signs and extended differential diagnosis, Radiology **124**:659-665, 1977.

Yeh, H.C., and Wolf, B.S.: Radiographic anatomical landmarks of the metacarpophalangeal joints, Radiology **122**:353-355, 1977.

1978 Hayes, N., Gerard, F.M., and Burkhalter, W.E.: Air gap magnification techniques in upper extremity fractures, Clin. Orthop. **131**:173-175, 1978.

Kaye, J.J.: Fractures and dislocations of the hand and wrist. Semin. Roentgenol. **13**:109-116, 1978.

Kaye, J.J., and Lister, G.D.: Another use for the Brewerton view, J. Hand Surg. **3**:603, 1978.

Rogers, L.F.: Fractures and dislocations of the elbow, Semin. Roentgenol. **13**:97-107, 1978.

1979 Khanna, K.K., and Kiran, S.: Radiological study at wrist and elbow–epiphyseal fusion with diaphysis, Indian J. Med. Sci. **33**:121-125, 1979.

Silberstein, M.J., Brodeur, A.E., and Graviss, E.R.: Some vagaries of the capitellum, J. Bone and Joint Surg. **61**:244-247, 1979.

1980 Danzig, L.A., Greenway, G., and Resnick, D.: The Hill-Sachs lesion: an experimental study, Am. J. Sports Med. **8**:328,332, 1980.

Desautels, J.E., Radomsky, J.W., and Erickson, L.M.; Evaluation of mammography unit and rare earth screens for high resolution hand radiography, J. Can. Assoc. Radiol. **31**:185-186, 1980.

1980 Fodor, J., and Malott, J.C.: Radiography of the carpal navicular, Radiol. Technol. **52**:175-180, 1980.

Jones, R.P., and Leach, R.E.: Fracture of the ulnar sesamoid bone of the thumb, Am. J. Sports Med. **8**:446-447, 1980.

Rosenthal, D., Murray, W.T., and Smith, R.J.: Finger arthrography, Radiology **137**:647-651, 1980.

1981 De Smet, A.A., et al.: Radiographic projections for the diagnosis of arthritis of the hands and wrists, Radiology **139**:577-581, 1981.

Lower extremity

1907 Haenisch, H.: Diskussionsbemerkung, Verhandl. Deutsch. Röentgengesell. **3**:54, 1907.

1909 Settegast, H.: Fraktur des calcaneus und röntgenographische Diagnose derselben, Verhandl. Deutsch. Röentgengesell. **5**:114-117, 1909.

1910 Kuchendorf: Drei Fälle von Längsbrüchen der Kniescheibe mittels schräger Durchleuchtung festgestellt, Fortschr. Roentgenstr. **15**:368-369, 1910.

1922 Walters, R.A.: Radiography of the os calcis, J. Radiol. **3**:493-494, 1922.

1923 Scott, E.: Technique radiography of the knee joint, Arch. Radiol. Electrol. **28**:57-58, 1923.

1924 Béclère, H.: La radiographie des films courbes, Paris, 1924, Amédée Legrand.

Marchand, J.H.: La radiographie sur films courbes, Paris theses, 1924.

Schütze, T.: Die isolierte Darstellung der distalen Fusswurzel und der Mittelfussknochen bei der Röntgenaufnahme, Fortschr. Roentgenstr. **32**:121, 1924.

1925 Belot, J., Talon, and Nadal: A propos des films courbes, J. Radiol. Electrol. **9**:454, 1925.

1926 Conn, A.R.: Fractures of the os calcis, Radiology **6**:228-235, 1926.

Slomann, H.C.: On the demonstration and analysis of calcaneonavicular coalition by roentgen examination, Acta Radiol. **5**:304-312, 1926.

1927 Altschul, W.: Some new methods in roentgenography, A.J.R. **17**:659-666, 1927.

Badgley, C.E.: Coalition of the calcaneus and the navicular, Arch. Surg. **15**:75-88, 1927.

Lillienfeld, L.: Anordnung der normalisierten Röntgenaufnahmen des menschlichen Körpers, ed. 4, Berlin, 1927, Urban & Schwarzenberg, Inc., p. 36.

1929 Hülten, O.: Ueber die indirekten Bröche des Tibiakopfes nebst Beiträgen zur Röntgenologie des Kniegelenks, Acta Chir. Scandinav. **15**(suppl.):66, 1929.

1930 Petrignani, R.: Étude radiologique de la maladie de Pellegrini-Stieda, J. Radiol. **14**:544, 1930.

1931 Doub, H.P.: A useful position for examining the foot, Radiology **16**:764-766, 1931.

1932 Colaneri and Laguiere: Les fractures du scaphoide tarsien, J. Radiol. Electrol. **16**:68, 1932.

Dittmar, O.: Der Kniegelenks-Meniskus im Röntgenbilde, Röntgenpraxis **4**:442-445, 1932.

Frik, K.: Neue Röntgenuntersuchungen am Kniegelenk, Verhandl. Deutsch. Röntgengesell. **24-25**:155, 1932.

Grasman: Die exacte Messung der Malleolengabelverbreitung, München. Med. Woch. **79**:1721, 1932.

Popovic, L., and Doric, L.: Beitrag zur Röntgenuntersuchung des Kniegelenks, Röntgenpraxis **4**:905-910, 1932.

Regele-Bozen, H.: Die Verletzungen des inneren Seitenbandes des Kniegelenks, München. Med. Woch. **79**:1474-1476, 1932.

Stankiewics, Z.: A propos d'un cas d'ostéochondrite de l'os sésamoide du gros orteil, J. Radiol. **16**:65, 1932.

1935 Danelius, G., and Miller, F.L.: Roentgen examination of the intercondyloid fossa of the knee joint, Radiology **25**:605-608, 1935.

Felsenreich, F.: Darstellung des verletzten Meniscus medialis im Röntgenbild bei veralterter Kreuzbandund Seitenbandverletzung, Röntgenpraxis **7**:331-333, 1935.

Hellmer, H.: Röntgenologische Beobachtungen über die Ossifikationen der Patella, Acta Radiol. **27**(suppl.):112-114, 1935.

Hill, et al.: Radiography of wrist and ankle, Radiogr. Clin. Photogr. **11**:14-15, 1935.

Kaiser, R.: Die röntgenologische Darstellung der Fossa intercondyloidea und ihre Bedeutung für die Kniegelenkediagnostik (Frik's method), Bruns' Beitr. Klin. Chir. **161**:528, 1935.

1936 Allen, N.S.: Radiography of the os calcis, Radiology **2**:145-146, 1936.

Laarman, A.: Darstellung des Knieinnern im Röntgenbild, Arch. Klin. Chir. **187**:234-251, 1936-1937.

Thomsen, W.: Vorrichtung für Aufnahme des Fusskelettes unter Belastung zum Messen der Weichteile, Röntgenpraxis **8**:241-242, 1936.

Widmann, B.P., and Stecher, W.R.: Roentgenographic demonstration of the true articular space, Radiology **27**:541-544, 1936.

1937 Holmblad, E.C.: Postero-anterior x-ray view of the knee in flexion, J.A.M.A. **109**:1196-1197, 1937.

Lachman, E.: Roentgen anatomy of the knee joint, Radiology **29**:455, 1937.

Scott, V.M.: Radiography of the os calcis, Radiology **3**:28-30, 1937.

Zweifel, C.: Zur Röntgendiagnostik der Patella, Röntgenpraxis **9**:313-318, 1937.

1938 Guntz, E.: Ein Gerät für sämtliche Röntgenaufnahmen der Füsse mit und ohne Belastung in genauer Einstellung, Röntgenpraxis **10**:17-23, 1938.

Holmgren, B.S.: Variationem im Röntgenbild des normalen ersten Metatarsophalangealgelenks bedingt durch kleine Änderungen in der Richtung des Zentralstrahls, Acta Radiol. **19**:67-72, 1938.

Lewis, R.W.: Non-routine views in roentgen examination of the extremities, Surg. Gynecol. Obstet. **69**:38-45, 1938.

Löhr, R., and Hellpap, W.: Der Kniegelenkspalt im Röntgenbild, Fortschr. Roentgenstr. **58**:45-56, 1938.

Piotrowski, Brother D.: Oblique view of the ankle joint and foot, A.J.R. **45:**127-128, 1938.

Wordhein, Y.: Eine neue Methode, den Gelenkknorpel besonders die Kniegelenks-Menisken, roentgenologisch darzustellen, Fortschr. Roentgenstr. **57:**479-495, 1938.

1939 Alexander, O.M.: The utility of the curved cassette, Radiography **5:**57, 1939.

Genders, R.A.: The os calcis, Xray Techn. **11:**60, 1939.

Holmblad, E.C.: Improved x-ray technic in studying knee joints, South. Med. J. **32:**240-243, 1939.

Kite, J.H.: Principles involved in the treatment of congenital clubfoot, J. Bone Joint Surg. **21:**595-606, 1939.

1940 Evans, W.A.: Roentgenological demonstration of true articular space, A.J.R. **43:**860, 1940.

Lindblom, K.: Roentgenographic symptoms of meniscal lesion in the knee joint, Acta Radiol. **21:**274-285, 1940.

Piotrowski, Brother D.: The knee joint, Xray Techn. **12:**45-46, 1940.

1941 Knutsson, F.: Ueber die Röntgenologie des Femoropatellargelenks sowie eine gute Projection für das Kniegelenk, Acta Radiol. **22:**371-376, 1941.

Santora, P.J.: Anteroposterior view of the ankle joint and foot, A.J.R. **45:**127-128, 1941.

1942 Marique, P.: La réintégration non sanglante de l'astragale, Rev. Orthop. **28:**37-50, 1942.

1943 Anthonsen, W.: An oblique projection for roentgen examination of the talocalcaneal joint, particularly in intra-articular fracture of calcaneus, Acta Radiol. **24:**306-310, 1943.

Ball, R.P., and Egbert, E.W.: Ruptured ligaments of the ankle, A.J.R. **50:**770-771, 1943.

Cahoon, J.B.: Radiography of the foot, Xray Techn. **15:**13, 15, 1943.

Causton, J.: Projection of sesamoid bones in the region of the first metatarsophalangeal joint, Radiology **9:**39, 1943.

Gamble, F.O.: A special approach to foot radiography, Radiogr. Clin. Photogr. **19:**78-80, 1943.

Knish, M.: The knee, Xray Techn. **14:**200-201, 1943.

1944 Berridge, F.R., and Bonnin, J.B.: The radiographic examination of the ankle joint including arthrography, Surg. Gynecol. Obstet. **79:**383-389, 1944.

Camp, J.D., and Coventry, M.B.: Use of special views in roentgenography of the knee joint, U.S. Nav. Med. Bull. **42:**56-58, 1944.

Long, L.: Non-injection method for roentgenographic visualization of the internal semilunar cartilage, A.J.R. **52:**269-280, 1944.

Mohr, S.: Special consideration in radiography of the knee and ankle, Xray Techn. **16:**7-12, 1944.

Piotrowski, Brother D.: An instrument to facilitate the making of oblique views of the ankle joint, Xray Techn. **16:**62-65, 1944.

1945 Gershon-Cohen, J.: Internal derangements of the knee joint: the diagnostic scope of the soft tissue roentgen examinations and the vacuum technique demonstration of the menisci, A.J.R. **54:**337-347, 1945.

Grossman, J.D., and Minor, H.H.: Roentgen demonstration of the semilunar cartilages of the knee, A.J.R. **53:**454-465, 1945.

Marique, P.: L'examen radiographique du pied bot (Roentgenographic examination of club foot), Presse Méd. **53:**633-634, 1945.

Pendergrass, E.P., and Lafferty, J.O.: Roentgen study of the ankle in severe sprains and dislocations, Radiology **45:**40-45, 1945.

Simon, R.S.: A third routine x-ray exposure of the ankle joint, J. Bone Joint Surg. **27:**520, 1945.

1946 Bonnet, W.L., and Baker, D.R.: Diagnosis of pes planus by x-ray, Radiology **46:**36-45, 1946.

Cahoon, J.B.: Radiography of the foot, Radiogr. Clin. Photogr. **22:**2-9, 1946.

Hendelberg, T.: Roentgenographic examination of ankle joint in malleolar fractures, Acta Radiol. **27:**23-42, 1946.

Jones, H.: Radiography of the knee for internal derangement, Xray Techn. **17:**390-393, 408, 1946.

Moreau, H.M., Bertani, G.C. and Moreau, G.E.: Mediciones angulares en el estudio radiologico del valguismo y varismo del pie, Radiologica **9:**65-75, 1946.

Runge, R.K.: The roentgenographic examination of the knee joint, Xray Techn. **18:**97-100, 1946.

Wilner, D.: Diagnostic problems in fractures of the foot and ankle, A.J.R. **55:**594-616, 1946.

1947 Carter, D.R.: Radiographic examination of the knee joint, Xray Techn. **19:**77, 82, 1947.

Crawford, H.B., and Bridgman, C.F.: Radiography of injured lower extremities, Med. Radiogr. Photogr. **23:**31-33, 1947.

Weismann, J.C.: An improved technique for the roentgen demonstration of the semilunar cartilages of the knee, A.J.R. **58:**255-256, 1947.

1948 Harris, R.I., and Beath, T.: Etiology of peroneal spastic flatfoot, J. Bone Joint Surg. **30-B:**624-634, 1948.

Kestler, O.C.: Traumatic instability of the ankle joint, A.J.R. **60:**498-504, 1948.

Palmer, I.: The mechanism and treatment of fractures of the calcaneus, J. Bone Joint Surg. **30-A:**2-8, 1948.

1949 Broden, B.: Roentgen examination of the subtaloid joint in fractures of the calcaneus, Acta Radiol. **31:**85-91, 1949.

Odell, O.E.: Lateral knee technique, Xray Techn. **20:**274, 1949.

1950 Chambers, C.H.: Congenital anomalies of the tarsal navicular, Br. J. Radiol. **23:**580-586, 1950.

Coventry, M.B.: Flatfoot with special consideration of tarsal coalition, Minn. Med. **33:**1091-1097, 1950.

Vaughan, F.M.A.: Lateral knees, Radiography **16:**75-77, 1950.

Wilson, G.E.: Fractures of the calcaneus, J. Bone Joint Surg. **32-A:**59-70, 1950.

1951 Alexander, O.M.: Routine lateral radiography of the knee and ankle joints, Radiography **17:**10-11, 1951.

1952 Burdick, A.V.: Calcaneus, Xray Techn. **23:**276-277, 1952.

Kandel, B.: The suroplantar projection in the congenital clubfoot of the infant, Acta Orthop. Scand. **22:**161-173, 1952.

1953 Vaughan, W.H., and Segal, G.: Tarsal coalition with special reference to roentgenographic interpretation, Radiology **60:**855-863, 1953.

1954 Lauge-Hansen, N.: Fractures of the ankle, A.J.R. **71:**456-471, 1954.

Sonnenschein, A.: Roentgenographic visualization of the patella, J. Bone Joint Surg. **36-A:**109-112, 1954.

1955 Davis, L.A., and Hatt, W.S.: Congenital abnormalities of the feet, Radiology **64:**818-825, 1955.

Denny, J.C., and Lyons, N.J.: Radiography of the talocalcaneal articulations, Xray Techn. **26:**245-248, 1955.

Holly, E.W.: Radiography of the tarsal sesamoid bones, Med. Radiogr. Photogr. **31:**73, 1955.

1956 March, H.C., and London, R.I.: The os sustentaculi, A.J.R. **76:**1114-1118, 1956.

Wentzlik, G.: Zur Einstelltechnik des oberen Sprung-gelenkes, Fortschr. Roentgenstr. **84:**362-365, 1956.

1958 Denny, J.C., and Lyons, N.J.: Radiography of the knee, Xray Techn. **30:**87-91, 1958.

Kreppert, L.C.: A modified axial view of the patella, Xray Techn. **29:**375-377, 1958.

1960 Funke, T.: Radiography of the knee joint, Med. Radiogr. Photogr. **36:**1-37, 1960.

Scheller, S.: Roentgenographic studies on epiphyseal growth and ossification in the knee, Acta Radiol. **195**(suppl.):12-16, 1960.

1961 Isherwood, I.: A radiological approach to the subtalar joint, J. Bone Joint Surg. **43-B:**566-574, 1961.

Kleiger, B., and Mankin, H.J.: A roentgenographic study of the development of the calcaneus by means of posterior tangential view, J. Bone Joint Surg. **43-A:**961-969, 1961.

1962 Feist, J.H., and Mankin, H.J.: The tarsus: basic relationships and motions in the adult and definition of optimal recumbent oblique projection, Radiology **79:**250-263, 1962.

Graham, D., and Rorrison, J.: Radiography of the tarsal bones, Radiography **28:**156-163, 1962.

339

1964   Kite, J.H.: The clubfoot, New York, 1964, Grune & Stratton, Inc.

Willets, C., and Gerdes, R.A.: Radiographic improvement through application of anatomical stress, Radiol. Technol. **36**:176-178, 1964.

1965   Harris, J.: Radiography of the lower limb, Radiography **31**:235-248, 1965.

Templeton, A.W., et al.: Standardization of terminology and evaluation of osseous relationships in congenitally abnormal feet. A.J.R. **93**:374-381, 1965.

1968   Ahlbäck, S.: Osteoarthrosis of the knee: a radiographic investigation, Acta Radiol. [Diagn.] **277**(suppl.):7-72, 1968.

1969   Conway, J.J., and Cowell, H.R.: Tarsal coalition: clinical significance and roentgenographic demonstration, Radiology **92**:799-811, 1969.

1970   Freiberger, R.H., Hersh, A., and Harrison, M.O.: Roentgen examination of the deformed foot, Semin. Roentgenol. **5**:341-353, 1970.

James, A.E., Jr.: Tarsal coalitions and peroneal spastic flat foot, Australas. Radiol. **14**:80-83, 1970.

Leach, R.E., Gregg, T., and Siber, F.J.: Weight-bearing radiography in osteoarthritis of the knee, Radiology **97**:265-268, 1970.

Meschan, I.: Radiology of the normal foot, Semin. Roentgenol. **5**:327-340, 1970.

Zatkin, H.R.: Trauma to the foot, Semin. Roentgenol. **5**:419-435, 1970.

1971   Mandell, J.: Isolated fractures of the posterior tibial lip at the ankle as demonstrated by an additional projection, the "poor" lateral view, Radiology **101**:319-322, 1971.

1973   Dalinka, M.K., Gohel, V.K., and Rancier, L.: Tomography in the evaluation of the anterior cruciate ligament, Radiology **108**:31-33, 1973.

Gattereau, A., et al.: An improved radiological method for the evaluation of achilles tendon xanthomatosis, Can. Med. Assoc. J. **108**:39-42, 1973.

1974   Anderson, P.W., and Maslin, P.: Tomography applied to knee arthrography, Radiology **110**:271-275, 1974.

Blass, B.C., Imanuel, H.M., and Marcus, S.: Technique for radiographic digital isolation, J. Am. Podiatry Assoc. **64**:870-873, 1974.

Merchant, A.C., et al.: Roentgenographic analysis of patellofemoral congruence, J. Bone Joint Surg. **56**:1391-1396, 1974.

1975   Flynn, M., Moulton, A., and Rose, G.K.: A simple method of obtaining a lateral radiograph of the head and neck of the femur, Injury **6**:246-247, 1975.

Gamble, F.O., and Yale, I.: Clinical foot roentgenology, Huntington, N.Y., 1975, R.E. Krieger Publishing Co., Inc.

Resnick, D.: The interphalangeal joint of the great toe in rheumatoid arthritis, J. Can. Assoc. Radiol. **26**:255-262, 1975.

1976   Cobey, J.C.: Posterior roentgenogram of the foot, Clin. Orthop. **118**:202-207, 1976.

Elstrom, J., et al.: The use of tomography in the assessment of fractures of the tibial plateau, J. Bone Joint Surg. **58**:551-555, 1976.

1977   Goergen, T.G., et al.: Roentgenographic evaluation of the tibiotalar joint, J. Bone Joint Surg. **59**:874-877, 1977.

Horsman, A., et al.: Effect of rotation on radiographic dimensions of the humerus and femur, Br. J. Radiol. **50**:23-28, 1977.

McCrea, J.D., et al.: Effects of radiographic technique on the metatarsophalangeal joints, J. Am. Podiatry Assoc. **67**:837-840, 1977.

Moore, T.H., and Meyers, M.H.: Apparatus to position knees for varus-valgus stress roentgenograms, J. Bone Joint Surg. **59**:984, 1977.

Winiecki, D.G., and Biggs, E.W.: Xeroradiography and its application in podiatry, J. Am. Podiatry Assoc. **67**:393-400, 1977.

1978   Diamond, M.J.: The uprite lateral exposure: a new view for podiatric radiology, J. Am. Podiatry Assoc. **68**:47-52, 1978.

Edeiken, J., and Cotler, J.M.: Ankle injury: the need for stress films. J.A.M.A. **240**:1182-1184, 1978.

Kehr, L.E.: Radiology: a simplified axial view, J. Am. Podiatry Assoc. **68**:130-131, 1978.

Rogers, L.F., and Campbell, R.E.: Fractures and dislocations of the foot, Semin. Roentgenol. **13**:157-166, 1978.

Throckmorton, J.K., and Gudas, C.J.: Radiographic axial sesamoid projection in the diagnosis of sesamoid fractures: two case reports, J. Am. Podiatry Assoc. **68**:96-100, 1978.

1979   Laurin, C.A., Dussault, R., and Levesque, H.P.: The tangential x-ray investigation of the patello-femoral joint: x-ray technique, diagnostic criteria, and their interpretation, Clin. Orthop. **144**:16-26, 1979.

1980   Newberg, A.H., and Seligson, D.: The patellofemoral joint: 30 degrees, 60 degrees, and 90 degrees views, Radiology **137**:57-60, 1980.

Norfray, J.F., et al.: Common calcaneal avulsion fracture, A.J.R. **134**:119-123, 1980.

1981   Bradley, W.G., and Ominsky, S.H.: Mountain view of the patella, A.J.R. **136**:53-58, 1981.

Protas, J.M., and Kornblatt, B.A.: Fractures of the lateral margin of the distal tibia: the Tillaux fracture, Radiology **138**:55-57, 1981.

Extremities—general

1915   Case, J.T.: Bone and joint lesions: necessity for constant technique in roentgenography, Interstate Med. J. **22**:584-597, 1915.

McKendrick, A.: Radiography of normal parts, Arch. Radiol. Electrol. **20**:243-259, 285-295, 1915-1916.

1918   Laquerrière and Pierquin: De la nécessité d'employer une technique radiographique spéciale pour obtenir certains détails squelettiques, J. Radiol. Electrol. **3**:145-148, 1918.

1924   Marchand, J.H.: Technique de l'examen des articulations sur film courbe, Paris thèses 102, chap. 2, Paris, 1924, Amédée Legrand.

1927   Altschul, W.: Some new methods in roentgenography, A.J.R. **17**:659-666, 1927.

1930   Dittmar, O.: Weitere Mitteilungen über Schrägaufnahmen von Knochen und Gelenken, Röntgenpraxis **2**:1022, 1930.

1932   Leman, R.M.: General technique for radiography of the joints, Br. J. Radiol. **5**:501-512, 1932.

Thompson, M.: Variations of standard positions in taking radiographs, Xray Techn. **4**:18-20, 1932.

1933   Longervy, T., and Stecher, W.R.: Useful procedures in radiologic practice, Radiology **20**:225-230, 1933.

1935   Baer, A.: Cast problem in radiography, Xray Techn. **7**:66-67, 93, 1935.

1936   Eller, V.H.: Extremities, Xray Techn. **7**:114-117, 135, 1936.

Thompson, M.: Technic and position in radiography of the skeleton, Xray Techn. **8**:9-10, 31, 1936.

1937   Thomas, M.A.: The importance of a thorough examination in radiographic diagnosis, Xray Techn. **8**:103-106, 1937.

Wolcott, R.: Technics for unusual cases, Xray Techn. **9**:38-42, 1937.

1938   Garland, H.L.: The roentgen diagnosis of fractures and dislocations, Diagn. Roentgenol. **2**:827-854, 1938.

Leman, R.M.: Some radiographic techniques, Radiology **4**:41-44, 1938.

Lewis, R.W.: Nonroutine views in roentgen examination of the extremities, Surg. Gynecol. Obstet. **67**:38-45, 1938.

Nordhein, Y.: Eine neue Methode, den Gelenkknorpel, besonders die Kniegelenks-Menisken, roentgenologisch darzustellen, Fortschr. Roentgenstr. **57**:479-495, 1938.

Potter, C.F.: Roentgenologic considerations of certain joint injuries, Am. J. Surg. **42**:785-790, 1938.

1939   Rubin, E.L.: The delineation of articular cartilage by x-rays without the aid of contrast media, Br. J. Radiol. **12**:649-657, 1939.

1940   Kahle, L.M.: Solutions to some problems in x-ray technique, Xray Techn. **11**:172-174, 206, 1940.

1941   Larsen, R.M.: Radiography of extremities, Xray Techn. **12**:215-216, 1941.

Thvelkeld, A.: Routine for fracture clinics, Xray Techn. **13**:110-111, 141, 1941.

1942   Ashwin, C.: Economy in radiography, Radiology **8**:121, 1942.

Colson, D.H.: Inventive radiographic positions, Xray Techn. **14**:59-61, 1942.

1943   Eller, V.H.: Special multiple views as diagnostic aid to the radiologist, Xray Techn. **15**:51-54, 1943.

Lewis, R.W.: El estudio roentgenográfico de tejidos blandos en un hospital para ortopedia, Rev. Radiol. Fis. **10:**147-155, 1943.

1944 Zintheo, C.J.: Extremity radiography with no-screen film, Xray Techn. **16:**115, 1944.

1945 Champness, L.J.: Variations of routine techniques, Radiography **11:**17-20, 1945.

1947 Garland, H.L.: The roentgen diagnosis of fractures and dislocations. In Golden, R., editor: Diagnostic roentgenology, ed. 3, vol. 2, New York, 1947, Thomas Nelson & Sons.

Hodges, P.C., Phemister, D.B., and Brunschwig, A.: The roentgen-ray diagnosis of diseases of bones. In Golden, R., editor: Diagnostic roentgenology, ed. 3, vol. 1, New York, 1947, Thomas Nelson & Sons.

1949 Forsyth, H.H.: Some clinical examples of the value of supplemental radiographs, Med. Radiogr. Photogr. **25:**34-40, 1949.

1964 Willets, C., and Gerdes, R.A.: Radiographic improvement through application of anatomical stress, Radiol. Technol. **36:**176-178, 1964.

1967 Parlee, D.E., Freundlick, I.M., and McCarty, D.J.: A comparative study of roentgenographic techniques for detection of calcium pyrophosphate dihydrate deposits (pseudogout) in human cartilage, A.J.R. **99:**688-694, 1967.

1969 Wolfe, J.N.: Xeroradiography of bones, joints and soft tissues, Radiology **93:**583-587, 1969.

1970 Rogers, L.F.: The radiography of epiphyseal injuries, Radiology **96:**289-299, 1970.

1975 Genant, H.K., Doi, K., and Mall, J.C.: Optical versus radiographic magnification for fine-detail skeletal radiography, Invest. Radiol. **10:**160-172, 1975.

1976 Genant, H.K., Doi, K., and Mall, J.C.: Comparison of non-screen techniques (medical vs. industrial film) for fine detail skeletal radiography, Invest. Radiol. **11:**486-500, 1976.

1977 Genant, H.K., et al.: Direct radiographic magnification for skeletal radiology: an assessment of image quality and clinical application, Radiology **123:**47-55, 1977.

Goodman, D.A., Wells, C.A., and Weston, P.J.: An evaluation of some screen film combinations for use in radiography of the extremities, Radiography **43**(515):253-255, 1977.

1978 Resnick, D.: Skeletal aches and pains, Radiol. Clin. North Am. **16:**37-47, 1978.

1979 Spencer, J.D., and Hill, I.D.: Imaging factors for xeroradiography of the extremities, Br. J. Radiol. **52:**51-55, 1979.

Long bone measurement

1924 Hickey, P.M.: Teleoroentgenography as an aid in orthopedic measurements, A.J.R. **11:**232-233, 1924.

1937 Millwee, R.H.: Slit scanography, Radiology **28:**483-486, 1937.

1942 Gill, G.G., and Abbott, L.C.: Practical method of predicting growth of femur and tibia in the child, Arch. Surg. **45:**286-315, 1942.

Merrill, O.E.: A method for the roentgen measurement of the long bones, A.J.R. **48:**405-406, 1942.

1944 Gill, G.G.: A simple roentgenographic method for the measurement of bone growth: modification of Millwee's method of slit scanography, J. Bone Joint Surg. **26:**767-769, 1944.

1946 Green, W.T., Wyatt, G.M., and Anderson, M.: Orthoroentgenography as a method of measuring the bones of the lower extremities, J. Bone Joint Surg. **28:**60-65, 1946.

Rush, W.A., and Steiner, H.A.: A study of lower extremity length inequality, A.J.R. **56:**616-623, 1946.

1949 Cartwright, L.J.: Orthoroentgenography as applied to the lower extremities of children, Radiography **15:**234-235, 1949.

Mueller, W.K., and Higganson, J.M.: Spot scanography: a method of determining bone measurement, A.J.R. **61:**402-403, 1949.

1950 Bell, J.S., and Thomson, W.A.L.: Modified spot scanography, A.J.R. **63:**915-916, 1950.

Goldstein, L.A., and Dreisinger, F.: Spot orthoroentgenography: a method for measuring the length of the bones of the lower extremity, J. Bone Joint Surg. **32-A:**449-452, 1950.

1952 Sandaa, E.: Orthoroentgenographic measurement of long bones, Acta Orthop. Scand. **22:**76-79, 1952.

Sevastikoglou, J.: A simple application of orthoroentgenography, Acta Orthop. Scand. **22:**80-84, 1952.

1953 Farill, J.: Orthoradiographic measurement of shortening of the lower extremity, Med. Radiogr. Photogr. **29:**32-38, 1953.

1954 Kumpel, K.: Bone length radiography, Xray Techn. **25:**265-267, 1954.

Kunkle, H.M., and Carpenter, E.B.: A simple technique for x-ray measurement of limb-length discrepancies, J. Bone Joint Surg. **36-A:**152-154, 1954.

1955 Lewis, M.G.: Investigation of scanography, Xray Techn. **26:**327-333, 1955.

1961 Holohan, F.: Modified spot scanography, Xray Techn. **33:**106-112, 1961.

1966 Pugh, D.G., and Winkler, N.T.: Scanography of leg-length measurement: an easy satisfactory method, Radiology **87:**130-133, 1966.

Woodruff, J.H., Jr., and Lane, G.: A technique for slit scanography, A.J.R. **96:**907-912, 1966.

1977 Gore, D.R., et al.: Roentgenographic measurement after Muller total hip replacement, J. Bone Joint Surg. **59:**948-953, 1977.

Horsman, A., et al.: Effect of rotation on radiographic dimensions of the humerus and femur. Br. J. Radiol. **50:**23-28, 1977.

1979 Ogata, K., and Goldsand, E.M.: A simple, biplanar method of measuring femoral anteversion and neck-shaft angle, J. Bone Joint Surg. **61:**846-851, 1979.

1980 Weiner, D.S., and Cook, A.J.: Practical considerations in the use of computed tomography in the measurement of femoral anteversion, Isr. J. Med. Sci. **16:**288-294, 1980.

Contrast arthrography

1905 Robinsohn and Werndorff: Ueber eine neue röntgenologische Methode (Sauerstoffinsufflation) zur Untersuchung der Gelenke und Weichteile, Verhandl. Deutsch. Röntgengesell. **1:**161, 1905.

1907 Kaisin: Emploi du gaz oxygène pour la radiographie des articulations, J. Belg. Radiol. **1:**61-69, 1907.

1931 Bircher, E.: Pneumoradiographie des Knies und der anderen Gelenke, Schweiz. Med. Wochenschr. **61:**1210-1211, 1931.

1933 Bircher, E.: Ueber Binnenverletzungen des Kniegelenks, Arch. Clin. Chir. **177:**290-359, 1933.

1936 Simon, T., Hamilton, S.A., and Farrington, L.C.: Pneumography of the knee, Radiology **27:**533-539, 1936.

1937 Leveuf, J., and Bertrand, P.: L'arthrographie dans la luxation congénitale de la hanche, Presse Méd. **23:**437-440, 1937.

1938 Lindblom, K.: Arthrographic appearance of the ligaments of the knee joint, Acta Radiol. **19:**582-600, 1938.

Oberholzer, J.: Röntgendiagnostik des Gelenkes mittels Doppelkontrast-methode, Leipzig, 1938, Georg Thieme.

1939 Lindblom, K.: Arthrography and roentgenography in ruptures of the tendons of the shoulder joint, Acta Radiol. **20:**548-562, 1939.

1941 Axen, O.: Ueber den Wert des Arthrographie des Schultergelenkes, Acta Radiol. **22:**269, 1941.

Hansson, C.J.: Arthrographic studies of the ankle joint, Acta Radiol. **22:**281-287, 1941.

1944 Andersen, J.: Some experiences with a new method for arthrography, Acta Radiol. **25:**33-39, 1944.

Berridge, F.R., and Bonnin, J.B.: The radiographic examination of the ankle joint including arthrography, Surg. Gynecol. Obstet. **79:**383-387, 1944.

Glazebrook, L.: Air arthrography of the knee joint, Radiography **10:**43-44, 1944.

Hauch, P.P.: Pneumoroentgenography of the knee joint, Br. J. Radiol. **17:**70-74, 1944.

Nørgaard, F.: Arthrography of the mandible joint, Acta Radiol. **25:**679-685, 1944.

1945 Brooke, H.W., Mackenzie, W.C., and Smith, J.R.: Pneumoroentgenography with oxygen in the diagnosis of internal derangements of the knee joint, A.J.R. **54:**462-469, 1945.

McGaw, W.H., and Weckesser, E.G.: Pneumoarthrograms of the knee, J. Bone Joint Surg. **27:**432-445, 1945.

341

1946 Jacobsen, H.H.: On the normal arthrogram of the mandibular joint, Acta Radiol. 27:93-97, 1946.

Somerville, E.W.: Air arthrography as an aid to the diagnosis of lesions of the menisci of the knee joint, J. Bone Joint Surg. 28:451-465, 1946.

1947 Meschan, I., and McGaw, W.H.: New methods of pneumoarthrography of the knee with an evaluation of the procedure in 315 operated cases, Radiology 49:675-711, 1947.

Nørgaard, F.: Temporomandibular arthrography, Copenhagen, 1947, E. Munksgaard Publishing Co.

1948 Andersen, K.: Pneumoarthrography of the knee joint with particular reference to the semilunar cartilages, Acta Orthop. Scand. 4(suppl.):3-108, 1948.

Lindblom, J.: Arthrography of the knee: roentgenographic and anatomic study, Acta Radiol. 74(suppl.):1-112, 1948.

1949 Kilikian, H., and Lewis, E.K.: Arthrograms, Radiology 52:465-487, 1949.

1950 Sachs, M.D., McGaw, W.H., and Rizzo, R.P.: Studies in the scope of pneumoarthrography of the knee as a diagnostic aid, Radiology 54:10-31, 1950.

1951 Leroux, G.F.: L'examen des articulations au moyen des produits de contraste, J. Radiol. Electrol. 32:210-224, 1951.

1953 Archimbaud, J.: L'arthrographie du genou, J. Radiol. Electrol. 34:623-633, 1953.

Candardjis, G., and Saegesser, F.: L'arthrographie du genou par la methode du double contraste, Radiol. Clin. 22:521, 1953.

Kelly, F.: The technique of pneumoarthrography, Xray Techn. 24:399-401, 1953.

1955 Wolfe, T.F.: Fundamentals and technique of arthrography, Xray Techn. 27:171-174, 1955.

1957 Kerwein, G.A., Roseberg, B., and Sneed, W.R.: Arthrographic studies of the shoulder joint, J. Bone Joint Surg. 39-A:1267-1279, 1957.

1959 Philippon, J.: Étude des malformations congénitales méniscales par arthropneumographie, J. Radiol. 40:1-6, 1959.

1960 Andrén, L., and Wehlin, L.: Double-contrast arthrography of knee with horizontal roentgen ray beam, Acta Orthop. Scand. 29:307-314, 1960.

1961 Kessler, I., Silberman, Z., and Nissim, F.: Arthrography of the knee: a critical study of errors and their sources, A.J.R. 86:359-365, 1961.

Samilson, R.L., et al.: Shoulder arthrography, J.A.M.A. 175:773-778, 1961.

Wadi, H.: Ueber die Anwendung eines einfachen Gerätes bei der Kniegelenksarthrographie, Fortschr. Roentgenstr. 95:407-409, 1961.

1962 Heiser, S., Labriola, J.H., and Meyers, M.H.: Arthrography of the knee, Radiology 79:822-828, 1962.

1963 Aye, R.C., Dorr, T.W., and Drewry, G.R.: Arthrography of the knee in office practice, Radiology 80:829-836, 1963.

1965 Fleischer, H.: Die Arthrographie des Daumengrundgelenks, Roentgenblaetter 18:64-66, 1965.

1966 Freiberger, R.H., Killoran, P.J., and Cardona, G.: Arthrography of the knee by double contrast method, A.J.R. 97:736-747, 1966.

Liljedahl, S.O., Lindvall, N., and Wetterfors, J.: Roentgen diagnosis of rupture of anterior cruciate ligament, Acta Radiol. [Diagn.] 4:225-239, 1966.

Vialla, M., et al.: Arthrography of the hip with intra-articular pressure measurements in adults, J. Radiol. 47:593-597, 1966. (In French.) Abstract: Radiology 89:183, 1967.

1967 Haage, H.: Arthrography of the ankle joint, Radiologe 7:137-142, 1967.

Olson, R.W.: Knee arthrography, A.J.R. 101:897-914, 1967.

Wiener, S.N.: Contrast arthrography of the knee joint: comparison of positive and negative methods, Radiology 89:1083-1086, 1967.

1969 Butt, W.P., and McIntyre, J.L.: Double-contrast arthrography of the knee, Radiology 92:487-499, 1969.

Olson, R.W.: Arthrography of the ankle: its use in the evaluation of ankle sprains, Radiology 92:1439-1446, 1969.

Schawelson, R.T.: Double contrast knee arthrography with horizontal beam, Radiol. Technol. 41:98-103, 1969.

Weston, W.J.: The normal arthrograms of the metacarpophalangeal, metatarsophalangeal and interphalangeal joints, Australas. Radiol. 13:211-218, 1969.

1970 Callaghan, J.E., Percy, E.C., and Hill, R.O.: The ankle arthrogram, J. Can. Assoc. Radiol. 21:74-84, 1970.

Haverson, S.B., and Rein, B.I.: Lateral discoid meniscus of the knee: arthrographic diagnosis, A.J.R. 109:581-586, 1970.

Nicholas, J.A., Freiberger, R.H., and Killoran, P.J.: Double-contrast arthrography of the knee: its value in the management of two hundred and twenty-five knee derangements, J. Bone Joint Surg. 52-A:203-220, 1970.

Turner, A.F., and Budin, E.: Arthrography of the knee, Radiology 97:505-508, 1970.

1971 Angell, F.L.: A restraint device for arthrography of the knee, Radiology 98:186-187, 1971.

Harrison, M.O., Freiberger, R.H., and Ranawat, C.S.: Arthrography of the rheumatoid wrist joint, A.J.R. 112:480-486, 1971.

1972 Fordyce, A.J.W., and Horn, C.V.: Arthrography in recent injuries of the ligaments of the ankle, J. Bone Joint Surg. 54-B:116-121, 1972.

Horns, J.W.: Single contrast knee arthrography in abnormalities of the articular cartilage, Radiology 105:537-540, 1972.

Mittler, S., Freiberger, R.H., and Harrison-Stubbs, M.: A method of improving cruciate ligament visualization in double-contrast arthrography, Radiology 102:441-442, 1972.

1974 Anderson, P.W., and Maslin, P.: Tomography applied to knee arthrography, Radiology 110:271, 1974.

Hall, F.M.: Epinephrine-enhanced knee arthrography, Radiology 111:215-217, 1974.

Toller, P.A.: Opaque arthrography of the temporomandibular joint, Int. J. Oral Surg. 3:17-28, 1974.

Weston, W.J.: Arthrography of the acromioclavicular joint, Australas. Radiol. 18:213-214, 1974.

1975 Clark, J.M.: Arthrography in the diagnosis of synovial cysts of the knee, Radiology 115:480-481, 1975.

Eto, R.T., Anderson, P.W., and Harley, J.D.: Elbow arthrography with the application of tomography, Radiology 115:283-288, 1975.

Neviaser, J.S.: Arthrography of the shoulder, Springfield, Ill., 1975, Charles C Thomas, Publisher.

Wershba, M., et al.: Double contrast knee arthrography in the evaluation of osteochondritis dissecans, Clin. Orthop. 107:81-86, 1975.

1976 Katzberg, R.W., Burgener, P.A., and Fischer, H.W.: Evaluation of various contrast agents for arthrography, Invest. Radiol. 11:528-533, 1976.

Wilson, E.S.: Positive contrast shoulder arthrography, J. Med. Soc. N.J. 73:933-938, 1976.

1977 Dalinka, M.K.: A simple aid to the performance of shoulder arthrography, A.J.R. 129:942, 1977.

Dirkheimer, Y., Ramsheyi, A., and Reolon, M.: Positive arthrography of the craniocervical joints, Neuroradiology 12:257-260, 1977.

1978 Lee, K.R., and Sanders, W.F.: A practical stress device for knee arthrography, Radiology 127:542, 1978.

Lindholmer, E., Foged, N., and Jensen, J.T.: Arthrography of the ankle: value in diagnosis of rupture of the lateral ligaments, Acta Radiol. 19:585-598, 1978.

Spataro, R.F., et al.: Evaluation of epinephrine for arthrography, Invest. Radiol. 13:286-290, 1978.

1979 Katzberg, R.W., et al.: Arthrotomography of the temporomandibular joint: new technique and preliminary observations, A.J.R. 132:949-955, 1979.

Pavlov, H., Ghelman, B., and Warren, R.F.: Double-contrast arthrography of the elbow, Radiology 130:87-95, 1979.

Silverbach, S.: Simple method for marking knee arthrograms, A.J.R. 133:155, 1979.

Ward, M.D.: Fluroscopic technique for double contrast knee arthrography, Radiol. Technol. 50:675-681, 1979.

1980 Dalnika, M.K., editor: Arthrography, New York, 1980, Springer-Verlag.

Freiberger, R.H., and Kaye, J.J.: Arthrography, New York, 1980, Appleton-Century-Crofts.

Goldman, A.B.: Arthrography of the hip joint, CRC Crit. Rev. Diagno. Imaging 13:111-171, 1980.

Mink, J.H., and Dickerson, R.: Air or CO_2 for knee arthrography? A.J.R. **134:**991-993, 1980.

Neviaser, T.J.: Arthrography of the shoulder, Orthop. Clin. North Am. **11:**205-217, 1980.

Rosenthal, D., Murray, W.T., and Smith, R.J.: Finger arthrography, Radiology **137:**647-651, 1980.

Watt, I., and Tasker, T.: Pitfalls in double contrast knee arthrography, Br. J. Radiol. **53:**754-759, 1980.

1981 Franji, S.M.: New radiographic technique utilizing arthrotomography for studying shoulder derangements, Radiol. Technol. **52:**384, 1981.

Hall, F.M., et al.: Morbidity from shoulder arthrography: etiology, incidence, and prevention, A.J.R. **136:**59-62, 1981.

Goldberg, R.P., Hall, F.M., and Wyshak, G.: Pain in knee arthrography: comparison of air vs. CO_2 and reaspiration vs. no aspiration, A.J.R. **136:**377-379, 1981.

Shoulder girdle

1915 Iselin, H.: Die Röntgenuntersuchung der Schulter in zwei zueinander senkrechten Richtungen, Bruns' Beiträge **97:**473, 1915.

Lawrence, W.S.: New position in radiographing the shoulder joint, A.J.R. **2:**728-730, 1915.

1917 Lorenz: Die röntgenographische Darstellung des subskapularen Raumes und des Schenkelhalses im Querschnitt, Fortschr. Roentgenstr. **25:**342-343, 1917-1918.

1918 Bailleul, L.C., and Dubois-Roquebert: Le décalage dans les fractures de l'humérus, J. Radiol. Electrol. **3:**251-256, 1918.

George, F.D.: Importance of the upper arm in the detection of roentgenological shadows in the region of the shoulder joint, A.J.R. **5:**187-188, 1918.

Laquerrière and Pierquin: De la nécessité d'employer une technique radiographique spéciale pour obtenir certains details squelettiques, J. Radiol. Electrol. **3:**145-148, 1918.

Lawrence, W.S.: Method of obtaining accurate lateral roentgenogram of the shoulder joint, A.J.R. **5:**193-194, 1918.

1920 Arcelin, F.: L'exploration radiologique des grandes articulations, Lyon Chir. **17:**669-686, 1920.

Chassard, M.: Résultats de l'exploration radiologique de l'articulation scapulo-humérale, J. Radiol. Electrol. **4:**68-70, 1920.

1922 Béclère, H.: Radiographie de profil de l'omoplate, Bull. Soc. Radiol. Med. Paris **10:**53-55, 1922.

1924 Behn, O.: Schulter-und Hüftaufnahmen in der Frontalebene, Fortschr. Roentgenstr. **32:**123, 1924.

Buxton, D., and Knox, R.: A radiographic survey of normal joints. Part I. The shoulder, Br. J. Radiol. **29:**115-134, 1924.

Marko, D.: Isolierte Schlüsselbeinaufnahme, Fortschr. Roentgenstr. **32:**442, 1924.

1925 Pilz, W.: Zur Röntgenuntersuchung der habituellen Schulterverrenkung, Arch. Klin. Chir. **135:**1-22, 1925.

1926 Quesada, F.: Technique for the roentgen diagnosis of fractures of the clavicle, Surg. Gynecol. Obstet. **42:**424-428, 1926.

1927 King, J.M., and Homes, G.W.: Review of 450 roentgen ray examinations of the shoulder, A.J.R. **17:**214-218, 1927.

Mauclaire: Radiographies de profil et radiographies a pic de la hanche et de l'épaule, Arch. Prov. Chir. **30:**677-694, 1927.

1928 Dittrich, R.: Eine neue Stellung zur röntgenologischen Erfassung der Schultergegend, Fortschr. Roentgenstr. **37:**526-529, 1928.

1929 Cohoon, C.W.: Lateral transthoracic roentgenogram as a diagnostic aid in fractures of the upper end of the humerus, A.J.R. **21:**174-175, 1929.

Didiée, J.: Une position nouvelle pour la radiographie de la tête humérale: son intérêt dans l'étude de la luxation récidivante de l'épaule, Bull. Soc. Radiol. Med. Paris **17:**150-154, 1929.

Williams, H.H.: Oblique views of the clavicle, Radiogr. Clin. Photogr. **5:**191-192, 1929.

1930 Didiée, J.: Le radiodiagnostic dans la luxation récidivante de l'épaule, J. Radiol. Electrol. **14:**209-218, 1930.

Wahl, R.: Ueber eine neue Scapulaaufnahme, Röntgenpraxis **2:**652-657, 1930.

1933 Berent, F., and von Hecker, H.: Zur axialen Aufnahmetechnik des Schultergelenks, Der Chir **5:**210, 1933.

Wijnbladh, H.: Zur Röntgendiagnose von Schulterluxationen, Der Chir **5:**702-704, 1933.

1934 Fergusson, N.J.: An improved technique for the examination of the shoulder, Br. J. Radiol. **7:**33-42, 1934.

Freedman, E.: Radiography of the shoulder, Radiogr. Clin. Photogr. **10:**8-9, 1934.

Timpano, M.: Aspetti radiografici dell'articolazione coraco-clavicolare, Ann. Radiol. Fis. Med. **8:**491, 1934.

1935 Henry, L.S.: Roentgenographic evidence in the tuberosity of the humerus of recent and old injuries to the supraspinatus tendon attachment, A.J.R. **33:**486, 1935.

Jordan, H.: New technique for the roentgen examination of the shoulder joint, Radiology **25:**480-484, 1935.

Philips, H.B.: A lateral view of the clavicle, J. Bone Joint Surg. **17:**202-203, 1935.

Schoen, H.: Zur Technik der axialen Schulterfernaufnahme, Röntgenpraxis **7:**264, 1935.

1936 Jones, M.L.: Radiographic examination of the shoulder, Xray Techn. **7:**104-105, 134-135, 1936.

Pearson, G.R.: Radiographic technic for acromioclavicular dislocation, Radiology **27:**239, 1936.

1937 Blackett, C.W., and Healy, T.R.: Roentgen studies of the shoulder, A.J.R. **37:**760-766, 1937.

Fray, W.W.: Effect of position on the production of cystlike shadows around the shoulder joints, Radiology **28:**673-682, 1937.

Liberson, F.: The value and limitation of the oblique view as compared with the ordinary anteroposterior exposure of the shoulder, A.J.R. **37:**498-509, 1937.

Moreau, L.: Remarques sur quelques radiographies osseuses de profil, Bull. Soc. Radiol. Med. Paris **25:**49-50, 1937.

1938 Codman, E.A.: Rupture of the supraspinatus, Am. J. Surg. **42:**603, 1938.

Holmblad, E.C.: X-ray examination of the clavicles and acromioclavicular joints, Am. J. Surg. **42:**791-797, 1938.

Massa, J.: Une nouvelle position pour l'examen radiologique de l'épaule de profil, Gaz. Méd. France (suppl. Cah. Radiol.) **45:**363, 1938.

Mullins, S.A.: Technique for radiography of the luxations of joints, Radiology **4:**94-96, 1938.

Scaglietti, O: The obstetrical shoulder trauma, Surg. Gynecol. Obstet. **66:**868-877, 1938.

Wehl, G.F.: A useful and easily obtained view of the scapula, Radiography **4:**174-175, 1938.

1939 Pinelli, I.: Frattura della spina della scapola: sua proiezione e immagine radiografica, Quad. Radiol. **4:**92-97, 1939.

Williams, H.H.: An oblique view of the clavicle, Radiography **5:**191-192, 1939.

1940 Gunson, E.F.: Technical procedure in the x-ray examination of the scapula, Xray Techn. **11:**165-167, 203, 1940.

Hill, H.A., and Sachs, M.D.: Grooved defect of the humeral head, Radiology **35:**690-700, 1940.

Perry, E.C.: Radiography of the shoulders, Xray Techn. **11:**168-169, 193, 1940.

Watson, W.: An abnormal view of the shoulder, Radiography **6:**76-77, 1940.

1941 Alexander, O.M.: Simple technique for obtaining a lateral view of the upper end of the humerus, Radiology **7:**31-32, 1941.

Bosworth, B.M.: Examination of the shoulder for calcium deposits, J. Bone Joint Surg. **23:**567-577, 1941.

Cleaves, E.N.: A new film holder for roentgen examination of the shoulder, A.J.R. **45:**288-290, 1941.

Devvis et Proux, Ch.: Sur une technique de radiographie de l'épaule de profil, J. Radiol. Electrol. **24:**111-112, 1941.

Rendich, R.H., and Poppel, M.H.: Roentgen diagnosis of the posterior dislocation of the shoulder, Radiology **36:**42-45, 1941.

Sachs, M.D., Hill, H.A., and Chuinard, E.L.: Further studies of the shoulder joint with special reference to the bicipital groove, Radiology **36:**731-735, 1941.

1942 Johnson, D.R.: Lateral projection of the scapula, Radiogr. Clin. Photogr. **18:**47-48, 1942.

343

Jones, L.: The shoulder joint: observations on the anatomy and physiology, Surg. Gynecol. Obstet. **75**:433-444, 1942.

1943 Alexander, S.: Study of the shoulder with special reference to the humerus, Xray Techn. **14**:147-150, 1943.

1944 Oppenheimer, A.: Lesions of the acromioclavicular joint causing pain and disability of the shoulder, A.J.R. **51**:699-706, 1944.

1945 Howorth, B.M.: Calcification of tendon cuff of shoulder, Surg. Gynecol. Obstet. **80**:337-345, 1945.

1946 Soule, A.B.: Ossification of the coraco-clavicular ligament following dislocation of the acromioclavicular articulation, A.J.R. **56**:607-615, 1946.

1947 Lane, R.G.: A technique for radiography of the humerus in the lateral view, Xray Techn. **19**:129, 168, 1947.

1948 Alexander, O.M.: Radiography of the acromioclavicular joint, Radiography **54**:139-141, 1948.

Bosworth, B.M.: Acromioclavicular dislocations, Ann. Surg. **127**:98-111, 1948.

Fengler, K.: Special projections for the coracoid process and clavicle, A.J.R. **59**:435-438, 1948.

Howes, W.E., and Alicandri, B.B.: A method of roentgenologic examination of the shoulder, Radiology **50**:569-580, 1948.

Knutsson, F.: An axial projection of the shoulder joint, Acta Radiol. **30**:214-216, 1948.

Porcher, P.: Précis de technique radiographique, ed. 2, Paris, 1948, Gauthier-Villars.

Warrick, C.K.: Posterior dislocation of the shoulder joint, J. Bone Joint Surg. **30-B**:651-655, 1948.

1950 Tarrant, R.M.: The axial view of the clavicle, Xray Techn. **21**:358-359, 1950.

1952 McLaughlin, H.L.: Posterior dislocation of the shoulder, J. Bone Joint Surg. **34-A**:584-590, 1952.

1953 Mazujian, M.: Lateral profile view of the scapula, Xray Techn. **25**:24-25, 1953.

1954 Alexander, O.M.: Radiography of the acromioclavicular articulation, Med. Radiogr. Photogr. **30**:34-39, 1954.

1956 O'Connor, S.J., and Jacknow, A.S.: Posterior dislocation of the shoulder, Arch. Surg. **72**:479-491, 1956.

1957 Brown, W.H., et al.: Posterior dislocation of the shoulder, Radiology **69**:815-822, 1957.

Schönbauer, H.R.: Zur Röntgentechnik des Schlüsselbeinbruches, Fortschr. Roentgenstr. **86**:349-351, 1957.

1958 Barraco, N.R.: A lateral projection of the shoulder joint to permit an evaluation of the degree of dislocation, Xray Techn. **29**:221-224, 1958.

Funke, T.: Tangential view of the scapular spine, Med. Radiogr. Photogr. **34**:41-43, 1958.

1959 Conklin, W.A., and Atwill, J.H., Jr.: Lateral radiography of the scapula with the patient supine, Med. Radiogr. Photogr. **35**:46-47, 1959.

Seyss, R.: Zur Röntgentechnik des Schlüsselbeinbruches, Fortschr. Reontgenstr. **90**:768-769, 1959.

1960 Berens, D.L., and Lockie, L.M.: Ossification of the coracoacromial ligament, Radiology **74**:802-805, 1960.

1961 Künlen, H.: Projection of the clavicle in a second plane, Fortschr. Roentgenstr. **94**:739-750, 1961. (In German.) Abstract: Radiology **78**:848, 1962.

1962 Golding, F.C.: The shoulder—the forgotten joint, Br. J. Radiol. **35**:149-158, 1962.

Nobel, W.: Posterior traumatic dislocation of the shoulder, J. Bone Joint Surg. **44-A**:523-538, 1962.

1963 Stripp, W.J.: Radiographs of the scapulothoracic region, Xray Focus **4**:8-12, 1963.

Stripp, W.J.: The clavicle and the acromioclavicular joint, Xray Focus **4**:21-26, 1963.

1964 Stripp, W.J.: Sternoclavicular joint and the bicipital groove, Xray Focus **5**:11-13, 1964.

1965 Fisk, C.: Adaptation of the technique for radiography of the bicipital groove, Radiol. Technol. **37**:47-50, 1965.

Warrick, C.K.: Posterior dislocation of the shoulder joint, Br. J. Radiol. **38**:758-761, 1965.

1966 Figiel, S.J., et al.: Posterior dislocation of the shoulder, Radiology **87**:737-740, 1966.

1967 Bloom, M.H., and Obata, W.G.: Diagnosis of posterior dislocation of the shoulder with the use of Velpeau axillary and angle-up roentgenographic views, J. Bone Joint Surg. **49-A**:943-949, 1967.

1970 ViGario, G.D., and Keats, T.E.: Localization of calcific deposits in shoulder, A.J.R. **108**:806-811, 1970.

1971 Zanca, P.: Shoulder pain: involvement of the acromioclavicular joint, A.J.R. **112**:493-506, 1971.

1974 Kimberlin, G.E.: Radiography of injuries to the region of the shoulder girdle: revisited, Radiol. Technol. **46**:69-83, 1974.

Rubin, S.A., Gray, R.L., and Green, W.R.: The scapular "Y": a diagnostic aid in shoulder trauma, Radiology **110**:725-726, 1974.

Weston, W.J.: Arthrography of the acromioclavicular joint, Australas. Radiol. **18**:213-214, 1974.

1975 Protass, J.J., Stampfli, F.V., and Osmer, J.C.: Coracoid process fracture diagnosis in acromioclavicular separation, Radiology **116**:61-64, 1975.

Reichmann, S., et al.: Soft tissue xeroradiography of the shoulder joint, Acta Radiol. **16**:572-576, 1975.

1976 Wilson, E.S.: Positive contrast shoulder arthrography, J. Med. Soc. N.J. **73**:933-938, 1976.

1978 Froimson, A.I.: Fracture of the coracoid process of the scapula, J. Bone Joint Surg. **60**:710-711, 1978.

Pavlov, H., and Freiberger, R.H.: Fractures and dislocations about the shoulder, Semin. Roentgenol. **13**:85-96, 1978.

1979 Cockshott, W.P.: The coracoclavicular joint, Radiology **131**:313-316, 1979.

Slivka, J., and Resnick, D.: An improved radiographic view of the glenohumeral joint, J. Can. Assoc. Radiol. **30**:83-85, 1979.

1980 De Smet, A.A.: Anterior oblique projection in radiography of the traumatized shoulder, A.J.R. **134**:515-518, 1980.

De Smet, A.A.: Axillary projection in radiography of the non-traumatized shoulder, A.J.R. **134**:511-514, 1980.

Franji, S.M., and El-Khoury, G.Y.: A new radiographic technique utilizing multidirectional tomography with double contrast arthrography for studying the glenoidal labrum, Radiol. Technol. **52**:143-147, 1980.

Horsfield, D., and Renton, P.: The "other view" in the radiography of shoulder trauma, Radiography **46**(549):213-214, 1980.

Neviaser, R.J.: Anatomic considerations and examination of the shoulder, Orthop. Clin. North Am. **11**:187-195, 1980.

Bony thorax
Sternum

1919 Drüner, L.: Ueber die Röntgenologie des Brustbeins, Fortschr. Roentgenstr. **27**:54, 1919-1921.

1920 Delherm and Chaperon: Radiographie du sternum en position oblique antérieure droite, J. Radiol. Electrol. **4**:227-228, 1920.

1924 Pfahler, G.E.: Study of the sternum by roentgen rays, A.J.R. **9**:311, 1924.

1929 Pendergrass, R.C.: Roentgenographic demonstration of sternal injury, Radiology **13**:451-455, 1929.

1936 Blumensaat, C.: Zur Röntgendarstellung des Brustbeins, Bruns' Beitr. Klin. Chir. **163**:120, 1936.

Holman, C., and Stober, E.: Technic for radiography of the sternum, Radiology **26**:757-758, 1936.

1937 Jönsson, G.: Method of obtaining structural pictures of the sternum, Acta Radiol. **18**:336-339, 1937.

1939 Zimmer, E.A.: Das Brustbein und seine Gelenke, Fortschr. Roentgenstr. **58**:1939.

1940 Dixon, F.L.: Technic for roentgenography of the sternum, Xray Techn. **12**:8-12, 1940.

Kraft, E.: Respiratory blurring in routine roentgenography, Quart. Bull. Sea View Hosp. **5**:167-174, 1940.

Mullans, S.A.: Technique for radiography of the sternum, Radiography **6**:12-13, 1940.

Weinbren, M.: Tomography of the spine and the sternum, Br. J. Radiol. **8**:325-336, 1940.

1942 Holly, E.W.: Some radiographic techniques in which movement is utilized, Radiogr. Clin. Photogr. **18**:78-83, 1942.

Runge, R.K.: A technique for roentgenography of the sternum, Xray Techn. **13**:153-154, 175, 1942.

1946 Jensen, C.: Radiographic examination of the sternum—posterior-anterior position, Xray Techn. **18**:18, 41, 1946.

1953 Benmussa, M.: Technique d'examen radiographique du sternum, J. Radiol. Electrol. **34**:646-648, 1953.

1955 Russell, D.A., and Albrecht, L.: A new technic for radiology of the bony thorax and sternum, Radiology **64**:721-723, 1955.

1956 Balzarini, E., and Pompili, G.: Tecnica e anatomia radiografica normale dello sterno, Radiol. Med. **42**:625-637, 1956.

1959 Saudan, Y.: Aspects radiologiques de quelques lésions sternales, Radiol. Clin. **28**:313-319, 1959.

1981 Destouet, J.M., et al.: Computed tomography of the sternoclavicular joint and sternum, Radiology **138**:123-128, 1981.

Sternoclavicular articulation

1937 Schnorr, A.: Die Darstellung des Sternum und der Sternoklavikulargelenke im Tomogramm, Röntgenpraxis **9**:622-629, 1937.

1938 Leman, R.M.: Some radiographic techniques, Radiography **4**:41-44, 1938.

1939 Zimmer, E.A.: Das Brustbein und seine Gelenke, Fortschr. Roentgenstr. **58**:1939.

1943 Gunson, E.F.: Radiography of the sternoclavicular articulation, Radiogr. Clin. Photogr. **19**:20-24, 1943.

1946 Kurzbauer, R.: The lateral projection in roentgenography of the sternoclavicular articulation, A.J.R. **56**:104-105, 1946.

1947 Ritvo, M., and Ritvo, M.: Roentgen study of the sternoclavicular region, A.J.R. **58**:644-650, 1947.

1949 Blocklage, M.H.: A comparison of roentgenographic examinations of the sternum and sternoclavicular joints, Xray Techn. **21**:19-27, 1949.

1964 Pretorius, R.: Radiography of the sternoclavicular joints—a new technique, Radiography **30**:26-27, 1964.

Stripp, W.J.: Sternoclavicular joint and the bicipital groove, Xray Focus **5**:11-13, 1964.

1968 Hobbs, D.W.: Sternoclavicular joint: a new axial radiographic view, Radiology **90**:801, 1968.

1973 Kattan, K.R.: Modified view for use in roentgen examination of the sternoclavicular joints, Radiology **108**:8, 1973.

1975 Morag, B., and Shahin, N.: The value of tomography of the sterno-clavicular region, Clin. Radiol. **26**:57-62, 1975.

1979 Abel, M.S.: Symmetrical anteroposterior projections of the sternoclavicular joints with motion studies, Radiology **132**:757-759, 1979.

Levinsohn, E.M., Bunnell, W.P., and Yuan, H.A.: Computed tomography in the diagnosis of dislocations of the sternoclavicular joint, Clin. Orthop. **140**:12-16, 1979.

1980 Resnick, D.: Sternocostoclavicular hyperostosis, A.J.R. **135**:1278-1280, 1980.

1981 Destouet, J.M., et al.: Computed tomography of the sternoclavicular joint and sternum, Radiology **138**:123-128, 1981.

Ribs

1920 Knox, R.: Special points in technique for the radiograph of the clavicle and lateral aspect of the ribs for detection of injuries, Arch. Radiol. Electrol. **24**:248-252, 1920.

1931 Perry, L.M., and Newton, E.S.: Rib position and radiographic technic of mid-axillary and mid-clavicular lines, Xray Techn. **2**:74-75, 1931.

1933 Ernst, G.: Einfache Einstellungstechnik zur Darstellung zeitlicher Rippenbrüche im Bereich der unterem Brusthälfte, Röntgenpraxis **5**:154, 1933.

1939 Bloom, A.R.: A new technique of taking roentgenographs of the upper ribs, Radiology **33**:648-649, 1939.

1942 Bartsch, G.W.: Radiographic examination of the ribs, Xray Techn. **14**:18-22, 29, 1942.

1943 Rogers, N.J.S.: A technique of x-ray examination of the ribs, Radiography **9**:7, 1943.

Sanborn, R.L.: Radiography of the ribs, Xray Techn. **14**:202-203, 1943.

1945 Kalsbeek, A.: Tube angle rib technique, Xray Techn. **16**:147-148, 1945.

1947 Liberson, F.: Fractures of the ribs (with comparison of the standard and the one-film two-exposure technic), A.J.R. **57**:349-354, 1947.

1956 Bridgeman, C.F., Holly, E.W., and Zariquiey, M.O.: Radiography of the ribs and costovertebral joints, Med. Radiogr. Photogr. **32**:38-60, 1956.

1963 Agnesia, Sister M.: A wide-angle rib technique, Xray Techn. **34**:289-290, 1963.

Berlin, H.S., et al.: Wide-angle roentgenography, A.J.R. **90**:189-197, 1963.

1966 Reynolds, J., and Davis, J.T.: Injuries of the chest wall, pleura, pericardium, lungs, bronchi, and esophagus, Radiol. Clin. North Am. **4**:383-401, 1966.

1970 Hohmann, D., and Gasteiger, W.: Roentgen diagnosis of the costovertebral joints, Fortschr. Roentgenstr. **112**:783-789, 1970.

Morris, L., and Bailey, J.: A simple method to demonstrate the ribs and sternum, Clin. Radiol. **21**:320-322, 1970.

1974 Wolstein, D., Rabinowitz, J.G., and Twersky, J.: Tuberculosis of the rib, J. Can. Assoc. Radiol. **25**:307-309, 1974.

Pelvic bones and upper femora

1897 Cowl: Ein Sagittal nebst Frontalbild eines anomalen coxalen Femurendes, Fortschr. Roentgenstr. **1**:136, 1897-1898.

1900 Lauenstein, C.: Das Röntgenbild einer Luxato femoris infraglenoidalis, Fortschr. Roentgenstr. **3**:186, 1900-1901.

1916 Arcelin, F.: Rapport mensuel des services d'électroradiologie de la XIV region, December 1916.

Hickey, P.M.: Value of the lateral view of the hip, A.J.R. **3**:308-309, 1916.

1917 Lilienfeld, L.: Die seitliche Aufnahme des Hüftgelenkes, Deutsche Med. **43**:294-296, 1917.

Lorenz: Die röntgenographische Darstellung des subskapularen Raumes und des Schenkelhalses im Querschnitt, Fortschr. Roentgenstr. **25**:342-343, 1917-1918.

Salmond, A.W.R.: Technique for the lateral view of the upper end of the femur, Arch. Radiol. Electrol. **22**:297-300, **1917-1918.**

1918 Prentiss, H.J.: Standardization of roentgenography of the shoulder and hip joint, J. Roentgenol. **1**:145-150, 1918.

1919 Lilienfeld, L.: Die axiale Aufnahme der Regio pubica, Fortschr. Roentgenstr. **26**:285-290, 1919.

Staunig, K.: Die axiale Aufnahme der Regio pubica, Fortschr. Roentgenstr. **27**:514-517, 1919-1921.

1920 Arcelin, F.: Technique et résultats de l'exploration radiographique de profil de l'extremité supérieure du fémur, J. Radiol. Electrol. **4**:12-18, 1920.

Kisch, E.: Eine neue Methode für röntgenologische Darstellung des Hüftgelenks in frontaler Ebene, Fortschr. Roentgenstr. **27**:309, 1920.

1921 Arcelin, F., and Duchene Marullaz, L.: L'exploration radiologique de profil de la hanche, Bull. Soc. Radiol. Méd. Paris **9**:40-45, 1921.

Bouchacourt: Des avantages et des inconvenients respectifs des radiographies de la hanche en position de profil et en position de trois quarts obliques, Bull. Soc. Radiol. Méd. Paris **9**:90, 1921.

1923 Chassard and Lapiné: Étude radiographique de l'arcade pubienne chez la femme enceinte: une nouvelle méthode d'appreciation du diamètre bi-ischiatique, J. Radiol. Electrol. **7**:113-124, 1923.

1927 Béclère, H., and Porcher, P.: La radiographie latérale de la hanche, J. Radiol. Electrol. **10**:97-105, 1926. Abstract: A.J.R. **17**:132, 1927.

Regner and LeFloch: Radiographie du profil de la hanche dans les luxations congénitales, J. Radiol. Electrol. **11**:167-170, 1927.

1928 Philips, H.B.: New roentgenographic demonstration of the fractured neck of the femur, Am. J. Surg. **5**:392-393, 1928.

1929 Schertlein, A.: Die Bestimmung des Schenkelhalstorsionswinkels mit Hilfe der Röntgenstrahlen, Fortschr. Roentgenstr. **39**:304-318, 1929.

1930 Paschetta, V.: La méthode des radiographies en trois positions dans les fractures du col du femur, Arch. Electr. Méd. **38**:12-17, 1930.

1931 Kniper, E.: Röntgenaufnahmen des Oberschenkelhalses bei seitlicher Strahlenrichtung, Röntgenpraxis **3**:909-911, 1931.

1932 Johansson, S.: Zur Technik der Osteosynthese der Fraktur colli femoris, Zbl. Chir. **59**:2019, 1932.

Johnson, C.R.: A new method for roentgenographic examination of the upper end of the femur, J. Bone Joint Surg. **30**:859-866, 1932.

Leonard, R.D., and George, A.W.: Cassette with convex curve, A.J.R. **28**:261-263, 1932.

Wittek-Saltzberg, R.: Ueber seitliche Aufnahmen des Schenkelhalses und Trochanterregion, Röntgenpraxis **4**:965-968, 1932.

1933 Jones, L.: Intracapsular fracture of the neck of the femur, Ann. Surg. **97**:237-246, 1933.

1934 George, A.W., and Leonard, R.D.: Ununited intracapsular fractures of the femoral neck roentgenologically considered, A.J.R. **31**:433, 1934.

1935 Erlacher, J.: Eine zweite Röntgenaufnahme des Hüftgelenkes, Zbl. Chir. **62**:731-734, 1935.

Jones, L.: Lateral roentgenography of the neck of the femur, A.J.R. **33**:504-510, 1935.

Manfredi, M., and Swenson, P.C.: Lateral roentgenography of the hip, A.J.R. **34**:404-405, 1935.

1936 Danelius, G., and Miller, L.: Lateral view of the hip, A.J.R. **35**:282-284, 1936.

Friedman, L.J.: Lateral roentgen ray study of the hip joint, Radiology **27**:240-241, 1936.

Gaenslen, F.J.: Fracture of the neck of the femur, J.A.M.A. **107**:105-114, 1936.

Hsieh, C.K.: Posterior dislocation of the hip, Radiology **27**:450-455, 1936.

Pletz, F.: Lateral roentgenography of the hip, Xray Techn. **8**:60-61, 1936.

1937 Kewesch, E.L.: De l'examen radiologique de l'articulation de la hanche et du col du femur dans la projection latérale, Vestn. Rentgen. Radiol. **18**:71-73, 1937.

Polgar, F.: Die Incisura acetabuli im Röntgenbilde des Hüftgelenks, Fortschr. Roentgenstr. **56**:521, 1937.

1938 Cleaves, E.N.: Observations on lateral views of the hips, A.J.R. **34**:964-966, 1938.

Danelius, G., and Miller, L.: Lateral view of the hip, Xray Techn. **9**:176-178, 1938.

Dooley, E.A., Caldwell, C.W., and Glass, G.A.: Roentgenography of the femoral neck, A.J.R. **39**:834-837, 1938.

Douglas, J.J.: Further notes on hip technique, Xray Techn. **10**:134, 138, 1938.

Douglas, J.J.: Modified lateral hip technique, Xray Techn. **10**:77-78, 1938.

Grasser, C.H.: Hilfsmethoden zur Darstellung des Hüftgelenks und des Schenkelhalses, Röntgenpraxis **10**:544-551, 1938.

Teufel, S.: Eine gezielte Aufsichtsaufnahme der Hüftgelenkspfanne, Röntgenpraxis **10**:398-402, 1938.

1940 Dooley, E.A., Caldwell, C.W., and Glass, G.A.: Roentgenografía del cuello del femur: técnica para obtener vistas lateral y anteroposterior verdaderas, Rev. Radiol. Fis. **7-8**:49, 1940.

Hovious, C.: X-ray technic for fractures of the hip, Xray Techn. **12**:90-91, 1940.

1941 Taylor, R.: Modified anteroposterior projection of the anterior bones of the pelvis, Radiogr. Clin. Photogr. **17**:67-69, 1941.

1942 Wolcott, R.E.: Technique for securing lateral roentgenograms of the femoral neck in the operating room, Xray Techn. **13**:155-158, 181, 1942.

1943 Barnard, V.L.: A new surgical table top and cassette holder for surgical roentgenographic examinations of the hip, Radiology **40**:599-602, 1943.

1945 Lane, R.G.: Radiographic technique for lateral hip position with the Potter-Bucky diaphragm, Xray Techn. **16**:175-176, 1945.

Massa, J.: Contribution à l'étude de la radiographie de la hanche de profil, chez les traumatisés du col fémoral, J. Radiol. Electrol. **26**:288-291, 1944-1945.

Wood, F.G., Camb, M.B., and Wilkinson, M.C.: The x-ray examination of the hip in tuberculous disease, Br. J. Radiol. **18**:332-334, 1945.

1948 Donaldson, S.W., Badgley, C.E., and Hunsberger, W.G.: Lateral view of the pelvis in examination for hip dislocation, J. Bone Joint Surg. **30-A**:512-514, 1948.

Urist, M.R.: Fracture-dislocation of the hip joint, J. Bone Joint Surg. **30-A**:699-727, 1948.

1950 Bridgman, C.F.: Radiography of the hip joint, Med. Radiogr. Photogr. **26**:2-17, 70-83, 1950.

1951 Bridgman, C.F.: Radiography of the hip joint, Med. Radiogr. Photogr. **27**:2-13, 34-38, 70-80, 1951.

de Cuveland, E., and Hueck, F.: Osteochondropathie der Spina iliaca anterior inferior unter Berücksichtigung der Ossifikationsvorgänge der Apophyse des lateralen Pfannenrandes, Fortschr. Roentgenstr. **75**:430-445, 1951.

Mitton, K.L., and Auringer, E.M.: Roentgenological study of the femoral neck, A.J.R. **66**:639-641, 1951.

Raap, G.: A position of value in studying the pelvis and its contents, South. Med. J. **44**:95-98, 1951.

Williams, A.J.: Roentgenographic study of the hip joint in the lateral projection, A.J.R. **66**:459-460, 1951.

1952 Bridgman, C.F.: Radiography of the hip bone, Med. Radiogr. Photogr. **28**:38-46, 1952.

1953 Colonna, P.C.: A diagnostic roentgen view of the acetabulum, Surg. Clin. North Am. **33**:1565-1569, 1953.

Dunlap, K., Swanson, A.B., and Penner, R.S.: A new method for determination of torsion of the femur, J. Bone Joint Surg. **35-A**:289-311, 1953.

Laage, H., et al.: Horizontal lateral roentgenography of the hip in children, J. Bone Joint Surg. **35-A**:387-398, 1953.

1954 Martz, C.D., and Taylor, C.C.: The 45-degree angle roentgenographic study of the pelvis in congenital dislocation of the hip, J. Bone Joint Surg. **36-A**:528-532, 1954.

1955 Broderick, T.F.: Complementary roentgenographic view of the hip, J. Bone Joint Surg. **37-A**:295-298, 1955.

1956 Dunlap, K., Swanson, A.B., and Penner, R.S.: Studies of the hip joint by means of lateral acetabular roentgenograms, J. Bone Joint Surg. **38-A**:1218-1230, 1956.

Magilligan, D.J.: Calculation of the angle of anteversion by means of horizontal lateral roentgenography, J. Bone Joint Surg. **38-A**:1231-1246, 1956.

1958 Fisk, C., and Fry, M.J.: Femoral torsion and the Shands technique, Xray Techn. **29**:225, 1958.

Shands, A.R., and Steele, M.K.: Torsion of the femur: a follow-up report on the use of the Dunlap method for its determination, J. Bone Joint Surg. **40-A**:803-816, 1958.

1962 Fisk, C.: A review of the clinical and radiographic studies of dislocated hips, Xray Techn. **34**:66-69, 1962.

Voorhis, C.C.: A cassette holder to be used in pinning hips, Surg. Gynecol. Obstet. **115**:359-360, 1962.

1964 Fisk, C.: Acetabular fractures—where? Radiol. Technol. **35**:330-333, 1964.

1965 Berkebile, R.D., Fischer, D.L., and Albrecht, L.F.: The gull-wing sign: value of the lateral view of the pelvis in fracture dislocation of the acetabular rim and posterior dislocation of the femoral head, Radiology **84**:937-939, 1965.

1966 Mounts, R.J., and Schloss, C.D.: Injuries to the bony pelvis and hip, Radiol. Clin. North Am. **4**:307-322, 1966.

Liliequist, B.: Roentgenologic examination of the acetabular part of the os coxae, Acta Radiol. [Diagn.] **4**:289-292, 1966.

1967 Gibson, R.D.: Anteversion of the femoral neck: a method of measurement, Australas. Radiol. **11**:163-169, 1967.

1970 Angell, F.L., and Watts, F.B., Jr.: Total hip replacement: roentgen appearance of current devices, A.J.R. **110**:787-792, 1970.

Martel, W., and Poznanski, A.K.: The value of traction during roentgenography of the hip, Radiology **94**:497-503, 1970.

1971 Martel, W., Poznanski, A.K., and Kuhns, L.R.: Further observations on the value of traction during roentgenography of the hip, Invest. Radiol. **6**:1-8, 1971.

1973 Pepper, H.W., and Noonan, C.D.: Radiographic evaluation of total hip arthroplasty, Radiology **108**:23-29, 1973.

1974 Wiltse, L.L.: Internal rotation for the diagnosis of impacted fracture of the hip, Clin. Orthop. **103**:20, 1974.

1975 Hooper, A.C., and Ormond, D.J.: A radiographic study of hip rotation, Ir. J. Med Sci. **144**:25-29, 1975.

Rogers, L.F., Novy, S.B., and Harris, N.F.: Occult central fractures of the acetabulum, A.J.R. **124**:96-101, 1975.

1976 Salvati, E.A., et al.: Radiology of total hip replacements, Clin. Orthop. **121**:74-82, 1976.

1978 Armbuster, T.G., et al.: The adult hip: an anatomic study. Part I: the bony landmarks, Radiology **128**:1-10, 1978.

Chuinard, E.G.: Lateral roentgenography in the diagnosis and treatment of dysplasia/dislocation of the hip, Orthopedics **1**:130-140, 1978.

Fredensborg, N., and Nilsson, B.E.: The joint space in normal hip radiographs, Radiology **126**:325-326, 1978.

Thaggard, A., III, Harle, T.S., and Carlson, V.: Fractures and dislocations of bony pelvis and hip, Semin. Roentgenol. **13**:117-134, 1978.

Whitehouse, G.H.: Radiological aspects of posterior dislocation of the hip, Clin. Radiol. **29**:431-441, 1978.

1979 Katz, J.F.: Precise identification of radiographic acetabular landmarks, Clin. Orthop. **141**:166-168, 1979.

Naimark, A., Kossoff, J., and Schepsis, A.: Intertrochanteric fractures: current concepts of an old subject, A.J.R. **133**:889-894, 1979.

1980 Clements, R.W., and Nakayama, H.K.: Radiographic methods in total hip arthroplasty, Radiol. Technol. **51**:589-600, 1980.

Resnick, D., and Guerra, J., Jr.: Stress fractures of the inferior pubic ramus following hip surgery, Radiology **137**:335-338, 1980.

1981 Eisenberg, R.L., Hedgecock, M.W., and Akin, J.R.: The 40° cephalad view of the hip, A.J.R. **136**:835-836, 1981.

Vertebral column

Occipitocervical articulations

1920 Massimo, L.: Contributo allo studio dell'anatomia radiografica delle prime vertebre cervicali e del cranio, Radiol. Med. **7**:393-407, 1920.

1926 Goldhamer, K.: Beitrag zur röntgenographischen Darstellung des Atlas und der Pars lateralis occipitis, Fortschr. Roentgenstr. **35**:627-629, 1926-1927.

1942 Englander, O.: Non-traumatic occipito-atlanto-axial dislocation: a contribution to the radiology of the atlas, Br. J. Radiol. **15**:341-345, 1942.

1961 Lombardi, G.: The occipital vertebra, A.J.R. **86**:260-269, 1961.

1977 Dirkheimer, Y., Ramsheyi, A., and Reolon, M.: Positive arthrography of the craniocervical joints, Neuroradiology **12**:257-260, 1977.

Atlas and axis

1910 Albers-Schönberg, H.E.: Die Röntgentechnik, ed. 3, Hamburg, 1910, Gräfe & Sillem.

1919 George, A.W.: Method for more accurate study of injuries to the atlas and axis, Boston Med. Surg. J. **181**:395-398, 1919.

1931 Fuchs, A.W.: Regional radiographic technique, Radiogr. Clin. Photogr. **7**:12-13, 1931.

1937 Kukka, Z.: Transkranielle Aufnahme des ersten Halswirbels, Röntgenpraxis **9**:128-129, 1937.

1938 Plaut, H.F.: Fractures of the atlas resulting from automobile accidents, A.J.R. **40**:867, 1938.

1939 Kasabach, H.H.: A roentgenographic method for the study of the second cervical vertebra. A.J.R. **42**:782-785, 1939.

1940 Pancoast, H.K., Pendergrass, E.P., and Schaeffer, J.P.: The head and neck in roentgen diagnosis, Springfield, Ill., 1940, Charles C Thomas, Publisher.

1942 Dariaux: Radiographie de face de la colonne cervicale en incidence antérieure, J. Radiol. Electrol. **25**:28, 1942.

1943 Judd, G.: A useful view of the odontoid process of the axis vertebra, Radiography **9**:46, 1943.

1950 Schunk, F.: Radiography of the first cervical ring (atlas), Xray Tchn. **21**:219-220, 1950.

Walters, B.: An additional technique for the roentgen demonstration of the first cervical vertebra, A.J.R. **63**:739-740, 1950.

1951 Buetti, C.: Zur Darstellung der Atlanto-epistropheal Gelenke bzw. der Procc. transversi atlantis und epistrophei, Radiol. Clin. **20**;168-172, 1951.

1956 Jacobson, G., and Adler, D.C.: Examination of the atlanto-axial joint following injury, A.J.R. **76**:1081-1094, 1956.

1962 Herrmann, E., and Stender, H.S.: Eine einfache Aufnahmetechnik zur Darstellung der Dens axis, Fortschr. Roentgenstr. **96**:115-119, 1962.

1969 Gabrielsen, T.O.: Roentgenographic examination of foramen transversarium of axis: practical considerations, A.J.R. **105**:361-364, 1969.

Lame, E.L., and Redick, T.J.: Autotomography applied to the pharynx and dens, A.J.R. **105**:359-360, 1969.

Wackenheim, A., and Lopez, F.: Radiographic study of the movements of C1 and C2 during flexion and extension of the head, J. Belg. Radiol. **52**:117-120, 1969.

1978 Apuzzo, M.L., Weiss, M.H., and Heiden, J.S.: Transoral exposure of the atlantoaxial region, Neurosurgery **3**:201-207, 1978.

1979 Farman, A.G., Nortjé, C.J., and Joubert, J.J.: Radiographic profile of the first cervical vertebra, J. Anat. **128**:595-600, 1979.

Kattan, K.R.: Two features of the atlas vertebra simulating fractures by tomography, A.J.R. **132**:963-965, 1979.

1980 Harrison, R.B., et al.: Pseudosubluxation of the axis in young adults, J. Can. Assoc. Radiol. **31**:176-177, 1980.

Mellström, A., Grepe, A., and Levander, B.: Atlantoaxial arthrography, a postmortem study, Neuroradiology **20**:135-144, 1980.

Cervical vertebrae

1916 Hobbs, A.L.: A method of showing the lower cervical vertebrae, A.J.R. **3**:233, 1916.

1923 Feil, A.: Comment doit-on radiographier la colonne cervicale quand on soupçonne l'existence d'une anomalie? J. Radiol. Electrol. **7**:125-133, 1923.

1925 Grandy, C.C.: A new method for making radiographs of the cervical vertebrae in lateral position, Radiology **4**:128-129, 1925.

1926 Barsóny, T., and Koppenstein, E.: Eine neue Methode zur Roentgenuntersuchung der Halswirbelsäule, Fortschr. Roentgenstr. **35**:593-594, 1926-1927.

1929 Barsóny, T., and Koppenstein, E.: Beitrag zur Aufnahmetechnik der Halswirbelsäule: Darstellung der Foramina intervertebralia, Röntgenpraxis **1**:245-249, 1929.

Erdélyi, J.: Neues Verfahren zur seitlichen Aufnahme der Halswirbel, Röntgenpraxis **1**:138-140, 1929.

Gally and Bernard: Technique particulière pour la radiographie de profil de la colonne cervicale, Bull. Mém. Soc. Radiol. Méd. Paris **17**:288-289, 1929.

Ottonello, P.: Nuevo método para la radiografía de la columna cervical completa en proyección sagital ventrodorsal, Anal. Radiol. (Havana) **1**:57-58, 1929.

1930 Ottonello, P.: New method for roentgenography of the entire cervical spine in ventrodorsal projection, Rev. Radiol. Fis. Med. **2**:291-294, 1930.

Schneider, C.C.: Mechanical devices for immobilizing the head and hand, Xray Techn. **1**:70-71, 1930.

1931 Arskussky, J.: Eine vereinfachte Methode der Röntgenaufnahme des oberen Halswirbel, Röntgenpraxis **3**:953-957, 1931.

Pélissier, G.: Radiographie de face de la colonne cervicale dans son ensemble technique nouvelle, Bull. Mém. Soc. Radiol. Méd. Paris **19**:360-361, 1931.

1935 Lupacciolu, G.: Fratture del rachide cervicale all'indagine radiologica, Radiol. Med. **22**:529-562, 1935. Abstract: A.J.R. **37**:135, 1937.

1938 Gaudentia, Sister M.: The cervical vertebrae, Xray Techn. **10**:74-75, 86, 1938.

Jacobs, L.: Roentgenography of the cervical second vertebra by Ottonello's method, Radiology **31**:412-413, 1938.

Kovács, Á.: Röntgendarstellung und Diagnostik der zervicalen Zwischenwirbellöcher, Röntgenpraxis **10**:478-484, 1938.

Oppenheimer, A.: The swollen atrophic hand, Surg. Gynecol. Obstet. **67**:446-454, 1938.

1940 Fuchs, A.W.: Cervical vertebrae, Radiogr. Clin. Photogr. **16**:2-17, 34-41, 1940.

1942 Beatrice, Sister M.: Roentgenography of the cervical spine, Xray Techn. **13**:147-149, 1942.

Belot, J.: A propos de la radiographie de la colonne vertebrale, J. Radiol. Electrol. **25**:135-136, 1942-1943.

1943 Garthright, E.G.: Technique for roentgenography of the upper cervical vertebrae, Xray Techn. **14**:241-242, 1943.

1944 Hadley, L.A.: Roentgenographic studies of the cervical spine, A.J.R. **52**:173-195, 1944.

1946 Pollino, W.W.: Method for obtaining optimum visualization of the seventh cervical vertebra in lateral projections, Roentgenography **1**:10-11, 1946.

1948 Marchand, J.H., Djian, A., and Fétiveau: Radiographie de la colonne cervicale en double obliquité, J. Radiol. Electrol. **29**:291-295, 1948.

1950 Marks, J.L., and Parks, S.L.: A simplified position for demonstrating the cervical intervertebral foramina, A.J.R. **63**:575-577, 1950.

1954 Albers, D.: Eine Studie über die Funktion der Halswirbelsäule bei dorsaler und ventraler Flexion, Fortschr. Roentgenstr. **81**:606-615, 1954.

1955 Bumstead, H.D.: Routine examination of the cervical spine, Xray Techn. **27**:247-250, 1955.

1957 Boylston, B.F.: Oblique roentgenographic views of the cervical spine in flexion and extension: an aid in the diagnosis of cervical subluxations and obscure dislocations, J. Bone Joint Surg. **39-A**:1302-1309, 1957.

Dorland, P., and Frémont, J.: Aspect radiologique normale du rachis postérieur cervicodorsal (vue postérieure ascendante) Semaine Hapit., pp. 1457-1464, 1957.

Gersh, M., and Vincent, P.J.: Anteroposterior projection of the cervical vertebrae on one film, Med. Radiogr. Photogr. **33**:2-3, 1957.

1958 Abel, M.S.: Moderately severe whiplash injuries of the cervical spine and their roentgenologic diagnosis, Clin. Orthop. **12**:189-208, 1958.

Dorland, P., et al.: Technique d'examen radiologique de l'arc postérieur des vertèbres cervico-dorsales, J. Radiol. Electrol. **39**:509-519, 1958.

Hartley, J.: Modern concepts of whiplash injury, N.Y. J. Med. **58**:3306-3310, 1958.

1961 Conklin, W.A.: Radiographic studies of the cervical spine, Xray Techn. **33**:181-185, 1961.

1962 Coupe, C.W.: Cervicodorsal region: lateral projection. Xray Techn. **33**:256-257, 1962.

1963 Beatson, T.R.: Fractures and dislocations of the cervical spine, J. Bone Joint Surg. **45-B**:21-35, 1963.

1964 Cahoon, J.B., Jr.: All in one, C-1 and you see seven, Radiol. Technol. **35**:252-258, 1964.

Hagen, D.E.: Introduction to the pillar projection of the cervical spine, Radiol. Technol. **35**:239-242, 1964.

1969 Vines, F.S.: The significance of "occult" fractures of the cervical spine, A.J.R. **107**:493-504, 1969.

1970 Ott, H., et al.: Radiologic examination of the cervical spine in rheumatoid arthritis, Schweiz. Med. Wochenschr. **100**:1726-1730, 1970. (In German.) Abstract: Radiology **100**:233, 1971.

1971 Li, C.P., and Paull, D.: A new head rotation method for cervical spine radiography, Radiology **98**:568, 1971.

1972 Cancelmo, J.J., Jr.: Clay shoveler's fracture: a helpful diagnostic sign, A.J.R. **115**:540-543, 1972.

1975 Smith, G.R., and Abel, M.S.: Visualization of the posterolateral elements of the upper cervical vertebrae in the anteroposterior projection, Radiology **115**:219-220, 1975.

1976 Kattan, K.R.: The notched articular process of C7, A.J.R. **126**:612-616, 1976.

1977 Dolan, K.D.: Cervical spine injuries below the axis, Radiol. Clin. North Am. **15**:247-259, 1977.

Furuse, M., et al.: Orthopantomography of the cervical spine, Radiology **124**:517-520, 1977.

Jergens, M.E., Morgan, M.T., and McElroy, C.E.: Selective use of radiography of the skull and cervical spine, West. J. Med. **127**:1-4, 1977.

Tenney, R.F., and Kerekes, E.S.: Cervical spine lateral horizontal beam technique, Radiology **124**:520, 1977.

1979 Braun, J.P., et al.: The transverse cervical canal: anatomical-radiological comparison with a review of the values and limitations of different radiographic techniques, J. Neuroradiol. **6**:327-334, 1979.

Park, W.M., O'Neill, M., and McCall, I.W.: The radiology of rheumatoid involvement of the cervical spine, Skeletal Radiol. **4**:1-7, 1979.

Yelton, R.: Cervica spine protocol for emergency room use, Radiol. Technol. **50**:693-698, 1979.

1980 Cerisoli, M., Vernizzi, E., and Giulioni, M.: Cervical spine changes following laminectomy, J. Neurosurg. Sci. **24**:63-70, 1980.

De Luca, S.A., and Rhea, J.A.: Radiographic anatomy of the cervical vertebrae, Med. Radiogr. Photogr. **56**:18-24, 1980.

Shmueli, G., and Herold, Z.H.: Prevertebral shadow in cervical trauma, Isr. Med. Sci. **16**:698-700, 1980.

Thoracic vertebrae

1925 Badolle, M.: La radiographie de la colonne dorsale chez l'adulte en positions obliques, Lyon Méd. **135**:224-232, 1925.

1926 Alberti, O.: Tecnica radiografica per la proiezione esattamente laterale delle prime vertebre dorsali, Radiol. Med. **13**:212-214, 1926.

1927 Barsóny, T., and Koppenstein, E.: Eine neue Methode zur Röntgenuntersuchung der oberen Brustwirbelsäle, Fortschr. Roentgenstr. **36**:338-341, 1927.

1928 Alberti, O.: Tecnica radiografica per la proiezione esattamente laterale delle prime vertebre dorsali, Atti Congresso Ital. Radiol. Med. **8**:340-345, 1928.

Dall'Acqua, V.: Nuovo metodo per la proiezione laterale delle ultime vertebre cervicali e delle prime dorsali, Radiol. Med. **15**:843-845, 1928.

Gutzeit: Aufnahmetechnik der oberen Brustwirbelsäule in frontaler Richtung, Fortschr. Roentgenstr. **37**:400, 1928.

1929 Pawlov, M.K.: Zur Frage über die seitliche Strahlenrichtung bei den Aufnahmen der unteren und oberen Brustwirbel, Röntgenpraxis **1**:285-288, 1929.

Sgalitzer, M.: Zur Technik der Röntgenuntersuchung der 4 obersten Brustwirbel in seitlicher Richtung, Fortschr. Roentgenstr. **40**:267-271, 1929.

1933 Corlay, G.: Contribution à l'étude radiologique de la region cervico-dorsale, Paris theses, 1933.

1937 Barsóny, T., and Winkler, K.: Beiträge zur Röntgenologie der Wirbelsäule: die "elektive" Profil-Röntgenaufnahme der Brustwirbelsäule, Röntgenpraxis **9**:601-608, 1937.

Twining, E.W.: Lateral view of the lung apices, Br. J. Radiol. **10**:123-131, 1937.

1938 Bartsch, G.W.: Radiography of the upper dorsal spine, Xray Techn. **10**:135-138, 1938.

Fletcher, J.: Radiography of the upper vertebrae, Radiogr. Clin. Photogr. **14**:10-12, 1938.

Oppenheimer, A.: The apophyseal intervertebral articulations roentgenologically considered, Radiology **30**:724-740, 1938.

1940 Clarke, E.K.: Visualization of the first and second dorsal and the fifth lumbar vertebrae in lateral or slightly semilateral positions, Xray Techn. **12**:5-7, 1940.

Horwitz, T., and Smith, R.M.: An anatomical, pathological and roentgenological study of the intervertebral joints of the lumbar spine and of the sacroiliac joints, A.J.R. **43**:173-186, 1940.

1941 Eller, V.H.: Radiography of the thoracic spine, Xray Techn. **13**:18-20, 36, 1941.

Fuchs, A.W.: Thoracic vertebrae, Radiogr. Clin. Photogr. **17**:2-13, 42-51, 1941.

1944 Desgrez and Pioux: Contribution à létude des premières vertèbres dorsales en profil vrai, J. Radiol. Electrol. **26**:29, 1944-1945.

1946 Oregeron, E.A.: An additional technique for the demonstration of the cervical and upper thoracic spine in a lateral position, Xray Techn. **17**:385-386, 1946.

1950 Guerreiro, G.: Lateral roentgenographic examination of the thoracic spine, J. Bone Joint Surg. **32-A**:192, 1950.

1976 McAllister, V.L., and Sage, M.R.: The radiology of thoracic disc protrusion, Clin. Radiol. **27**:291-299, 1976.

1980 Scher, A.T.: The diagnostic value of the antero-posterior radiograph for thoracolumbar injuries, S. Afr. Med. J. **58**:415-417, 1980.

Lumbar vertebrae

1917 Hammes, J.: Ueber die Technik und den Wert seitlicher Wirbelaufnahmen, Fortschr. Roentgenstr. **25**:1, 1917-1918.

Hickey, P.M.: Lateral roentgenology of the spine, A.J.R. **4**:101-106, 1917.

1919 Gage, H.C.: La radiographie de lésions suspectés de la colonne vertébrale par la methode latérale, J. Radiol. Electrol. 3:219-221, 1918-1919.

1924 Magnuson, P.B.: Reasons for lack of positive roentgen findings in many cases of low back pain, A.J.R. 12:15-23, 1924.

1929 Dittmar, O.: Die sagittal und lateral flexorische Bewegung der menschlichen Lendeniwirbelsäule im Röntgenbild, Z. Ges. Anat. (Abt. I) 92:644-667, 1929.

Samuel, M.: Ueber Ausbau und Bedeutung einer röntgenologischen Darstellung der Bechengelenke, Röntgenpraxis 1:944-947, 1929.

1931 Bell, M.E.: Lateral spine technic, Xray Techn. 2:91-96, 1931.

Hibbs, R.A., Risser, J.C., and Ferguson, A.B.: Scoliosis treated by the fusion operation: an end result study of 360 cases, J. Bone Joint Surg. 13:91-104, 1931.

Hubney, M.J.: The oblique projection in examination of the lumbar spine, Radiology 16:720-724, 1931.

Meyer-Burgdorff, H.: Untersuchungen über das Wirbelgleiten, Leipzig, 1931, Georg Thieme.

1933 Ghormley, R.K.: Low back pain with special reference to articular facets with presentation of an operative procedure, J.A.M.A. 101:1773-1777, 1933.

1935 Files, G.: La radiografia de la espina lumbar, Rev. Radiol. Fis. 4:22-37, 1935.

1937 Hodges, F.J., and Peck, W.S.: Clinical and roentgenological study of low back pain with sciatic radiation, A.J.R. 37:461, 1937.

Jordan, H.: Roentgen analysis of the spine, Radiology 28:714-724, 1937.

Morton, S.A.: Value of the oblique view in radiographic examination of lumbar spine, Radiology 29:568-573, 1937.

1939 Eller, V.H.: Various positions for the x-ray examination of the lumbar spine, Xray Techn. 11:57-59, 1939.

Elward, J.F.: Motion in the vertebral column, A.J.R. 42:91-99, 1939.

1940 Horwitz, T., and Smith, M.R.: An anatomical, pathological and roentgenological study of the intervertebral joints of the lumbar spine and of the sacroiliac joints, A.J.R. 43:173, 1940.

1941 Doub, H.P., and Camp. J.D.: Oblique radiography of the spine, Radiology 37:232-233, 1941.

Gibson, M.: The use of diaphragms in radiography of the lumbar spine, Xray Techn. 12:128-129, 145, 1941.

1942 Cornwell, W.S.: Lumbar vertebrae, Radiogr. Clin. Photogr. 18:2-11, 30-35, 54-61, 1942.

Cornwell, W.S.: Some aspects of radiography of the lumbar vertebrae, Xray Techn. 14:77-83, 88, 1942.

Duncan, W., and Hoen, T.: A new approach to the diagnosis of herniation of the intervertebral disc, Surg. Gynecol. Obstet. 75:257-267, 1942.

Morgan, F.E.: Technical considerations in x-raying the lumbar and sacral spine, Xray Techn. 13:228-230, 245, 1942.

Scott, W.G.: Low back pain resulting from arthritis and subluxations of the apophyseal joints and fractures of the articular facets of the lumbar spine, A.J.R. 48:491-509, 1942.

1943 Gunson, E.F.: Technique for oblique radiography of the spine, Xray Techn. 14:188-193, 210, 1943.

Maltson, S.: Technique for spot radiography, Xray Techn. 14:233-235, 247, 1943.

Scott, W.G.: Dolor en la parte inferior de la espalda debido a artritis y a subluxaciones de las articulaciones apofisarias y fracturas de las facetas articulares de la columna lumbar, Rev. Radiol. Fis. 10:55-72, 1943.

1944 Copleman, B.: The roentgenographic diagnosis of the small central protruded intervertebral disc, A.J.R. 52:245-260, 1944.

Gianturco, C.: A roentgen analysis of the motion of the lower lumbar vertebrae in normal individuals and in patients with low back pain, A.J.R. 52:261-268, 1944.

Knutsson, F.: The instability associated with disk degeneration in the lumbar spine, Acta Radiol. 25:593-609, 1944.

1945 Slauson, D.B.: A new principle in the roentgenography of the lateral lumbar spine, Radiography 44:280-282, 1945.

1946 Meschan, I.: A radiographic study of spondylolisthesis with special reference to stability determination, Radiology 47:249-262, 1946.

Slauson, D.B.: A new principle in roentgenography of the lateral lumbar spine, Xray Techn. 17:383-384, 400, 1946.

1947 Boyland, K.G.: True lateral positioning of lumbar spine and pelvis, Radiography 13:44, 1947.

Melamed, A., and Ansfield, D.J.: Posterior displacement of lumbar vertebrae, A.J.R. 58:307-328, 1947.

1949 Etter, L.E., and Carabello, N.C.: Roentgen anatomy of oblique views of the lumbar spine, A.J.R. 61:699-705, 1949.

1950 Kovács, A.: X-ray examination of the exit of the lowermost lumbar root, Radiol. Clin. 19:6-13, 1950.

1951 Kröker, P.: Ueber die Röntgenuntersuchung beim lumbalem Bandscheibenvorfall mit Hilfe der lumboinguinalen Einstellung von Kovács, Fortschr. Roentgenstr. 74:519, 1951.

1952 Hasner, E., Schalimtzek, M., and Snorrason, E.: Roentgenological examination of the function of the lumbar spine, Acta Radiol. 37:141-149, 1952.

1953 Lyons, N.J.: Dynamic views of the lumbar spine, Xray Techn. 24:402-407, 1953.

1961 Stevens, R., and Bauer, D.: Posteroanterior view of the lumbar spine, Xray Techn. 32:603-608, 1961.

1963 Holohan, F.: Simplified positioning of the scoliotic spine, Xray Techn. 34:347-351, 1963.

1971 Dehner, J.R.: Seatbelt injuries of the spine and abdomen, A.J.R. 111:833-843, 1971.

Hellems, H.K., and Keats, T.E.: Measurement of normal lumbosacral angle, A.J.R. 113:642-645, 1971.

Rogers, L.F.: The roentgenographic appearance of transverse or chance fractures of the spine: the seat belt fracture, A.J.R. 111:844-849, 1971.

1973 Barnhard, H.J., and Dodd, D.: Radiographic anatomy of the lumbar vertebrae, Med. Radiogr. Photogr. 49:7-20, 1973.

1976 Hanley, E.N., Matteri, R.E., and Frymoyer, J.W.: Accurate roentgenographic determination of lumbar flexion-extension, Clin. Orthop. 115:145-148, 1976.

1978 Rosomoff, H.L., Post, M.J., and Quencer, R.M.: Axial radiology of the lumbar spine, Clin. Neurosurg. 25:251-265, 1978.

1979 MacGibbon, B., and Farfan, H.F.: A radiologic survey of various configurations of the lumbar spine, Spine 4:258, 266, 1979.

1980 Carrera, G.F., et al.: Computed tomography in sciatica, Radiology 137:433-437, 1980.

Rhea, J.T., et al.: The oblique view: an unnecessary component of the initial adult lumbar spine examination, Radiology 134:45-47, 1980.

Wagner, A.C.: "Spurious" defect of the lumbar vertebral body, A.J.R. 135:1095-1096, 1980.

1981 Scavone, J.G., Latshaw, R.F., and Weidner, W.A.: Anteroposterior and lateral radiographs: an adequate lumbar spine examination, A.J.R. 136:715-717, 1981.

Lumbosacral region

1905 Ludloff, K.: Verletzungen der Lendenwirbelsäule und des Kreuzbeins, Fortschr. Roentgenstr. 9:175, 1905.

1920 Marcel, Galland, and de Berck: La radiographie de face de la Ve vertèbre lombaire, Rev. Méd. Francaise, October 1920.

1921 Garcin, J.: Radiographie de la Ve vertèbre lombaire, J. Radiol. Electrol. 5:410-412, 1921.

1924 LeWald, L.T.: Lateral roentgenography of the lumbosacral region, A.J.R. 12:362-367, 1924.

1929 Dittmar, O.: Halbseitliche Aufnahme des Lendenwirbel-Kreuzbeinabschnittes, Fortschr. Roentgenstr. 39:864-865, 1929; 40:99-107, 1929.

Galland, M., and Las Casas, H.: La dynamique lombo-sacrée, J. Radiol. Electrol. 13:529-547, 1929.

Samuel, M.: Ueber Ausbau und Bedeutung einer röntgenologischen Darstellung der Beckengelenke, Röntgenpraxis 1:944-947, 1929.

349

Warner, F.: Studien zur Pathologie des Lumbosakralgebietes, Verhandl. Deutsch. Ges. Unfallheilkunde, September 1929.

1931 Belden, W.W.: Fifth lumbar vertebra roentgenologically demonstrated, Radiology **16**:905-932, 1931.

Harttung, H.: Technisches zur Röntgenaufnahme des Lenden-Kreuzbeinwinkels, Zbl. Chir. **58**:453, 1931.

Reisner, A.: Unterscheidungs-merkmale normaler, entzündlicher und post-traumalischer Zustände an der Wirbelsäule, Fortschr. Roentgenstr. **44**:726-751, 1931.

1932 Barsóny, T., and Schulhoff, O.: Die Aufnahmetechnik zur Sagitallen. Darstellung des lumbo-sakro-iliakalen Gebietes im Röntgenbilde, Röntgenpraxis **4**:594-598, 1932.

Samuel, M.: Technisches zur Röntgenaufnahme des Lenden-Kreuzbeinwinkels, Zbl. Chir. **59**:661, 1932.

1933 Warner, F.: Der 5. Lendenwirbel, Arch. Orthop. Unfall-Chir. **33**:279-306, 1933.

1934 Ferguson, A.B.: The clinical and roentgenographic interpretation of lumbosacral anomalies, Radiology **22**:548, 1934.

Ghormley, R.K., and Kirklin, B.R.: The oblique view for demonstration of the articular facets in lumbosacral backache and sciatic pain, A.J.R. **31**:173-176, 1934.

1935 Williams, P.C., and Wigby, P.E.: Technique for the roentgen examination of the lumbosacral articulation, A.J.R. **33**:511-515, 1935.

1937 Chamberlain, W.E.: Low back pain, J. Proc. Calif. Acad. Med., 1937-1938.

Gage, C.: A new position for the examination of the lumbosacral area, Radiology **28**:495, 1937.

1938 Petsing, H.C.: The fifth lumbar body and lumbosacral junction, Xray Techn. **9**:187-190, 1938.

1939 Geissenberger, H.: Roentgenography of the lumbar and lumbosacral spine, Xray Techn. **10**:174-176, 196, 1939.

1941 Ferguson, A.B.: Roentgen diagnosis of the extremities and spine, enlarged ed. 1, New York, 1941, Harper & Row, Publishers.

1943 Cornwell, W.S.: The lumbosacral junction, Radiogr. Clin. Photogr. **19**:30-39, 58-69, 1943.

1944 Cornwell, W.S.: The lumbosacral junction, Radiogr. Clin. Photogr. **20**:2-11, 1944.

1945 Wilsey, R.B., Holly, E.W., and Cornwell, W.S.: Special problems in lateral radiography of the lumbar and lumbosacral region, Radiogr. Clin. Photogr. **21**:2-8, 1945.

1946 Bonfilia, Sister M.: Some aspects of radiography of the lumbosacral region, Xray Techn. **17**:381-382, 1946.

1949 Kovács, Á.: Vertebral ligaments on native roentgenograms, Acta Radiol. **32**:287-303, 1949.

1953 Holly, E.W., and Weingartner, G.: Oblique lateroposterior radiography of the lumbosacral junction, Med. Radiogr. Photogr. **29**:91-92, 1953.

1961 Sparks, O.J.: Lumbosacral oblique: improvement by longitudinal deviation, Xray Techn. **33**:93-99, 1961.

1975 Curran, J.T.: New approach to positioning for lumbosacral junction in lateral projection, Radiol. Technol. **46**:294-297, 1975.

1979 Eisenberg, R.L., Akin, J.R., and Hedgcock, M.W.: Single, well-centered lateral view of lumbosacral spine: is coned view necessary? A.J.R. **133**:711-713, 1979.

Sacroiliac joints

1911 Fischer, W.: Der letzte Lendenwirbel: eine Röntgenstudie, Fortschr. Roentgenstr. **8**:346-359, 1911-1912.

1923 Allen, H.R.: The iliosacral joint, Indianapolis Med. J. **26**:151-155, 1923.

1924 Darling, B.C.: The sacro-iliac joint: its diagnosis as determined by x-ray, Radiology **3**:486-491, 1924.

1927 Pincherle, P.: La sacro-ileite, Radiol. Med. **14**:153-167, 1927.

1930 Chamberlain, W.E.: The symphysis pubis in the roentgen examination of the sacro-iliac joint, A.J.R. **24**:621-625, 1930.

1932 Chamberlain, W.E.: The x-ray examination of the sacro-iliac joint, Delaware State Med. J. **4**:195-200, 1932.

1934 Ghormley, R.K., and Kirklin, B.R.: The oblique view for demonstration of the articular facets in lumbosacral backache and sciatic pain, A.J.R. **31**:173-176, 1934.

1935 Kovács, Á.: Die sakroiliale Spaltenaufnahme, Röntgenpraxis **7**:763-768, 1935.

1936 Logroscino, D.: L'anca e la sacro-illiaca in una nuova proiezione radiografica, Boll. Ass. Med. Trieste **27**:82-89, 1936; Röntgenpraxis **8**:433-445, 1936.

Logroscino, D.: Das Hüftgelenk und das Sakroiliakalgelenk in günstiger röntgenographischer Projektion, Röntgenpraxis **8**:433-445, 1936.

1937 Coliez, R.: La radiographie de l'articulation sacroiliaque, Bull. Soc. Radiol. Méd. Paris **25**:263, 1937.

Nemours-Auguste: A propos de la radiographie de l'articulation sacro-iliaque, Bull. Soc. Radiol. Méd. Paris **25**:181-183, 1937.

Tillier, H., and Coriat, P.: Anatomie radiographie de l'articulation sacro-iliaque dans les incidences de face et de trois quarts, Bull. Soc. Radiol. Méd. Paris **25**:449, 1937.

1940 Horowitz, T., and Smith, M.R.: An anatomical, pathological and roentgenological study of the intervertebral joints of the lumbar spine and of the sacroiliac joints, A.J.R. **43**:173-186, 1940.

Ruwett, L.H.: Technic in radiography of the sacro-iliac joint: an evaluation of the symphysis pubis method, Xray Techn. **11**:214-218, 1940.

1953 Bridgman, C.F., and Cornwell, W.S.: Radiography of the sacroiliac articulation, Med. Radiogr. Photogr. **29**:78-90, 1953.

1956 Meese, T.: Die dorso-ventrale Aufnahme der Sacroiliacalgelenke, Fortschr. Roentgenstr. **85**:601-603, 1956.

1957 Kamieth, H.: What do spot films of the sacroiliac joint accomplish? Pathology of the sacroiliac joint, Radiol. Clin. **26**:139-157, 1957.

1974 Johannsen, A., Jepsen, O.L., and Winge, J.: Radiological and scintigraphical examination of the sacroiliac joints in the diagnosis of sacroiliitis, Dan. Med. Bull. **21**:246-250, 1974.

1978 Dory, M.A., and Francois, R.J.: Craniocaudal axial view of the sacroiliac joint, A.J.R. **130**:1125-1131, 1978.

1980 De Carvalho, A., and Graudal, H.: Sacroiliac involvement in classical or definite rheumatoid arthritis, Acta Radiol. **21**:417-423, 1980.

Sacrum and coccyx

1917 Lilienfeld, L.: Die seitliche Kreuzbeinaufnahme, München. Med. Wochenschr. **64**:211-214, 1917.

1930 Nölke, W.: Axiale Aufnahmen zur Darstellung des Sakralkanalquerschnittes und des Beckens, Röntgenpraxis **2**:742-748, 1930.

1933 Zochert, R.W.: The sacrum and coccyx: location and technic for radiography, Xray Techn. **4**:118-120, 1933.

1935 Hoing, M.: A new technic of coccyxography, Xray Techn. **7**:68-72, 89, 1935.

1936 Sabat, B.: Intrarectal radiography, Fortschr. Roentgenstr. **53**:143-165, 1936. Abstract: Yearbook of Radiology, p. 354, 1936.

1937 Guarini, C.: La radiografia del coccige, Arch. Radiol. **13**:228-235, 1937.

1957 Ruttimann, A.: Eine einfache Methode zur Verbesserung der Steissbeinaufnahmen, Fortschr. Roentgenstr. **86**:511-514, 1957.

1975 Northrop, C.H., Eto, R.T., and Loop, J.W.: Vertical fracture of the sacral ala: significance of the noncontinuity of the anterior superior sacral foraminal line, A.J.R. **124**:102-106, 1975.

1976 Bucknill, T.M., and Blackburne, J.S.: Fracture-dislocations of the sacrum, J. Bone Joint Surg. (Br.) **58-B**(4):467-470, 1976.

1977 Fountain, S.S., Hamilton, R.D., and Jameson, R.M.: Transverse fractures of the sacrum, J. Bone Joint Surg. **59**:486-489, 1977.

1981 Turner, M.L., Mulhern, C.B., and Dalinka, M.K.: Lesions of the sacrum: differential diagnosis and radiological evaluation, J.A.M.A. **245**:275-277, 1981.

Vertebral column—entire

1909 Simon, M.: Ueber die Röntgenanatomie der Wirbelsäule, und die Röntgendiagnose von Wirbelverletzungen, Fortschr. Roentgenstr. **14**:353-419, 1909.

1910 Putti, V.: Die angeborenen Deformitäten der Wirbelsäule, Fortschr. Roentgenstr. **15**:65-92, 1910.

1921 Suggars, H.J.: Thesis upon the subject of radiographing the spine and the pelvis, Arch. Radiol. Electrol. **26**:382-396, 1921-1922.

1924 George, A.W., and Leonard, R.D.: Fundamental facts relative to the study of the vertebrae in industrial accident cases, Radiology **2**:197-213, 1924.

1926 Kloiber: Fehlerquelle bei Röntgenaufnahmen der Wirbelsäule, Fortschr. Roentgenstr. **35**:451-454, 1926.

1929 George, A.W., and Leonard, R.D.: The vertebrae roentgenologically considered, Ann. Roentgenol. **8**:1929.

1930 Ferguson, A.B.: The study and treatment of scoliosis, South. Med. J. **23**:116-120, 1930.

1931 Jaeger, W.: Ueber Fernaufnahmen der Wirbelsäule, Verhandl. Deutsch. Röntgengesell. **23**:1931; Röntgenpraxis **4**:193-209, 1932.

Meyer-Burgdorff, H.: Untersuchungen über das Wirbelgleiten, Leipzig, 1931, Georg Thieme.

Thoma, E.: Die Zwischenwirbellöcher im Röntgenbild, ihre normale und pathologische Anatomie, Z. Orthop. Chir. **55**:55-115, 1931.

1932 Dittmar, O.: Die Wirbelsäule, Fortschr. Roentgenstr. **43**:1932.

Jaeger, W.: Distant roentgenography of the spinal column, Röntgenpraxis **4**:193-209, 1932. Abstract: Yearbook of Radiology, p. 327, 1932.

Schmorl, G.: Die gesunde und die kranke Wirbelsäule im Röntgenbild, Leipzig, 1932, Dr. Werner Klinkhardt.

1933 Jaeger, W.: Beobachtungen über den Achsenverlauf der Wirbelsäule, Fortschr. Roentgenstr. **47**:299, 1933.

Joyner, T.H.: Radiography of the spine, Xray Techn. **5**:11-14, 1933.

1934 Lange, M.: Die Wirbelgelenke, Z. Orthop. Chir. **61**(suppl.):1934.

Lapenna, M.: La radiologia delle affezioni e delle lesion: traumatiche vertebrale, Atti Congresso Ital. Radiol. Med. **11**:1-22, 1934.

1935 Lewis, R.W.: Certain aspects of roentgenology of the spine from the orthopedic viewpoint, A.J.R. **33**:491-503, 1935.

Pearson, G.R.: Technic for the use of a small cone in check radiographs of the spine, Radiology **24**:601-606, 1935.

Storck, H.: Die Röntgenraumbildmessung in der Orthopädie, Fortschr. Roentgenstr. **51**:369-379, 1935.

1936 Fuchs, A.W.: Radiography of the spine—a new method, Radiogr. Clin. Photogr. **12**:2-7, 1936.

Hadley, L.A.: Apophyseal subluxation, J. Bone Joint Surg. **34**:428, 1936.

Perry, E.C.: Spinal radiography, Xray Techn. **7**:108-109, 1936.

1937 Jordan, H.: Roentgen analysis of the spine, Radiology **28**:714-724, 1937.

Mensor, M.C.: Injuries to the accessory processes of the spinal vertebrae, J. Bone Joint Surg. **35**:381, 1937.

Oppenheimer, A.: Diseases affecting the intervertebral foramina, Radiology **28**:582-592, 1937.

1938 Brocher, J.E.W.: Der Kreutzschmerz in seiner Beziehung zur Wirbelsäule, Fortschr. Roentgenstr. **57**:1938.

Oppenheimer, A.: The apophyseal intervertebral articulations roentgenologically considered, Radiology **30**:724-740, 1938.

Palmer, P.E.: Fractures of the spine with injuries to the cord, Southwestern Med. **22**:360, 1938.

1939 Ferguson, A.B.: Roentgen diagnosis of the extremities and spine, New York, 1939, Harper & Row, Publishers.

1940 Krogdahl, T., and Torgersen, O.: Die "Unco-Vertebralgelenke" und die "Arthrosis deformans unco-vertebralis," Acta Radiol. **21**:234-235, 1940.

Oppenheimer, A.: The apophyseal intervertebral joints, Surgery **8**:699-712, 1940.

Stinchfield, F.E.: Fractures of the vertebrae, Surg. Gynecol. Obstet. **70**:378, 1940.

1941 McElvenny, R.T.: Principles underlying treatment of scoliosis, Surg. Gynecol. Obstet. **72**:228-236, 1941.

1943 Albu, Z.: Synopsis of spine radiography, Xray Techn. **14**:241-242, 1943.

Carey, E.: Anatomical and physiological considerations prerequisite to diagnosis of back trauma, Radiology **41**:554-559, 1943.

Gianturco, C.: Lateral roentgenography of the spine, A.J.R. **50**:695, 1943.

1946 Davis, A.G.: Fractures and dislocations of the spine. In Pillmore, G.U., editor: Clinical radiology, vol. 2, Philadelphia, 1946, F.A. Davis Co.

1948 Cobb, J.R.: Outline for study of scoliosis, Am. Acad. Orthop. Surg. **5**:261-267, 1948.

1966 Hanafee, W., and Crandall, P.: Trauma of the spine and its contents, Radiol. Clin. North Am. **4**:365-382, 1966.

1967 Board, R.F.: Radiography of the scoliotic spine, Radiol. Technol. **38**:219-224, 1967.

1970 Kittleson, A.C., and Lim, L.W.: Measurement of scoliosis, A.J.R. **108**:775-777, 1970.

Young, L.W., Oestreich, A.E., and Goldstein, L.A.: Roentgenology in scoliosis: contribution to evaluation and management, Radiology **97**:778-795, 1970.

1980 Ritter, E.M., et al.: Use of a gradient intensifying screen for scoliosis radiography, Radiology **135**:230-232, 1980.

1981 Bhatnagar, J.P.: X-ray doses to patients undergoing full-spine radiographic examination, Radiology **138**:231-233, 1981.

Farren, J.: Routine radiographic assessment the scoliotic spine, Radiography **47**(556):92-96, 1981.

BEDSIDE RADIOGRAPHY

1933 Bell, M.E.: Bedside unit technic, Xray Techn. **4**:75-79, 1933.

1935 Ottonello, P.: Technica radiografica and ampolla mobile, Ann. Radiol. Fis. Med. **9**:22-25, 1935.

1937 Moser, L.: Schönende Aufahmetechnik zur seitlichen Darstellung der unteren Hals- und Brustwirbelsäule, Röntgenpraxis **9**:488-490, 1937.

1939 Baker, W.E.: Bedside radiography, Radiography **5**:89-97, 1939.

1942 Estelle, Sister: Technique for radiographing the mandible at the bedside, Xray Techn. **14**:118-120, 133, 1942.

Rigler, L.G.: X-ray technique in emergency conditions (bedside technique), Xray Techn. **13**:183-187, 220, 1942.

1978 Barnhard, H.J.: The bedside examination: a time for analysis and appropriate action, Radiology **129**:539-540, 1978.

Cantwell, K.G., Press, H.C., and Anderson, J.E.: Bedside radiographic examinations: indications and contraindications, Radiology **129**:383-384, 1978.

1979 Colley, D.P.: Device for improving quality of bedside decubitus examinations, Radiol. Technol. **51**:88-89, 1979.

1980 Eisenberg, R.L., Akin, J.R., and Hedgecock, M.W.: Optimal use of portable and stat examination, A.J.R. **134**:523-524, 1980.

OPERATING ROOM RADIOGRAPHY

1931 Beer, E.: Roentgenological control of exposed kidneys in operations for nephrolithiasis with the use of special intensifying cassette, J. Urol. **25**:159-164, 1931.

Benjamin, E.W.: Notes on the technique of x-ray control in the operating room, J. Urol. **25**:165-171, 1931.

1942 Wolcott, R.E.: Technique for securing lateral roentgenogram of the femoral neck in the operating room, Xray Techn. **13**:155-158, 181, 1942.

1945 Minear, W.L.: Rapid roentgenography in the operating room, J. Bone Joint Surg. **27**:157-159, 1945.

Ritchie, D.: Radiography in the operating theatre, Radiography **11**:73-76, 1945.

1947 Judd, G.: Radiography—an auxiliary in surgery, Radiography **13**:49-50, 1947.

1948 Olsson, O.: Rubber cassette with intensifying screens designed for roentgen examination of operatively exposed organs, Acta Radiol. **30**:91-96, 1948.

1950 Crawford, H.B., Merrill, E.F., and Bridgman, C.F.: Radiography of the hip joint, Part III. Radiographic procedures during hip-joint operations, Med. Radiogr. Photogr. **26**:106-117, 1950.

1952 Bridgman, C.F.: Improving radiographic quality during hip-nailing operations, Xray Techn. **23**:406-409, 1952.

1954 Young, B.R., and Scanlan, R.L.: New explosion-proof and shock-proof mobile roentgenographic equipment for the operating room, A.J.R. **71**:873-877, 1954.

1957 Pyper, J.B.: An aid in the reduction of radiation hazard in the operating theatre, Lancet **2**:1204-1205, 1957.

1959 Madsen, E.T.: An adjustable mobile cassette holder for orthopaedic operations, J. Bone Joint Surg. **41-B**:774-775, 1959.

Nachlas, I.W., and Feldman, J.R.: X-ray control for operations on the hip, J. Bone Joint Surg. **41-A**:1339-1341, 1959.

351

1962 Voorhis, C.C.: A cassette holder to be used in pinning hips, Surg. Gynecol. Obstet. **115**:359-360, 1962.

1964 Leslie, C.G., and Deguire, F.: Helpful hint for operating room radiography, Radiol. Technol. **36**:70, 1964.

1969 Lindgren, E., and Fenz, K.J.: Concentra: a new overhead unit for roentgenography in the operation theatre, Acta Radiol. [Diagn.] **8**:251-256, 1969.

1976 Berci, G., and Zheutlin, N.: Improving radiology in surgery, Med. Instrum. **10**:110-114, 1976.

Carter, P.R.: Brief note: simple method of obtaining intraoperative x-rays of the hand. J. Bone Joint Surg. **58**:576, 1976.

1977 Pochaczevsky, R.: Kidney cassettes for intraoperative radiography, Radiology **123**:237-238, 1977.

1978 Berci, G., et al.: Operative fluoroscopy and cholangiography: the use of modern radiologic technics during surgery, Am. J. Surg. **135**:32-35, 1978.

1979 Forster, I.W., and Lindsay, J.A.: Image intensifier as an aid to insertion of the Zickel nail apparatus for proximal femoral fractures, Injury **11**:148-154, 1979.

1980 Sigel, B., et al.: Sterile, portable radiation shield for the operating room, Arch. Surg. **115**:347-348, 1980.

ANESTHETICS IN RADIOLOGY DEPARTMENTS

1944 Clark, L.H.: Some dangers involved in the use of anesthetics in x-ray departments, Radiography **10**:25-27, 1944.

Hadfield, C.F.: The use of anesthetics in x-ray departments, Radiography **10**:17-23, 1944.

1976 Aidinis, S.J., et al.: Anesthesia for brain computer tomography, Anesthesiology **44**:420-425, 1976.

1977 Korten, K.: Anesthesia for diagnostic procedures, Am. Fam. Physician **15**:103-107, 1977.

PEDIATRIC RADIOGRAPHY

1912 Benjamin, E., and Goett, T.: Interpretation of chest roentgenogram in the nursling, Deutsch. Arch. Klin. Med. **107**:508-517, 1912.

1915 Waldron, C.W.: Roentgenology of the accessory nasal sinuses with special reference to sinusitis in children, Interstate Med. J. **22**:1031, 1915.

1921 Blackfan, K.D., and Little, K.: Clinical and radiographic study of thymus in infants, Am. J. Dis. Child. **22**:459-470, 1921.

Gerstenberger, H.J.: Factor of position of diaphragm in roentgen-ray diagnosis of enlarged thymus, Am. J. Dis. Child. **21**:534-545, 1921.

Noback, G.I.: A contribution to the topographical anatomy of the thymus glands, Am. J. Dis. Child. **22**:120, 1921.

1922 Wimberger, H.: Technische Erfahrungen aus der Kinderröntgenologie, Fortschr. Roentgenstr. **29**:98, 1922.

1923 Evans, W.A.: The value of the roentgen study of mastoid disease in children under five, A.J.R. **10**:382, 1923.

1924 Allen, B.: Nasal accessory sinuses in infants and children, Radiology **3**:136-138, 1924.

Schultz, J.: Die Darstellung der Torsionswinkels vom Femur mit Helfe von Röntgenstrahlen, Z. Orthop. Chir. **44**:325-334, 1924.

1925 Wasson, W.W.: Radiography of the infant chest, Radiology **5**:365-396, 1925.

1926 Carter, T.M.: Technique and devices used in radiographic study of wrist bones of children, J. Educ. Psychol. **17**:237-247, 1926.

Noback, G.I.: The thymus in the newborn and early infancy, Radiology **7**:416, 1926.

Wasson, W.D.: The thymus gland, Arch. Otolaryngol. **4**:495-511, 1926.

1928 Bonar, B.E.: Thymus in childhood, Northwest Med. **27**:178-182, 1928.

1929 Martin, C.L.: Roentgenologic studies of mastoid in infants, A.J.R. **22**:431-439, 1929.

1930 Pancoast, H.K., and Pendergrass, E.P.: Roentgenologic diagnosis of diseases of the upper respiratory tract in children, A.J.R. **23**:241-264, 1930.

Stoloff, G.: The thymus. In The chest in children, Ann. Roentgenol. **12**:345-356, 1930.

1931 Allison, R.G.: Non-opaque foreign bodies in the air passages of infants, Xray Techn. **3**:53-55, 1931.

1932 Bowen, D.R.: Roentgen examination of the infant thorax, A.J.R. **27**:610-615, 1932.

Eley, C.R., and Vogt, E.C.: Encephalography in children, A.J.R. **27**:686-696, 1932.

Granger, A.: Infant mastoid. In Radiological study of the para-nasal sinuses and mastoid, Philadelphia, 1932, Lea & Febiger.

1933 Anderson, W.S.: The thymus and its radiographic technic, Xray Techn. **4**:116-117, 1933.

Freund, L.: Ueber die Zurichtung des Kleinkindes für das Röntgenverfahren, Röntgenpraxis **5**:112-121, 1933.

Herpel, F.K.: Roentgenologic examination of the nasal accessory sinuses in infants and children, Radiology **20**:181-185, 1933.

1934 Pottenger, F.M.: Tuberculosis in the child and in the adult, St. Louis, 1934, The C.V. Mosby Co., pp. 275-291.

Stunz, I.D.: X-ray technic for children, Radiology **22**:694-700, 1934.

1935 Hanner, D.D.: Chest radiography in infants and uncooperative children, Xray Techn. **7**:62-65, 91, 1935.

1937 Shields, D.G.: General roentgenologic technic for infants and children, Xray Techn. **9**:10-18, 42, 1937.

1939 Hart, C.: Intravenous pyelography in children, Xray Techn. **10**:212-213, 1939.

Loew, J.: Problems in mastoid radiography of infants, Xray Techn. **11**:10-11, 1939.

1940 Batt, C.C.: Technical procedure in the x-ray examination of the mastoids in children, Xray Techn. **11**:175-176, 1940.

1941 Wyatt, G.M.: Excretory urography for children, Radiology **36**:664-671, 1941.

1942 Harvey, R.A.: Restraining device and technical factors for chest roentgenography of infants, A.J.R. **47**:322-327, 1942.

1943 Shapiro, A.V., and Bell, L.: Study of the widened mediastinum in children and pitfalls in diagnosis, A.J.R. **49**:159-176, 1943.

1944 Alexander, O.M.: Radiographic techniques applicable to infants, Radiography **10**:77-80, 1944.

Alexander, O.M.: Radiographic techniques applicable to infants, Radiography **10**:81-84, 1944.

1945 Christiansen, H.: Some practical hints on the performance of urography on infants, Acta Radiol. **26**:46-48, 1945.

Freeth, D.H.: Dental radiography of children and some of its problems, Radiography **11**:65-69, 1945.

Hrdlicker, V.E., Watkins, C.G., and Robb, J.A.: Cholecystography for children, Am. J. Dis. Child. **70**:325, 328, 1945.

1946 Eilert, G.J.: The psychological and technical handling of children in the radiographic department, Xray Techn. **17**:396-398, 1946.

Schaper, M.: Intramuscular urography in children as carried out at the Children's Hospital of Pittsburgh, Xray Techn. **18**:71, 1946.

Shields, D.G.: Radiography of the mastoid portion of the temporal bone in infants and children, Xray Techn. **17**:426-431, 433, 1946.

1947 Fletcher, C.: X-ray examination of the thymus of the newborn infant, Xray Techn. **18**:172-174, 1947.

1948 Schoen, C.P.: X-ray technique in pediatric cases, Xray Techn. **19**:241-243, 1948.

Waldeier, Sister M.A.: Child psychology in the x-ray room, Xray Techn. **19**:191-194, 1948.

1949 Koiransky, H.G., et al.: Radiologic study of the mastoid bone in infants in conjunction with anatomic and pathologic investigations, N.Y. J. Med. **49**:1291-1292, 1949.

Scatchard, G.N.: Orthopedic x-ray problems in children, N.Y. J. Med. **49**:2545-2547, 1949.

1951 Crooks, M.L.: Roentgen examination of the urinary tract in children, Xray Techn. **23**:24-26, 1951.

1953 Dunlap, K., and Shands, A.R., Jr.: A new method for determination of torsion of the femur, J. Bone Joint Surg. **35-A**:289-311, 1953.

Laage, H., et al.: Horizontal lateral roentgenography of the hip in children, J. Bone Joint Surg. **35-A**:387-389, 1953.

1954 Billings, L.: Roentgen examination of the proximal femur end in children and adolescents; standardized technique also suitable for determination of collum-, anteversion-, and epiphyseal angles: study of slipped epiphysis and coxa plana, Acta Radiol. **110** (suppl.):1-80, 1954.

Cleaver, H.W.: An apparatus for the measurement of femoral torsion, Xray Techn. **25:**7-10, 1954.

Martz, C.D., and Taylor, C.C.: The 45-degree angle roentgenographic study of the pelvis in congenital dislocation of the hip, J. Bone Joint Surg. **36-A:**528-532, 1954.

1955 Chuinard, E.G.: Early weight-bearing and the correction of anteversion in the treatment of congenital dislocation of the hip, J. Bone Joint Surg. **37-A:**229-244, 1955.

Hope, J.W., and Campoy, F.: The use of carbonated beverages in pediatric excretory urography, Radiology **64:**66-71, 1955.

1956 Edgren, W., and Laurent, L.E.: A method of measuring the torsion of the femur in congenital dislocation of the hip in children, Acta Radiol. **45:**371-376, 1956.

Magilligan, D.J.: Calculation of the angle of anteversion by means of horizontal lateral roentgenography, J. Bone Joint Surg. **38-A:**1231-1246, 1956.

1957 Backman, S.: The proximal end of the femur: investigations with special reference to the etiology of femoral neck fractures: anatomical studies: roentgen projections, Acta Radiol. **146** (suppl.):35-42, 1957.

Budin, E., and Chandler, E.: Measurement of femoral neck anteversion, Radiology **69:**209-213, 1957.

Hope, J.W., et al.: Pediatric radiography, Med. Radiogr. Photogr. **33:**25-56, 1957.

Rossmann, B.: Einfache röntgenologische Aufnahmetechnik des Saüglingsohres, Fortschr. Roentgenstr. **86:**741-748, 1957.

Wolf, H.G.: The roentgen examination of the gastrointestinal tract in the newborn, with particular reference to examination without the use of an oral contrast medium, Fortschr. Roentgenstr. **86:**323-334, 1957. Abstract: Radiology **70:**128, 1958.

1958 Andrén, L., and Rosen, S.: The diagnosis of dislocation of the hip in newborns and the primary results of immediate treatment, Acta Radiol. **49:**89-95, 1958.

Antoine, M., et al.: Le diagnostic radiologique des fractures du crâne chez le nourrisson par la technique des incidences tangentielles, J. Radiol. Electrol. **39:**573-576, 1958.

Fisk, C., and Fry, M.J.: Femoral torsion and the Shands technique, Xray Techn. **29:**225, 1958.

Hope, J.W., and O'Hara, A.E.: Use of air as a contrast medium in the diagnosis of intestinal obstruction of the newborn, Radiology **70:**349-361, 1958.

1959 Billing, L., and Severin, E.: Slipping epiphysis of the hip: a roentgenological and clinical study based on a new roentgen technique, Acta Radiol. **174**(suppl.):15-18, 1959.

Darling, D.B.: A simple device for obtaining lateral acetabular views of the hip in infants, Radiology **73:**432-433, 1959.

1960 Barrett, A.F., and Verney, G.I.: Tomography and other radiological methods in the management of congenital dislocation of the hip, Br. J. Radiol. **33:**684-690, 1960.

Pius, Sister M.: The pede-ply: restraining device for pediatric radiography, Xray Techn. **31:**382-386, 1960.

1961 Andrén, L.: Aetiology and diagnosis of congenital dislocation of the hip in newborns, Radiology **1:**89-94, 1961.

Dunbar, J.S., et al.: An automatic device for voiding urethrography in infants and small children, Radiology **76:**467-471, 1961.

Green, R.I.: The radiology of speech defects, Radiology **27:**331-338, 1961.

Gugliantini, P.: Utilità delle incidenze oblique caudocraniali nello studio radiologico della stenosi congenita ipertrofica del piloro, Ann. Radiol. Diagn. **34:**56-69, 1961.

1962 Altman, W.S., and Morace, V.: Laminagraphy, an aid in accurate localization in congenital hip dysplasia, Radiology **78:**19-28, 1962.

Darling, D.B.: Radiography of infants and children, Springfield, Ill., 1962, Charles C Thomas, Publisher.

Hope, J.W., and Koop, C.E.: Abdominal tumors in infants and children, Med. Radiogr. Photogr. **38:**2-51, 1962.

Lyons, C.D.: A new device for lateral radiography of the hip in children, Xray Techn. **33:**251-255, 1962.

Owsley, W.C.: Palate and pharynx: roentgenographic evaluation in the management of cleft palate and related deformities, A.J.R. **87:**811-821, 1962.

Rosen, S.: Diagnosis and treatment of congenital dislocation of the hip joint in the newborn, J. Bone Joint Surg. **44-B:**284-291, 1962.

Shurtleff, F.E.: Children's radiographic technic, Philadelphia, 1962, Lea & Febiger.

1963 Anderson, M.L., and Zatz, L.M.: Voiding cystourethrography in children, Radiol. Technol. **35:**171-175, 1963.

Brünner, S., and Buchmann, G.: Anesthesiologic problems in pediatric radiology, A.J.R. **89:**1075-1079, 1963.

Pinck, R.L., et al.: Congenital dislocation of the hip: determination of the anterior-posterior position of the femoral head on the Chassard-Lapiné view, Radiology **80:**650-652, 1963.

1964 Franklyn, P.P.: Paediatric radiology, Radiography **30:**243-251, 1964.

Kreel, L., et al.: Pneumo-mediastinography by the transternal method, Clin. Radiol. **15:**219-223, 1964.

1965 O'Hara, A.E., et al.: Controlled pulmonary roentgenographic exposures in newborn infants, A.J.R. **95:**99-103, 1965.

Tausend, M.E., and Stern, W.Z.: Thymic patterns in the newborn, A.J.R. **95:**125-130, 1965.

1968 Berdon, W.E., et al.: The radiographic evaluation of imperforate anus: an approach correlated with current surgical concepts, Radiology **90:**466-471, 1968.

1969 Kelly, J.H.: Cine radiography in anorectal malformations, J. Pediatr. Surg. **4:**538-546, 1969.

1973 Oh, K.S., et al.: Positive-contrast peritoneography and herniography, Radiology **108:**647-654, 1973.

1975 Gooding, C.A., et al.: Adverse reactions to intravenous pyelography in children, A.J.R. **123:**802-804, 1975.

Haller, J.O., and Slovis, T.L.: Importance of horizontal beam for lateral view of skull in pediatric radiography, Radiol. Technol. **47:**150-152, 1975.

Holbert, C.L., et al.: Radiographic technique, safety, and interpretation in the newborn nursery, J. Pediatr. **87:**968-972, 1975.

Knake, J.E.: A device to aid in positioning for the Andren von Rosen hip view, Radiology **117:**735-736, 1975.

1976 Buckle, C.M.: Immobilization of the patient in pedicatric radiography, Radiography **42**(501): 195-196, 1976.

Poznanski, A.K.: Practical approaches to pediatric radiology, Chicago, 1976, Year Book Medical Publishing, Inc.

1977 Barry, J.F., et al.: Metrizamide in pediatric myelography, Radiology **124:**409-418, 1977.

Eklof, O., editor: Current concepts in pediatric radiology, New York, 1977, Springer-Verlag,

Hass, E.A., and Solomon, D.J.: Telling children about diagnostic radiology procedures, Radiology **124:**521, 1977.

Hirsch, D.J., et al.: Evaluation for hip dysplasia in infancy: the significance of x-ray in diagnosis, J. Med. Soc. N.J. **74:**528-532, 1977.

1978 American Academy of Pediatrics, Committee on Radiology: Water-soluble contrast material, Pediatrics **62:**114-116, 1978.

Hernandez, R., Gutowski, D., and Poznanski, A.K.: A simple method of using a shadow gonadal shield with closed incubators, Radiology **128:**821-822, 1978.

Merten, D.F.: Comparison radiographs in extremity injuries of childhood: current application in radiological practice, Radiology **126:**209-210, 1978.

1979 Cohen, M.D.: Intravenous urography in neonates and infants: what dose of contrast media should be used? Br. J. Radiol. **52:**942-944, 1979.

Kalender, W., Reither, M., and Schuster, W.: Reduction of dose in pelvic examinations of infants using modern x-ray techniques, Pediatr. Radiol. **8:**233-235, 1979.

1980 Lonnerholm, T.: Arthrography of the hip in children: technique, normal anatomy, and findings in unstable hip joints, Acta Radiol. **21:**279-292, 1980.

Swischuk, L.E.: Radiology of the newborn and young infant, Baltimore, 1980, The Williams & Wilkins Co.

1980 Wesenberg, R.L., et al.: Low-dose radiography of children, Radiol. Techol. **51**:641-648, 1980.

1981 Milne, E.N., and Gillan, G.G.: Technique for improving neonatal chest roentgenograms, Appl. Radiol. **10**:45-49, 1981.

TOMOGRAPHY

1922 Bocage, A.E.M.: French patent no. 536464, 1922.

1931 Vellebona, A.: Radiography with great enlargement (micro-diography) and a technical method for the radiographic dissociation of the shadow, Radiology **17**:340-341, 1931.

Ziedses des Plantes, B.G.: Special method of making roentgenograms of the cranium and spinal column, Nederl. Tijdschr. Geneesk. **75**:5218-5222, 1931. (In Dutch.)

1932 Ziedses des Plantes, B.G.: Eine neue Methode zur Differenzierung der Röntgengraphie, Acta Radiol. **13**:182-191, 1932.

1933 Bartelink, D.L.: Method of obtaining clear pictures of a limited area by blocking out superfluous parts, Fortschr. Roentgenstr. **47**:399-407, 1933.

Vellebona, A.: A method of taking roentgenograms which makes it possible to eliminate shadows, Fortschr. Roentgenstr. **48**:599-605, 1933.

1934 Kieffer, J.: United States patent, 1934.

Ziedses des Plantes, B.G.: Planigraphie: une méthode permettant en radiographie d'obtenir une image nette de la section d'un objet à un plan bien déterminé, J. Radiol. Electrol. **18**:73-76, 1934.

Ziedses des Plantes, B.G.: Planigraphy, a roentgenographic differentiation method, Utrecht, Netherlands, 1934, Kemink & Son N.V.

1935 Bozzetti, G.: La realizzazione practica della stratigrafia, Radiol. Med. **22**:257-267, 1935.

Grossmann, G.: Tomographie I and II, Fortschr. Roentgenstr. **51**:61-80, 191-209, 1935.

Grossmann, G.: Practical considerations of tomography, Fortscr. Roentgenstr. **52**:44, 1935.

1936 Andrews, J.R.: Planigraphy I. Introduction and history, A.J.R. **36**:575-587, 1936.

1937 Andrews, J.R., and Stava, R.T.: Planigraphy. II. Mathematical analyses of the methods: description of apparatus and experimental proof, A.J.R. **38**:145-151, 1937.

Ljvraga, P.: La roentgenstratigrafia nella sua concezione teorica ed applicazione practica, Arch. Radiol. **15**:7-22, 1937.

Twining, E.W.: Tomography by means of a simple attachment to the Potter-Bucky couch, Br. J. Radiol. **10**:332-347, 1937.

1938 Alexander, G.H.: A simple and inexpensive tomographic method, A.J.R. **39**:956-958, 1938.

Kieffer, J.: The laminagraph and its variations: applications and implications of the planigraphic principles, A.J.R. **39**:497-513, 1938.

Moore, S.: Body-section roentgenography with the laminagraph, A.J.R. **39**:514-522, 1938.

1939 Danelius, G.: Cross-sectional radiography of the heart, Radiology **32**:190-194, 1939.

Kieffer, J.: Analysis of laminagraphic motions and their values, Radiology **33**:560-585, 1939.

Kieffer, J.: Body-section radiographic technic, Xray Techn. **11**:12-16, 34, 1939.

Moore, S.: Body-section radiography, Radiology **33**:605, 1939.

Watson, W.: Differential radiography I, Radiography **5**:81-88, 1939.

Zintheo, C.J., Jr.: Planigraphy, Xray Techn. **10**:206-211, 1939.

1940 Watson, W.: Differential radiography II, Radiography **6**:161, 1940.

1941 Cahill, M.: Rectilinear body-section radiography, Xray Techn. **13**:16-17, 1941.

1943 Kieffer, J.: The general principles of body-section radiography, Radiogr. Clin. Photogr. **19**:2-9, 1943.

Watson, W.: Differential radiography. III. Body-section radiography in practice, Radiography **9**:33-38, 1943.

1944 Scott, W.G., and Botton, D S.: Laminographic studies of the aorta: their advantages and limitations. A.J.R. **51**:18-28, 1944.

Sundberg, C.G., and Lindholm, S.: Ueber die Anwendung des Schichtbildes in der Röntgendiagnostik, Acta Radiol. **25**:825-834, 1944.

1947 Frain, C., and Lacroix, F.: Courbe-enveloppe et coupes horizontales, J. Radiol. Electrol. **28**:142-143, 1947.

Lisi, F.J.: Laminography—some technical and practical aspects, Xray Techn. **18**:209-215, 1947.

Moore, S.: Development and applications of body-section radiography. In Golden, R. editor: Diagnostic roentgenology, ed. 3, vol.2, New York, 1947, Thomas Nelson & Sons.

1948 de Abreu, M.: Theory and techniques of simultaneous tomography, A.J.R. **60**:668-674, 1948.

Vallebona, A.: I nuovo orizzonti della stratigrafia nei vari campi della medicina: l'esplorazione stratigrafica tridimensionale, Inform. Med. (Genova) **22**:89-96, 1948.

Vallebona, A.: La stratigrafia assiale transverse, J. Radiol. Electrol. **29**:443, 1948.

White, E.W.: Stereoscopic planography, Xray Techn. **19**:238-240, 1948.

1949 Gebauer, A.: Körperschichtaufnahmen in transversalen (horizontalen) Ebenen, Fortschr. Roentgenstr. **71**:669-696, 1949.

Macarini, N., and Oliva, L.: Axial transverse stratigraphy, J. Belg. Radiol. **32**:187-213, 1949.

Takahashi, S., Imaoka, M., and Shinozaki, T.: Rotary cross-section radiography, Hirosaki Med. J. **1**:3, 1949.

Paatero, Y.V.: A new tomographic method for radiographing curved outer surfaces, Acta Radiol. **32**:177-184, 1949.

1950 Stevenson, J.J.: Horizontal body section radiography, Br. J. Radiol. **23**:319-334, 1950.

Tobb: Polytome de Messieurs Sans et Porcher, J. Radiol. Electrol. **31**:300-302, 1950.

1951 Gebauer, A.: Diagnostische Vorteile und Indikationsstellung der Körperschichtaufnahmen in transversalen Ebenen gegenüber denen in Vertikalen, Fortschr. Roentgenstr. **75**:9-21, 1951.

Watson, W.: Simultaneous multisection radiography, Radiography **17**:221-228, 1951.

1955 Amisano, P.: Three dimensional stratigraphic examination: axial transverse stratigraphy. Part II, A.J.R. **74**:777-790, 1955.

Vallebona, A.: Three dimensional stratigraphic examination: axial transverse stratigraphy. Part I, A.J.R. **74**:769-776, 1955.

1956 Epstein, B.S., and Sloven, J.: Body section radiography with special reference to the skeleton, Med. Radiogr. Photogr. **32**:2-12, 1956.

1957 Manfredi, R.A., and Kruse, F.J.: Laminography with cerebral pneumography, J. Neurosurg. **14**:374-381, 1957.

1958 Csákány, G., and Donáth, T.: Vergleichende röntgenanatomische Untersuchung der beiderseitigen Foramina jugularia, Fortschr. Roentgenstr. **88**:439-446, 1958.

1959 Mundnich, K., and Frey, K.W.: Das Roentgenschichtbild des Ohres, Stuttgart, 1959, Georg Thieme.

Roswitt, B., et al.: Transverse laminography: the third dimension in body section roentgenography: application in radiation therapy, A.J.R. **81**:130-139, 1959.

Watson, W.: Simultaneous multisection radiography, Xray Techn. **30**:265-271, 1959.

Wilk, S.P.: Axial transverse tomography of the chest, Radiology **72**:42-50, 1959.

1960 Edholm, P.: The tomogram: its formation and content, Acta Radiol. **193**(suppl.):1-109, 1960.

1962 Bistolfi, F., and Podesta, A.M.: Tomography of the limb joints with particular regard to the multidirectional technique, Panminerva Med. **4**:126-137, 1962.

Lapayowker, M.S., et al.: The use of plesiosectional tomography in the diagnosis of eighth nerve tumors, A.J.R. **88**:1187-1193, 1962.

McGann, M.J.: Plesiosectional tomography of the temporal bone: a new multi-screen cassette, A.J.R. **88**:1183-1186, 1962.

Smith, G.V.: Autotomography of the cerebral ventricular system, Xray Techn. **34**:5-7, 1962.

Watson, W.: Axial transverse tomography, Radiography **28**:179-190, 1962.

Westra, D.: Zonographie, die Tomographie mit sehr geringer Verwischung, Fortschr. Roentgenstr. **87**:605-618, 1962.

1963 Goree, J.A., et al.: The pineal tomogram, A.J.R. **89**:1209-1211, 1963.

Hodes, P.J., et al.: Body-section radiography, fundamentals, Radiol. Clin. North Am. **1**:229-244, 1963.

Littleton, J.T., et al.: Polydirectional body section roentgenography, A.J.R. **89**:1179-1193, 1963.

Updegrave, W.J.: Panoramic dental radiography, Med. Radiogr. Photogr. **36**:75-83, 1963.

Valvassori, G.E.: Laminagraphy of the ear: normal roentgenographic anatomy, A.J.R. **89**:1155-1167, 1963.

1965 Greenwell, F.P., and Wright, R.W.: Rotational tomography, Clin. Radiol. **16**:377-389, 1965.

Landau, P.: La tomographie multiple simultanée unidirectionnelle: méthodes et possibilités nouvelles, J. Radiol. Electrol. **46**:299-305, 1965.

1966 Ettinger, A., and Fainsinger, M.H.: Zonography in daily radiological practice, Radiology **87**:82-86, 1966.

Liliequist, B.: Tomography with the Mimer in otosclerosis of the temporal bone, Acta Radiol. [Diagn.] **4**:639-644, 1966.

Ring, J.: Elements of sectional radiography, Radiol. Technol. **38**:17-22, 1966.

Westra, D.: Zonography: the narrow angle tomography, Amsterdam, 1966, Excerpta Medica Foundation.

1967 Lodin, H.: Tomography of the middle and lingular bronchi, Acta Radiol. [Diagn.] **6**:26-32, 1967.

1968 Inzinna, J.F., Salomon, H., and Vazir, A.: The synchroplanigraphic device: a new simultaneous tomographic device, A.J.R. **103**:678-680, 1968.

Rybadova, N.I., and Kuznetsov, A.A.: Concerning the method of tomographic examination of the bronchial tree, Vestn. Rentgen. Radiol. **43**:36-43, 1968. (In Russian.) Abstract: Radiology **91**:1249, 1968.

Wright, J.T., and Benjamin, B.: Cycloidal tomography of the temporal bone, Australas. Radiol. **12**:320-327, 1968.

1969 Brünner, S.: Roentgen anatomy of the temporal bone using the Polytome, Semin. Roentenol. **4**:118-121, 1969.

Conway, J.J., and Cowell, H.R.: Tarsal coalition: clinical significance and roentgenographic demonstration, Radiology **92**:799-811, 1969.

du Boulay, G., and Bostick, T.: Linear tomography in congenital abnormalities of the ear, Br. J. Radiol. **42**:161-183, 1969.

Kimber, P.M.: A thin-layer cassette for precision neuroradiology, Radiography **35**:183-184, 1969.

Lame, E.L., and Redick, T.J.: Automography applied to the pharynx and dens, A.J.R. **105**:359-360, 1969.

Mattsson, O.: Control of a tomographic system, Acta Radiol. [Diagn.] **8**:433-445, 1969.

Potter, G.D., and Trokel, S.L.: Tomography of the optic canal, A.J.R. **106**:530-535, 1969.

1970 Brünner, S., and Pedersen, C.B.: Roentgen examination of the facial canal, Acta Radiol. [Diagn.] **10**:545-552, 1970.

Chin, F.K., Anderson, W.B., and Gilbertson, J.D.: Radiation dose to critical organs during petrous tomography, Radiology **94**:623-627, 1970.

Crysler, W.E.: Tomoscopy and related matters, A.J.R. **109**:619-623, 1970.

Frimann-Dahl, J., and Kühl, H.B.: Immediate centering and tomographic cut localization by means of roentgen television, Acta Radiol. [Diagn.] **10**:236-240, 1970.

James, A.E., Jr.: Tarsal coalition and personal spastic flat foot, Australas. Radiol. **14**:80-83, 1970.

1971 Lockery, R.M.: Principles of body-section radiography, Radiol. Technol. **42**:335-345, 1971.

Smith, W.V.J.: A review of tomography and zonography, Radiography **37**:5-15, 1971.

Ziedses des Plantes, B.G.: Body-section radiography: history, image information, various techniques and results, Australas. Radiol. **15**:57-64, 1971.

1972 El Gammal, T., and King, G.E.: Patient positioning device for hypocycloidal tomography of the midline ventricles of the brain, Radiology **102**:206-207, 1972.

Potter, G.D.: Tomography of the orbit, Radiol. Clin. North Am. **10**:21-38, 1972.

Reichmann, S.: Modified theory of the development of tomographic blurring, Acta Radiol. **12**:457-468, 1972.

1973 Amplatz, K.: Autotomography, A.J.R. **117**:896-902, 1973.

Berrett, A.: Modern thin-section tomography, Springfield, Ill., 1973, Charles C Thomas, Publisher.

Dalinka, M.K., Gohel, V.K., and Rancier, L.: Tomography in the evaluation of the anterior cruciate ligament, Radiology **108**:31-33, 1973.

Greig, J.H., and Musaph, F.W.: A method of radiological demonstration of the temporomandibular joints using the orthopantomograph, Radiology **106**:307-310, 1973.

Littleton, J.T., Crosby, E.H., and Durizch, M.L.: Adjustable- versus fixed-fulcrum tomographic systems, A.J.R. **117**:910-929, 1973.

1974 Anderson, P.W., and Maslin, P.: Tomography applied to knee arthrography, Radiology **110**:271-275, 1974.

Berger, P., Gildersleeve, S., and Poznanski, A.: The feasibility of the PA projection for tomography of the petrous bone: significant reduction in radiation dose to the lens of the eye, A.J.R. **122**:67-69, 1974.

Bosniak, M.A.: Nephrotomography: a relatively unappreciated but extremely valuable diagnostic tool, Radiology **113**:313-321, 1974.

1975 Freedman, G.S., Putman, C.E., and Potter, G.D.: Critical review of tomography in radiology and nuclear medicine, CRC Crit. Rev. Clin. Radiol. Nucl. Med. **6**:253-294, 1975.

Norman, A.: The use of tomography in the diagnosis of skeletal disorders, Clin. Orthop. **107**:139-145, 1975.

Welander, V.: Layer formation in narrow beam rotation radiography, Acta Radiol. **16**:529-540, 1975.

1976 Harding, G., and Day, M.J.: Blurring quality in spiral tomography, Acta Radiol. (Ther.) **15**:465-480, 1976.

Littleton, J.T.: Tomography: physical principles and clinical application, Baltimore, 1976, The Williams & Wilkins Co.

Polga, J.P., and Watnick, M.: Whole lung tomography in metastatic disease, Clin. Radiol. **27**:53-56, 1976.

Stanson, A.W., and Baker, H.L.: Routine tomography of the temporomandibular joint, Radiol. Clin. North Am. **14**:105-127, 1976.

1977 Helander, C.G., Reichmann, S., and Astrand, K.: Xeroradiographic tomography, Acta Radiol. **18**:369-382, 1977.

Wayrynen, R.E., Holland, R.S., and Schwenker, R.P.: Film-screen sharpness in complex motion tomography, Invest. Radiol. **12**:195-198, 1977.

1978 Durizch, M.L.: Technical aspects of tomography, Baltimore, 1978, The Williams & Wilkins Co.

1979 Palmer, A., and Munro, L.: The principles of tomographic positioning with particular reference to skull tomography, Radiography **45**(531):51-60, 1979.

1980 Farber, A.L.: Advantages of variant section of thickness relative to specific anatomy, Radiol. Technol. **51**:793-796, 1980.

Littleton, J.T., Durizch, M.L., and Callahan, W.P.: Linear vs. pluridirectional tomography of the chest: correlative radiographic anatomic study, A.J.R. **134**:241-248, 1980.

1981 Bein, M.E., and Stone, D.N.: Full lung linear and pluridirectional tomography: a preliminary evaluation of nodule detection, A.J.R. **136**:1013-1015, 1981.

FOREIGN BODY LOCALIZATION

1904 Poirier de Clisson, H.: Sur un procède simple de localisation des projectiles par la radioscopie, Paris, 1904.

1915 Coleschi, L.: Il più semplice e il più rapido metodo de apparecchio per la localizzazione dei corpi estranei mediante i raggi röntgen, Radiol. Med. **2**:49-59, 1915.

Grier, G.W.: Roentgen examination of foreign bodies, A.J.R. **2**:109-122, 1915.

Weber, A.: Localisation des projectiles de guerre au moyen des rayons X, Paris, 1915, Le Francois.

Weski, O.: Die röntgenologische Lagebestimmung von Fremdkörpern: ihre schulgemäse Methodik dargestellt an kriegschirurgischen Material, Stuttgart, 1915, Ferdinand Enke.

355

1916 Heyl, W.: Ueber röntgenologische Lokalisation metallischer Fremdkörper, Berlin, 1916, E. Ebering.

Renard, L.P.E.: Contribution à l'étude de la localisation anatomique et repérage rigoureux des projectiles par le radio stéréometre Tauleigne-Mazo, Paris, 1916, Ollier-Henry.

1917 Beck, E.G.: Stereo-clinic: localization of foreign bodies with steroscopic roentgenograms, and methods of their removal, Troy, 1917, Southworth Co.

Blaine, E.S.: The caliper method of foreign body localization, A.J.R. **4**:545-550, 1917.

Cole, L.G.: Localization of foreign bodies, A.J.R. **4**:455-461, 1917.

Skinner, E.H.: The Sutton method of foreign body localization, A.J.R. **4**:350, 1917.

Wilkins, W.A.: The localization of foreign bodies, A.J.R. **4**:343, 1917.

1918 Bowen, D.R.: Localization of foreign bodies, A.J.R. **5**:59-76, 1918.

Case, J.T.: A brief history of the development of foreign body localization by means of the X-ray, A.J.R. **5**:113-124, 1918.

Lilienfeld, L: Methodik der Fremdkörperlokalisation. In Holzknecht: Röntgenologie, 1918.

1919 Gage, H.: X-ray observations for foreign bodies and their localization, London, 1919.

1920 Case, J.T.: Localization and extraction of foreign bodies under x-ray control, Oxford Loose-Leaf Surg. **5**:449-488, 1920.

1921 de Abreu, M.D.: La localisation et l'extraction des corps étrangers par la double projection, Paris, 1921, Bourse de Commerce.

1932 Lewis, R.: A roentgenographic study of glass and its visibility as a foreign body, A.J.R. **27**:853-857, 1932.

1934 Thompson, B.: The localization of foreign bodies with the roentgenoscope, A.J.R. **32**:412-413, 1934.

1935 Béclère, H.: La radiographie sur films cintrés pour la recherche des corps étrangers du genou, Presse Méd. **43**:1839-1845, 1935.

Kimble, H.E.: Un método mecano simplificado para la medicon radiografia y la localización, Rev. Radiol. Fis. **2**:20-28, 1935. Taken from Radiology **24**:39-46, 1935.

1936 Lea, P.: Localization of a foreign body with x-ray, Xray Techn. **7**:150-152, 1936.

Schmitz, E.: Die röntgenologische Festellung von Fremdkörpern, Bonn, 1936, A. Brand.

1937 Ulrich, K.: Zur Splitterlokalisation im Rücken, Röntgenpraxis **9**:770-773, 1937.

1938 Reid, E.K., et al.: Foreign body localization in military roentgenology, Radiology **31**:567-583, 1938.

1939 Brailsford, J.F.: Simple radiographic method for the localization of foreign bodies, Br. J. Radiol.**12**:65-75, 1939.

Clark, K.C.: Radiographic depth localization of foreign bodies, Radiography **5**:195-211, 1939.

Roberts, R.I.: Visualization of non-metallic foreign bodies, Br. J. Radiol. **12**:680-684, 1939.

1940 Clark, K.C.: Localization of a metallic foreign body in the buttock, Radiography **6**:105-106, 1940.

Sayman, I.: A new method for localization of foreign bodies, Radiology **35**:87-88, 1940.

Watson, W.: Simple triangulation and localization, Radiography **6**:107-109, 1940.

1941 Westermark, N.: A simple method of localizing foreign bodies, Acta Radiol. **22**:490-492, 1941.

1942 DeLorimier, A.A.: Foreign body localization as provided with the United States army table unit, A.J.R. **47**:307-313, 1942.

1946 Mannheimer, B.: Visualization of foreign bodies of low radio-opacity, Br. J. Radiol. **19**:469-470, 1946.

Rudisill, H., Jr.: Foreign bodies other than those in the eye. In Pillmore, G.U., editor: Clinical radiology, vol. 2, Philadelphia, 1946, F.A. Davis Co.

1948 Hassell, M.K., and Wilson, E.J.: Foreign body localization—double parallel film method, Xray Techn. **19**:227-229, 1948.

1972 Randall, P.A.: Percutaneous removal of iatrogenic intracardia foreign body, Radiology **102**:591-595, 1972.

Woesner, M.E., and Sanders, I.: Xeroradiography: significant modality in the detection of nonmetallic foreign bodies in soft tissues, A.J.R. **115**:636-640, 1972.

1974 Muroff, L.R., and Seaman, W.B.: Normal anatomy of the larynx and pharynx and the differential diagnosis of foreign bodies, Semin. Roentgenol. **9**:267-272, 1974.

1975 McArthur, D.R., and Taylor, D.F.: A determination of the minimum radiopacification necessary for radiographic detection of an aspirated or swallowed object, Oral Surg. **39**:329-338, 1975.

Meyer, W.G.: Sequel technique for localization and extraction of radiopaque foreign bodies in various anatomic sites, Ohio State Med. J. **71**:15-18, 1975.

Taupman, R.E., and Martin, J.E.: The detection of non-opaque foreign bodies by xeroradiography, South. Med. J. **68**:1186-1187, 1975.

1977 Bowers, D.G., Jr., and Lynch, J.B.: Xerodiography for non-metallic foreign bodies, Plast. Reconstr. Surg. **60**:470-471, 1977.

1978 Thompson, D.H., Stasney, C.R., and Miller, T.: Xeroradiographic detection of foreign bodies, Laryngoscope **88**:254-259, 1978.

1979 Kjhns, L.R., et al.: An in vitro comparison of computed tomography, xeroradiography, and radiography in the detection of soft-tissue foreign bodies, Radiology **132**:218-219, 1979.

EXPOSURE TECHNIQUES

1896 MacIntyre, J.: X-ray demonstration with special reference to the soft tissues, Br. Med. J. **1**:750, 1094, 1896.

1926 Files, G.W.: The relation, radiographically, of Kv. P. to time or exposure, Radiology **7**:255, 1926.

1927 Bronkhorst, W.: Kontrast und Schärfe im Röntgenbild, Leipzig, 1927, Georg Thieme.

1930 Files, G.W.: Soft tissue differentiation, Xray Techn. **1**:65-69, 1930.

1931 Bouwers, A.: Ueber die Technik der Momentaufnahmen, Acta Radiol. **12**:175-182, 1931.

Laurell, H.: Eine Methode, beim Röntgenphotographieren den grösseren Teil der Schädlichen Sekundärstrahlung auszuschalten, Acta Radiol. **12**:574-579, 1931.

1932 Bassett, S.: Soft tissue differentiation, Xray Techn. **4**:59-61, 1932.

Hunsberger, H.S.: Adaption of techniques to individual cases, Radiology **18**:320-323, 1932.

1933 Loughery, T.P., and Stecher, W.R.: Useful procedures in radiologic practice, Radiology **20**:225-230, 1933.

Newman, H.: Relation of kilovolts to thickness of part: X-ray technic, Xray Techn. **5**:21-26, 1933.

Weyl, C., Warren, S.R., and O'Neill, D.B.: Scientific control of radiographic results, Radiology **21**:546-555, 1933.

1934 Benassi, E.: Realazione sui nuovi mezzi di contrasto in radiologia, Atti Congresso Ital. Radiol. Med. **11**:1934.

Fuchs, A.W.: Radiography of the entire body, Radiogr. Clin. Photogr. **10**:9-14, 1934.

Kirklin, B.R.: Old principles and new radiography, Xray Techn. **6**:56-62, 1934.

1935 Files, G.W.: La diferenciacíon de tejidos blandos, Rev. Radiol. Fis. **4**:38-49, 1935.

Files, G.W.: Maximum tissue differentiation, Xray Techn. **7**:17-24, 1935.

1936 Carty, J.R.: Roentgenographic diagnosis of soft tissue tumors excluding the breast, A.J.R. **36**:932-935, 1936.

Carty, J.R.: Soft tissue roentgenography, A.J.R. **35**:474-484, 1936.

Franke, H.: Ein röntgen-photographisches Verfahren zur gleichzeitigen Darstellung der Weichteile und Knochenpartien des Profilschädels, Röntgenpraxis **8**:43-46, 1936.

Fuchs, A.W.: A radiographic view-finder, Radiogr. Clin. Photogr. **12**:2-7, 1936.

Gratz, C.M.: Air injections of the fascial spaces: new method of soft tissue roentgenography, A.J.R. **35**:750-751, 1936.

Lingeman, L.R.: Infection of soft tissues by gas-producing organisms: early recognition by roentgenogram, N.Y. J. Med. **36**:259-263, 1936.

1937 Files, G.W.: Non-screen procedure with Potter-Bucky diaphragm, Radiology **29**:582-595, 1937.

Zintheo, C.J.: The specification of roentgenographic technique, A.J.R. **38**:352-361, 1937.

Zintheo, C.J.: Transferring of x-ray technic from one laboratory to another, Xray Techn. **9**:77-81, 114, 1937.

1938 Bettelheim, F.: Concerning roentgenographic details, A.J.R. **40**:401-404, 1938.

Carty, J.R.: Some important considerations in roentgenographic demonstration of tissues, normal and pathological, having a relatively low differential absorption, Radiology **30**:417-419, 1938.

Fuchs, A.W.: Higher kilovoltage technic with high-definition screens, Radiogr. Clin. Photogr. **14**:2-8, 1938.

Hötterman, C.: Die Augenlieder im Röntgenbild, Röntgenpraxis **10**:377-384, 1938.

1939 Files, G.W.: Estudios recientes relativos a la manera de mejorar el detalle radiografico, Rev. Radiol. Fis. **6**:28-33, 1939.

Files, G.W.: Factores que influyen in la nitidez de detalle o definicíon: efecto del área focal del tubo de rayos X en la nitidez de detalle, Rev. Radiol. Fis. **6**:284-296, 1939.

1940 Allen, P.E., and Calder, H.W.: Soft tissue radiography, Br. J. Radiol. **13**:422-427, 1940.

Fuchs, A.W.: Balance in radiographic image, Xray Techn. **12**:81-84, 118, 1940.

Hulpien, E.: X-ray technic charts, Xray Techn. **11**:224-226, 1940.

Melter, T.B.: Technic of soft tissue radiography, Xray Techn. **11**:229, 1940.

Newey, M.: Soft tissue radiography, Radiography **6**:29-40, 1940.

1941 Lingley, J.R., and Elliott, W.J.: Soft tissue roentgenography. In Golden, R. editor: Diagnostic roentgenology, ed. 2, vol.2, New York, 1941, Thomas Nelson & Sons.

Melot, G.J.: Roentgenologic examination of the soft tissues, A.J.R. **46**:189-196, 1941.

1942 Cahoon, J.B., Jr.: Uses of opaque plastic filters in radiography of the lateral lumbodorsal spine, lateral cervicodorsal spine, and cases of suspected placenta previa, Xray Techn. **13**:242-243, 246, 1942.

Doyle, M.: Hundred factors in high-class radiography, Radiology **8**:12-16, 1942.

Gould, D.R.: In defence of orthodox radiography: a consideration of the total tissue differentiation, Radiology **8**:78-79, 1942.

Jaffke, R.C.: Tissue thickness measurements technique, Xray Techn. **13**:150-152, 180, 1942.

Lewis, R.W.: Roentgenographic soft tissue study in orthopedic hospital, A.J.R. **48**:634-642, 1942.

1943 Davis, F.G., and Fagen, M.: Factores que influyen en la densidad y en el contraste de la radiografía, Rev. Radiol. Fis. **10**:88-90, 1943.

Mahoney, H.O., and Thomas, J.B.: Factores que influyen en la densidad y en el contraste de la radiografía: la opacidad de los tejidos, Rev. Radiol. Fis. **10**:37-39, 1943.

1944 Altman, W.S.: The advantage of increased filtration, A.J.R. **52**:344, 1944.

Brill, E.: Close-range radiography, Xray Techn. **16**:97-100, 1944.

1945 Arendt, J.: Close range technic in diagnostic roentgenology, Radiology **44**:177-180, 1945.

Champness, L.J.: Variations of routine techniques, Radiography **11**:17-20, 1945.

Dawdy, E.B.: Consideration of distance as a technical factor, Xray Techn. **16**:131-133, 1945.

Henderson, E.: Helpful aids in chest work, Xray Techn. **16**:196-198, 1945.

Holly, E.W.: Balsawood accessory for chest radiography, Radiogr. Clin. Photogr. **21**:38-39, 1945.

1946 Alexander, S.: A sinple method of radiography of chests which presents marked variations in density, Xray Techn. **18**:57-61, 1946.

Carty, J.R.: Soft tissue radiography. In Pillmore, G.U., editor: Clinical radiology, vol. 2, Philadelphia, 1946, F.A. Davis Co.

1947 Alexander, S.: A simple method for roentgenography of the chest presenting marked variations in density, A.J.R. **57**:532-535, 1947.

Avery, G.: Changing extremity technique to compensate for aluminum filter, Xray Techn. **19**:24-27, 37, 1947.

Bannen, J.E.: Radiographic technique and its relationship to pathology and injury, Radiography **13**:28-31, 1947.

Guyant, M.: Roentgenograms of surgical and post mortem specimens, Xray Techn. **18**:164-165, 1947.

Hulbert, M.H.E.: Radiography as an aid to dose control in the radium treatment of the cervix, J. Obstet. Gynaec. Br. Emp. **54**:137, 1947.

Lingley, J.R., and Elliott, W.J.: Soft tissue roentgenography. In Golden, R. editor: Diagnostic roentgenology, ed. 3, vol.2, New York, 1947, Thomas Nelson & Sons.

Piatrowski, Brother D.: Double tilt technique, Xray Techn. **18**:286-288, 1947.

Torp, I.M.: Problems of mass chest x-ray in industry, Xray Techn. **18**:216-219, 1947.

1948 Alexander, S.: Fundamentals of soft tissue radiography, Xray Techn. **19**:174-179, 205, 1948.

Terzo, C.: Long scale radiography, Roentgenography **1**:17, 21, 1948.

1951 Holman, C.B., and Camp, J.D.: Identification of right and left sides in roentgenograms by a permanent cassette marker, Radiology **56**:260-263, 1951.

Pearson, G.R.: Radiographic projection studies, Xray Techn. **23**:1-9, 1951.

Updegrave, W.J.: Higher fidelity in intraoral roentgenography, J. Am. Dent. Assoc. **62**:1-8, 1951.

1952 Gilardoni, A., and Schwarz, G.S.: Magnification of radiographic images in clinical roentgenology and its present day limit, Radiology **59**:866-878, 1952.

1954 Lofstrom, J.E., and Warren, C.R.: Magnification techniques in radiography: their practical value, Xray Techn. **26**:161-165, 1954.

1958 Fuchs, A.W.: Principles of radiographic exposure and processing, ed. 2, Springfield, Ill., 1958, Charles C Thomas, Publisher.

1961 Cahoon, J.B., Jr.: Radiographic technique: its origin, concept, practical application and evaluation of radiation dosage, Xray Techn. **32**:354-364, 1961.

Mahoney, G.J., and Rule, I.: The design of optical density filters for long film radiology of the lower extremities, Xray Techn. **33**:103-105, 1961.

1962 Isard, H.J., Ostrum, B.J., and Cullinan, J.E.: Magnification roentgenography, Med. Radiogr. Photogr. **38**:92-109, 1962.

Morgan, J.A.: The art and science of medical radiography, St. Louis, 1962, Catholic Hospital Association.

1963 Agnesia, Sister, M.: A wide-angle rib technique, Xray Techn. **34**:289-290, 1963.

Berlin, H.S., et al.: Wide-angle roentgenography, A.J.R. **90**:189-197, 1963.

1964 Horenstein, R., et al.: The subtraction method, Acta Radiol. [Diagn.] **2**:264-272, 1964.

1965 Cahoon, J.B., Jr.: Formulating x-ray technics, ed. 6, Durham, N.C., 1965, Duke University Press.

Chynn, K-Y: Simplified subtraction technique, A.J.R. **95**:970-975, 1965.

1966 Greissberger, H.: Wedge-shaped filters for improved radiography of the thoracic vertebrae and the foot, Med. Radiogr. Photogr. **42**:6-8, 1966.

1968 Cullinan, J.E.: Fractional-focus x-ray tubes: newer clinical and research applications, Radiol. Technol. **39**:333-338, 1968.

1969 DePoto, D.W., and Barnes, M.R.: The value of Polaroid radiography today—a reappraisal, A.J.R. **107**:881-883, 1969.

Friedman, P.J., and Greenspan, R.H.: Observation on magnification radiography: visualization of small blood vessels and determination of focal spot size, Radiology **92**:549-557, 1969.

1970 Rao, G.U.V., and Clark, R.L.: Radiographic magnification versus optical magnification, Radiology **94**:196, 1970.

1971 Bookstein, J.J., and Voegeli, E.: A critical analysis of magnification radiography, Radiology **98**:23-30, 1971.

Edholm, P.R., and Jacobson, B.: Primary x-ray dodging, Radiology **99**:694-696, 1971.

1973 Melson, G.L., Staple, T.W., and Evens, R.G.: Soft tissue radiographic techniques, Semin. Roentgenol. **8**:19-24, 1973.

Wolfe, J.N.: Xeroradiography: image content and comparison with film roentgenograms, A.J.R. **117**:690-695, 1973.

1974 Christensen, E.E., Bull, K.W., and Dowdey, J.E.: Grid cut-off with oblique radiographic techniques, Radiology **111**:473-474, 1974.

Reichmann, S., and Helander, C.G.: High voltage radiography: theory and clinical applications, Acta Radiol. **15**:561-569, 1974.

1975 Eastman, T.R.: Technique charts: the key to radiographic quality, Radiol. Technol. **46**:365-368, 1975.

Hiss, S.S.: Technique management, Radiol. Technol. **46**:369-375, 1975.

Stein, J.A.: X-ray imaging with a scanning beam, Radiology **117**:713-716, 1975.

Sweeney, R.J.: Some factors affecting image clarity and detail perception in the radiograph, Radiol. Technol. **46**:443-451, 1975.

1976 Genant, H.K., Doi, K., and Mall, J.C.: Comparison of non-screen techniques (medical vs. industrial film) for fine detail skeletal radiography, Invest. Radiol. **11**:486-500, 1976.

Rossi, R.P., Hendee, W.R., and Athrens, C.R.: An evaluation of rare earth screen/film combinations, Radiology **121**:465-471, 1976.

1977 Castle, J.W.: Sensitivity of radiographic screens to scattered radiation and its relationship to image contrast, Radiology **122**:805-809, 1977.

Harms, A.A., and Zeilinger, A.: A new formulation of total unsharpness in radiography, Phys. Med. Biol. **22**:70-80, 1977.

Moyer, R.F.: The mysterious wall around exposure, Radiol. Technol. **48**:707-710, 1977.

Stables, D.P., et al.: The application of fast screen-film systems to excretory urography, A.J.R. **128**:617-619, 1977.

1978 Amplatz, K., Moore, R., and Korbuly, D.: The ''swinging'' tube: a new concept, Radiology **128**:783-785, 1978.

Newlin, N.: Reduction in radiation exposure: the rare-earth screen, A.J.R. **130**:1195-1196, 1978.

Rao, G.U., Fatouros, P.P., and James, A.E., Jr.: Physical characteristics of modern radiographic screen-film systems, Invest. Radiol. **13**:460-469, 1978.

Weaver, K.E., Barone, G.J., and Fewell, T.R.: Selection of technique factors for mobile capacitor energy storage x-ray equipment, Radiology **128**:223-228, 1978.

1979 Stopford, J.E.: Log$_{10}$ technique charts, Radiol. Technol. **51**:331-333, 1979.

Venema, H.W.: X-ray absorption, speed, and luminescent efficiency of rare-earth and other intensifying screens, Radiology **130**:765-771, 1979.

1980 Barnes, G.T., et al.: The scanning grid: a novel and effective bucky movement, Radiology **135**:765-767, 1980.

Ritter, E.M., et al.: Use of a gradient intensifying screen for scoliosis radiography, Radiology **135**:230-232, 1980.

Skucas, J., and Gorski, J.: Application of modern intensifying screens in diagnostic radiology, Med. Radiogr. Photogr. **56**:25-36, 1980.

Vyborny, C.J., Metz, C.E., and Doi, K.: Relative efficiencies of energy to photographic density conversions in typical screen-film systems, Radiology **136**:465-471, 1980.

1981 Brodeur, A.E., et al.: Three-tier rare-earth imaging system, A.J.R. **136**:755-758, 1981.

Franji, S.M., and El-Khoury, G.Y.: Applications of double screen roentgenography, Appl. Radiol. **10**:59-61, 1981.

STEREOSCOPY

1930 Wilsey, R.B.: Identification of right and left eye radiographs of a stereoscopic pair, Radiogr. Clin. Photogr. **6**:2-5, 1930.

1932 Kelly, J.F.: Stereoscopy, Xray Techn. **3**:93-98, 133-139, 1932.

Sweany, H.C., and Martinson, W.: A note on the principles of stereoroentgenography, Xray Techn. **3**:140-144, 1932.

Wilsey, R.B.: Stereoradiography and distortion, Radiogr. Clin. Photogr. **8**:(5):2-5, 1932.

Wilsey, R.B., and Fuchs, A.W.: Stereoradiography, Radiogr. Clin. Photogr. **8**:(4):2-8, 1932.

1933 Jarre, H.A., and Teschendorf, O.E.W.: Roentgenstereoscopy, Radiology **21**:139-155, 1933.

Wilsey, R.B.: Stereoradiography, Xray Techn. **5**:4-9, 1933.

1934 Gianturco, C.: Un metodo di radiografia stereoscopica con l'uso di una sola film: l'applicazione in radioscopia stereoscopica, Ann. Radiol. Fis. Med. **8**:311-313, 1934.

1963 Hodges, P.C.: Technic of stereoscopic radiography, Postgrad. Med. **33**:A61-A65, 1963.

1973 Rothman, S.L., Allen, W.E., and Kier, E.L.: Stereo roentgenography in craniofacial injuries, Radiol. Clin. North Am. **11**:683-696, 1973.

AUTOTOMOGRAPHY

1929 Ottonello, P.: Nuevo método para la radiografía de la columna cervical completa en proyección sagital ventro-dorsal, Anal. Radiol. (Havana) **1**:57-58, 1929.

1937 Barsóny, T., and Winkler, K.: Die ''elective'' Profilaufnahme der Brustwirbelsäule, Röntgenpraxis **9**:9, 1937.

Jönsson, G.: Method of obtaining structural pictures of the sternum, Acta Radiol. **18**:336-340, 1937.

1938 Barsóny, T., and Winkler, K.: Beiträge zur Röntgenologie der Wirbelsäule; ''Gasfreie'' Aufnahmen durch Atmung, Röntgenpraxis **10**:384-390, 1938.

Weiser, M.: ''Tomographie'' ohne Tomographen, Röntgenpraxis **10**:28, 1938.

1939 Bloom, A.R.: A new technic of taking roentgenographs of the upper ribs, Radiology **33**:648-649, 1939.

1942 Holly, E.W.: Some radiographic technics in which movement is utilized, Radiogr. Clin. Photogr. **18**:78-83, 1942.

1977 Forman, W.H.: Autotomography: a means of improving visualization of the upper cervical spine, Radiology **123**:800-801, 1977.

CONTRAST MEDIA

1897 Williams, F.H.: A study of the adaptation of the x-rays to medicine, Reports of the Boston City Hospital, January 1897.

1898 Cannon, W.B.: Movements of the stomach studied by means of the roentgen ray, Am. J. Physiol. **1**:359-382, 1898.

1910 Bachem, C., and Günther, H.: Bariumsulfat als schattenbildendes Kontrastmittel bei Röntgenuntersuchungen, Z. Röntgenk. Radiumforsch. **12**:369, 1910.

1918 Cameron, D.F.: Sodium and potassium iodides in roentgenography, J.A.M.A. **70**:1516, 1918.

Dandy, W.E.: Ventriculography following the injection of air into the cerebral ventricles, Ann. Surg. **68**:5-11, 1918.

Weld, E.H.: The use of sodium bromide in radiography, J.A.M.A. **71**:1111-1112, 1918.

1919 Dandy, W.E.: Roentgenography of the brain after the injection of air into the spinal canal, Ann. Surg. **70**:397-403, 1919.

1920 Schanz, R.T.: Iodide and bromide pastes as used in roentgenography, J.A.M.A. **74**:316, 1920.

1922 Sicard, J.A., and Forestier, J.: Méthode générale d'exploration radiologique par l'huile iodée (Lipiodol), Bull. Soc. Méd. Hôp. Paris **46**:463-469, 1922.

1923 Rowntree, L.G., et al.: Roentgenography of the urinary tract during excretion of sodium iodide, J.A.M.A. **80**:368-373, 1923.

1924 Graham, E.A., and Cole, W.H.: Roentgenologic examination of gall bladder, new method utilizing intravenous injection of tetrabromphenophthalein, Ann. Surg. **80**:473-477, 1924.

1925 Graham, E.A., Cole, W.H., and Copher, G.H.: Cholecystography: the use of dodium tetraiodophenolphthalein, J.A.M.A. **84**:1175-1177, 1925.

1926 Sicard, J.A., and Forestier, J.E.: Radiological exploration with iodized oil, Br. J. Radiol. **31**:239, 1926.

1927 Levyn, L., and Aaron, H.H.: Cholecystography by oral administration of sodium tetraiodophenolphthalein, A.J.R. **18**:557-559, 1927.

1928 Levyn, L., and Aaron, H.H.: Simplified method of oral colecystography, N.Y. J. Med. **28**:264, 1928.

Odin and Rundstrom: Iodized oils, Acta Radiol. **7**:(suppl.): 1928.

1929 Radt, P.: Eine Methode zur röntgenologischen Kontrastdarstellung vom Milz und Leber, Klin. **8**:2128, 1929.

Roseno, A., and Jephins, H.: Intravenous pyelography, Fortschr. Roentgenstr. **39:**859-863, 1929. Abstract: A.J.R. **22:**685-686, 1929.

Swick, M.: Darstellung der Niere und Harnwege im Röntgenbild durch intravenose Einbringung eines neuen Kontrastoffes, des Uroselectans, Klin. Wochenschr. **8:**2087-2089, 1929. Abstract: A.J.R. **23:**686-687, 1930.

1930 Swick, M.: Intravenous urography by means of the sodium salt 5-iodo-2-pyradon-N-acetic acid, J.A.M.A. **95:**1403, 1930.

1933 Swick, M.: Excretion urography with particular reference to newly developed compound: sodium orthoiodohippurate, J.A.M.A. **101:**1843, 1933.

1934 Egas Moniz, A.C.: L'angiographie cérébrale: ses applications et résultats en anatomie, physiologie et clinique, Paris, 1934, Masson & Cie.

1938 Green, A.B.: The chemistry of contrast media used in radiography, Xray Techn. **9:**231-237, 1938.

Robb, G.P., and Steinberg, I.: Practical method of visualization of chambers of the heart, the pulmonary circulation, and the great blood vessels in man, J. Clin. Invest. **17:**507, 1938.

1939 Robb, G.P., and Steinberg, I.: Visualization of the chambers of the heart, the pulmonary circulation, and the great blood vessels in man, A.J.R. **41:**1-18, 1939.

1940 Alexander, O.M.: The use of differential media in radiography, Radiography **6:**121-138, 1940.

Dohrn, M., and Diedrich, P.: Ein neues Röntgenkontrastmittel der Gallenblase, Deutsch. Med. Wochenschr. **66:**1133-1134, 1940.

Lauer-Schmaltz, W.: Erfahrungen über perorale Cholezystographie mit dem neuen Kontrastmittel Biliselectan, München Med. Wochenschr. **87:**1139, 1940.

1941 Anderson, H.T.: The use of iodized oil in roentgenography, A.J.R. **46:**362, 1941.

Rating, B.: Ueber ein neues Kontrastmittel zur Röntgendarstellung der Gallenblase (Biliselectan), Fortschr. Roentgenstr. **63:**99-110, 1941.

1942 Modell, W.: Pharmacology of beta (3, 5 diiodo-4-hydroxy phenyl) alpha phenyl propionic acid, J. Lab. Clin. Med. **27:**1376-1384, 1942.

1943 Einsel, I.H., and Einsel, T.H.: Gall bladder visualization with beta (3, 5 di-iodo-4-hydroxy-phenyl) alphaphenyl-propionic acid (Priodax), A.J. Dig. Dis. **10:**206-208, 1943.

Marshall, W.A.: Some observations on Priodax, A.J.R. **50:**680-682, 1943.

Wasch, M.G.: A new medium for gall bladder visualization, A.J.R. **50:**677-679, 1943.

1944 Hefke, H.W.: Cholecystography with Priodax: a report on 600 examinations, Radiology **42:**233, 1944.

Ochsner, H.C.: A new cholecystographic preparation, A.J.R. **51:**326-327, 1944.

Ramsay, G.H., French, J.D., and Strain, W.H.: Iodinated organic compounds as contrast media for radiographic diagnoses. IV. Pantopaque myelography, Radiology **43:**236-240, 1944.

Ramsay, G.H., and Strain, W.H.: Pantopaque: a new contrast medium for myelography, Radiogr. Clin. Photogr. **20:**25-33, 1944.

1945 Rigler, L.G.: The development of roentgen diagnosis, Radiology **45:**467-502, 1945.

1946 Epstein, B.S., Natelson, S., and Kramer, B.: A new series of radiopaque compounds, A.J.R. **56:**201-207, 1946.

1947 Unfug, G.A.: A comparative clinical investigation of cholecystographic preparations, Radiology **46:**489-495, 1947.

1952 Eubank, M.C.: Properties and uses of contrast media, Xray Techn. **23:**255-264, 1952

1953 Mattsson, O.: A simple method for ensuring correct concentration of barium contrast media, Acta Radiol. **39:**501-506, 1953.

Okell, E.: Opaque media, Xray Techn. **24:**337-350, 1953.

1958 Garfinkel, B., and Furst, N.J.: Simultaneous roentgen examination of the urinary and biliary tracts with Duografin, Radiology **70:**243-245, 1958.

1962 Sanen, F.J.: Considerations of cholecystographic contrast media, A.J.R. **88:**797-802, 1962.

1964 Pattinson, J.N.: Iodine compounds in the alimentary tract, Radiography **30:**103-109, 1964.

Strain, W.H., et al.: Radiologic diagnostic agents: a compilation, Med. Radiogr. Photogr. **40:**(suppl.):1-110, 1964.

1965 Miller, R.E.: Barium sulfate suspensions, Radiology **84:**241-251, 1965.

1966 Shehadi, W.H.: Clinical problems and toxicity of contrast agents, A.J.R. **97:**762-771, 1966.

1968 Embring, G., and Mattsson, O.: Barium contrast agents, Acta Radiol. [Diagn.] **7:**245-256, 1968.

1969 Mattsson, O.: Areometer for estimating the concentration of modern barium meals, Acta Radiol. [Diagn.] **8:**446-448, 1969.

1973 Metrizamide: a non-ionic water-soluble contrast medium, Acta Radiol. **335**(suppl.):1-390, 1973.

1974 Lalli, A.F.: Urographic contrast media reactions and anxiety, Radiology **112:**267-271, 1974.

1975 Jekell, K., Ohlson, T., and Widebeck, J.: Physical characteristics of barium contrast media and their influence on roentgen image information, Acta Radiol. [Diagn.] **16:**263-272, 1975.

Sargent, N.E., et al.: A new contrast medium for cholangio-cholecystography: meglumine iodoxamate, A.J.R. **125:**251-258, 1975.

Shehadi, W.H.: Adverse reactions to intravascularly administered contrast media, A.J.R. **124:**145-152, 1975.

1976 Andrews, E.J.: The vagus reaction as a possible cause of severe complications of radiological procedures, Radiology **121:**1-4, 1976.

Bentson, J.R., and Wilson, G.H.: Clinical comparison of three contrast agents used in cerebral angiography, Invest. Radiol. **11:**602-604, 1976.

Berk, R.N., and Loeb, R.M.: Pharmacology and physiology of the biliary radiographic contrast materials, Semin. Roentgenol. **11:**147-156, 1976.

Robbins, A.H., et al.: Double-blind comparison of meglumine iodoxamate (Cholevue) and meglumine iodipamide (Cholegrafin), A.J.R. **127:**257-260, 1976.

1977 Lindgren, E., editor: Metrizamide—Amipaque: the non-ionic water-soluble contrast medium, Acta Radiol. **355**(suppl.):1-432, 1977.

Loeb, P.M., Barnhart, J.L., and Berk, R.N.: Iotroxamide—a new intravenous cholangiographic agent, Radiology **125:**323-329, 1977.

Miller, R.E., and Skucas, J.: Radiographic contrast agents, Baltimore, 1977, University Park Press.

Shehadi, W.H.: Contrast media in diagnostic radiology: recommendations for labels, package inserts, and dosage determination, A.J.R. **129:**167-170, 1977.

1978 Johansen, J.G.: Assessment of a nonionic contrast medium (Amipaque) in the gastrointestinal tract, Invest. Radiol. **13:**523-527, 1978.

Kieffer, A.A., et al.: Contrast agents for myelography: clinical and radiological evaluation of Amipaque and Pantopaque, Radiology **129:**695-705, 1978.

Pizzolato, N.F., Arcomano, J.P., and Baum, A.E.: A new contrast agent for oral cholecystography: iopronic acid (Oravue), A.J.R. **130:**845-847, 1978.

1979 Gelmers, H.J.: Adverse side effects of metrizamide in myelography, Neuroradiology **18:**119-123, 1979.

1980 Bush, W.H., Mullarkey, M.F., and Webb, D.R.: Adverse reactions to radiographic contrast material, Western J. Med. **132:**95-98, 1980.

Grainger, R.G.: Osmolality of intravascular radiological contrast media, Br. J. Radiol. **53:**739-746, 1980.

Harnish, P.P., et al.: Drugs providing protection from severe contrast media reactions, Invest. Radiol. **15:**248-259, 1980.

Index